NURSING DIAGNOSIS REFERENCE MANUAL

FIFTH EDITION

NURSING DIAGNOSIS REFERENCE MANUAL

FIFTH EDITION

Sheila M. Sparks, RN, DNSc, CS

Associate Professor, Division of Nursing
Shenandoah University
Winchester, Va.

Cynthia M. Taylor, RN, MS, CNAA

Health Consultant and Parish Nurse
Rockville, Md.

SPRINGHOUSE CORPORATION

Springhouse, Pennsylvania

STAFF

Publisher
Judith A. Schilling McCann, RN, MSN

Design Director
John Hubbard

Editorial Director
David Moreau

Editors
Cynthia C. Breuninger, Margaret Eckman

Copy Editors
Jaime Stockslager (supervisor), Virginia Baskerville, Priscilla DeWitt, Heather Ditch, Mary T. Durkin, Shana Harrington, Kimberly A. J. Johnson, Pamela Wingrod, Helen Winton

Designers
Arlene Putterman (associate design director), Susan Sheridan (project manager), Joseph John Clark, Donna Morris

Projects Coordinator
Liz Schaeffer

Electronic Production Services
Diane Paluba (manager), Joyce Rossi Biletz

Manufacturing
Deborah Meiris (director), Patricia K. Dorshaw (manager), Otto Mezei (book production manager)

Editorial and Design Assistants
Tom Hasenmayer, Beverly Lane, Beth Janae Orr, Elfriede Young

Indexer
Manjit Sahai

Printed in the United States of America.

NDRM5- D

03 02   10 9 8 7 6 5 4

Library of Congress Cataloging-in-Publication Data
Sparks, Sheila M.
   Nursing diagnosis reference manual / Sheila M.
Sparks, Cynthia M. Taylor. — 5th ed.
      p.; cm.
   Includes bibliographical references and index.
   1. Nursing diagnosis — Handbooks, manuals, etc.
   I. Taylor, Cynthia M. II. Title.
   [DNLM: 1. Nursing Diagnosis — Handbooks.
   2. Patient Care Planning — Handbooks.
WY 49 S736na 2000]
RT48.6 .S66 2000
610.73 — dc21
   ISBN 1-58255-072-7 (alk. paper)   00-056307

CONTENTS

CONTRIBUTORS

Patricia Anasiewicz, RN, MSN
Director of Enrollment and Development
Center for Life and Learning
Gwynedd Mercy College
Gwynedd Valley, Pa.

Lynne Hutnick Conrad, RN,C, MSN, MBA, MHA
Patient Progressions Coordinator
Albert Einstein Healthcare Network
Philadelphia

Linda Carman Copel, RN,CS, PhD, DAPA, ACFE, CGP, CFLE
Psychotherapist (private practice)
Associate Professor
Villanova (Pa.) University

Susan B. Dickey, RN,C, PhD, MSN
Assistant Professor, Department of Nursing
Temple University
Philadelphia

Louama K. Driscoll, RN, MSN
Veterans Affairs Medical Center
New Orleans

Janice S. DuBrueler, RN, MSN
Assistant Professor, Division of Nursing
Shenandoah University
Winchester, Va.

Janyce G. Dyer, RN, DNSc, CS
Assistant Professor, School of Nursing
University of Pittsburgh

Kathryn M. Ganske, RN, MSN
Clinical Instructor
Shenandoah University
Winchester, Va.

Laurel S. Garzon, RN, DNSc, CPNP
Director, Advanced Maternal Child
Graduate Programs
Associate Professor, School of Nursing
Old Dominion University
Norfolk, Va.

Pauline McKinney Green, RN, PhD, MSN
Associate Professor, College of Pharmacy,
Nursing, and Allied Health Sciences
Howard University
Washington, D.C.

Betty Glenn Harris, RN, PhD
Assistant Professor, School of Nursing
University of North Carolina at Chapel Hill

Teri J. Harrison, RN, MSN, CDE
Pediatric Clinical Nurse Specialist
Methodist Hospital of Indiana, Inc.
Indianapolis

Kathryn VanDyke Hayes, RN,C, DNSc
Associate Professor, Division of Nursing
Shenandoah University
Winchester, Va.

Jacqueline M. Himes, RN, BSN, SNP
School Nurse Practitioner
School District of Philadelphia

Susan L.W. Krupnick, RN, MSN, CCRN, CS
Psychiatric Consultation Liaison Nurse
University of Pennsylvania Hospital
Philadelphia

Ruth Anne McCormick, RN, DNSc
Day Treatment Center
Adventist Hospital
Takoma Park, Md.

Caroline Meyer, RN, BSN
Independent Nurse Consultant
New York

Carolyn D. Moore, RN, MSN, CNOR
Staff Nurse, Operating Room
The Arlington (Va.) Hospital

Marian Newton, RN, PhD, CS, NPP
Associate Professor, Division of Nursing
Shenandoah University
Winchester, Va.

Peggy Plunkett, RN, MSN, ARNP, CS
Psychiatric Liaison Clinical Nurse Specialist
Dartmouth-Hitchcock Medical Center
Lebanon, N.H.

Vanice W. Roberts, RN, DSN
Professor and Assistant Dean
Kennesaw (Ga.) State College

Patricia C. Seifert, RN, MSN, CNOR, CRNFA
Perioperative Educator and Consultant
Falls Church, Va.

Kathleen C. Sheppard, RN, PhD
Director of Nursing, Continuity of Care
University of Texas M.D. Anderson
Cancer Center
Houston

Vickie L. Stone, RN, MSN
Assistant Professor, Division of Nursing
Shenandoah University
Winchester, Va.

Susan S. Thomason, RN, MN, CS, CETN
Clinical Nurse Specialist
Veterans Affairs Medical Center
Tampa, Fla.

Diane M. Wieland, RN, MSN, CS
Assistant Professor, Department of Nursing
College of Allied Health Sciences
Thomas Jefferson University
Philadelphia

Judith G. Winterhalter, RN, DNSc, CS
Professor of Graduate Nursing, School of
Nursing
Gwynedd Mercy College
Gwynedd Valley, Pa.

Beryla Wolf, RN, PhD
Assistant Professor of Nursing, Department
of Nursing
Regis University
Denver

Stephanie Wright, RN, PhD, FNP
Assistant Professor, School of Nursing
Georgetown University
Washington, D.C.

Helen H. Zebarth, RN,C, BSN, MEd
Director of Wilkins Wellness Center
Assistant Professor of Nursing
Shenandoah University
Winchester, Va.

PREFACE

For student nurses as well as expert clinicians, *Nursing Diagnosis Reference Manual,* Fifth Edition, offers clearly written, authoritative plans of care to help meet patients' health care needs throughout the life span. For this new edition, the authors have expanded the book's focus to cover psychiatric and mental health, along with adult, adolescent, child, maternal-neonatal, geriatric, and community-based health. You will find the plans of care in this book invaluable in every health care setting you encounter throughout your career.

The nursing process is thoroughly integrated into the material on every page of this book. Providing care based on the nursing process offers benefits to both beginning and experienced nurses. The nursing process:
• provides a framework for independent nursing action
• promotes a consistent structure for professional practice
• helps you focus more precisely on each patient's health care needs.

Nursing Diagnosis Reference Manual provides the information you need to accurately apply the nursing process. It focuses on health problems that you can diagnose legally and treat independently. This manual incorporates all diagnoses approved by the North American Nursing Diagnosis Association (NANDA).

Nursing Diagnosis Reference Manual begins with an explanation of each step of the nursing process — assessment, nursing diagnosis, outcome identification, planning, implementation, and evaluation. Included in this introductory section are clear guidelines for writing a clinically accurate diagnostic statement. This section also clarifies the distinction between a nursing diagnosis and a medical diagnosis.

After this section come the manual's seven major parts: adult health, adolescent health, child health, maternal-neonatal health, geriatric health, psychiatric and mental health, and community-based health. Together, these parts include comprehensive plans of care for more than 300 nursing diagnostic statements. Each plan of care has been written and reviewed by leading nursing clinicians, educators, and researchers. Each one is complete and can be used independently to avoid searching for material in different places.

Plans of care
All plans of care contain the following sections:
• *Diagnostic statement.* Each diagnostic statement includes a NANDA-approved label and, in most cases, a related etiology. This edition of the *Nursing Diagnosis Reference Manual* contains all the diagnostic labels approved by NANDA to date.
• *Definition.* This section offers a brief explanation of the diagnosis.
• *Assessment.* This section suggests parameters to use when collecting data to ensure an accurate diagnosis. Data may include health history, physical findings, psychosocial status, laboratory studies, patient statements, and other subjective and objective information.

• *Defining characteristics.* This section lists clinical findings that confirm the diagnosis. For diagnoses expressing the possibility of a problem, such as "Risk for injury," this section is labeled *Risk factors.*
• *Associated medical diagnoses.* Here you'll find examples of medical conditions that are commonly associated with the nursing diagnosis.
• *Expected outcomes.* Here you'll find realistic goals for resolving or ameliorating the patient's health problem, written in measurable behavioral terms. You should select outcomes that are appropriate to the condition of your patient. Outcomes are arranged to flow logically from admission to discharge of the patient.
• *Interventions and rationales.* This section provides specific activities you carry out to help attain expected outcomes. Each intervention contains a rationale, highlighted in *italic* type. Rationales receive typographic emphasis because they form the premise for every nursing action. You'll find it helpful to consider rationales before intervening. Understanding the why of your actions can help you see that carrying out repetitive or difficult interventions are essential elements of your nursing practice. More important, it can improve critical thinking and help avoid mistakes.
• *Evaluations for expected outcomes.* Here you'll find evaluation criteria for the expected outcomes. These criteria will help you determine whether expected outcomes have been attained or provide support for revising outcomes or interventions to meet changing patient conditions.
• *Documentation.* This section lists critical topics to include in your documentation — for example, patient perceptions, status, and response to treatment as well as nursing observations and interventions. Using the information provided in this section will enable you to write the careful, concise documentation required to meet professional nursing standards.

Cross-references
The manual includes several cross-references that will help you select appropriate nursing diagnoses for every clinical situation. The largest cross-reference lists nursing diagnoses for specific medical diagnoses. Other cross-references group diagnoses by Gordon's functional health patterns, Maslow's hierarchy of needs, and Orem's universal self-care demands.

Acknowledgments
We would like to express our sincere appreciation to the nurses who contributed to the *Nursing Diagnosis Reference Manual,* Fifth Edition. Their expertise and commitment to quality patient care made this work possible.

Finally, we dedicate this book to nursing students and clinicians who are striving to provide quality care in today's turbulent health care arena.

Sheila M. Sparks, RN, DNSc, CS
Cynthia M. Taylor, RN, MS, CNAA

NURSING DIAGNOSIS REFERENCE MANUAL

FIFTH EDITION

THE NURSING PROCESS

The cornerstone of clinical nursing, the nursing process is a systematic method for taking independent nursing action. Steps in the nursing process include:
• assessing the patient's problems
• forming a diagnostic statement
• identifying expected outcomes
• creating a plan to achieve expected outcomes and solve the patient's problems
• implementing the plan or assigning others to implement it
• evaluating the plan's effectiveness.

These phases of the nursing process — assessment, nursing diagnosis, outcome identification, planning, implementation, and evaluation — are dynamic and flexible; they often overlap.

Becoming familiar with this process has many benefits. It will allow you to apply your knowledge and skills in an organized, goal-oriented manner. It will also enable you to communicate about professional topics with colleagues from all clinical specialties and practice settings. Using the nursing process is essential to documenting nursing's role in the provision of comprehensive, quality patient care.

The growing recognition of the nursing process is an important development in the struggle for greater professional autonomy. By clearly defining problems a nurse may treat independently, the nursing process has helped to dispel the notion that nursing practice is based solely on carrying out doctor's orders.

Despite recent advances, nursing is still in a state of professional evolution. In the years ahead, researchers and expert practitioners will continue to develop a body of knowledge specific to the field. A strong foundation in the nursing process will enable you to better assimilate emerging concepts and to incorporate these concepts into your practice. (See *Nursing's approach to problem solving.*)

ASSESSMENT
The vital first phase in the nursing process, assessment, consists of the patient history, the physical examination, and laboratory studies. The other nursing process phases — nursing diagnosis formation, outcome identification, care planning, implementation, and evaluation — depend on the quality of the assessment data for their effectiveness.

A properly recorded initial assessment provides a:
• way to communicate patient information to other caregivers
• method of documenting initial baseline data
• foundation on which to build an effective plan of care.

Your initial patient assessment begins with the collection of data (patient history, physical examination findings, and laboratory data) and ends with a statement of the patient's actual or potential problem — the nursing diagnosis.

Building a database
The information you collect in taking your patient's history, performing a

Nursing's approach to problem solving

Dynamic and flexible, the phases of the nursing process resemble the steps that many other professions rely on to identify and correct problems. Here is how the nursing process phases correspond to the standard problem-solving method.

NURSING PROCESS	PROBLEM-SOLVING METHOD
Assessment • Collect and analyze subjective and objective data about the patient's health problem.	• Recognize that a problem exists. • Learn about the problem by obtaining facts.
Diagnosis • State the health problems.	• State the nature of the problem.
Outcome identification • Identify expected outcomes.	• Establish goals and a time frame for achieving them.
Planning • Write a plan of care that includes the nursing interventions designed to achieve expected outcomes.	• Think of and select ways to achieve goals and solve the problem.
Implementation • Put the plan of care into action. • Document the actions taken and their results.	• Act on ways to solve the problem.
Evaluation • Critically examine the results achieved. • Review and revise the plan of care as needed.	• Decide if the actions taken have effectively solved the problem.

physical examination, and analyzing laboratory test results serves as your assessment database. Your goal is to gather and record information that will be most helpful in assessing your patient. You can't, however, collect or use *all* the information that exists about your patient. To limit your database appropriately, ask yourself these questions: What data do I want to collect? How should I collect the information? How should I organize the data to make care planning decisions?

Your answers will help you to be selective in collecting meaningful data during patient assessment.

The well-defined database for a patient may begin with admission signs and symptoms, chief complaint, or medical diagnosis. It also may center on the type of patient care given in a specific nursing unit, such as the intensive care unit or the emergency department (ED). For example, you wouldn't ask a trauma victim in the ED if she has a family history of breast cancer, nor would you perform a routine breast examination on her.

You would, however, do these types of assessment during a comprehensive health checkup in an ambulatory care setting.

If you work in a setting where patients with similar diagnoses are treated, choose your database from information pertinent to this specific patient population. Even when addressing patients with similar diagnoses, however, complete a thorough assessment to make sure unanticipated problems don't go unnoticed.

Subjective and objective data

The assessment data you collect and analyze fall into two important categories, subjective and objective.

The patient's history, embodying a *personal perspective* of problems, provides *subjective data*. It's your most important assessment data source. Because it's also the most subjective source of patient information, it must be interpreted carefully.

In the *physical examination* of a patient — involving inspection, palpation, percussion, and auscultation — you collect *objective data* about your patient's health status or about the pathologic processes that may be related to his illness or injury. In addition to adding to your patient database, this information helps you interpret the patient's history more accurately by providing a basis for comparison. Use it to validate and amplify the historical data. However, don't allow the physical examination of your patient to assume undue importance.

The most objective form of assessment data, *laboratory test results* provide another source for interpreting your history and physical examination findings. The advanced technology used in laboratory tests enables you to assess anatomic, physiologic,

and chemical processes that neither your nor your patient's senses are capable of measuring. For example, if your patient complains of feeling tired (history) and you observe conjunctival pallor (physical examination), check his hemoglobin level and hematocrit (laboratory data).

You need both subjective and objective data for comprehensive patient assessment. They validate each other and together provide more data than either could provide alone.

Consider all three types of assessment information — history, physical examination, and laboratory data — in their appropriate relationships to one another. Performing an accurate physical examination requires technical skill that is in itself valuable. It becomes even more valuable, however, when you place the examination findings in perspective as one aspect of total patient assessment.

Taking a complete health history

This portion of the assessment consists of the subjective data you collect from the patient. Use your interviewing skills to help the patient describe biological, social, spiritual, and psychological responses to the particular anatomic, physiologic, and chemical processes involved in his illness or injury. In addition, the patient may recall events in his own life or in relatives' lives that may indicate an increased risk for certain pathologic processes.

A complete health history provides the following information about a patient:
• biographical data including ethnic, cultural, and spiritual factors
• chief complaint (or concern)
• history of present illness (or current health status)
• past health history

- family medical history
- psychosocial history
- activities of daily living (ADLs)
- review of systems.

Follow this orderly format in taking your patient's history, but allow for modifications based on your patient's chief complaint or concern. For example, the health history of a patient with a localized allergic reaction will be much shorter than that of a patient who complains vaguely of mental confusion and severe headaches.

If your patient has a chief complaint, use information from your health history to decide if his problems stem from physiologic causes or psychophysiologic maladaptation and how your nursing interventions may help. The depth of such a history depends on the patient's cooperation and your skill in asking insightful questions.

A patient who requests a complete physical checkup may not even have a chief complaint. Such a patient's health history would be comprehensive, with detailed information about lifestyle, self-image, family and other interpersonal relationships, and degree of satisfaction with current health status.

Be sure to record health history data in an organized fashion so that the information will be meaningful to everyone involved in a patient's care. Some health care facilities provide patient questionnaires or computerized checklists. (See *Using an assessment checklist,* page 6.) These forms make history-taking easier, but they aren't always available. Therefore, you must know how to take a comprehensive health history without them. This is easy to do if you develop an orderly and systematic method of interviewing. Ask the history questions in the same order every time. With experience, you'll know which types of questions to ask in specific patient situations.

Review of systems

When interviewing the patient, use this review of systems as a guide.

General: overall state of health, ability to carry out ADLs, weight changes, fatigue, exercise tolerance, fever, night sweats, repeated infections

Skin: changes in color, pigmentation, temperature, moisture, or hair distribution; eruptions; pruritus; scaling; bruising; bleeding; dryness; excessive oiliness; growths; moles; scars; rashes; scalp lesions; brittle, soft, or abnormally formed nails; cyanotic nail beds; pressure ulcers

Head: trauma, lumps, alopecia, headaches

Eyes: nearsightedness, farsightedness, glaucoma, cataracts, blurred vision, double vision, tearing, burning, itching, photophobia, pain, inflammation, swelling, color blindness, injuries (also ask about use of glasses or contact lenses, date of last eye examination, and past surgery to correct vision problems)

Ears: deafness, tinnitus, vertigo, discharge, pain, tenderness behind the ears, mastoiditis, otitis or other ear infections, earaches, ear surgery

Nose: sinusitis, discharge, colds, or coryza more than four times a year; rhinitis; trauma; sneezing; loss of sense of smell; obstruction; breathing problems; epistaxis

Mouth and throat: changes in color or sores on tongue, dental caries, loss of teeth, toothaches, bleeding gums, lesions, loss of taste, hoarseness, sore throats (streptococcal), tonsillitis, voice changes, dysphagia, date of last dental checkup, use of dentures, bridges, or other dental appliances

Using an assessment checklist

To ensure that you cover all key points during your health history interview, you may use an assessment checklist such as the one below. Although their format may vary from one facility to another, all guides include the same key elements.

❑ *Reason for hospitalization or chief complaint:* As patient sees it.
❑ *Duration of this problem:* As patient recalls it. Has it affected patient's lifestyle?
❑ *Other illnesses and previous experience with hospitalization:* Reason? When? Results? Impressions of previous hospitalizations? Problems encountered? Effect of this hospitalization on education? Family? Child care? Employment? Finances?
❑ *Observation of patient's condition:* Level of consciousness? Well-nourished? Healthy? Color? Skin turgor? Senses? Headaches? Cough? Syncope? Nausea? Seizures? Edema? Lumps? Bruises or bleeding? Inflammation? Integrity of skin? Pressure areas? Temperature? Range of motion? Unusual sensations? Paralysis? Odors? Discharges? Pain?
❑ *Mental and emotional status:* Cooperative? Understanding? Anxious? Language? Expectations? Feelings about illness? State of consciousness? Mood? Self-image? Reaction to stress? Rapport with interviewer and staff? Compatibility with roommate?
❑ *Review of systems:* Neurologic, EENT, Pulmonary, Cardiovascular, GI, GU, Skin, Reproductive, Musculo-skeletal, and so forth.
❑ *Allergies:* Food? Drugs? Type of reaction?
❑ *Medication:* Dosage? Why taken? When taken? Last dose? Does he have it with him? Any others taken occasionally? Recently? Why? Use of over-the-counter drugs or cough preparations? Use of alcohol or illegal drugs?
❑ *Prostheses:* Pacemaker? Intermit-tent positive-pressure breathing unit?

Tracheostomy tube? Drainage tubes? Feeding tube? Catheter? Ostomy appliance? Breast form? Hearing aid? Glasses or contacts? Dentures? False eye? Prosthetic leg? Cane? Brace? Walker? Does the patient have the device with him? Need anything?
❑ *Hygiene patterns:* Dentures? Gums? Teeth? Bath or shower? When?
❑ *Rest and sleep patterns:* Usual times? Aids? Difficulties?
❑ *Activity status:* Self-care? Ambulatory? Aids? Daily exercise?
❑ *Bladder and bowel patterns:* Continent? Frequency? Nocturia? Characteristics of stool and urine? Discharge? Pain? Ostomy? Appliances? Who cares for these? Laxatives? Medications?
❑ *Meals and diet:* Feeds self? Diet restrictions (therapeutic and cultural or preferential)? Frequency? Snacks? Allergies? Dislikes? Fad diets? Usual dietary intake?
❑ *Health practices:* Breast self-examination? Physical examination? Pap smear? Testicular self-examination? Digital rectal examination? Smoking? ECG? Annual chest X-ray? Practices related to other conditions, such as glaucoma testing, urine testing, weight control?
❑ *Lifestyle:* Parent? Family? Number of children? Residence? Occupation? Recreation? Diversion? Interests? Financial status? Religion? Sexuality? Education? Ethnic background? Living environment?
❑ *Typical day profile:* Have patient describe.
❑ *Informant:* From whom did you obtain this information? Patient? Family? Old records? Ambulance driver?

Neck: pain, stiffness, swelling, limited movement, or injuries

Breasts: change in development or lactation pattern, trauma, lumps, pain, discharge from nipples, gynecomastia, changes in contour or in nipples, history of breast cancer (also ask if the patient knows how to perform breast self-examination)

Cardiovascular: palpitations, tachycardia, or other rhythm irregularities; pain in chest; dyspnea on exertion; orthopnea; cyanosis; edema; ascites; intermittent claudication; cold extremities; phlebitis; orthostatic hypotension; hypertension; rheumatic fever (also ask if an electrocardiogram has been performed recently)

Respiratory: dyspnea, shortness of breath, pain, wheezing, paroxysmal nocturnal dyspnea, orthopnea (number of pillows used), cough, sputum, hemoptysis, night sweats, emphysema, pleurisy, bronchitis, tuberculosis (contacts), pneumonia, asthma, upper respiratory tract infections (also ask about results of chest X-ray and tuberculin skin test)

Gastrointestinal: changes in appetite or weight, dysphagia, nausea, vomiting, heartburn, eructation, flatulence, abdominal pain, colic, hematemesis, jaundice (pain, fever, intensity, duration, color of urine), stools (color, frequency, consistency, odor, use of laxatives), hemorrhoids, rectal bleeding, changes in bowel habits

Renal, genitourinary: color of urine, polyuria, oliguria, nocturia (number of times per night), dysuria, frequency, urgency, problem with stream, dribbling, pyuria, retention, passage of stones or gravel, venereal disease (discharge), infections, perineal rashes and irritations, incontinence (stress, functional, total, reflex, urge), protein or sugar ever found in urine

Reproductive: male — lesions, impotence, prostate problems (also ask about use of contraceptives and whether the patient knows how to perform a testicular self-examination); female — irregular bleeding, discharge, pruritus, pain on intercourse, protrusions, dysmenorrhea, vaginal infections (also ask about number of pregnancies; delivery dates; complications; abortions; onset, regularity, and amount of flow during menarche; last normal period; use of contraceptives; date of menopause; last Pap test)

Neurologic: headaches, seizures, fainting spells, dizziness, tremors, twitches, aphasia, loss of sensation, weakness, paralysis, numbness, tingling, balance problems

Psychiatric: changes in mood, anxiety, depression, inability to concentrate, phobias, suicidal or homicidal thoughts, hallucinations, delusions

Musculoskeletal: muscle pain, swelling, redness, pain in joints, back problems, injuries (such as broken bones, pulled tendons), gait problems, weakness, paralysis, deformities, range of motion, contractures

Hematopoietic: anemia (type, degree, treatment, response), bleeding, fatigue, bruising (also ask if patient is receiving anticoagulant therapy)

Endocrine, metabolic: polyuria, polydipsia, polyphagia, thyroid problem, heat or cold intolerance, excessive sweating, changes in hair distribution and amount, nervousness, swollen neck (goiter), moon face, buffalo hump

When documenting the health history, be sure to record negative findings as well as positive ones. Note the absence of symptoms that other history data indicate might be present. For example, if a patient reports pain and burning in his abdomen, ask him if he has experienced nausea and vomiting or noticed blood in his stools. Record the presence or absence of these symptoms.

Also remember that the information will be used by others who will be caring for the patient. It could even be used as a legal document in a liability case, a malpractice suit, or an insurance disability claim. With these considerations in mind, record history data thoroughly and precisely. Continue your questioning until you're satisfied that you've recorded sufficient detail. Don't be satisfied with inadequate answers, such as "a lot" or "a little." These words mean different things to different people and must be explained to be meaningful. If taking notes seems to make the patient anxious, explain the importance of keeping a written record. To facilitate accurate recording of your patient's answers, familiarize yourself with standard history data abbreviations.

When you complete your patient's health history, it becomes part of the permanent written record. It will serve as a subjective database with which you and other health care professionals can monitor the patient's progress. Remember that history data must be specific and precise. Avoid generalities. Instead, provide pertinent, concise, detailed information that will help determine the direction and sequence of the physical examination — the next phase in your patient assessment.

Physical examination

After taking your patient's health history, the next step in the assessment process is the *physical examination.* During this assessment phase, you obtain objective data that usually confirm or rule out suspicions raised during the health history interview.

You use four basic techniques to perform a physical examination: *inspection, palpation, percussion,* and *auscultation* (IPPA). These skills require you to use your senses of sight, hearing, touch, and smell — all necessary for an accurate appraisal of the structures and functions of body systems. If, after much careful study and practice, you learn to use IPPA skills effectively, you'll be less likely to overlook something important during the physical examination. In addition, each examination technique collects data that validate and amplify data collected through other IPPA techniques.

Accurate and complete physical assessments depend on two interrelated elements. One is the critical act of sensory perception, by which you receive and perceive external stimuli. The other element is the conceptual, or cognitive, process by which you relate these stimuli to your knowledge base. This two-step process gives meaning to your assessment data.

You need to develop a system for assessing patients that identifies their problem areas in priority order. By performing physical assessments systematically and efficiently instead of in a random or indiscriminate manner, you'll save time and identify priority problems quickly.

Choosing an examination method. The most commonly used methods for completing a total systematic physical assessment are *head to toe* and *major body systems.*

Using the head-to-toe method, you systematically assess your patient — as the name suggests — beginning at the head and working toward the toes. Examine all parts of one body region before progressing to the next region to save time and energy for yourself and your patient. Proceed from left to right within each region so you can make symmetrical comparisons. Don't examine the patient's left side from head to toe, and then examine his right side.

The major-body-systems method involves systematically assessing your patient by examining each body system in priority order or in a pre-designated sequence.

Both the head-to-toe and the major-body-systems methods are systematic and provide a logical, organized framework for collecting physical assessment data. They also provide the same information; therefore, neither is more correct than the other. Choose the method (or a variation of it) that works well for you and is appropriate for your patient population. Follow this routine whenever you assess a patient, and try not to deviate from it.

To decide which method to use, first determine whether the patient's condition is life-threatening. Identifying the *priority* problems of a patient suffering from a life-threatening illness or injury — for example, severe trauma, a heart attack, or GI hemorrhage — is essential to preserve his life and function and prevent additional damage.

Next, identify the *patient population* to which the patient belongs, and take the common characteristics of that population into account in choosing an examination method. For example, elderly or debilitated patients tire easily; for a patient in either category, you would select a method that requires minimal position changes. Also, you would probably defer parts of the examination to avoid tiring your patient.

Try to view your patient as an integrated whole rather than as a collection of parts, regardless of the examination method you use. Remember, the integrity of a body *region* may reflect adequate functioning of many body *systems,* both inside and outside this particular region. For example, the integrity of the chest region may provide important clues about the functioning of the cardiovascular and respiratory systems. Similarly, the integrity of a body *system* may reflect adequate functioning of many body *regions* and of the various systems within these regions.

You may want to plan your physical examination around your patient's *chief complaint* or *concern.* To do this, begin by examining the body system or region that corresponds to the chief complaint. This allows you to identify priority problems promptly and reassures your patient that you are paying attention to his primary reason for seeking health care.

Consider the following example. Your patient, Sarah Clemson, is a 65-year-old, active, well-nourished woman who appears younger than her chronologic age. She complains of having difficulty breathing on exertion; she also has a dry, frequent, painful cough. Intermittent chills have persisted for 3 days. First, you would record her vital signs: temperature, 103° F (39.4° C); pulse rate, 106 beats/minute; respiratory rate, 29 to 30 breaths/minute; blood pressure, 128/82 mm Hg.

Because Mrs. Clemson's chief complaints are difficulty breathing, a cough, and chills, your physical examination would initially focus on her respiratory system. You would examine the patency of her airways, observe the color of her lips and extremities, and systematically palpate her lung fields for symmetry of expansion, crepitus, increased or decreased fremitus, and areas of tenderness. After auscultating her lung fields for abnormal or adventitious sounds (such as crackles, rhonchi, or wheezing), you would percuss her lung fields for increased or decreased resonance.

Next, you would examine Mrs. Clemson's cardiovascular system, looking for further clues to the cause of her signs and symptoms. You would inspect her neck veins for distention and her extremities for edema, venous engorgement, and pigmented areas. Then you would palpate her chest to see if you could feel the heart's apical impulse at the fifth intercostal space, in the midclavicular line. You would also palpate for a precordial heave and for valvular thrills. After determining her apical pulse rate, you would auscultate for any abnormal heart sounds.

At this point in the examination, you would probably be aware of Mrs. Clemson's level of consciousness, motor ability, and ability to use her muscles and joints. You probably wouldn't need to perform a more thorough musculoskeletal or neurologic examination. You would, however, proceed with an examination of her GI, genitourinary, and integumentary systems, modifying the examination sequence depending on your findings and Mrs. Clemson's tolerance. If her signs and symptoms worsened during the examination, you would interrupt the procedure to report her condition to her doctor. Then you would plan to come back and finish the examination after her condition stabilized.

Documenting physical examination findings. Physical examination findings are crucial to arriving at a nursing diagnosis and, ultimately, to developing a sound nursing plan of care. Record your examination results thoroughly, accurately, and clearly.

Although some examiners don't like to use a printed form to record physical assessment findings, preferring to work with a blank paper, others believe that standardized data collection forms can make recording physical examination results easier. These forms simplify comprehensive data collection and documentation by providing a concise format for outlining and recording pertinent information. They also remind you to include all essential assessment data.

When documenting, describe exactly what you've inspected, palpated, percussed, or auscultated. Don't use general terms, such as *normal, abnormal, good,* or *poor.* Instead, be specific. Include positive and negative findings. Try to document as soon as possible after completing your assessment. Remember that abbreviations aid conciseness. (See *Documentation tips.*)

NURSING DIAGNOSIS

According to the North American Nursing Diagnosis Association (NANDA), the nursing diagnosis is a "clinical judgment about individual, family, or community responses to actual or potential health problems or life processes. Nursing diagnoses provide the basis for selection of nursing interventions to achieve outcomes for which the nurse is accountable." The nursing diagnosis must be supported by clinical information obtained during patient assessment. (See *Nursing diagnoses and the nursing process,* page 12.)

Each nursing diagnosis describes a patient problem that a nurse can legally manage. Becoming familiar with nursing diagnoses will enable you to better understand how nursing

Documentation tips

Remember these rules about documenting your initial assessment:

• Always document your findings as soon as possible after you take the health history and perform the physical examination.
• Always document your assessment away from the patient's bedside. Jot down only key points while you're with the patient.
• Always answer every question on the assessment form if you're using one. If a question doesn't apply to your patient, write "N/A" or "not applicable" in the space.
• Always focus your questions on areas that relate to the patient's chief complaint. Record information that has significance and will help you build a plan of care.
• If you delegate the job of filling out the first section of the form to another

nurse or an aide, remember — you must review the information gathered and validate it if you aren't sure it's correct.
• Always accept accountability for your assessment by signing your name to the areas you have completed.
• Always directly quote the patient or family member who gave you the information if you fear that summarizing will make it lose some of its meaning.
• Always write or print legibly, in ink.
• Always be concise, specific, and exact when you describe your physical findings.
• Always go back to the patient's bedside to clarify or validate information that seems incomplete.

practice is distinct from medical practice. Although the identification of problems commonly overlaps in nursing and medicine, the approach to treatment clearly differs. Medicine focuses on curing disease; nursing focuses on holistic care that includes cure and comfort. Nurses can independently diagnose and treat the patient's response to illness, certain health problems, and the need for patient education. Nurses comfort, counsel, and care for patients and their families until they are physically, emotionally, and spiritually ready to provide self-care.

Developing your diagnosis
The nursing diagnosis expresses your professional judgment of the patient's clinical status, responses to treatment, and nursing care needs. You perform this step so that you can develop your

plan of care. In effect, the nursing diagnosis *defines* the practice of nursing. Translating the history, physical examination, and laboratory data about a patient into a nursing diagnosis involves organizing the data into clusters and interpreting what the clusters reveal about your patient's ability to meet basic needs. In addition to identifying the patient's needs in coping with the effects of illness, consider what assistance the patient requires to grow and develop to the fullest extent possible.

Your nursing diagnosis describes the cluster of signs and symptoms indicating an actual or potential health problem that you can identify — and that your care can resolve. Nursing diagnoses that indicate potential health problems can be identified by the words "risk for," which appear in the diagnostic label. There are also

Nursing diagnoses and the nursing process

When first described, the nursing process included only assessment, planning, implementation, and evaluation. However, during the past three decades, several important events have helped to establish diagnosis as a distinct part of the nursing process.

• The American Nurses Association (ANA), in its 1973 publication *Standards of Nursing Practice,* mentioned nursing diagnosis as a separate and definable act performed by the registered nurse. In 1991, the ANA published its revised standards of clinical practice, which continued to list nursing diagnosis as a distinct step of the nursing process.

• Individual states passed nurse practice acts that listed diagnosis as part of the nurse's legal responsibility.

• In 1973, the North American Nursing Diagnosis Association (NANDA) began a formal effort to classify nursing diagnoses. NANDA continues to meet biennially to review proposed new nursing

diagnoses and examine applications of nursing diagnoses in clinical practice, education, and research. Their most recent meeting was held in April 2000 in Orlando, Florida. NANDA also publishes *NANDA Nursing Diagnoses: Definitions and Classification 1999-2000,* a complete list of nursing diagnoses, definitions, and defining characteristics. Currently, members of NANDA are working in cooperation with the ANA and the International Council of Nurses to develop an International Classification of Nursing Practice.

• The emergence of the computer-based patient record has underscored the need for a standardized nomenclature for nursing.

---

nursing diagnoses that focus on prevention of health problems and enhanced wellness.

Creating your nursing diagnosis is a logical extension of collecting assessment data. In your patient assessment, you asked each history question, performed each physical examination technique, and considered each laboratory test result because it provided evidence of how your patient could be helped by your care or because the data could affect nursing care.

To develop the nursing diagnosis, use the assessment data you've collected to develop a problem list. Less formal in structure than a fully developed nursing diagnosis, this list describes your patient's problems or needs. It's easy to generate such a list if you use a conceptual model or an accepted set of criterion norms. Ex-

amples of such norms include normal physical and psychological development, Maslow's hierarchy of needs, Orem's universal self-care demands, and Gordon's functional health patterns. (See appendices, pages 662 to 720.)

You can identify the patient's problems and needs with simple phrases, such as *poor circulation, high fever,* or *poor hydration.* Next, prioritize the problems on the list and then develop the working nursing diagnosis.

Writing a nursing diagnosis

Some nurses are confused about how to document a nursing diagnosis because they think the language is too complex. By remembering the following basic guidelines, however, you can ensure that your diagnostic statement is correct:

• Use proper terminology that reflects the patient's *nursing* needs.
• Make your statement concise so it's easily understood by other health team members.
• Use the most precise words possible.
• Use a problem–cause format, stating the problem and its related cause.

Whenever possible, use the terminology recommended by NANDA. NANDA diagnostic headings, when combined with suspected etiology, provide a clear picture of the patient's needs. Thus, for clarity in charting, start with one of the NANDA categories as a heading for the diagnostic statement. The category can reflect an actual or potential problem. Consider this sample diagnosis:

Heading: Mobility impairment
Etiology: Related to pain and discomfort following surgery
Signs and symptoms: "I can't walk without help." Patient hasn't ambulated since surgery on (give date and time). Range of motion limited to 10 degrees flexion in the right hip. Patient can't walk 3' from the bed to the chair without the help of two nurses.

This format links the patient's problem to the etiology without stating a direct cause-and-effect relationship (which may be hard to prove). Remember to state only the patient's problems and the probable origin. Omit references to possible solutions. (Your solutions will derive from your nursing diagnosis, but they aren't part of it.)

Avoiding common errors
One major pitfall in developing a nursing diagnosis is writing one that nursing interventions can't treat. Errors can also occur when nurses take shortcuts in the nursing process, either by omitting or hurrying through

assessment or by basing the diagnosis on inaccurate assessment data.

Keep in mind that a nursing diagnosis is a statement of a health problem that a nurse is licensed to treat — a problem for which you'll assume responsibility for therapeutic decisions and accountability for the outcomes. A nursing diagnosis is *not* a:
• diagnostic test ("schedule for cardiac angiography")
• piece of equipment ("set up intermittent suction apparatus")
• problem with equipment ("the patient has trouble using a commode")
• nurse's problem with a patient ("Mr. Jones is a difficult patient; he's rude and won't take his medication.")
• nursing goal ("encourage fluids up to 2,000 ml per day")
• nursing need ("I have to get through to the family that they must accept the fact that their father is dying.")
• medical diagnosis ("cervical cancer")
• treatment ("catheterize after each voiding for residual urine").

At first, these distinctions may not be clear. The following examples should help clarify what a nursing diagnosis is:
• Don't state a need instead of a problem.
    Incorrect: *Fluid replacement related to fever*
    Correct: *Fluid volume deficit related to fever*
• Don't reverse the two parts of the statement.
    Incorrect: *Lack of understanding related to noncompliance with diabetic diet*
    Correct: *Noncompliance with diabetic diet related to lack of understanding*
• Don't identify an untreatable condition instead of the actual problem it indicates (which can be treated).

Incorrect: *Inability to speak related to laryngectomy*

Correct: *Social isolation related to inability to speak because of laryngectomy*

• Don't write a legally inadvisable statement.

Incorrect: *Skin integrity impairment related to improper positioning*

Correct: *Skin integrity impairment related to immobility*

• Don't identify as unhealthful a response that would be appropriate, allowed for, or culturally acceptable.

Incorrect: *Anger related to terminal illness*

Correct: *Ineffective management of therapeutic regimen related to anger over terminal illness*

• Don't make a tautological statement (one in which both parts of the statement say the same thing).

Incorrect: *Pain related to alteration in comfort*

Correct: *Pain related to postoperative abdominal distention and anxiety*

• Don't identify a nursing problem instead of a patient problem.

Incorrect: *Difficulty suctioning related to thick secretions*

Correct: *Ineffective airway clearance related to thick tracheal secretion*

How nursing and medical diagnoses differ

You assess your patient to obtain data for making a nursing diagnosis, just as the doctor examines a patient to establish a medical diagnosis. Learn the differences between the two, and remember that sometimes they overlap. You perform a complete patient assessment to identify patient problems that your nursing interventions can help resolve; your nursing diagnoses state these problems. (Some may occur secondary to medical treatment.) If you plan your care of a patient around only the medical aspects of his illness, you'll probably overlook significant problems.

For example, suppose your patient's medical diagnosis is a fractured femur. In your assessment, take a careful history. Include questions to determine if the patient has adequate financial resources to cope with prolonged disability. To assess the patient's capacity to adjust to the physical restrictions caused by the disability, gather data about his previous lifestyle.

Suppose your physical examination of this patient — in addition to uncovering signs and symptoms pertaining to the medical diagnosis — reveals actual or potential skin breakdown secondary to immobility. Your nursing diagnoses, in that case, may include home maintenance management impairment, diversional activity deficit (related to prolonged immobility), and risk for skin integrity impairment.

The plan of care you prepare for this patient should include the nursing interventions suggested by your nursing diagnoses as well as the nursing actions necessary to fulfill the patient's medical treatment plan. When integrated into a plan of care, the nursing and medical diagnoses describe the complete nursing care your patient needs.

Study the examples here to better understand the difference between medical and nursing diagnoses.
1. Frank Smith, age 67, complains of "stubborn, old muscles." He has difficulty walking, as you can see by his shuffling gait. During the interview, Mr. Smith speaks in a monotone and seems very depressed. Physical examination shows a pill-rolling hand

tremor. Laboratory tests reveal a decreased dopamine level.

Medical diagnosis
Parkinson's disease
Nursing diagnoses
• Mobility impairment related to decreased muscle control
• Body image disturbance related to physical alterations
• Knowledge deficit related to lack of information about progressive nature of illness
2. For 5 consecutive days, Judy Wilson, age 26, has had sporadic abdominal cramps of increasing intensity. Most recently, the pain has been accompanied by vomiting and a slight fever. Your examination reveals rebound tenderness and muscle guarding.
Medical diagnosis
Appendicitis
Nursing diagnoses
• Pain related to biological agents
• Fluid volume deficit related to vomiting
3. During an extensive bout with respiratory tract infections, Tom Bradley, age 7, complains of throbbing ear pain. Tom's mother notes his hearing difficulty and his fear of the pain and possible hearing loss. On inspection, his tympanic membrane appears red and bulging.
Medical diagnosis
Acute suppurative otitis media
Nursing diagnoses
• Pain related to swollen tympanic membrane
• Fear related to progressive hearing loss
• Sensory or perceptual alteration (auditory) related to obstructed middle ear.

Outcome identification
During this phase of the nursing process, you identify expected outcomes for the patient. Expected outcomes are measurable, patient-focused goals that are derived from the patient's nursing diagnoses. These goals may be short- or long-term. Short-term goals include those of immediate concern that can be achieved quickly. Long-term goals take more time to achieve and usually involve prevention, patient teaching, and rehabilitation.

In many cases, you can identify expected outcomes by converting the nursing diagnosis into a positive statement. For instance, for the nursing diagnosis "mobility impairment related to a fracture of the right hip," the expected outcome might be "The patient will ambulate independently before discharge."

When writing the plan of care, state expected outcomes in terms of the patient's behavior — for example, "the patient correctly demonstrates turning, coughing, and deep breathing." Also identify a target time or date by which the expected outcomes should be accomplished. The expected outcomes will serve as the basis for evaluating your nursing interventions.

Keep in mind that each expected outcome must be stated in measurable terms. If possible, consult with the patient and family when establishing expected outcomes. As the patient progresses, expected outcomes should be increasingly directed toward planning for discharge and follow-up care.

Outcome statements should be tailored to your practice setting. For example, in the intensive care unit you may focus on maintaining hemodynamic stability, whereas on a rehabilitation unit you would focus on maximizing the patient's independence and preventing complications.

Tips for writing expected outcome statements

When writing expected outcomes in your plan of care, always start with a specific action verb that focuses on your patient's behavior. By telling your reader how your patient should *look, walk, eat, drink, turn, cough, speak,* or *stand,* for example, you give a clear picture of how to evaluate progress.

Avoid starting expected outcome statements with *allow, let, enable,* or similar verbs. Such words focus attention on your own and other health team members' behavior — not on the patient's.

With many documentation formats, you won't need to include the phrase "The patient will..." with each expected outcome statement. You will, however, have to specify which person the goals refer to when family, friends, or others are directly concerned.

Make sure target dates are realistic. Be flexible enough to adjust the date if your patient needs more time to respond to your interventions.

PLANNING

The nursing plan of care refers to a written plan of action designed to help you deliver quality patient care. It includes relevant nursing diagnoses, expected outcomes, and nursing interventions. Keep in mind that the plan of care usually forms a permanent part of the patient's health record and will be used by other members of the nursing team. The plan of care may be integrated into an interdisciplinary plan for the patient. In this instance, clear guidelines should outline the role of each member of the health care team in providing care.

Reviewing the planning stages

Planning involves three stages:
• assigning priorities to the nursing diagnoses
• selecting appropriate nursing actions (interventions)
• documenting the nursing diagnoses, expected outcomes, nursing interventions, and evaluations on the plan of care.

Assigning priorities. Any time you develop more than one nursing diagnosis for your patient, you must assign priorities to them and begin your plan of care with those having the highest priority. High-priority nursing diagnoses involve the patient's most urgent needs (such as emergency or immediate physical needs). Intermediate-priority diagnoses involve nonemergency needs, and low-priority diagnoses involve needs that don't directly relate to the patient's specific illness or prognosis. (To help establish priorities, you may want to refer to *Nursing diagnoses and Maslow's hierarchy of needs,* pages 714 and 715.)

Selecting appropriate nursing interventions. You must develop one or more nursing interventions to achieve each of the expected outcomes identified for your patient. For example, if one expected outcome statement reads "The patient will transfer to chair with assistance," the appropriate nursing interventions include placing the wheelchair facing the foot of the bed and assisting the patient to stand and pivot to the chair. If another expected outcome statement reads "The patient will express feelings related to recent injury," appropriate interventions might include spending time with the patient each shift, conveying an open and nonjudgmental attitude, and asking open-ended questions.

Reviewing the second part of the nursing diagnosis statement (the part describing etiologic factors) may help guide your choice of nursing interventions. For example, for the nursing diagnosis *Risk for injury related to inadequate blood glucose levels,* you would determine the best nursing interventions for maintaining an adequate blood glucose level. Typical interventions for this goal include observing the patient for evidence of hypoglycemia and providing an appropriate diet.

Try to think creatively during this step in the nursing process. It's an opportunity to describe exactly what you and your patient would like to have happen and to establish the criteria against which you'll judge further nursing actions.

Documenting your plan. The planning phase culminates when you write the plan of care and document the nursing diagnoses, expected outcomes, nursing interventions, and evaluations for expected outcomes. Write your plan of care in concise, specific terms so that other health team members can follow it. Keep in mind that because the patient's problems and needs will change, you'll have to review your plan of care frequently and modify it when necessary.

Benefits of writing a plan of care

To provide quality care for each patient, you must plan and direct that care. Writing a plan of care lets you document the scientific method you have used throughout the nursing process. On the plan of care, you summarize the patient's problems and needs (as nursing diagnoses) and identify appropriate nursing interventions and expected outcomes. A plan of care that is well conceived and properly written helps decrease the risk of incomplete or incorrect care by:

• giving direction
• providing continuity of care
• establishing communication between you and nurses on other shifts, between you and health-team members in other departments, and between you and your patient
• serving as a key for patient care assignments.

Giving direction. A written plan of care gives direction by showing colleagues the goals you have set for your patient and giving clear instructions for helping to achieve them. It also makes clear exactly what to document on the patient's progress notes. For instance, it lists what observations to make and how often, what nursing measures to take and how to implement them, and what to teach the patient and family before discharge.

Providing continuity. A written plan of care identifies the patient's needs to each shift and tells what must be done to meet those needs. With this information, nurses on each shift can adjust their routines to meet the patient's care demands. A plan of care also provides each shift with specific instructions on patient care, eliminating the confusion that can exist between shifts. If your patient is discharged from your health care facility to another, your plan of care can help ease this transition.

Establishing communication. By soliciting your patient's input as you develop the plan of care, you build a rapport that lets the patient know you value his opinions and feelings. By reviewing the plan of care with other health-team members, and with other nurses during change-of-shift reports, you can regularly evaluate your patient's response or lack of response to the nursing care and medical regimen.

Guiding patient care assignments. If you're a team leader, you may want to delegate some specific routines or duties described in each nursing intervention — not all of them need your professional attention.

What your plan of care should include

Care-planning formats vary from one health care facility to another. For example, you may write your plan of care on a form supplied by the hospital or you can use software that is approved by your agency. Nearly all care-planning formats include space in which to document the nursing diagnoses, expected outcomes, and nursing interventions. In many health care facilities, you may also document assessment data and discharge planning on the plan of care.

No matter which format you use, be sure to write the plan of care in ink (and sign it), even though you may have to make revisions if your nursing interventions don't work. Remember — your patient's plan of care becomes part of the permanent record and shouldn't be erased or destroyed. If you write it in pencil — so you can erase to revise — you make it seem unimportant. The information must remain intact, enabling you and other health-team members to readily refer to nursing interventions used in the past. (See *Guidelines for writing the plan of care.*)

Be specific when writing your plan of care. By discussing specific problems, expected outcomes, nursing interventions, and evaluations for expected outcomes, you leave no doubt as to what needs to be done by other health-team members. When listing

nursing interventions, for example, be sure to include *when* the action should be implemented, *who* should be involved in each aspect of implementation, and the *frequency, quantity,* and *method* to be used. Specify dates and times when appropriate. List target dates for each expected outcome.

If your nursing interventions have resolved the problem on which you've based the nursing diagnosis, write "discontinued" next to the diagnostic statement on the plan of care, and list the date you discontinued the interventions. If your nursing interventions haven't resolved the problem by the target date, reevaluate your plan and do one of the following:
• Extend the target date and continue the intervention until the patient responds as expected.
• Discontinue the intervention and select a new one that will achieve the expected outcome.

Keeping the plan of care current

You'll need to update and modify a patient's plan of care as problems (or their priorities) change and resolve, new assessment information becomes available, and you evaluate the patient's responses to nursing interventions.

Care planning for students

Developing a plan of care helps the nursing student improve problem-solving technique, learn the nursing process, and improve written and verbal communication and organizational skills. More important, it shows how to apply classroom and textbook knowledge to practice.

Because it aims to teach the care-planning process, the student plan of care is longer than the standard plan

Guidelines for writing the plan of care

Keeping these tips in mind will help you write a plan of care that is accurate and useful.

• Write your patient's plan of care in ink. It's a part of the permanent record. Sign your name.
• Be specific; don't use vague terms or generalities on the plan of care.
• Never use abbreviations that may be confused with ones meaning something different.
• Take time to review all your assessment data *before* you select an approach for each problem. (*Note:* If you can't complete the initial assessment, immediately note "insufficient database" on your records.)
• Write down a specific expected outcome for each problem you identify, and record a target date for its completion.
• Avoid setting an initial goal that is too high to be achieved. For example, suppose the outcome for a newly admitted patient with cerebrovascular accident says, "Patient will ambulate with assistance." Several patient outcomes will need to be achieved before this goal can be addressed.
• Consider the following three phases of patient care when writing nursing in-

terventions: what observations to make and how often, what nursing measures to do and how to do them, and what to teach the patient and family before discharge.
• Make each nursing intervention specific.
• Make sure nursing interventions match the resources and capabilities of the staff. Combine what is necessary to correct or modify the problem with what is reasonably possible in your setting.
• Be creative when you write your patient's plan of care; include a drawing or an innovative procedure if either will make your directions more specific.
• Don't overlook any of the patient's problems or concerns. Include them on the plan of care so they won't be forgotten.
• Make sure your plan of care is implemented correctly.
• Evaluate the results of your plan of care, and discontinue any nursing diagnoses that have been resolved. Select new approaches, if necessary, for problems that haven't been resolved.

used in most health care facilities. In a step-by step manner, it progresses from assessment to evaluation. However, some teaching institutions model the student plan of care on the plan used by the affiliated health care institution, adding a space for the scientific rationale for each nursing intervention selected.

Writing out all of your planned actions enables you to review planned nursing activities with your clinical instructor. This is an opportunity to consider whether or not you have complete assessment data to support

your diagnoses and interventions and if you've taken into consideration all the problems that a more experienced nurse is likely to identify.

IMPLEMENTATION

During this phase, you put your plan of care into action. Implementation encompasses all nursing interventions directed toward solving the patient's nursing problems and meeting health care needs. While you coordinate implementation, you also seek help from other caregivers, the patient, and the patient's family.

Nursing interventions: Three types

Knowing the three types of nursing interventions will help you document implementation appropriately.

1. *Independent interventions.* These interventions fall within the purview of nursing practice and don't require a doctor's direction or supervision. Most nursing actions required by the patient's plan of care are independent interventions. Examples include patient teaching, health promotion, counseling, and helping the patient with activities of daily living.
2. *Dependent interventions.* Based on written or oral instructions from another professional — usually a doctor — dependent interventions include administering medication, inserting indwelling urinary catheters, and obtaining specimens for laboratory tests.
3. *Interdependent interventions.* Performed in collaboration with other professionals, interdependent interventions include following a protocol and carrying out standing orders.

Implementation requires some (or all) of the following interventions:
• assessing and monitoring (for example, recording vital signs)
• therapeutic interventions (for example, giving medications)
• making the patient more comfortable and helping him with activities of daily living
• supporting his respiratory and elimination functions
• providing skin care
• managing the environment (for example, controlling noise to ensure a good night's sleep)
• providing food and fluids
• giving emotional support
• teaching and counseling
• referring the patient to appropriate agencies or services.

Elements of implementation

Incorporate these elements into the implementation stage:
• *Reassessing.* Although it may be brief or narrowly focused, reassessment should confirm that the planned interventions remain appropriate.
• *Reviewing and modifying the plan of care.* Never static, an appropriate plan of care changes with the patient's condition. As necessary, update the assessment, nursing diagnoses, implementation, and evaluation sections. (Entering the new data in a different color of ink alerts other staff members to the revisions.) Date the revisions.
• *Seeking assistance.* Determine, for example, whether you need help from other staff members or additional information before you can intervene.

Documentation

Implementation isn't complete until you've documented each intervention, the time it occurred, the patient's response, and any other pertinent information. Make sure each entry relates to a nursing diagnosis. Remember that any action not documented may be overlooked during quality assurance monitoring or evaluation of care. Another good reason for thorough documentation: It offers a way for you to take rightful credit for your contribution in helping a patient achieve the highest possible level of wellness. After all, nurses use a unique and worthwhile combination of interpersonal, intellectual, and technical skills when providing care. (See *Nursing interventions: Three types.*)

EVALUATION

In this phase of the nursing process, you assess the effectiveness of the plan of care by answering questions such as:
• How has the patient progressed in terms of the plan's projected outcomes?
• Does the patient have new needs?
• Does the plan of care need to be revised?

Evaluation also helps you determine whether the patient received high-quality care from the nursing staff and the health care facility. Your facility bases its own nursing quality assurance system on nursing evaluations.

Steps in the evaluation process

Include the patient, family members, and other health care professionals in the evaluation. Then follow these steps:
• *Select evaluation criteria.* The plan of care's projected outcomes — the desired effects of nursing interventions — form the basis for evaluation.
• *Compare the patient's response to the evaluation criteria.* Did the patient respond as expected? If not, the plan of care may need revision.
• *Analyze your findings.* If your plan wasn't effective, determine why. You may conclude, for example, that several nursing diagnoses were inaccurate.
• *Modify the plan of care.* Make revisions (for example, change inaccurate nursing diagnoses) and implement the new plan.
• *Reevaluate.* Like all steps in the nursing process, evaluation is ongoing. Continue to assess, plan, implement, and evaluate for as long as you care for the patient.

Questions to answer

When evaluating and documenting your patient's care, collect information from all available sources — for example, the patient's medical record, family members, other caregivers, and the patient. Also include your own observations.

During the evaluation process, ask yourself these questions:
• Has the patient's condition improved, deteriorated, or remained the same?
• Were the nursing diagnoses accurate?
• Have the patient's nursing needs been met?
• Did the patient meet the outcome criteria documented in the plan of care?
• Which nursing interventions should I revise or discontinue?
• Why did the patient fail to meet some goals (if applicable)?
• Should I reorder priorities? Revise expected outcomes?

NURSING DIAGNOSES AND CRITICAL PATHWAYS

In a growing number of health care settings — inpatient and outpatient, acute and long-term care — critical pathways are being used to guide the process of care for a patient. Critical pathways describe the course of a specific health-related condition. A critical pathway may used along with or instead of a nursing plan of care, depending on the standards set by the individual health care facility. These tools may also be referred to as clinical pathways, care maps, collaborative care plans, or multidisciplinary action plans (MAPs). (See *Developing a critical pathway*.)

The concept of the critical pathway evolved out of the growth of managed care and the development of the case management model in the early 1990s. Pressure from managed care organizations to control costs led to the evolution of case management.

In case management, one professional — usually a nurse or a social worker — assumes responsibility for coordinating care so that patients move through the health care system in the shortest time and at the lowest cost possible.

Early on, case managers used the nursing process and based their plans on nursing diagnoses. Over time, however, it became evident that a multidisciplinary approach was needed to adequately monitor length of stay and reduce overall costs. This led to the development of the critical pathway concept.

In critical pathways, a time line is defined for each condition and for the achievement of expected outcomes. By reading the critical pathway, caregivers can determine on any given day where the patient should be in his progress toward optimal health.

The critical pathway provides a method for doctors and nurses to standardize and organize care for routine conditions. These pathways also make it easier for case managers to track data needed to:
• streamline utilization of material resources and labor
• ensure that patients receive quality care
• improve the coordination of care
• reduce the cost of providing care.

The most successful critical pathways have been developed for medical diagnoses with predictable outcomes, such as hip replacement, mastectomy, myocardial infarction, and cardiac catheterization. Critical pathways work best with high volume, high risk, high cost conditions or procedures for which there are predictable outcomes.

THE IMPORTANCE OF NURSING DIAGNOSES

Using a critical pathway can be helpful, especially for nursing students and new graduates. You may be assigned to provide care to a particular patient for only 1 or 2 days. Seeing the entire pathway and examining the outcomes the patient is expected to achieve will help you obtain a broader clinical perspective on care.

Using a critical pathway as a guide for delivering care doesn't, however,

Developing a critical pathway

An interdisciplinary tool, the critical pathway requires the collaborative efforts of all disciplines involved in patient care. The interdisciplinary team must decide on a diagnosis, select a set of achievable outcomes, and agree on a plausible time line for achieving the desired outcomes. Note that when establishing standard practices for treatment of a given condition, it has often proved difficult for doctors to achieve consensus.

Establishing a time line

Time intervals allocated on a critical pathway vary according to the type of condition and its acuity. For a hip replacement, the time line extends over days; for a cardiac catheterization procedure, time intervals are expressed in hours. In the postanesthesia period, a critical pathway can be defined in minutes.

Average length of stay is an important concept in developing a critical pathway. If agency data indicate that the average length of stay for an inpatient who has had a modified radical mastectomy with reconstruction is 4 days, then the team begins planning around a 4-day stay.

Building the pathway

The interdisciplinary team must choose a framework for developing outcomes and interventions. Some agencies build pathways around nursing diagnoses. If interdisciplinary collaboration is strong, an agency may build pathways around general aspects of care; for example, pain, activity, nutrition, assessment, medications, psychosocial status, treatments, teaching, and discharge planning.

In an acute care setting, outcomes and interventions for each aspect of care are determined for each day of an expected length of stay. In long-term care and other community-based settings, progress may be measured in longer intervals.

---

negate the need to formulate and utilize nursing diagnoses. Nursing diagnoses continue to define the primary responsibility of nursing — to diagnose and treat human responses to actual or potential health problems. The full nursing care needs of any patient are unlikely to be documented on a critical pathway. When using a pathway, always keep in mind that your patient may require nursing intervention beyond what is specified in the critical pathway.

For example, a patient enters a hospital for a hip replacement and can't communicate verbally because of a recent stroke. The critical pathway wouldn't include measures to assist the patient to make his needs known. Therefore, you would develop a nursing plan of care around the diagnosis *Verbal communication impairment related to decreased circulation to the brain.*

Even if you practice in a clinical setting that relies on critical pathways to fill documentation requirements, the *Nursing Diagnosis Reference Manual,* Fifth Edition, will prove to be a valuable resource for identifying and treating each patient's unique nursing needs. Creating a plan of care based on carefully selected nursing diagnoses and using it along with a critical pathway will enable you to provide your patients with high-quality collaborative care that includes a strong nursing component.

ADULT HEALTH

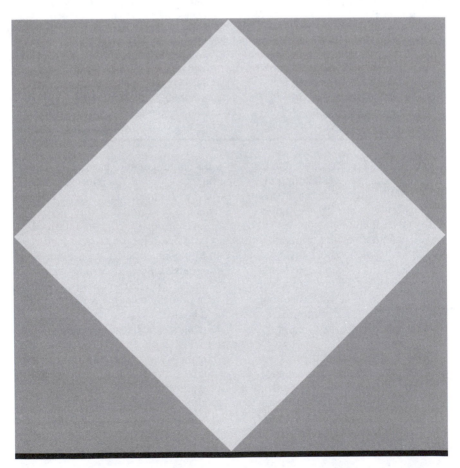

INTRODUCTION

This section includes approximately 200 alphabetically organized diagnostic labels and associated plans of care that identify adult health problems amenable to independent nursing action. Many of them focus on meeting the patient's actual physiologic needs. For example, you'll find plans of care for ensuring the survival of a patient with decreased cardiac output, for helping an injured patient maintain joint range of motion, and for teaching an immunosuppressed patient measures to prevent infection. In addition, you'll find plans for warding off potential health problems, such as risk for infection or injury.

Other plans of care focus on the psychological and psychosocial problems of adulthood. For example, if a patient with a chronic illness experiences related emotional difficulties, look up such diagnostic labels as *hopelessness, role performance alteration,* and *body image disturbance* to help pinpoint his needs. If a patient lacks adequate financial, social, or spiritual resources, appropriate plans of care provide instructions for documenting such hardships and interventions for ameliorating them.

Still other plans of care focus on more specialized patient problems. For instance, you'll find plans for patients undergoing surgery.

In sum, the diagnostic labels and associated plans of care in this section cover the full range of nursing responsibilities. To make full use of this broad database, you'll need to perform a complete and careful nursing assessment. When appropriate, include questions about the patient's cultural background. Ask about self-concept, stressors, daily living habits, and coping mechanisms. Discuss the patient's health goals. How well does the patient understand his condition? Will family members or friends take an active role in his care? Add information from your own observations.

Use information gathered during assessment to select an accurate diagnostic statement and an appropriate plan of care. That way, you can ensure your adult patient comprehensive, individualized, and consistent nursing care.

■ Activity intolerance

related to imbalance between oxygen supply and demand

Definition
Extreme fatigue or other physical symptoms caused by simple activity

Assessment
• History of circulatory disease, respiratory disease, or both
• Patient's perception of tolerance for activity
• Respiratory status, including arterial blood gas analysis, pulmonary function studies, and respiratory rate, depth, and pattern both at rest and with activity
• Cardiovascular status, including blood pressure, complete blood count, exercise electrocardiogram (ECG) results, and heart rate and rhythm both at rest and with activity
• Knowledge, including understanding of present condition, perception of need to maintain or restore an activity level consistent with capabilities, and physical, mental, and emotional readiness to learn

Defining characteristics
• Abnormal heart rate or blood pressure in response to activity, arrhythmia or ischemic changes on ECG, and exertional discomfort or dyspnea
• Verbal report of fatigue or weakness

Associated medical diagnoses (selected)
Acute respiratory failure, anemias, aortic insufficiency, aortic stenosis, asthma, bone marrow transplantation, chronic bronchitis, chronic obstructive pulmonary disease, congenital heart disease, coronary artery disease, cor pulmonale, Cushing's syndrome, cystic fibrosis, emphysema, endo-carditis, end-stage cardiac disease, heart failure, hyperthyroidism, hypothyroidism, interstitial pulmonary fibrosis, lung cancer, Lyme disease, mitral insufficiency, mitral stenosis, multiple myeloma, myocardial infarction, peripheral vascular disease, pregnancy-induced hypertension, pulmonary edema, pulmonary embolus, sarcoidosis

Expected outcomes
• Patient will state desire to increase activity level.
• Patient will state understanding of the need to increase activity level gradually.
• Patient will identify controllable factors that cause fatigue.
• Blood pressure and pulse and respiratory rates will remain within prescribed limits during activity.
• Patient will state sense of satisfaction with each new level of activity attained.
• Patient will demonstrate skill in conserving energy while carrying out daily activities to tolerance level.
• Patient will explain illness and connect symptoms of activity intolerance with deficit in oxygen supply or use.

Interventions and rationales
• Discuss with patient the need for activity, *which will improve physical and psychosocial well-being.*
• Identify activities patient considers desirable and meaningful *to enhance their positive impact.*
• Encourage patient to help plan activity progression, being sure to include activities the patient considers essential. *Participation in planning helps ensure patient compliance.*
• Instruct and help patient to alternate periods of rest and activity *to reduce the body's oxygen demand and prevent fatigue.*

• Identify and minimize factors that decrease patient's exercise tolerance *to help increase activity level.*
• Monitor physiologic responses to increased activity (including respirations, heart rate and rhythm, and blood pressure) *to ensure return to normal a few minutes after exercising.*
• Teach patient how to conserve energy while performing activities of daily living — for example, sitting in a chair while dressing, wearing lightweight clothing that fastens with Velcro or a few large buttons, and wearing slip-on shoes. *These measures reduce cellular metabolism and oxygen demand.*
• Teach patient exercises for increasing strength and endurance, *which will improve breathing and gradually increase activity level.*
• Support and encourage activity to patient's level of tolerance. *This helps develop the patient's independence.*
• Before discharge, formulate a plan with patient and caregivers that will enable the patient either to continue functioning at maximum activity tolerance or to gradually increase tolerance. For example, teach patient and caregivers to monitor patient's pulse during activities; to recognize need for oxygen, if prescribed; and to use oxygen equipment properly. *Participation in planning encourages patient satisfaction and compliance.*

Evaluations for expected outcomes
• Patient states a desire to increase activity level.
• Patient identifies a plan to increase activity level.
• Patient lists factors that cause fatigue.
• Patient's blood pressure, pulse, and respiratory rates remain within normal parameters.

• Patient expresses satisfaction with increase in activity level.
• Patient is proficient in conserving energy while performing activities of daily living.
• Patient demonstrates an understanding of relationship between signs and symptoms of activity intolerance and deficit in oxygen supply or use.

Documentation
• Patient's perception of need for activity
• Patient's priorities in performing selected activities
• Patient's description of physical effects of various activities
• Observations made while patient performs activities
• Skills demonstrated by patient in conserving energy during activity
• New activities patient was able to perform
• Evaluations for expected outcomes

■ Activity intolerance
related to immobility

Definition
Extreme fatigue or other physical symptoms caused by simple activity

Assessment
• History of present illness
• Past experience with prolonged bed rest
• Neurologic status, including level of consciousness, orientation, motor status, and sensory status
• Respiratory status, including arterial blood gas analysis, breath sounds, and rate, depth, and pattern of respiration both at rest and with activity
• Cardiovascular status, including blood pressure, skin color, hemoglo-

bin and hematocrit, and heart rate and rhythm both at rest and with activity
• Musculoskeletal status, including range of motion and muscle size, strength, and tone

Defining characteristics
• Abnormal heart rate or blood pressure in response to activity, arrhythmia or ischemic changes on electrocardiogram, and exertional discomfort or dyspnea
• Verbal report of weakness or fatigue

Associated medical diagnoses (selected)
Bone sarcomas, bursitis, encephalitis, fractures, gout, Guillain-Barré syndrome, head injury, osteoarthritis, Parkinson's disease, rheumatoid arthritis, spinal cord injury, tendinitis

Expected outcomes
• Patient will regain and maintain muscle mass and strength.
• Patient will maintain maximum joint range of motion.
• Patient will perform isometric exercises.
• Patient will help perform self-care activities.
• Heart rate, rhythm, and blood pressure will remain within expected range during periods of activity.
• Patient will state understanding of and willingness to cooperate in maximizing activity level.
• Patient will perform self-care activities to tolerance level.

Interventions and rationales
• Perform active or passive range-of-motion exercises to all extremities every 2 to 4 hours. *These exercises foster muscle strength and tone, maintain joint mobility, and prevent contractures.*
• Turn and reposition patient at least every 2 hours. Establish a turning schedule for the dependent patient. Post schedule at bedside and monitor frequency. *Turning and repositioning prevents skin breakdown and improves breathing.*
• Maintain proper body alignment at all times *to avoid contractures and maintain optimal musculoskeletal balance and physiologic function.*
• Encourage active exercise:
– Provide a trapeze or other assistive device whenever possible. *Such devices simplify moving and turning for many patients and also allow them to strengthen some upper-body muscles.*
– Teach isometric exercises *to allow patient to maintain or increase muscle tone and joint mobility.*
– Have patient perform self-care activities. Begin slowly and increase daily, as tolerated. *Activities will help patient regain health.*
• Provide emotional support and encouragement *to help improve patient's self-concept and motivation to perform activities of daily living.*
• Involve patient in care-related planning and decision making *to improve compliance.*
• Monitor physiologic responses to increased activity level, including respirations, heart rate and rhythm, and blood pressure *to ensure they return to normal within a few minutes after exercising.*
• Teach caregivers to assist patient with self-care activities in a way that maximizes patient's potential. *This enables caregivers to participate in patient's care and also encourages them to support patient's independence.*

Evaluations for expected outcomes
• Patient regains and maintains preillness muscle mass and strength, as demonstrated by increased activity level.

• Patient demonstrates maximum joint range of motion.
• Patient performs isometric exercise _____ times per day.
• Patient assists caregiver in performing self-care activities.
• Patient's blood pressure, pulse rate, and rhythm remain within normal parameters.
• Patient verbalizes understanding of need to maximize activity level.
• Patient performs self-care activities at optimal level within restrictions imposed by illness.

Documentation
• Patient's perceptions about the importance of maintaining optimal levels of activity within restrictions imposed by the illness
• Activities performed by patient
• Observations of physical findings in response to activity
• Teaching activities performed with patient or caregivers
• Evaluations for expected outcomes

◼ Activity intolerance, risk for

related to immobility

Definition
Accentuated risk of extreme fatigue or other physical symptoms following simple activity

Assessment
• History of present illness
• Past experience with immobility or prescribed bed rest
• Cardiovascular status, including blood pressure, heart rate and rhythm at rest and with activity, complete blood count, skin temperature and color, edema, and chest pain or discomfort
• Respiratory status, including arterial blood gas analysis, auscultation of breath sounds, pain or discomfort associated with respiration, and rate, rhythm, depth, and pattern of respirations at rest and with activity
• Neurologic status, including level of consciousness, orientation, and mental, sensory, and motor status
• Musculoskeletal status, including range of motion, muscle size, strength, tone, and functional mobility as follows:
0 = completely independent
1 = requires use of equipment or device
2 = requires help, supervision, or teaching from another person
3 = requires help from another person and equipment or device
4 = dependent; doesn't participate in activity

Risk factors
• Circulatory or respiratory problems
• History of previous intolerance
• Inexperience with a particular activity
• Poor physical condition

Associated medical diagnoses (selected)
Cerebrovascular accident, dermatomyositis, head injury, heart failure, hip fracture, multiple sclerosis, polymyositis

Expected outcomes
• Patient will maintain muscle strength and joint range of motion.
• Patient will carry out isometric exercise regimen.
• Patient will communicate understanding of rationale for maintaining activity level.
• Patient will avoid risk factors that may lead to activity intolerance.

• Patient will perform self-care activities to tolerance level.
• Blood pressure, pulse, and respiratory rate will remain within prescribed range during periods of activity (specify).

Interventions and rationales
• Position patient to maintain proper body alignment. Use assistive devices as needed *to maintain joint function and prevent musculoskeletal deformities.*
• Turn and position the patient at least every 2 hours. Establish turning schedule for dependent patient. Post at bedside and monitor frequency. *Turning helps prevent skin breakdown by relieving pressure.*
• Assess patient's level of functioning using the functional mobility scale *to determine patient's capabilities.*
• Communicate patient's level of functioning to all staff. *Communication among staff members ensures continuity of care and enables patient to preserve identified level of independence.*
• Unless contraindicated, perform range-of-motion exercises every 2 to 4 hours. Progress from passive to active, according to patient tolerance. *Range-of-motion exercises prevent joint contractures and muscular atrophy.*
• Encourage active movement by helping patient use trapeze or other assistive devices *to improve muscle tone and enhance self-esteem.*
• Teach patient how to perform isometric exercises *to maintain and improve muscle tone and joint mobility.*
• Assist patient in carrying out self-care activities. Increase patient's participation in self-care, as tolerated, *to foster independence and improve mobility.*

• Encourage patient to become involved in planning care and making decisions related to treatment. *Participation in planning enhances compliance.*
• Teach patient, family member, or other caregiver methods to maximize patient's participation in self-care. *Informed caregivers can encourage patient to become more independent.*
• Assess patient's physiologic response to increased activity (blood pressure, respirations, heart rate, and rhythm). *Monitoring vital signs helps to assess tolerance for increased exertion and activity.*
• Teach patient symptoms of overexertion, such as dizziness, chest pain, and dyspnea, *to help patient take responsibility for monitoring activity level.*
• Explain rationale for maintaining or improving activity level. Discuss factors that increase risk of activity intolerance. *Education will help patient avoid activity intolerance.*
• Encourage patient to carry out activities of daily living. Provide emotional support and offer positive feedback when patient displays initiative. *Offering emotional support will enhance patient's self-esteem and motivation.*

Evaluations for expected outcomes
• Functional mobility scale indicates that muscle strength and joint range of motion remain stable.
• Patient demonstrates isometric exercises.
• Patient explains rationale for maintaining activity level.
• Patient states at least five risk factors for activity intolerance.
• Patient performs self-care activities in preparation for discharge.
• Patient doesn't exhibit evidence of cardiovascular or respiratory complications during or after activity.

Documentation
• Patient's expressions of motivation to maintain maximum activity level within restrictions imposed by illness
• Activities performed by patient
• Teaching instructions provided to patient and family member or other caregivers
• Patient's physiologic response to increased activity
• Evaluations for expected outcomes

■ Adjustment impairment

related to disability

Definition
Inability to modify lifestyle or behavior consistent with changed health status

Assessment
• Nature and impact of medical diagnosis
• Behavioral responses, including verbal or nonverbal, engagement or disengagement, interest or apathy, acceptance or denial, and independence or dependence
• Knowledge of health condition
• Past experiences with family, friends, and media
• Psychosocial factors, such as age, sex, ethnic and cultural background, religious preference and beliefs, values, occupation, family support, and coping style
• Nutritional status, including modifications in diet and weight changes

Defining characteristics
• Demonstration of denial of health status change
• Failure to achieve optimal sense of control

• Failure to take action to prevent further health problems

Associated medical diagnoses (selected)
Amputation, chronic pain, colitis, dependent personality disorder, diabetes mellitus, lupus erythematosus, multiple sclerosis, muscular dystrophy, myocardial infarction, paralysis, spinal cord defects, spinal cord injury

Expected outcomes
• Patient will identify inability to cope and will adjust adequately.
• Patient will express understanding of the illness or disease.
• Patient will participate in health care regimen and will plan care activities.
• Patient will demonstrate ability to manage health problem.
• Patient will show ability to accept and adapt to a new health status and integrate learning.
• Patient will demonstrate new coping strategies.

Interventions and rationales
• Encourage patient to express feelings in a safe, nonthreatening environment. *This allows the patient to gain insight into and rationally define fears, goals, and potential problems.*
• Allow patient to grieve. *After working through denial and isolation, anger, bargaining, and depression, patient will progress toward acceptance.*
• Provide reassurance that the patient's feelings are normal *to promote coping.*
• Begin teaching patient and caregivers the skills needed to adequately manage care *to encourage compliance and adjustment to optimum wellness.*
• Spend 15 minutes per shift listening to patient's feelings. *This will help re-*

assure patient you're interested and care.
• Help patient identify areas where it's possible to maintain control. *This avoids feelings of powerlessness and lets patient feel part of a team effort.*
• Encourage patient to plan care activities, such as time of treatment, personal hygiene, and rest periods, *to help give patient a better sense of control.*
• Arrange for others who have suffered similar health problems to speak with patient and family. *This exposes patient to suitable role models and may allow a trusting, supportive relationship to develop.*
• Discuss health problems and implications with family members *to enable them to participate in patient's care and to foster a trusting relationship.*
• Obtain a consultation with a mental health specialist if patient develops severe depression or other psychiatric problems. *Although trauma or illness commonly causes some depression, consultation with a mental health professional may help minimize it.*

Evaluations for expected outcomes
• Patient recognizes necessity of learning to live with impairment.
• Patient understands that grieving is a normal response to impairment.
• Patient meets learning objectives before discharge.
• Patient identifies and contacts sources of continued psychological support, if needed.
• Patient identifies two areas in which he can maintain control despite altered health status.
• Patient meets with individual who has similar health problem and reports results of meeting.

Documentation
• Patient's nonverbal behaviors
• Patient's verbal expressions of denial, anger, or guilt because of the illness or disease process
• Patient's ability or inability to participate in care
• Evaluations for expected outcomes

■ Airway clearance, ineffective

related to decreased energy or fatigue

Definition
Anatomic or physiologic obstruction of the airway that interferes with normal ventilation

Assessment
• History of present illness
• Patient's perception of ability to clear airway
• Knowledge of physical condition
• Neurologic status, including level of consciousness, orientation, sensory status, and motor status
• Respiratory status, including symmetry of chest expansion; use of accessory muscles; cough (productive or nonproductive); respiratory rate, depth, and pattern; sputum characteristics (color, consistency, amount, odor, and changes from patient's norm); palpation for fremitus; percussion of lung fields; auscultation for breath sounds; pulse oximetry; chest X-ray; arterial blood gas (ABG) values; and hemoglobin (Hb) and hematocrit
• Pulmonary function studies
• Psychosocial status, including interest, motivation, and knowledge

Defining characteristics
• Adventitious breath sounds, such as crackles, rhonchi, and wheezes
• Changes in respiratory rate and rhythm
• Cyanosis
• Diminished breath sounds
• Difficulty vocalizing
• Dyspnea
• Ineffective or absent cough
• Orthopnea
• Restlessness
• Sputum

Associated medical diagnoses (selected)
Asthma, chest trauma, chronic bronchitis, emphysema, Guillain-Barré syndrome, heart failure, lung cancer, meningitis, multiple sclerosis, pneumonia

Expected outcomes
• Airway will remain patent.
• Adventitious breath sounds will be absent.
• Chest X-ray will show no abnormality.
• Oxygen level will be in normal range.
• Patient will breathe deeply and cough to remove secretions.
• Patient will expectorate sputum.
• Patient will demonstrate controlled coughing techniques.
• Ventilation will be adequate.
• Patient will demonstrate skill in conserving energy while attempting to clear airway.
• Patient will state understanding of changes needed to diminish oxygen demands.

Interventions and rationales
• Assess respiratory status at least every 4 hours or according to established standards *to detect early signs of compromise.*

• Turn patient every 2 hours. Always position for maximal aeration of lung fields and mobilization of secretions. *This prevents pooling and stasis of respiratory secretions.*
• When helping patient cough and deep-breathe, use whatever position best ensures cooperation and minimizes energy expenditure, such as high Fowler's position or sitting on side of bed. *Such positions promote chest expansion and ventilation of basilar lung fields.*
• Suction, as ordered, to stimulate cough and clear airways. Be alert for progression of airway compromise. *These steps prevent respiratory distress.*
• Perform postural drainage, percussion, and vibration to facilitate secretion movement. Monitor sputum, noting amount, odor, and consistency. *Sputum amount and consistency may indicate hydration status and effectiveness of therapy. Foul-smelling sputum may indicate respiratory infection.*
• Teach patient an easily performed cough technique *to clear airways without fatigue.*
• Encourage sputum expectoration *to remove pathogens and prevent spread of infection.* Provide tissues and paper bags for hygienic disposal.
• Give expectorants, bronchodilators, and other drugs, as ordered, and record effectiveness. Also encourage fluids to help liquefy secretions. *These measures enhance clearance of secretions from airways.*
• Provide bronchodilator treatments before chest physiotherapy *to optimize results.*
• Administer oxygen, as ordered, *to help relieve respiratory distress.*
• Monitor ABG values and Hb *to assess oxygenation and ventilatory sta-*

tus; report deviations from baseline levels.
• If conservative measures fail to maintain partial pressure of arterial oxygen (Pao_2) within an acceptable range, prepare for endotracheal intubation, as ordered, *to maintain artificial airway and optimize Pao_2 level.*
• Assess patient's learning needs and provide appropriate information *to help prevent recurrence of obstruction and promote change in daily activities to reduce oxygen demands.*

Evaluations for expected outcomes
• Patient's airway remains clear and allows for adequate ventilation.
• Auscultation of patient's lung fields doesn't reveal crackles, rhonchi, wheezes, or stridor.
• Patient's chest X-ray is normal.
• Patient's oxygen level remains within normal range.
• Patient coughs and deep-breathes to expectorate secretions.
• Patient expectorates sputum.
• Patient performs controlled coughing techniques.
• Patient doesn't experience dyspnea or change in respiratory pattern.
• Patient performs energy conservation techniques.
• Patient demonstrates understanding of changes needed to diminish oxygen demands.

Documentation
• Patient's perceptions of ability to cough
• Observations of physical findings
• Effectiveness of medications
• Patient's attempts to clear airway
• Maneuvers performed to clear airway
• Evaluations for expected outcomes

■ Airway clearance, ineffective

related to presence of tracheobronchial obstruction or secretions

Definition
Anatomic or physiologic obstruction of the airway that interferes with normal ventilation

Assessment
• History of respiratory disorder
• Respiratory status, including rate and depth of respiration, fever, symmetry of chest expansion, use of accessory muscles, cough, sputum (color, consistency, amount, odor, and changes from patient's norm related to infection, irritation, dehydration, or exposure to pollutants), palpation for fremitus, percussion of lung fields, auscultation for breath sounds, pulse oximetry, arterial blood gas (ABG) values, and chest X-ray
• Neurologic status, including level of consciousness, orientation, and mental status
• Knowledge, including understanding of physical condition and skill in performing maneuvers to clear airway

Defining characteristics
• Adventitious breath sounds, such as crackles, rhonchi, and wheezes
• Changes in respiratory rate and rhythm
• Cyanosis
• Difficulty vocalizing
• Diminished breath sounds
• Dyspnea
• Ineffective or absent cough
• Orthopnea
• Restlessness
• Sputum
• Widened eyes

Associated medical diagnoses (selected)
Adult respiratory distress syndrome, amyotrophic lateral sclerosis, asthma, atelectasis, bronchiectasis, cerebral aneurysm, cerebrovascular accident, chronic bronchitis, chronic obstructive pulmonary disease, cor pulmonale, craniotomy, cystic fibrosis, emphysema, Guillain-Barré syndrome, head or neck cancer, infant respiratory distress syndrome, lung abscess, myasthenia gravis, pneumonia, pulmonary edema, seizure disorders, shock, spinal cord injury, thoracic surgery, tuberculosis

Expected outcomes
• Patient will cough effectively.
• Patient will expectorate sputum.
• Adventitious breath sounds will be absent.
• Chest X-ray will reveal no abnormality.
• Patient will produce normal sputum.
• Patient will drink 3 to 4 L (3⅛ to 4¼ qt) of fluid daily.
• ABG levels will remain at baseline.
• Airway will remain patent.
• Patient will understand and be able to explain the need for adequate hydration, sputum monitoring, and taking medications as ordered.
• Patient will demonstrate controlled coughing techniques.
• Patient will perform chest physiotherapy, particularly postural drainage.
• Patient will report symptoms that indicate need for medical intervention.

Interventions and rationales
• Assess respiratory status at least every 4 hours or according to established standards *to detect early signs of compromise.*
• Place patient in Fowler's position and support upper extremities *to aid breathing and chest expansion and to ventilate basilar lung fields.*
• Help patient turn, cough, and deep-breathe every 2 to 4 hours *to help prevent pooling of secretions and to maintain airway patency.*
• Suction as needed *to stimulate cough and clear airways.* Be alert for progression of airway compromise.
• Provide adequate humidification *to loosen secretions.*
• Encourage fluids (at least 3,000 ml daily) *to ensure adequate hydration and loosen secretions,* unless contraindicated.
• Monitor patient's daily weight *to assess fluid balance.*
• Perform postural drainage, percussion, and vibration every 4 hours or as ordered *to enhance mobilization of secretions that interfere with oxygenation.* Monitor sputum *to gauge effectiveness of therapy.*
• Mobilize patient to full capabilities *to facilitate chest expansion and ventilation.*
• Avoid supine position for extended periods. Encourage lateral, sitting, prone, and upright positions as much as possible *to enhance lung expansion and ventilation.*
• Provide tissues and paper bags for hygienic sputum disposal *to prevent spreading infection.*
• Monitor and document sputum characteristics every shift *to gauge therapy's effectiveness and detect possible respiratory infection.*
• Teach patient about:
– maintaining adequate hydration
– daily monitoring of sputum and reporting changes
– taking prescribed drugs and avoiding over-the-counter respiratory drugs
– controlled coughing and postural drainage
– the need to remain active.

These steps involve patient in own health care.

Evaluations for expected outcomes
• Patient clears airway using controlled coughing techniques.
• Patient expectorates sputum.
• Auscultation of patient's lung fields doesn't reveal crackles, rhonchi, wheezes, or stridor.
• Patient's chest X-ray is normal.
• Patient's sputum is thin, white, odorless, and moderate in quantity.
• Patient drinks 3 to 4 L (3⅛ to 4¼ qt) of fluid daily.
• Patient's ABG values are within normal limits.
• Patient's airway remains clear.
• Patient understands necessity of adequate hydration, sputum monitoring, and taking medications as ordered.
• Patient performs controlled coughing.
• Patient performs chest physiotherapy, especially postural drainage.
• Patient lists symptoms that indicate a need for medical intervention.

Documentation
• Patient's statement of ability to clear airway and comfort in doing so
• Respiratory status, including cough and sputum
• Need for suctioning and its effectiveness
• Effectiveness of medications
• Teaching about airway clearance; response to interventions
• Evaluations for expected outcomes

■ Altered protection
related to myelosuppression and immunosuppression

Definition
A decrease in the ability to guard the self from internal or external threats such as illness or injury

Assessment
• Vital signs
• Health maintenance, including high-risk behaviors and health-promoting activities
• Patient's knowledge of present condition, including diagnosis, treatment, prevention of complications, and management of adverse effects
• Coping skills, including physical, psychosocial, and spiritual strengths
• Mobility status
• Comfort level, including symptom management
• Activities of daily living, including rest, sleep, and exercise
• Cardiovascular status, including heart rate, rhythm, heart sounds, blood pressure, peripheral pulses, and electrocardiogram results
• Neurologic status, including sensory perception, decision-making abilities, and thought processes
• Respiratory status, including gas exchange and breathing patterns
• Nutritional status, including food preferences, modifications in diet, and weight changes
• Bowel and bladder elimination patterns
• Protective mechanisms, including immune, hematopoietic, integumentary, and sensorimotor systems
• Laboratory studies, including white blood cell count and differential, erythrocyte sedimentation rate, immunoelectrophoresis, enzyme-linked im-

munosorbent assay, and cultures of blood, body fluid, sputum, urine, and wound exudate
• Sexuality patterns

Defining characteristics
• Altered clotting
• Deficient immunity
• Dyspnea
• Immobility
• Impaired healing
• Insomnia
• Itching
• Maladaptive stress response
• Neurosensory alteration
• Perspiring
• Pressure ulcers
• Restlessness
• Weakness

Associated medical diagnoses (selected)
Acquired immunodeficiency syndrome, anemias, hemophilia, Hodgkin's disease, leukemia, lymphomas, pressure ulcers, rheumatoid arthritis, sickle cell disease; disorders that require treatment with organ or bone marrow transplant, chemotherapy, or radiation therapy

Expected outcomes
• Patient will not experience chills, fever, or other signs and symptoms of illness.
• Patient will demonstrate use of protective measures, including conservation of energy, maintenance of balanced diet, and obtainment of adequate rest.
• Patient will demonstrate effective coping skills.
• Patient will demonstrate personal cleanliness and will maintain clean environment.
• Patient will maintain safe environment.
• Patient will demonstrate increased strength and resistance.

• Patient's immune system response will improve.

Interventions and rationales
• Spend as much time as possible with patient *to provide comfort and support.*
• Promote personal and environmental cleanliness *to decrease threat from microorganisms.*
• Monitor vital signs. *This allows for early detection of complications.*
• Institute safety precautions *to reduce risk of falls, cuts, or other injuries and subsequent infection, bleeding, and impaired healing.*
• Teach protective measures, including the need to conserve energy, obtain adequate rest, and eat a balanced diet. *Adequate sleep and nutrition enhance immune function. Energy conservation can help to decrease the weakness caused by anemia.*
• Provide relief for symptoms (fever, chills, myalgias, weakness). *Discomfort interferes with rest, disturbs nutritional intake, and places added stress on patient.*
• Teach patient coping strategies, including stress management and relaxation techniques. *Relaxation and decreased stress can increase immune function, thereby improving strength and resistance.*

Evaluations for expected outcomes
• Patient doesn't develop petechiae, epistaxis, melena, hematuria, fever, cough, redness, drainage, pallor, headache, weakness, or dizziness. Vital signs remain within normal limits.
• Patient demonstrates a normal pattern of rest, activity, and sleep. He consumes an adequate diet.
• Patient reports being able to cope effectively.

• Patient demonstrates personal cleanliness and maintains clean environment.
• Patient uses safety precautions to avoid falls and other injuries.
• Patient demonstrates increased strength and resistance.
• Patient's immune system response improves.

Documentation
• Patient's understanding of abnormal blood profiles
• Patient's description of measures to prevent or manage complications
• Observations of patient's behavior, including health-promoting and high-risk activities
• Signs and symptoms of decreased immune resistance in body systems assessed (cardiopulmonary, neurologic, GI, genitourinary, and integumentary)
• Observations of infection or bleeding
• Interventions to assist with coping strategies and health maintenance and promotion
• Patient's response to interventions
• Evaluations for expected outcomes

■ Anxiety

related to obsessive-compulsive behavior

Definition
Feeling of threat or danger to self arising from an unidentifiable source

Assessment
• Physical status, including skin breakdown, excoriation of skin tissue, alopecia, fatigue, weight loss, sleeplessness, and other physical indications of anxiety
• Psychological status, including patient's explanation of problem; onset and duration of problem; precipitating events; past coping strategies; present coping strategies (such as use of repression and undoing as psychological defenses); insight; motivation to change; level of anxiety (+1, +2, +3, +4); secondary gains (what kind of secondary gains patient receives and from whom); acting-out behavior (such as compulsive gambling); current stressors; mental status examination (especially psychomotor behavior, thought content, concentration, judgment, affect, communication style, impulse control, and presenting appearance); and personal abilities, talents, and strengths
• Sociologic status, including support systems, hobbies, interests, and work history
• Family status, including roles of members, evidence of harmony or disharmony, family coping mechanisms, and evidence of reinforcement of patient's problem by family members
• Medication history (response, effectiveness, and adverse reactions)

Defining characteristics
• Anguish
• Decreased perceptual field
• Distress
• Excitability
• Fear of unspecific consequences
• Insomnia
• Preoccupation
• Rumination
• Scanning and vigilance
• Sleep disturbance

Associated medical diagnoses (selected)
Affective disorders, obsessive-compulsive disorder, schizophrenia, self-destructive behavior, suicidal behavior

Expected outcomes
- Patient will reduce amount of time spent each day on obsessing and ritualizing.
- Patient will perform activities of daily living (ADLs).
- Patient's ritualistic behavior will not produce harmful effects.
- Patient will maintain nutritional status.
- Patient will obtain adequate rest.
- Patient will exhibit no signs of skin breakdown.
- Patient will express feelings of anxiety as they occur.
- Patient will express anger in socially acceptable ways.

Interventions and rationales
- Identify your own feelings toward patient *to prevent prejudices from interfering with treatment.*
- Understand that anxiety is the cause of patient's problem, and accept patient's need to obsess or ritualize. *An accepting attitude will nurture feelings of sympathy and minimize feelings of disapproval.* Don't attempt to thwart ritualistic behavior. *Forcing patient to change behavior can lead to panic and possibly psychosis.*
- Help patient identify situations that trigger ritualistic behaviors. *Patient must know what situations trigger behaviors before he can stop behaviors.*
- When possible, help patient channel ritualistic behavior into constructive outlets, such as writing, painting, and physical activity, *to develop patient's self-esteem.*
- Allow patient sufficient time to engage in rituals. *Rushing patient may increase anxiety and create hostility.*
- Don't attempt to reason with patient about his obsession. *Patient already recognizes the irrationality of his symptoms. Your explanations may increase feelings of inadequacy.*

- Avoid criticizing patient's behavior, either verbally or by attitude. Only discuss ritualistic behavior if patient brings it up first. *Criticism will further damage patient's already low self-esteem.*
- Develop a relationship with patient that encourages open expression of emotions *to help patient cope effectively with feelings that usually remain repressed.*
- Promote patient's self-esteem by encouraging participation in activity. Begin with simple objectives and progress to larger goals. Praise patient's efforts frequently. *Feelings of accomplishment increase patient's sense of worth and decrease anxiety, thus decreasing need for rituals.*
- If needed, set consistent limits on self-destructive behavior *to promote patient's physical safety. Consistent limits will help prevent patient from vacillating.*
- Assess what secondary gain patient achieves through ritualistic behavior. When possible, preempt the ritual by providing this gain when patient is not ritualizing. For example, if patient seeks attention through ritual behavior, ignore ritual behavior but pay ample attention to patient at other times. *This may help patient realize gains can be achieved without ritual behavior. Remember that, if ignored, negative behavior is less likely to be repeated.*
- If rituals interfere with nutrition, place patient on an established feeding schedule *to promote health and prevent patient from becoming indecisive about meals.*
- If patient practices washing or "picking" rituals, take steps to prevent skin breakdown. Provide hand lotion and rubber gloves, bandage hands, and keep fingernails trimmed. *These*

measures will prevent skin break-down.
• Teach relaxation techniques *to counteract anxiety.*
• Teach assertiveness skills. *Learning to say no to other people's demands can help patient manage anger.*
• Assess patient's readiness to overcome ritual behavior. Patient can begin to change when able to manage anxiety without resorting to rituals. When patient is ready, assist in setting goals for limiting unwanted behavior *to help motivate patient to change.*

Evaluations for expected outcomes
• Patient shows less evidence of ritualizing and reports that obsessive thoughts are less frequent.
• Patient performs ADLs efficiently, unhampered by distracting rituals.
• Patient shows no evidence of harmful effects from ritualistic behavior.
• Patient eats at least 80% of meals without being distracted by obsessive thoughts or rituals.
• Patient achieves 6 to 8 hours of uninterrupted sleep each night.
• Patient's skin remains intact and supple.
• Patient expresses anxiety.
• Patient voices anger appropriately or expresses it through writing, painting, physical activity, or other healthy outlets.

Documentation
• Observations of ritualistic behavior
• Statements indicating obsessive thoughts
• Interventions performed to reduce anxiety and to increase coping
• Patient's response to nursing interventions, including ability to relax; willingness to think flexibly, socialize, and engage in diversions; and efforts to maintain physical health

• Patient's weight, food intake, and skin condition
• Patient's ability to accept less control over self and environment
• Patient's achievement of mutually established goals
• Evaluations for expected outcomes

■ Anxiety
related to situational crisis

Definition
Feeling of threat or danger to self arising from an unidentifiable source

Assessment
• Current health status
• Patient's perception of problem, onset of problem, recent stressors, life changes, and other precipitants
• Mental status, including orientation to time, place, and person; insight regarding current situation; judgment; abstract thinking; general information; mood; affect; recent and remote memory; thought processes; and thought content
• Coping and problem-solving ability
• Ability to perform activities of daily living
• Sleep habits
• Dietary and nutritional status
• Available support systems, including family members, friends, clergy, and health care agencies

Defining characteristics
• Fear
• Fidgeting
• Forgetfulness
• Glancing about
• Insomnia
• Impaired attention
• Preoccupation
• Restlessness

- Trembling, hand tremors
- Worry

Associated medical diagnoses (selected)

Any patient can experience anxiety. It appears most often in patients with conditions that require surgery, diseases that pose a threat to self-concept, diseases that require use of high-technology devices or techniques, or newly diagnosed chronic or terminal diseases.

Examples of medical diagnoses include abruptio placentae, affective disorders, Alzheimer's disease, angina pectoris, anorexia nervosa, anxiety disorder, asthma, atelectasis, bulimia nervosa, cellulitis, coronary artery disease, Crohn's disease, detached retina, duodenal ulcer, encephalitis, endocarditis, endometriosis, gastric ulcer, glaucoma, Guillain-Barré syndrome, hydrocephalus, hyperparathyroidism, hypoparathyroidism, labor, lung abscess, maternal psychological stress, multisystem trauma, myocardial infarction, panic disorder, passive-aggressive personality disorder, pericarditis, peritonitis, placenta previa, postpartum hemorrhage, rheumatic fever, seizure disorders, self-destructive behavior, spinal cord injury, suicidal behavior, trigeminal neuralgia, urinary calculi, and urinary incontinence.

Expected outcomes

- Patient will identify factors that elicit anxious behaviors.
- Patient will discuss activities that tend to decrease anxious behaviors.
- Patient will practice progressive relaxation techniques a specified number of times each day.
- Patient will cope with current medical situation without demonstrating severe signs of anxiety.

Interventions and rationales

- Spend 10 minutes with patient twice a shift. Convey a willingness to listen. Offer verbal reassurance; for example, "I know you're frightened. I'll stay with you." *Specific amount of uninterrupted, non-care-related time spent with anxious patient builds trust and reduces tension. Active listening helps patient ventilate feelings.*
- Give patient clear, concise explanations of anything about to occur. Avoid information overload; an anxious patient can't assimilate many details. *Anxiety may impair patient's cognitive abilities.*
- Listen attentively; allow patient to express feelings verbally. *This may allow patient to identify anxious behaviors and discover source of anxiety.*
- Make no demands on patient. *Anxious patient may respond to excessive demands with hostility and abuse.*
- Identify and reduce as many environmental stressors (including people) as possible. *Anxiety often results from lack of trust in the environment.*
- Have patient state what kinds of activities promote feelings of comfort, and encourage patient to perform them. *This gives patient a sense of control.*
- Remain with patient during severe anxiety. *Anxiety is often related to fear of being left alone.*
- Include patient in decisions related to care when feasible. *Anxious patient may mistrust own abilities; involvement in decision making may reduce anxious behaviors.*
- Support family members in coping with patient's anxious behavior. *Involving family members in process of reassurance and explanation allays patient's anxiety as well as their own.*
- Allow extra visiting periods with family if this seems to allay patient's

anxiety. *This allows anxious patient and family to support each other according to their abilities and at their own pace.*
• Teach patient relaxation techniques to be performed at least every 4 hours, such as guided imagery, progressive muscle relaxation, and meditation. *These measures can restore psychological and physical equilibrium by decreasing autonomic response to anxiety.*
• Refer patient to community or professional mental health resources *to provide ongoing mental health assistance.*

Evaluations for expected outcomes
• Patient describes at least two situations that increase tension.
• Patient states at least two ways to eliminate or minimize anxious behaviors.
• Patient demonstrates progressive relaxation exercises and practices them a specified number of times each day.
• Patient reports being able to cope with current situation without experiencing severe anxiety.

Documentation
• Patient's statement of anxiety and feelings of relief
• Statements about observable signs of patient's anxiety
• Interventions to reduce patient's anxiety
• Effectiveness of nursing interventions that can be observed
• Evaluations for expected outcomes

■ Aspiration, risk for

related to absence of protective mechanisms

Definition
State of being at risk for aspiration of GI or oropharyngeal secretions, food, or fluids into tracheobronchial passages

Assessment
• Neurologic status, including level of consciousness (LOC), orientation, and mental status
• GI status, including gag and swallow reflexes, inspection of abdomen, abdominal girth, auscultation of bowel sounds, palpation for masses and tenderness, percussion of abdomen, and medications
• Nutritional status, including continuous and intermittent tube feeding
• Respiratory status, including skin color, rate and depth of respiration, cough (productive or nonproductive), auscultation of breath sounds, palpation for fremitus, sputum characteristics (color, consistency, amount, and odor), arterial blood gas values, and chest X-ray
• Vital signs
• Laboratory studies, such as white blood cell (WBC) count and sputum culture

Risk factors
• Decreased GI motility
• Delayed gastric emptying
• Depressed cough and gag reflexes
• Feeding or GI tubes
• Impaired swallowing
• Incompetent lower esophageal sphincter
• Increased gastric residual
• Increased intragastric pressure
• Medication administration

- Reduced LOC
- Situations hindering elevation of upper body
- Surgery or trauma to face, mouth, or neck
- Tracheostomy or endotracheal tube
- Wired jaws

Associated medical diagnoses (selected)
Achalasia, acute respiratory failure, amyotrophic lateral sclerosis, asphyxia, brain abscess, cerebrovascular accident, chest trauma, esophageal cancer, head injury, hemorrhage, intestinal obstruction, intoxication, neuromuscular trauma, Parkinson's disease, pneumonia, poisoning

Expected outcomes
- Patient will tolerate ___ ml of tube feeding.
- Patient's temperature and WBC count will remain normal.
- Pathogens will not appear in cultures.
- Respiratory secretions will be clear and odorless.
- Auscultation will reveal no adventitious breath sounds.
- Patient will have normal bowel sounds.
- Patient will discuss measures to prevent aspiration with caregiver.

Interventions and rationales
- Assess respiratory status at least every 4 hours *for signs of possible aspiration (increased respiratory rate, cough, sputum production, or diminished breath sounds).*
- Monitor and record neurologic status *to detect altered LOC, which could affect intake of food or saliva.*
- Monitor and record vital signs *to detect signs of aspiration or impaired gas exchange due to aspiration.*
- Suction as needed *to keep airway clear.*

- Assess patient for gag and swallow reflexes. *Decreased gag or swallow reflex may cause aspiration.*
- Encourage patient to cough and expectorate sputum *to mobilize secretions.* Provide tissues and paper bags for hygienic sputum disposal *to prevent spreading infection.*
- Auscultate for bowel sounds every shift and report changes. *Delayed gastric emptying and elevated intragastric pressure may promote regurgitation of stomach contents.*
- If patient is receiving tube feedings:
– Assess cuff inflation for patient with artificial airway and adjust appropriately *to protect lower airways from oropharyngeal secretions.*
– Add food coloring to tube feeding if patient has altered state of consciousness, diminished gag reflex, or history of aspiration *to help monitor gastric secretions for aspiration.*
– Begin regimen with a small, diluted amount as tolerated and ordered to allow adjustment to formula osmolality and avoid nausea, vomiting, and diarrhea.
– Elevate head of bed during and after feedings unless contraindicated *to prevent aspiration.*
– Check for residual tube feeding every shift and record amount. If more than 50 ml remains, withhold feeding *to prevent vomiting and aspiration.* Report findings to doctor.
– Place tube properly before feeding or giving medication *to protect airway.*
– Stop feeding immediately if you suspect aspiration; then apply suction as needed, and turn patient on side *to avoid further aspiration.*
- Assess need for antiemetic drug *to reduce nausea and vomiting.* Administer if ordered and monitor effectiveness.

• Review test results *to identify signs of infection;* report abnormalities.
• Explain treatment to patient and caregivers *to encourage compliance.*

Evaluations for expected outcomes
• Patient tolerates ____ ml of tube feeding.
• Patient's temperature and WBC count remain within normal parameters.
• No pathogens appear in patient's cultures.
• Patient's respiratory secretions remain clear and odorless.
• Auscultation of lungs reveals no adventitious breath sounds.
• Auscultation of abdomen reveals normal bowel sounds.
• Patient and caregiver discuss measures necessary to prevent aspiration.

Documentation
• Verification of tube placement
• Tolerance of tube feedings
• Residuals of tube feedings
• Vomiting or aspiration
• Breath sounds
• Patient's indication of situations that may lead to aspiration
• Observations of physical findings
• Interventions performed to prevent aspiration
• Evaluations for expected outcomes

■ Body image disturbance

Definition
Negative perception of self that makes healthy functioning more difficult

Assessment
• Physiologic changes
• Behavioral changes
• Patient's and family's perception of patient's present health problem
• Patient's usual pattern of coping with stress
• Marital status
• Patient's role in the family
• Patient's past experiences with health problems
• Sleep pattern
• Appetite
• Hobbies and interests
• Occupational history
• Ethnic background and cultural perceptions

Defining characteristics
• Actual change in structure or function
• Behaviors of avoiding, monitoring, or acknowledging one's body
• Expressing an actual or perceived change in appearance, structure, or function
• Hiding or overexposing body part (intentional or unintentional)
• Missing body part
• Nonverbal response to actual or perceived change in structure or function
• Not looking at or touching body part
• Trauma to nonfunctioning part

Associated medical diagnoses (selected)
Adrenal insufficiency; anorexia nervosa; atrophic senile vaginitis; Bell's palsy; blindness; brain abscess; breast cancer requiring mastectomy; bulimia nervosa; burns; cerebrovascular accident; cervical cancer; chronic renal failure; colitis; conditions requiring amputation, colostomy, craniotomy, hemodialysis, ileostomy, peritoneal dialysis, prostatectomy, or kidney transplantation; Cushing's disease; diabetes mellitus; gout; head injury; head or neck cancer; hydrocephalus; hyperpituitarism; hyperthyroidism; hypothyroidism; impotence; melanoma; orthopedic injuries; osteoarthritis; osteomyelitis; Parkinson's disease; pemphigus; psoriasis;

rheumatoid arthritis; sarcoidosis; spinal cord injury; testicular cancer; uterine prolapse

Expected outcomes
• Patient will acknowledge change in body image.
• Patient will participate in decision making about his care (specify).
• Patient will communicate feelings about change in body image.
• Patient will express positive feelings about self.
• Patient will talk with someone who has experienced the same problem.
• Patient will demonstrate ability to practice two new coping behaviors.

Interventions and rationales
• While assisting with self-care measures, involve patient in discussions that will provide further insights into patient's coping patterns and self-esteem. *Patient's usual coping patterns and self-perception provide baseline data for assessing potential threat of current situation.*
• Accept patient's perception of self *to validate patient's self-perception and provide reassurance that he can successfully overcome crisis.*
• Assess patient's readiness for decision making; then involve him in making choices and decisions related to care. *This gives patient sense of control over environment.*
• Encourage patient to participate actively in performing care. *This gives patient sense of independence.*
• Give patient opportunities to voice feelings. *This helps patient ventilate doubts and resolve concerns.*
• Provide positive reinforcement to patient's efforts to adapt *to increase probability that healthy adaptation will continue.*
• Arrange for patient to interact with others who have similar problems. *A*

support group allows patient to share mutual support and caring with others who can fully understand.
• Refer patient to a mental health professional for further counseling. *Referral to psychiatric liaison nurse is indicated when patient is adapting poorly to situation.*
• Teach patient coping strategies (specify) *to help overcome maladaptive coping behaviors.*
• Have patient provide feedback about coping behaviors that seem to work. Reinforce the practice of these behaviors. *This allows you to evaluate patient's adaptive abilities. Positive feedback reinforces adaptability and encourages similar behaviors in future.*

Evaluations for expected outcomes
• Patient acknowledges change in body image.
• Patient takes an active role in planning aspects of care (specify).
• Patient expresses emotions associated with change in body image.
• Patient expresses at least one positive feeling about self daily.
• Patient participates in discussions with support group composed of individuals with a similar change in body image (specify).
• Patient uses at least two healthy coping skills to deal with change in body image.

Documentation
• Words patient uses to describe self, prostheses, adaptive equipment, and limitations
• Body parts that patient focuses on or ignores
• Observations related to change in structure or function of body part
• Observed responses of patient to change in body part, such as touching or not touching

• Health education or counseling provided to help patient cope with altered body image
• Patient's response to nursing interventions
• Evaluations for expected outcomes

■ Breathing pattern, ineffective

related to decreased energy or fatigue

Definition
Change in rate, depth, or pattern of breathing that alters normal gas exchange

Assessment
• History of respiratory disorder
• Respiratory status, including rate and depth of respiration, symmetry of chest expansion, use of accessory muscles, presence of cough, anterior-posterior chest diameter, palpation for fremitus, percussion of lung fields, auscultation of breath sounds, and pulmonary function studies
• Cardiovascular status, including heart rate and rhythm, blood pressure, and skin color, temperature, and turgor
• Neurologic and mental status, including level of consciousness and emotional level
• Knowledge, including current understanding of physical condition and physical, mental, and emotional readiness to learn

Defining characteristics
• Accessory muscle use
• Altered chest excursion
• Altered respiratory rate or depth or both
• Assumption of three-point position

• Decreased inspiratory or expiratory pressure
• Decreased minute ventilation
• Decreased vital capacity
• Dyspnea
• Increased anterior-posterior diameter
• Nasal flaring
• Orthopnea
• Prolonged expiration phase
• Pursed-lip breathing
• Shortness of breath

Associated medical diagnoses (selected)
Acoustic neuroma, adult respiratory distress syndrome, amyotrophic lateral sclerosis, anemias, asphyxia, asthma, brain abscess, bronchiectasis, cerebrovascular accident, chronic bronchitis, chronic obstructive pulmonary disease, cirrhosis, cor pulmonale, craniotomy, cystic fibrosis, emphysema, food poisoning, Guillain-Barré syndrome, heart failure, Hodgkin's disease, hyperparathyroidism, infant respiratory distress syndrome, lung cancer, lupus erythematosus, meningitis, metabolic acidosis, metabolic alkalosis, mitral valve prolapse, Parkinson's disease, pneumonia, pulmonary edema, pulmonary fibrosis, sarcoidosis, seizure disorders, spinal tumor, tuberculosis

Expected outcomes
• Patient's respiratory rate will stay within ±5 of baseline.
• Arterial blood gas (ABG) levels will return to baseline.
• Patient will report feeling comfortable when breathing.
• Patient will report feeling rested each day.
• Patient will demonstrate diaphragmatic pursed-lip breathing.
• Patient will achieve maximum lung expansion with adequate ventilation.

• Patient will demonstrate skill in conserving energy while carrying out activities of daily living (ADLs).

Interventions and rationales

• Assess and record respiratory rate and depth at least every 4 hours *to detect early signs of respiratory compromise.* Also assess ABG levels according to facility policy *to monitor oxygenation and ventilation status.*
• Auscultate breath sounds at least every 4 hours *to detect decreased or adventitious breath sounds;* report changes.
• Assist patient to a comfortable position, such as by supporting upper extremities with pillows, providing overbed table with a pillow to lean on, and elevating head of bed. *These measures promote comfort, chest expansion, and ventilation of basilar lung fields.*
• Help patient with ADLs, as needed, *to conserve energy and avoid overexertion and fatigue.*
• Administer oxygen as ordered. *Supplemental oxygen helps reduce hypoxemia and relieve respiratory distress.*
• Suction airway as needed *to remove secretions.*
• Schedule necessary activities to provide periods of rest. *This prevents fatigue and reduces oxygen demands.*
• Teach patient about:
– pursed-lip breathing
– abdominal breathing
– performing relaxation techniques
– taking prescribed medications (ensuring accuracy of dose and frequency and monitoring adverse effects)
– scheduling activities to avoid fatigue and provide for rest periods.
These measures allow patient to participate in maintaining health status and improve ventilation.
• Refer patient for evaluation of exercise potential and development of in-dividualized exercise program. *Exercise conditions patient and gives him sense of well-being.*

Evaluations for expected outcomes

• Patient's respiratory rate remains within established limits.
• Patient's ABG levels return to and remain within established limits.
• Patient indicates, either verbally or through behavior, feeling comfortable when breathing.
• Patient reports feeling rested each day.
• Patient performs diaphragmatic pursed-lip breathing.
• Patient demonstrates maximum lung expansion with adequate ventilation.
• When patient carries out ADLs, breathing pattern remains normal.

Documentation

• Patient's expressions of comfort in breathing, emotional state, understanding of medical diagnosis, and readiness to learn
• Physical findings from pulmonary assessment
• Interventions carried out and patient's responses to them
• Evaluations for expected outcomes

■ Breathing pattern, ineffective

related to pain

Definition

Change in the rate, depth, or pattern of breathing that alters normal gas exchange

Assessment

• History of medical or surgical problem that causes ineffective breathing

• Respiratory status, including rate and depth of respiration, symmetry of chest expansion, use of accessory muscles, presence of cough, anterior-posterior chest diameter, palpation for fremitus, percussion of lung fields, auscultation of breath sounds, and arterial blood gas (ABG) levels
• Cardiovascular status, including heart rate and rhythm and blood pressure
• Neurologic status, including level of consciousness and sensory and motor status
• Psychosocial status, including willingness to cooperate with treatment, coping mechanisms, and knowledge level (current understanding of physical condition)

Defining characteristics
• Accessory muscle use
• Altered chest excursion
• Altered respiratory rate or depth or both
• Assumption of three-point position
• Decreased inspiratory or expiratory pressure
• Decreased minute ventilation
• Decreased vital capacity
• Dyspnea
• Increased anterior-posterior diameter
• Nasal flaring
• Orthopnea
• Prolonged expiration phase
• Pursed-lip breathing
• Shortness of breath

Associated medical diagnoses (selected)
Aortic aneurysm, cerebral aneurysm, chest trauma, empyema, fractures, hemothorax, lung abscess, pleural effusion, pleurisy, pneumothorax, pulmonary embolus, thoracic surgery, urinary diversion

Expected outcomes
• Patient's respiratory rate will stay within ±5 of baseline.
• ABG levels will remain normal.
• Patient will achieve comfort without depressing respirations.
• Patient will demonstrate correct use of incentive spirometer.
• Auscultation will reveal no adventitious breath sounds.
• Patient will state importance of taking deep breaths periodically.
• Patient will practice relaxation techniques ___ times per day.
• Patient will report ability to breathe comfortably.

Interventions and rationales
• Assess and record respiratory status at least every 4 hours *to detect early signs of compromise.* Also assess ABG levels according to facility policy *to monitor oxygenation and ventilation status.*
• Assess for pain every 3 hours. *Pain reduces respiratory effort and ventilation.*
• Give pain medication, as ordered, *to allow maximal chest expansion.* Record effectiveness, and monitor respiratory depression induced by narcotic analgesic *to guide further therapy.*
• Assist patient to a comfortable position that also allows for maximal chest expansion; for example, use Fowler's position or have patient lean on overbed table with pillow *to enhance chest expansion.*
• Assist patient in using incentive spirometer or other device, as ordered, *to ensure proper use and help prevent atelectasis.*
• Teach patient how to splint chest while coughing. Keep extra pillow for patient's use. *Splinting reduces pain during coughing.*

• Perform chest physiotherapy to aid mobilization and secretion removal, if ordered. *Percussion, vibration, and postural drainage enhance airway clearance and respiratory effort.*
• Provide rest periods between breathing enhancement measures *to avoid fatigue.*
• Encourage patient to use incentive spirometer independently. Praise patient's efforts *to encourage compliance.*
• Provide oxygen, as ordered, *to help relieve respiratory distress caused by hypoxemia.*
• Teach relaxation techniques to help reduce anxiety. Guided imagery, progressive muscle relaxation, breathing exercises, and meditation *reduce pain and anxiety and enhance patient's sense of self-control.*
• Change patient's position frequently *to maximize comfort.*
• Encourage patient to discuss fears *to help reduce anxiety.*

Evaluations for expected outcomes
• Patient's respiratory rate remains within set limits (specify).
• Patient's ABG levels remain within set limits (specify).
• Patient doesn't express feelings of pain, either verbally or through behavior.
• Patient uses incentive spirometer or other respiratory device unassisted every 2 hours, or as ordered.
• Patient's breath sounds remain clear.
• Patient explains why periodic deep breathing is important to maintaining respiratory status.
• Patient practices relaxation techniques ___ times daily.
• Patient reports breathing comfortably, either verbally or through behavior.

Documentation
• Patient's reports of pain
• Patient's perception of need to take deep breaths and cough
• Patient's expression of the effectiveness of pain medication
• Observations of physical findings
• Effectiveness of medications
• Descriptions of patient's efforts to take deep breaths and cough
• Interventions performed to enhance patient's ability to breathe effectively
• Evaluations for expected outcomes

■ Cardiac output, decreased

related to reduced stroke volume as a result of electrophysiologic problems

Definition
Cardiovascular or respiratory symptoms resulting from insufficient blood being pumped by the heart

Assessment
• History of cardiac disorder
• Mental status, including orientation and level of consciousness
• Cardiovascular status, including history of arrhythmias and syncope, jugular vein distention, hepatojugular reflux, heart rate and rhythm, heart sounds, blood pressure, peripheral pulses, electrocardiogram (ECG), exercise ECG, echocardiogram, phonocardiogram, serum digoxin levels, and skin color, temperature, turgor, and capillary refill time
• Respiratory status, including respiratory rate and depth, breath sounds, chest X-ray, and arterial blood gas values

• Renal status, including weight, intake and output, urine specific gravity, and serum electrolytes

Defining characteristics
• Abnormal chest X-ray and cardiac enzymes
• Altered mental state
• Arrhythmias, ECG changes, and increased heart rate
• Audible S_3 or S_4 heart sounds
• Chest pain, coughing and wheezing, fatigue, restlessness, and cold, clammy skin
• Crackles
• Edema
• Decreased cardiac output and peripheral pulses
• Dyspnea, increased respiratory rate, orthopnea, and paroxysmal nocturnal dyspnea
• Ejection fraction less than 40%
• Elevated pulmonary artery pressure
• Jugular vein distention
• Mental status changes
• Mixed venous oxygen saturation
• Oliguria
• Skin color changes
• Variations in blood pressure readings
• Weight gain

Associated medical diagnoses (selected)
Cardiac arrhythmias, digitalis toxicity, heart failure, hyperthyroidism, hypoparathyroidism, hypothyroidism, myocardial infarction, sarcoidosis

Expected outcomes
• Pulse will not be less than _____ and not greater than _____; blood pressure will not be less than _____ and not greater than _____.
• Patient's skin will remain warm and dry.
• Patient will experience few or no dyspneic episodes.

• Patient will show no signs of dizziness or syncope.
• Patient will not complain of chest pain.
• Patient will practice stress-reduction techniques every 2 hours.
• Patient's cardiac output will remain adequate.
• Patient will have no arrhythmias.
• Patient will verbalize reportable signs and symptoms.
• Patient will understand diet, medication regimen, and prescribed activity level.

Interventions and rationales
• Monitor apical and radial pulses at least every 4 hours *to better detect arrhythmias.* Immediately report abnormal pulse rates.
• Note pulse rhythm at least every 4 hours and report irregularities. *Arrhythmias may indicate cardiac arrest or other complications.*
• Assess skin temperature every 4 hours. *Cool, clammy skin may indicate decreased cardiac output.*
• Assess respiratory status at least every 4 hours. Report complaints of dyspnea or restlessness. *Adventitious breath sounds or dyspnea may indicate fluid buildup in lungs and pulmonary capillary bed (as in heart failure).*
• Administer oxygen, as ordered, *to increase supply to myocardium.*
• Report complaints of dizziness or syncope promptly; *these may indicate cerebral hypoxia.*
• Tell patient to report chest pain right away *because it may signal myocardial hypoxia or injury.*
• Plan patient's care to avoid overexertion, *which increases myocardial oxygen demand.*
• Change patient's position frequently *to promote comfort and avoid tachy-*

cardia and other sympathetic responses.
• Teach patient how to perform stress-reduction techniques, such as deep breathing and meditation, *to allay anxiety and avoid cardiac complications.*
• Remind patient to practice stress-reduction techniques every 2 hours while awake *to help internalize learned techniques.*
• Give antiarrhythmic drugs as prescribed *to reduce or eliminate arrhythmias.* Monitor for adverse effects.
• Instruct patient to avoid straining during bowel movements, *which may cause bradycardia and decreased cardiac output.*
• Administer stool softeners as prescribed *to reduce straining during defecation.*
• Carry out the medical plan of care as ordered. *Collaborative practice enhances care.*
• Teach patient about reportable symptoms (chest pain, palpitations, weakness, dizziness, and syncope), prescribed diet, medications (name, dosage, frequency, and therapeutic and adverse effects), and activity level. *These measures let patient and caregivers participate in patient's care and help patient make informed decisions about health status.*

Evaluations for expected outcomes
• Patient's pulse rate and blood pressure remain within set limits.
• Patient's skin remains warm and dry.
• Patient experiences fewer dyspneic episodes.
• Patient doesn't experience dizziness or syncope.
• Patient doesn't report experiencing chest pain.

• Patient practices stress-reduction techniques every 2 hours.
• Patient's cardiac output remains adequate.
• No arrhythmias are noted during monitoring or physical examination of patient.
• Patient lists signs and symptoms of decreased cardiac output (dizziness, syncope, cool or clammy skin, fatigue, and dyspnea).
• Patient expresses understanding of importance of following prescribed diet, taking medications, and maintaining activity level.

Documentation
• Patient's symptoms
• Observation of physical findings
• Incidents of chest pain, including location, character, duration, and treatment
• Patient's tolerance for activity
• Interventions to control or monitor symptoms and patient's response
• Patient teaching
• Evaluations for expected outcomes

■ Cardiac output, decreased

related to reduced stroke volume as a result of mechanical or structural problems

Definition
Cardiovascular or respiratory symptoms resulting from insufficient blood being pumped by the heart

Assessment
• Mental status, including orientation and level of consciousness
• Cardiovascular status, including history of valvular disorder, capillary heart disease, or myopathy; skin col-

or, temperature, turgor, and capillary refill time; jugular vein distention; hepatojugular reflux; heart rate and rhythm; heart sounds; blood pressure; peripheral pulses; electrocardiogram (ECG); exercise ECG; echocardiogram; and phonocardiogram
• Respiratory status, including respiratory rate and depth, breath sounds, chest X-ray, and arterial blood gas values
• Renal status, including weight, intake and output, and urine specific gravity

Defining characteristics
• Abnormal chest X-ray and cardiac enzymes
• Altered mental state
• Arrhythmias, ECG changes, and increased heart rate
• Audible S_3 or S_4 heart sounds
• Chest pain, coughing and wheezing, fatigue, restlessness, and cold, clammy skin
• Crackles
• Edema
• Decreased cardiac output and peripheral pulses
• Dyspnea, increased respiratory rate, orthopnea, and paroxysmal nocturnal dyspnea
• Ejection fraction less than 40%
• Elevated pulmonary artery pressure
• Jugular vein distention
• Mental status changes
• Mixed venous oxygen saturation
• Oliguria
• Skin color changes
• Variations in blood pressure readings
• Weight gain

Associated medical diagnoses (selected)
Acute renal failure, acute respiratory failure, anaphylactic shock, anemia, angina pectoris, aortic insufficiency, aortic stenosis, bone marrow transplantation, cardiogenic shock, congenital heart disease, coronary artery disease, cor pulmonale, cyanotic maternal cardiac disease, diabetes mellitus, disseminated intravascular coagulation, endocarditis, end-stage cardiac disease, heart failure, hypertension, lupus erythematosus, mitral insufficiency, mitral stenosis, mitral valve prolapse, myocardial infarction, pericarditis, peritonitis, pulmonary edema, pulmonary embolus, Reiter's syndrome, rheumatic fever, shock

Expected outcomes
• Pulse will not be less than _____ and not greater than _____; blood pressure will not be less than _____ and not greater than _____.
• Patient will exhibit no arrhythmias.
• Skin will remain warm and dry.
• Patient will exhibit no pedal edema.
• Patient will perform activity within limits of prescribed heart rate.
• Patient will express sense of physical comfort after activity.
• Heart's workload will diminish.
• Patient will maintain adequate cardiac output.
• Patient will perform stress-reduction techniques every 4 hours while awake.
• Patient will verbalize reportable signs and symptoms.
• Patient will understand diet, medication regimen, and prescribed activity level.

Interventions and rationales
• Monitor and record level of consciousness, heart rate and rhythm, and blood pressure at least every 4 hours, or more often if necessary, *to detect cerebral hypoxia possibly resulting from decreased cardiac output.*
• Auscultate for heart and breath sounds at least every 4 hours. Report abnormal sounds as soon as they de-

velop. *Extra heart sounds may indicate early cardiac decompensation; adventitious breath sounds may indicate pulmonary congestion and diminished cardiac output.*
• Measure and record intake and output accurately. *Decreased urine output without lowered fluid intake may indicate decreased renal perfusion, possibly from decreased cardiac output.*
• Promptly treat life-threatening arrhythmias, as ordered, *to avoid crisis.*
• Weigh patient daily before breakfast *to detect fluid retention.*
• Inspect for pedal or sacral edema *to detect venous stasis and reduced cardiac output.*
• Provide skin care every 4 hours *to enhance skin perfusion and venous flow.*
• Gradually increase patient's activities within limits of prescribed heart rate *to allow heart to adjust to increased oxygen demand.* Monitor pulse rate before and after activity *to compare rates and gauge tolerance.*
• Plan patient's activities *to avoid fatigue and increased myocardial workload.*
• Maintain dietary restrictions, as ordered, *to reduce risk of cardiac disease.*
• Teach patient stress-reduction techniques *to reduce patient's anxiety and provide a sense of control.*
• Explain all procedures and tests *to enhance understanding and reduce anxiety.*
• Teach patient and family about chest pain and other reportable symptoms, prescribed diet, medications (name, dosage, frequency, therapeutic effects, and adverse effects), prescribed activity level, simple methods for lifting and bending, and stress-reduction techniques. *These measures involve patient and family in care.*

• Carry out medical plan of care, as ordered. *Collaborative practice enhances overall care.*
• Administer oxygen, as prescribed, *to increase supply to myocardium.*

Evaluations for expected outcomes
• Patient's pulse rate and blood pressure remain within set limits.
• Patient doesn't exhibit arrhythmias during monitoring or physical examination.
• Patient's skin remains warm and dry to touch.
• Inspection and palpation don't reveal pedal edema.
• Patient carries out activities of daily living without heart rate exceeding or dropping below set limits.
• Patient doesn't indicate, either verbally or through behavior, chest pain, dyspnea, fatigue, or other forms of discomfort after activity.
• Patient performs stress-reduction techniques every 4 hours.
• Patient describes signs and symptoms of decreased cardiac output, such as dizziness, syncope, clammy skin, fatigue, and dyspnea.
• Patient understands importance of following prescribed diet, taking medications as ordered, and maintaining activity level.

Documentation
• Patient's needs and perception of problem
• Observations of physical findings
• Patient's response to activity
• Development of skills related to diet, medication, activity, and stress management
• Evaluations for expected outcomes

■ Caregiver role strain

related to discharge of a family member with significant home care needs

Definition
Caregiver's perceived difficulty in providing care

Assessment
• Caregiver's physical and mental status, including chronic health problems, self-care abilities, mobility limitations, and level of cognitive function
• Care recipient's physical and mental status, including illness, self-care limitations, mobility limitations, and level of cognitive function
• Support systems, including financial resources, family members and friends, community services, health-related services such as geriatric daycare, and home health aides
• Home environment, including layout of home, structural barriers, need for equipment or assistive devices, and availability of transportation
• Cultural, ethnic, and religious background
• Perceived and actual obligations of caregiver
• Caregiver's personal strengths, including coping and problem-solving abilities and participation in diversional activities or hobbies

Defining characteristics
• Altered caregiving activities
• Altered health status (hypertension, cardiovascular disease, diabetes, headaches, GI upset, weight changes, or rashes)
• Difficulty or inability to perform specific caregiving activities
• Preoccupation with care routine

• Worrying about such possibilities as care recipient's deteriorating health, institutionalization of the care recipient, or the inability to continue to provide care

Associated medical diagnoses (selected)
Acquired immunodeficiency syndrome (AIDS), Alzheimer's disease, amyotrophic lateral sclerosis, cerebrovascular accident, chronic obstructive pulmonary disease, dementia, end-stage disease (cardiac or renal), heart failure, Huntington's disease, multiple sclerosis, muscular dystrophy, paralysis, schizophrenia

Expected outcomes
• Caregiver will describe current stressors.
• Caregiver will identify stressors that can and can't be controlled.
• Caregiver will identify formal and informal sources of support.
• Caregiver will show evidence of using support systems.
• Caregiver will report increased ability to cope with stress.

Interventions and rationales
• Help caregiver to identify current stressors *to evaluate the causes of role strain.*
• Using a nonjudgmental approach, help caregiver evaluate which stressors are controllable and which aren't *to begin to develop strategies to reduce stress.*
• Encourage caregiver to discuss coping skills used to overcome similar stressful situations in the past *to build confidence for managing the current situation.*
• Encourage caregiver to participate in a support group. Provide information on organizations such as Alzheimer's Association, Children of Aging Parents, or the referral service of

the community AIDS task force *to foster mutual support and provide an opportunity for caregiver to discuss personal feelings with empathetic listeners.*

• Help caregiver identify informal sources of support, such as family members, friends, church groups, and community volunteers, *to provide resources for obtaining an occasional or regularly scheduled respite.*

• Help caregiver to identify available formal support services, such as home health agencies, municipal or county social services, hospital social workers, doctors, clinics, and day-care centers, *to enhance coping by providing a reliable structure for support.*

• If caregiver seems overly anxious or distraught, gently point out facts about care recipient's mental and physical condition. *Many times, especially when care recipient is a family member, caregiver's perspective is clouded by a long history of emotional involvement. Your input may help caregiver view the situation more objectively.* If you believe that excessive emotional involvement is hindering caregiver's ability to function, consider recommending Codependents Anonymous, a support group for people whose preoccupation with a relationship leads to chronic suffering and diminished effectiveness, *to provide support.*

• Suggest ways for caregiver to use time more efficiently. For example, caregiver may save time by filling out insurance forms while visiting and chatting with care recipient. *Better time management may help caregiver reduce stress.*

Evaluations for expected outcomes

• Caregiver identifies and develops a realistic appraisal of each stressful situation.

• Caregiver describes emotional response to each stressful situation.
• Caregiver uses resources identified.
• Caregiver uses available support systems.
• Caregiver uses appropriate coping skills for each stressful situation.

Documentation

• Stressors (perceived and actual) identified by caregiver
• Observations of caregiver's response to stressful situations
• Referrals provided
• Caregiver's use of informal and formal support systems
• Coping strategies identified by caregiver and nurse
• Evidence of improvement in caregiver's ability to cope
• Evaluations for expected outcomes

■ Caregiver role strain, risk for

Definition
Caregiver's vulnerability to experiencing difficulty in providing care

Assessment
• Caregiver's physical and mental status, including chronic health problems, self-care abilities, mobility limitations, and level of cognitive function
• Care recipient's physical and mental status, including illness, self-care limitations, mobility limitations, and level of cognitive function
• Support systems, including financial resources, family members and friends, community services, health-related services such as geriatric day-care, and home health aids
• Home environment, including structural barriers, layout of home, need

for presence of equipment or assistive devices, and availability of transportation
• Cultural, ethnic, and religious background
• Perceived and actual obligations of caregiver
• Caregiver's personal strengths, including usual coping and problem-solving abilities and participation in diversional activities or hobbies

Risk factors
• Unreadiness for caregiver role (for example, young adult who must unexpectedly care for a middle-aged parent)
• Evidence of drug or alcohol addiction in caregiver or care recipient, health impairment of caregiver, severity or unpredictable course of illness, or instability of care recipient's health
• Evidence of codependency; deviant, bizarre behavior of care recipient; dysfunctional family coping patterns that existed before the caregiving situation
• Situational factors, such as close relationship between caregiver and patient; discharge of family member with significant home care needs; inadequate environment or facilities for providing care; isolation, inexperience, or overwork of caregiver; presence of abuse or violence; simultaneous occurrence of other events that cause stress for family (significant personal loss, natural disaster, economic hardship, or major life events)

Associated medical diagnoses (selected)
Alzheimer's disease, cerebrovascular accident, end-stage cardiac disease, heart failure, muscular dystrophy

Expected outcomes
• Caregiver will identify current stressors.

• Caregiver will identify appropriate coping strategies and will state plans to incorporate strategies into daily routine.
• Caregiver will state intention to contact formal and informal sources of support.
• Caregiver will state intention to incorporate recreational activities into daily routine.
• Caregiver will report satisfaction with ability to cope with stress caused by caregiving responsibilities.

Interventions and rationales
• Help caregiver identify current stressors. Ask whether stress is likely to increase or decrease in the future *to evaluate the risk for caregiver role strain.*
• Encourage caregiver to discuss coping skills used to overcome similar stressful situations in the past *to reinforce caregiver's confidence in ability to manage current situation and explore ways to apply coping strategies before caregiver becomes overwhelmed.*
• Help caregiver identify informal sources of support, such as family members, friends, church groups, and community volunteers, *to plan for an occasional or regularly scheduled respite.*
• Help caregiver to identify available formal support services, such as home health agencies, municipal or county social services, hospital social workers, doctors, clinics, and day-care centers, *to help caregiver and thereby lessen risk of strain.*
• Encourage caregiver to discuss hobbies or diversional activities. *Incorporating enjoyable activities into the daily or weekly schedule will discipline caregiver to take needed breaks from caregiving responsibilities and thereby diminish stress.*

• Encourage caregiver to participate in a support group. Provide information on organizations such as Alzheimer's Association, Children of Aging Parents, or the referral service of the community task force for acquired immunodeficiency syndrome *to foster mutual support and provide an outlet for expressing feelings before frustration becomes overwhelming.*

• If caregiver seems overly anxious or distraught, gently point out facts about care recipient's mental and physical condition. *Many times, especially when care recipient is a family member, caregiver's perspective is clouded by a long history of emotional involvement. Your input may help caregiver view the situation more objectively.* If you believe that excessive emotional involvement is hindering caregiver's ability to function, consider recommending Codependents Anonymous, a support group for people whose preoccupation with a relationship leads to chronic suffering and diminished effectiveness, *to provide support.*

• Suggest ways for caregiver to use time efficiently; for example, caregiver may save time by filling out insurance forms while visiting and chatting with care recipient. *Better time management may help caregiver reduce stress.*

Evaluations for expected outcomes

• Caregiver identifies and develops a realistic appraisal of each stressful situation.

• Caregiver describes coping strategies used in stressful situations.

• Caregiver uses available support systems.

• Caregiver incorporates recreational activities into daily routine.

• Caregiver reports satisfaction in coping with stress.

Documentation

• Current stressors identified by caregiver

• Risk factors (developmental, pathophysiologic, psychological, and situational) for caregiver role strain identified by nurse

• Caregiver's statements indicating intention to take action to minimize stress, such as seeking help from support services, participating in a caregiver support group, and scheduling time for recreational activities

• Coping strategies identified by caregiver and nurse

• Observations of caregiver's response to stressful situations

• Referrals provided

• Evaluations for expected outcomes

■ Confusion, acute

Definition

Abrupt onset of changes in attention span, cognition, psychomotor activity, level of consciousness (LOC), or sleep-wake cycle

Assessment

• Age, sex, level of education, occupation, and recent immigration status

• Health history, including use of medications, recent surgery, allergies, history of alcoholism, drug abuse, and depression

• Neurologic status, including LOC, orientation, thought and speech, mood, affect, memory, visual and spatial ability, judgment and insight, psychomotor activity, and perceptions; delusions, illusions, and hallucinations; pain level; recent behavioral changes; and history of transient is-

chemic attacks (TIAs), head injury, early dementia, acquired immunodeficiency syndrome, or schizophrenia
• Cardiovascular status, including vital signs, skin color, auscultation of carotid artery and heart sounds, and history of coronary artery disease or hypertension
• Respiratory status, including rate, depth, and pattern of respirations; auscultation for breath sounds; smoking history; shortness of breath; and history of chronic obstructive pulmonary disease, cancer, or tuberculosis
• Sensory status, including results of vision and hearing examination, use of corrective lenses or hearing aid, and history of eye or ear disorders
• Nutritional status, including typical daily food intake and weight loss
• Sleep status, including recent change in sleep pattern or environment (recent hospitalization)

Defining characteristics
• Fluctuations in LOC, psychomotor activity, cognition, and sleep-wake cycle
• Hallucinations
• Impaired perceptive ability
• Increased agitation
• Lack of motivation to initiate and follow through with goal-directed behavior

Associated medical diagnoses (selected)
Cerebrovascular accident, dementia, drug or alcohol addiction, head injury, sepsis, TIAs

Expected outcomes
• Patient will not experience injury.
• Patient's neurologic status will not deteriorate.
• Family members will report an improved ability to cope with the patient's confused state.

• Patient will start to participate in activities of daily living (ADLs).
• Patient will report feeling increasingly calm.
• Patient and family members will state the causes of acute confusion.
• Patient and family members will express an understanding of the importance of informing other health care providers about episodes of acute confusion.

Interventions and rationales
• Assess patient's LOC and changes in behavior *to provide baseline for comparison with ongoing assessment findings.*
• Have a staff member stay at patient's bedside, if necessary, *to protect patient from harm.*
• Enlist the aid of family member *to help calm patient.*
• Limit noise and environmental stimulation *to prevent patient from becoming more confused.*
• Monitor neurologic status on a regular basis *to detect any improvement or decline in patient's neurologic function.*
• Use appropriate safety measures *to protect patient from injury.* Avoid physical restraints *to prevent agitating patient.*
• Address patient by name and tell him your name *to foster his awareness of self and environment.*
• Give patient short, simple explanations each time you perform a procedure or task *to decrease confusion.*
• Schedule nursing care to provide quiet times for patient *to help avoid sensory overload.*
• Mention time, place, and date frequently throughout day. Have a clock and a calendar where patient can easily see them. Refer to these aids when orienting him *to foster awareness of self and environment.*

• Keep patient's possessions in the same place as much as possible. *A consistent, stable environment reduces confusion and frustration and aids completion of ADLs.*

• Ask family members to bring labeled family photos and other favorite articles *to create a more secure environment for patient.*

• Plan patient's routine and be as consistent as possible in following it. *A consistent routine aids task completion and reduces confusion.*

• Speak slowly and clearly and allow patient ample time to respond *to reduce his frustration and promote task completion.*

• Encourage patient to perform ADLs, dividing tasks into small, critical units. Be patient and specific in providing instructions. Allow time for patient to perform each task. *These measures enhance his self-esteem as well as help prevent complications related to inactivity.*

• Encourage family members to share stories and discuss familiar people and events with patient. *Sharing stories and familiar subjects promotes a sense of continuity, aids memory, and creates a sense of security and comfort.* Note that even if patient's short-term memory is impaired, his remote memory still may be intact.

• Support family members' attempts to interact with patient *to provide positive reinforcement.*

• Allow time before and after visits for family members to express feelings. *Listening to family members in an open and nonjudgmental manner will help them cope with patient's illness. Listening to their opinions may also help you assess and monitor patient's condition.*

• Reassure patient and family that confusion will be temporary *to help relieve their anxiety.* Always include patient in discussions.

• Confer with doctor about diagnostic test results, patient's progress in behavior, and patient's LOC. *A collaborative approach to treatment helps ensure high-quality care and continuity of care.*

• Discuss episodes of acute confusion with patient and family members *to make sure they understand the cause of confusion.*

• Review measures family members can take at home to help patient if he begins to exhibit signs of confusion. Tell them to give patient short explanations of activities; remind him of time, place, and date frequently; speak slowly and clearly and allow patient time to respond; and provide patient with a consistent routine. *Teaching empowers patient and family members to take greater responsibility for their health care needs.*

• Stress to patient and family that, in the future, they should inform health care providers about episodes of acute confusion *to help ensure continuity of care.*

Evaluations for expected outcomes

• Patient doesn't experience injury during episodes of acute confusion.

• Patient exhibits a mental status within the normal range.

• Family members report an increased ability to cope with the patient's confused state.

• Patient performs ADLs to the extent possible.

• Patient reports feelings of increased calm.

• Patient and family members express an understanding of episodes of acute confusion.

• Patient and family members express an understanding of the importance of telling future health care providers about episodes of acute confusion.

Documentation
• Description of episodes of acute confusion
• Factors that precipitate and ameliorate periods of acute confusion
• Teaching sessions and referrals
• Evaluations for expected outcomes

■ Confusion, chronic

Definition
An irreversible, long-standing, or progressive deterioration of intellect and personality characterized by decreased ability to interpret environmental stimuli; decreased capacity for thought; and disturbances of memory, orientation, and behavior

Assessment
• Age and sex
• Neurologic status, including level of consciousness (LOC), orientation, thought and speech, mood, affect, memory, visual and spatial ability, judgment and insight, psychomotor activity, and perceptions; recent behavior changes; lethargy, restlessness, short-term or long-term memory loss, and sleep disturbance; and history of multiple infarctions, transient ischemic attacks, Parkinson's disease, cerebral infarctions, seizures, and alcohol or drug abuse
• Self-care status, including ability to perform instrumental or routine activities of daily living (ADLs)
• Family status, including marital status, economic status, living arrangements, presence of caregiver and relationship to patient, and caregiver's perception of patient's abilities

Defining characteristics
• Altered interpretation and response to stimuli
• Altered personality
• Clinical evidence of organic impairment
• Impaired short-term and long-term memory
• Impaired socialization
• No change in LOC
• Progressive or long-standing cognitive impairment

Associated medical diagnoses (selected)
Acquired immunodeficiency syndrome, Alzheimer's disease, cerebrovascular accident, dementia, head injury

Expected outcomes
• Patient's cognitive abilities, behavior, and self-care status will be monitored.
• Patient will exhibit no signs of depression.
• Patient will maintain weight.
• Family members will discuss their ability to provide care for the patient.
• Patient will be provided with a structured environment to ensure maximum functioning.
• Family members or caregiver will describe strategies to help patient cope with chronic confusion.
• Patient will participate in selected activities to extent possible.
• Family members will maintain safety of patient's home environment.
• If necessary, patient and family members will prepare for relocation to long-term care facility.
• Patient will receive adequate emotional support to help him cope with stress of moving to a new environment.
• Staff at patient's new residence will receive clear instructions regarding

measures to help patient cope with chronic confusion.

Interventions and rationales

• Assess patient's cognitive abilities and changes in behavior *to provide baseline data for comparison with ongoing assessment findings.*
• Encourage family members to watch you perform mental status assessments *to give them a more accurate view of patient's abilities.*
• Evaluate patient's ability to care for himself, including his ability to function alone and drive a car. *Safety is a primary concern.*
• Assess patient for depression *to determine need for treatment.*
• Weigh patient, document your findings, and include instructions for regular weighing as part of plan of care *to monitor patient's nutritional status.*
• Ask family members about their ability to provide care for patient *to assess their need for assistance.* Project an attentive, nonjudgmental attitude when listening to them *to help ensure that you receive accurate information.*
• Take steps to provide a stable physical environment and consistent daily routine for patient. *Stability and consistency enhance functioning.*
• Teach family members or caregiver strategies to help patient cope with his condition:
– Place an identification bracelet on patient *to promote safety.*
– Touch patient to *convey acceptance.*
– Avoid unfamiliar situations when possible *to help ensure a consistent environment.*
– Provide structured rest periods *to prevent fatigue and reduce stress.*
– Avoid asking questions patient can't answer — for example, questions that test his orientation to time, place, per-

son, or situation — *to avoid frustrating him.*
– Provide finger foods if patient won't sit and eat *to ensure adequate nutrition.*
– Select activities based on patient's interests and abilities and praise him for participating in activities *to enhance his sense of self-worth.*
– Use television and radio carefully *to avoid sensory overload,* which may exacerbate confusion.
– Limit choices patient has to make *to provide structure and avoid confusion.*
– Label familiar photos with names of individuals pictured *to provide a sense of security.*
– Use symbols, rather than written signs, to identify patient's room, bathroom, and other facilities *to help patient identify surroundings.*
– Place patient's name in large block letters on clothing and other belongings *to help patient recognize his belongings and prevent them from becoming lost.*
• If possible, make a home visit *to assess safety of patient's living environment.*
• Assist family members in contacting appropriate community services. If necessary, act as an advocate for patient within health care system *to help secure services needed for ongoing care.*
• Provide family members with information concerning long-term health care facilities. If necessary, assist family members in moving patient to a nursing home or other long-term care setting. *A patient with chronic confusion may require ongoing skilled nursing care.*
• If patient is to be moved to a long-term care facility, explain to him the decision in as simple and gentle terms as possible *to facilitate comprehen-*

sion. Allow patient to express his feelings regarding the move *to facilitate grieving over loss of independence.* Provide psychological support to patient and family members *to alleviate stress they may experience during relocation.*

• Communicate all aspects of the discharge plan to staff members at patient's new residence, including measures to ensure a stable environment and consistent routine; need to monitor patient's ongoing ability to perform ADLs; measures to ensure adequate nutrition; and interventions to provide emotional support to patient and family members. *Documenting a discharge plan and communicating it to caregivers helps ensure continuity of care. Interventions should ensure patient's dignity and rights.*

Evaluations for expected outcomes

• Patient experiences no injury because of chronic confusion.
• Patient undergoes a complete diagnostic workup to rule out any reversible cause of confusion.
• Patient participates in appropriate activities.
• Patient functions to maximum ability in a stable and structured environment.
• Patient receives adequate nutrition.
• Patient receives adequate emotional support before, during, and after relocation to long-term care facility.
• Patient expresses feelings regarding living arrangement in the nursing home.
• Family members discuss openly their ability to provide for the patient.
• Family members describe strategies to help the patient cope with chronic confusion.
• Family members receive adequate information regarding long-term care

options to make informed decisions regarding the patient's future.
• Plan of care is communicated to staff at patient's new residence.

Documentation

• Assessment of patient's cognitive abilities, behavior, and self-care status
• Changes in patient's mental status as they occur
• Assistance given to family to help them cope with patient's confusion
• Any plans made to move patient to a long-term care facility
• Teaching sessions and referrals
• Evaluations for expected outcomes

■ Constipation

related to gastrointestinal obstruction

Definition
Interruption of normal bowel movements resulting in infrequent or absent stools

Assessment
• History of bowel disorder or surgery
• GI status, including nausea and vomiting, usual bowel elimination habits, change in bowel elimination habits, laxative use, stool characteristics (color, amount, size, and consistency), pain, inspection of abdomen, auscultation of bowel sounds, palpation for masses and tenderness, percussion for tympany and dullness, and results of upper GI series, barium enema, and sigmoidoscopy
• Nutritional status, including dietary intake, fiber intake, appetite, current weight, and change from normal weight
• Fluid and electrolyte status, including intake and output, skin turgor,

urine specific gravity, and serum electrolyte level
• History of ingesting nonfood items (in psychiatric patients)

Defining characteristics
• Abdominal tenderness or pain and feeling of rectal fullness or pressure
• Borborygmi, hypoactive or hyperactive bowel sounds, or abdominal dullness on percussion
• Bright red blood with stool; bark-colored or black, tarry stool; or hard, dry stool
• Change in elimination pattern
• Changes in mental status, urinary incontinence, unexplained falls, or elevated body temperature in older adults
• Decreased frequency and volume of stool
• Distended abdomen and increased abdominal pressure
• Inability to pass stool
• General fatigue, anorexia, headache, indigestion, nausea, or vomiting
• Oozing liquid stool
• Palpable rectal or abdominal mass
• Severe flatus
• Soft, pastelike stool in rectum
• Straining and possibly pain during defecation

Associated medical diagnoses (selected)
Colon and rectal cancer, diverticulitis, intestinal obstruction, ovarian cancer, salmonella, spinal cord injury

Expected outcomes
• Patient will return to usual bowel pattern.
• Patient will maintain fluid balance; intake equals output.
• Patient will display normal bowel sounds.
• Patient will express pain relief or comfort.
• Patient will stop vomiting through use of antiemetics or GI tube.
• Patient will state understanding of surgical procedure.
• Patient or caregiver will demonstrate use of ileostomy or colostomy equipment.
• Patient will discuss fears and anxieties associated with bowel diversion.
• Patient or caregiver will discuss effect of bowel diversion on lifestyle.
• Patient or caregiver will state intention to contact support group.
• Patient will maintain weight.
• Patient will perform oral hygiene.

Interventions and rationales
• Carefully monitor and record frequency and characteristics of stool *to form basis of effective treatment plan.*
• Record intake and output accurately *to ensure correct fluid replacement therapy.* Report any imbalance.
• Auscultate bowel sounds and record every 4 hours. Report significant changes. *Absent or diminished bowel sounds may indicate peritoneal irritation or intestinal obstruction.*
• Record patient's weight daily *to detect possible fluid retention, food malabsorption, or increased adaptation requirements on body processes.*
• Administer pain medication and antiemetics, as ordered. Monitor effectiveness *to determine need for alternative treatment.*
• Promote patient comfort during vomiting episodes by providing oral care and removing vomitus promptly. Carefully record amount and characteristics of vomitus *to ensure accurate intake and output records.*
• Provide oral and nasal care every 4 hours while GI tube is present. Keep nostrils clean and moist *to prevent irritation.*

• Prepare patient for surgery:
– Give preoperative instruction for abdominal surgery *to reduce patient's anxiety and increase trust.*
– Inform patient about ileostomy, colostomy, or colectomy, as indicated, *to reduce anxiety.*
• Instruct patient and caregivers in the use of ileostomy or colostomy equipment *to promote familiarity and establish therapeutic relationship.* Have patient and caregivers demonstrate use of equipment *to encourage feeling of shared responsibility.*
• Encourage patient and family to express feelings and concerns about changes in body image *to help them learn to cope.*
• Encourage visits to patient by persons from ileostomy or colostomy clubs and other support groups *to provide patient with additional health care resources.*

Evaluations for expected outcomes

• Patient exhibits a normal bowel elimination pattern.
• Patient drinks adequate amount of fluids, with intake equal to output.
• Patient displays normal bowel sounds.
• Patient states that pain medication is effective, and he doesn't experience increase in severity of pain.
• Patient doesn't vomit.
• Patient expresses understanding of surgical procedure, including need for ileostomy or colostomy.
• Patient or caregiver demonstrates care, changing, and irrigation of ileostomy or colostomy equipment.
• Patient states acceptance of bowel diversion.
• Patient comes to terms with effects of bowel diversion on lifestyle.
• Patient or caregiver identifies and contacts support group, if needed.

• Patient doesn't exhibit weight loss or gain. Weight is consistent with body weight chart.
• Patient's mouth is clear and free of odor, and nostrils are clean and moist.

Documentation

• Patient's expressions of concern about vomiting, GI tube, or surgery
• Observation of characteristics of vomitus and stool, intake and output, weight, bowel sounds, and condition of oral cavity
• Patient's reaction and adaptation to ileostomy or colostomy
• Patient's and caregivers' participation in care and response to instruction
• Evaluations for expected outcomes

■ Constipation

related to inadequate intake of fluid and bulk

Definition

Interruption of normal bowel movements resulting in infrequent or absent stools

Assessment

• History of bowel disorder or surgery
• GI status, including nausea and vomiting, usual bowel elimination habits, change in bowel elimination habits, laxative use, stool characteristics (color, amount, size, and consistency), pain, inspection of abdomen, auscultation of bowel sounds, palpation for masses and tenderness, and percussion for tympany and dullness
• Nutritional status, including dietary intake, fiber intake, appetite, current weight, and change from normal weight

• Fluid status, including fluid intake, urine output, urine specific gravity, and skin turgor
• Knowledge, including ability and motivation to change current patterns and understanding of relationship between intake, bulk, and constipation

Defining characteristics
• Abdominal tenderness or pain and feeling of rectal fullness or pressure
• Borborygmi, hypoactive or hyperactive bowel sounds, or abdominal dullness on percussion
• Bright red blood with stool; bark-colored or black, tarry stool; or hard, dry stool
• Change in bowel pattern
• Changes in mental status, urinary incontinence, unexplained falls, or elevated body temperature in older adults
• Decreased frequency and volume of stool
• Distended abdomen and increased abdominal pressure
• Inability to pass stool
• General fatigue, anorexia, headache, indigestion, nausea, or vomiting
• Oozing liquid stool
• Palpable rectal or abdominal mass
• Severe flatus
• Soft, pastelike stool in rectum
• Straining and possibly pain during defecation

Associated medical diagnoses (selected)
Anorexia nervosa, bipolar disorder (depressive phase), bulimia nervosa, burns, encephalitis, urinary diversion, or conditions requiring chemotherapy or restricted food or fluid intake

Expected outcomes
• Patient's elimination pattern will return to normal.
• Patient will experience bowel movement every ___ day(s).

• Patient will consume high-fiber or high-bulk diet, unless contraindicated.
• Patient will maintain oral fluid intake of 2,500 ml daily, unless contraindicated.
• Patient will state understanding of relationship of dietary intake and bulk to constipation.
• Patient will list foods needed to prevent recurrence of problem, such as fruit, fruit juices, whole grain bread, and cereals.

Interventions and rationales
• Monitor and record frequency and characteristics of stool. *Careful monitoring forms the basis of an effective treatment plan.*
• Record intake and output accurately *to ensure correct fluid replacement therapy.*
• Unless contraindicated, encourage fluid intake of 2,500 ml daily *to ensure correct fluid replacement therapy.*
• Place patient on bedpan or commode at specific times daily, as close to usual evacuation time (if known) as possible, *to aid adaptation to routine physiologic function.*
• Administer laxative or enema, as ordered, *to promote elimination of solids and gases from GI tract.* Monitor effectiveness.
• Teach patient to gently massage along the transverse and descending colon *to stimulate bowel's spastic reflex and aid stool passage.*
• Consult with dietitian about increasing fiber and bulk in diet to maximum prescribed by doctor. *This will improve intestinal muscle tone and promote comfortable elimination.*
• Instruct patient and family in the relationship of diet, exercise, and fluid intake to constipation. Develop plan and provide for mild exercise periods. *These measures promote muscle tone*

and circulation and discourage departure from prescribed diet.

Evaluations for expected outcomes
• Patient resumes regular bowel elimination schedule.
• Without using laxatives, enemas, or suppositories, patient has bowel movement every ____ day(s).
• Patient consumes fruit, bran, and other high-fiber foods.
• Patient drinks 2,500 ml of fluid daily, unless contraindicated.
• Patient expresses understanding of the effects of diet and fluid intake on constipation.
• Patient names foods that will help prevent recurrence of constipation.

Documentation
• Patient's expressions of concern about constipation, dietary changes, laxative use, and bowel pattern
• Observations of food and fluid intake and stool characteristics
• Patient's expression of understanding of relationship between constipation and dietary intake of fluid and bulk
• Patient's response to nursing interventions
• Evaluations for expected outcomes

■ Constipation

related to personal habits

Definition
Interruption of normal bowel movements resulting in infrequent or absent stools

Assessment
• History of bowel disorder or surgery
• GI status, including nausea and vomiting, usual bowel elimination habits, change in bowel elimination habits, stool characteristics (color, amount, size, and consistency), pain, inspection of abdomen, auscultation of bowel sounds, palpation for masses and tenderness, percussion for tympany and dullness, laxative or enema use, and medication use (iron or narcotics)
• Nutritional status, including dietary intake, fiber intake, appetite, current weight, and change from normal weight
• Activity status, type and duration of exercise, and occupation (sedentary, restricted access to bathroom)
• Knowledge, including understanding of need for regular bowel elimination habits, ability and motivation to change current patterns, and understanding of relationship between laxative and enema use, activity, and constipation

Defining characteristics
• Abdominal tenderness or pain and feeling of rectal fullness or pressure
• Borborygmi, hypoactive or hyperactive bowel sounds, or abdominal dullness on percussion
• Bright red blood with stool; bark-colored or black, tarry stool; or hard, dry stool
• Change in bowel pattern
• Changes in mental status, urinary incontinence, unexplained falls, or elevated body temperature in older adults
• Decreased frequency and volume of stool
• Distended abdomen and increased abdominal pressure
• Inability to pass stool
• General fatigue, anorexia, headache, indigestion, nausea, or vomiting
• Oozing liquid stool
• Palpable rectal or abdominal mass
• Severe flatus

• Soft, pastelike stool in rectum
• Straining and possibly pain during defecation

Associated medical diagnoses (selected)
Atonic colon, depression, diverticulosis, fecal impaction, hemorrhoids, spastic or irritable colon

Expected outcomes
• Patient's bowel elimination will return to normal.
• Patient will move bowels every ___ day(s) without laxative or enema.
• Patient will state understanding of causative factors of constipation.
• Patient will get regular exercise.
• Patient will describe changes in personal habits to maintain normal elimination pattern.
• Patient will state plans to seek help to resolve emotional or psychological problems.

Interventions and rationales
• Monitor and record frequency and characteristics of stool. *Careful monitoring forms the basis of an effective treatment plan.*
• Administer laxatives or enemas, as ordered, *to promote elimination.* Monitor effectiveness.
• Provide privacy for elimination. Encourage establishment of daily schedule *to aid adaptation to routine physiologic function.*
• Weigh patient weekly and record results *to detect fluid loss or retention, food malabsorption, or increased adaptation requirement on body processes.*
• Encourage intake of high-fiber foods, such as bananas, prunes, dates, figs, and whole grain cereals and breads, *to supply bulk for normal elimination.*
• Consult with dietitian and encourage adherence to a diet modification plan *to discourage departure from prescribed diet.*
• Teach patient about:
– effects of long-term laxative or enema use *to avoid damaging intestinal mucosa*
– need for diet high in fiber, bulk, and fluid *to soften stool and stimulate intestinal mucosa*
– importance of responding to defecation urge *to avoid pressure and discomfort in lower GI tract*
– selection of and adherence to regular exercise program *to promote muscle tone and circulation.*
• Make referral to psychiatric liaison nurse, community agencies, or support groups *to provide additional health care resources to patient and family.*

Evaluations for expected outcomes
• Patient resumes regular bowel elimination schedule.
• Without using laxatives, enemas, or suppositories, patient has bowel movement every ___ day(s).
• Patient states three ways to prevent constipation.
• Patient performs regular exercise.
• Patient states how he plans to change lifestyle and dietary habits to prevent constipation.
• Patient contacts at least one community resource for help with resolving psychological conflicts.

Documentation
• Patient's expressions of concern about change in diet, activity level, use of laxatives or enemas, and bowel elimination pattern
• Observations of characteristics of stool, diet, and activity tolerance
• Patient teaching about diet, exercise, and management of constipation
• Evaluations for expected outcomes

■ Constipation, perceived

Definition
State in which an individual makes a self-diagnosis of constipation and ensures daily bowel movements through use of laxatives, enemas, or suppositories

Assessment
• Family history of constipation
• History of psychiatric disorders
• Fluid and electrolyte status, including intake and output, skin turgor, urine specific gravity, and mucous membranes
• Marital status
• GI status, including bowel elimination habits, change in bowel elimination habits, stool characteristics (color, amount, size, and consistency), pain, auscultation of bowel sounds, laxative or enema use (time and duration), family habits concerning bowel movements, and rectal examination
• Nutritional status, including dietary intake and appetite
• Activity status
• Psychosocial status, including personality, stressors (finances, job, marital discord, and coping mechanisms), support systems (family and others), lifestyle, and knowledge level

Defining characteristics
• Expectation of passage of stool at same time each day, with resulting overuse of laxatives, enemas, and suppositories

Associated medical diagnoses (selected)
Acute emotional distress, chronic anxiety, laxative abuse

Expected outcomes
• Patient will decrease use of laxatives, enemas, or suppositories.
• Patient will state understanding of normal bowel function.
• Patient will discuss feelings about elimination pattern.
• Patient's elimination pattern will return to normal.
• Patient will experience bowel movement every _____ day(s) without laxatives, enemas, or suppositories.
• Patient will state understanding of factors causing constipation.
• Patient will get regular exercise.
• Patient will describe changes in personal habits to maintain normal elimination pattern.
• Patient will state intent to use appropriate resources to help resolve emotional or psychological problems.

Interventions and rationales
• Correct dietary habits to include adequate fluids, fresh fruits and vegetables, and whole grain cereals and breads, *which supply necessary bulk for normal elimination.*
• Encourage patient to engage in daily exercise, such as brisk walking, *to strengthen muscle tone and stimulate circulation.*
• Encourage patient to evacuate at regular times *to aid adaptation and routine physiologic function.*
• Urge patient to avoid taking laxatives if possible or to gradually decrease their use *to avoid further trauma to intestinal mucosa.*
• Inform patient not to expect a bowel movement every day or even every other day *to avoid use of poor health practices to stimulate elimination.*
• If not contraindicated, increase patient's fluid intake to about 3,000 ml daily *to increase functional capacity of bowel elimination.*
• Explain normal bowel elimination habits *so patient can better understand normal and abnormal body functions.*

• Reassure patient that normal bowel function is possible without laxatives, enemas, or suppositories *to give patient the necessary confidence for compliance.*
• Give information about self-help groups, as appropriate, *to provide additional resources for patient and family.*
• Establish and implement an individualized bowel elimination regimen based on patient's needs. *Knowledge of normal body functions will improve patient's understanding of problem.*
• Instruct patient to avoid straining during elimination *to avoid tissue damage, bleeding, and pain.*
• Instruct patient that abdominal massage may help relieve discomfort and promote defecation *because it triggers bowel's spastic reflex.*

Evaluations for expected outcomes
• Patient decreases use of laxatives, enemas, or suppositories.
• Patient describes normal bowel function and how fluid consumption, high-fiber diet, and exercise affect function.
• Patient expresses feelings about changes in elimination pattern.
• Patient's elimination pattern returns to normal.
• Without using laxatives, enemas, or suppositories, patient has bowel movement every ___ day(s).
• Patient lists factors that may cause constipation.
• Patient performs regular exercise
• Patient states plans to make changes in personal habits to prevent constipation.
• Patient makes contact with appropriate resources to help resolve psychological conflicts.

Documentation
• Patient's expressions of concern about change in diet, activity level, laxative and enema use, and bowel pattern
• Observations of diet, stool characteristics, and activity tolerance
• Patient teaching about diet, exercise, and constipation management
• Evaluations for expected outcomes

■ Constipation, risk of

Definition
Risk for interruption of normal bowel movement resulting in infrequent or absent stools

Assessment
• Age and sex
• Vital signs
• Health history, including bowel disorder or surgery, diabetic gastroparesis, immobility or inactivity, chronic debilitating disease, and episodes characterized by inability to swallow food and fluids
• GI status, including nausea and vomiting, usual bowel habits, change in bowel habits, laxative use, stool characteristics (color, amount, size, consistency), pain, inspection of abdomen, auscultation of bowel sounds, palpation for masses and tenderness, and percussion for tympany and dullness
• Nutritional status, including dietary intake, appetite, current weight, and changes from normal diet
• Fluid status, including intake and output and skin turgor
• Musculoskeletal status, including functional mobility, joint mobility, paralysis, paresis, and activity and exercise status

• Psychosocial status, including understanding of risk of constipation, motivation to change health habits, and understanding of relationship between intake, bulk, activity and mobility, and constipation

Risk factors
• Functional, such as habitual denial and ignoring urge to defecate, recent environmental changes, inadequate toileting (for example, timeliness, positioning for defecation, privacy), irregular defecation habits, insufficient physical activity, and abdominal muscle weakness
• Mechanical, such as rectal abscess or ulcer, pregnancy, rectal anal stricture, postsurgical obstruction, rectal anal fissures, megacolon (Hirschsprung's disease), electrolyte imbalance, tumors, prostate enlargement, rectocele, rectal prolapse, neurological impairment, hemorrhoids, and obesity
• Pharmacologic, such as phenothiazines, nonsteroidal anti-inflammatory agents, sedatives, aluminum-containing antacids, laxative overuse, iron salts, anticholinergics, antidepressants, anticonvulsants, antilipemic agents, calcium channel blockers, calcium carbonate, diuretics, sympathomimetics, opiates, and bismuth salts
• Physiologic, such as insufficient fiber intake, dehydration, inadequate dentition or oral hygiene, poor eating habits, insufficient fluid intake, change in usual foods and eating patterns, and decreased motility of GI tract
• Psychological, such as emotional stress, mental confusion, and depression

Associated medical diagnoses (selected)
This diagnosis may occur in any medical disorder characterized by restricted or altered food and fluid intake, inactivity, or immobility. Examples include anorexia nervosa, bulimia nervosa, cerebrovascular accident, depression, fractures (with traction or cast), neuromuscular disorders, severe head injury, and spinal cord injury. It may also be associated with some pharmacologic treatments and may occur in pregnancy and obesity, and in postoperative patients.

Expected outcomes
• Patient will not experience constipation.
• Patient will maintain bowel movement every _____ day(s).
• Patient will consume a high-fiber or high-bulk diet, unless contraindicated.
• Patient will maintain fluid intake of _____ ml daily (specify).
• Patient will express understanding of the relationship between constipation and dietary intake, bulk, and activity.
• Patient will express understanding of preventive measures, such as eating fruit and whole grain breads and cereals and engaging in mild activity, if appropriate.

Interventions and rationales
• Assess bowel sounds and check patient for abdominal distention. Monitor and record frequency and characteristics of stool *to develop an effective treatment plan for preventing constipation and fecal impaction.*
• Record intake and output accurately *to ensure accurate fluid replacement therapy.*
• Encourage fluid intake of 2.5 L (2½ qt) daily, unless contraindicated, *to promote fluid replacement therapy and hydration.*

• Initiate bowel program. Place patient on a bedpan or commode at specific times daily, as close to usual evacuation time (if known) as possible, *to aid adaptation to routine physiologic function.*
• Administer a laxative, an enema, or suppositories, as prescribed, *to promote elimination of solids and gases from GI tract.* Monitor effectiveness.
• Teach patient to gently massage along the transverse and descending colon *to stimulate the bowel's spastic reflex and aid in stool passage.*
• Consult with a dietitian about how to increase fiber and bulk in patient's diet to the maximum amount prescribed by the doctor *to improve intestinal muscle tone and promote comfortable elimination.*
• Instruct patient, family member, or caregiver in the relationship between diet, activity and exercise, and fluid intake and constipation *to discourage departure from prescribed diet and assist in promoting elimination.*
• Include a program of mild exercise in your plan of care *to promote muscle tone and circulation.*
• Review plan of care with patient, family member, or caregiver, emphasizing the relationship between the risk factors for constipation and preventive measures *to foster understanding.*

Evaluations for expected outcomes
• Patient doesn't experience constipation.
• Patient has bowel movement every _____ day(s).
• Patient consumes a high-fiber or high-bulk diet, unless contraindicated.
• Patient maintains fluid intake of _____ ml daily (specify).
• Patient expresses understanding of the relationship between constipation and dietary intake, bulk, and activity.

• Patient expresses understanding of preventive measures, such as eating fruit and whole grain breads and cereals and engaging in mild activity, if appropriate.

Documentation
• Patient's, family member's, or caregiver's statements regarding risk of constipation
• Presence of risk factors for constipation
• Observations of food and fluid intake, urine output, and stool characteristics
• Instructions regarding preventive care
• Patient's, family member's, or caregiver's statements indicating understanding of instructions
• Patient's response to preventive interventions
• Implementation, alteration, or continuation of bowel program
• Patient's, family member's, or caregiver's demonstrated ability to implement preventive measures
• Evaluations for expected outcomes

■ Coping, defensive
related to perceived threat to positive self-regard

Definition
Falsely positive self-evaluation based on a self-protective pattern that defends against underlying perceived threats to positive self-regard

Assessment
• Age
• Sex
• Developmental stage
• Family system, including marital status and sibling position

• Reason for hospitalization
• Past experience with illness
• Patient's perception of health problem
• Patient's perception of self, including self-worth, body image, problem-solving ability, and coping mechanisms
• Mental status, including general appearance, affect, mood, cognitive and perceptual functioning, and behavior
• Social interaction pattern
• Support systems, such as family and friends

Defining characteristics
• Denial of obvious problems
• Difficulty establishing or maintaining relationships
• Difficulty in reality-testing perceptions
• Extreme sensitivity to criticism
• Grandiosity
• Lack of follow-through or participation in treatment or therapy
• Projection of blame or responsibility
• Rationalization of failures
• Superior attitude toward and ridicule of others

Associated medical diagnoses (selected)
Any illness or injury resulting in chronic pain, permanent disability, or disfigurement (such as acquired immunodeficiency syndrome, anxiety disorder, chronic obstructive pulmonary disease, deafness, degenerative disease, drug or alcohol addiction, end-stage disease [cardiac or renal], melanoma)

Expected outcomes
• Patient will state reason for hospitalization.
• Patient will verbally describe self, including concept, body image, successes, and failures.
• Patient will participate in self-care.

• Patient will engage in decision making about treatment.
• Patient will accept responsibility for own behavior.
• Patient will demonstrate follow-through in decisions related to health care.
• Patient will interact with others in a socially acceptable manner.

Interventions and rationales
• Encourage patient to evaluate self, possibly by making a written list of positive and negative traits. *This helps patient identify aspects of self and relate changes to specific variables.*
• Have patient perform self-care to the extent possible *to provide a sense of control.*
• Provide a structured daily routine *to provide patient with alternatives to self-absorption.*
• Help patient make treatment-related decisions and encourage follow-through. *Ability to make decisions is principal component of autonomy.*
• Provide an opportunity for patient to meet with someone who's successfully coping with a similar problem. *This may encourage patient to work toward a positive outcome.*
• Arrange for interaction between patient and others and observe interaction pattern. *Studying patient's verbal and nonverbal interactions with others gives clues to patient's ability to communicate effectively.*
• Provide positive feedback when patient assumes responsibility for own behavior *to reinforce effective coping behaviors.*

Evaluations for expected outcomes
• Patient states reason for hospitalization.
• Patient uses at least two positive terms to describe self.

• Patient initiates and completes at least two self-care activities daily.
• Each day, patient makes at least one decision related to activities of daily living, self-care, or treatment.
• Patient expresses responsible attitude toward own behavior.
• Patient reports specific instances of following through on decisions.
• Each day, patient socializes with others.

Documentation
• Patient's perception of self
• Behavioral responses
• Social interaction patterns
• Patient's use of defense mechanisms
• Interventions used to facilitate effective coping
• Patient's responses to nursing interventions
• Evaluations for expected outcomes

■ Coping, family: Potential for growth
related to self-actualization needs

Definition
Effective managing of adaptive tasks by family members involved in the client's health problem

Assessment
• Family process, including normal pattern of interaction among family members, family's understanding and knowledge of patient's present condition, support systems available (financial, social, and spiritual), family's past response to crises (coping patterns), and communication patterns used to express anger, affection, and confrontation
• Patient's illness, including progression and severity of illness, patient's

perception of health problem, and problem-solving techniques used by patient to cope with life problems

Defining characteristics
• Interest of family member in making contact with others who have gone through similar situations
• Attempt by family member to describe impact of crisis on personal values, priorities, goals, or relationships
• Fostering by family member of a health-promoting and enriching lifestyle that supports and monitors maturational processes and audits and negotiates treatment programs

Associated medical diagnoses (selected)
Any disorder that results in long-term disability or incapacitation of family member, such as amyotrophic lateral sclerosis, asthma, cystic fibrosis, degenerative disease, hemophilia, multiple sclerosis, muscular dystrophy, and spinal cord defects

Expected outcomes
• Family members will discuss impact of patient's illness and feelings about it with health care professional.
• Family members will participate in treatment plan.
• Family members will establish a visiting routine beneficial to both patient and themselves.
• Family members will demonstrate care needed to maintain patient's health status.
• Family members will identify and use available support systems.

Interventions and rationales
• Allow time for family members to discuss impact of patient's illness and their feelings. Encourage expression of feelings *to allow family members*

to realistically adjust to patient's problems.

• Encourage family conferences; help family members identify key issues and select support services, if needed, *to develop sense of shared responsibility and feelings of safety, adequacy, and comfort.*

• Help patient and family establish a visiting routine that won't tax patient's or family's resources. Use patient's daily routine to aid in planning — for example, no visiting during treatments or during periods of uninterrupted sleep. *Involving family members reassures patient of their care and reduces family's fear and anxiety.*

• Reinforce family members' efforts to care for patient *to let them know they are doing their best and to ease adaptation and grieving process.*

• Demonstrate care procedures, and encourage participation in treatment and planning decisions (such as selecting times for pulmonary toilet for patient with cystic fibrosis). *Meeting others' needs promotes self-esteem.*

• Provide family members with clear, concise information about patient's condition. Be aware of what they have already been told and help them interpret information. *This information will help alleviate their concerns.*

• Ensure privacy for patient and family during visits *to foster open communication.*

• Help family support patient's independence. Encourage attendance at therapy sessions, and allow patient to demonstrate new skills and abilities. *Independence helps patient reach maximum functional level.*

• Provide emotional support to family by being available to answer questions. *Attentive listening conveys empathy, recognition, and respect for a person.*

• Inform family of community resources and support groups available to assist in managing patient's illness and providing emotional or financial support to caretakers, such as Easter Seals Association, Visiting Nurse Association, and Meals On Wheels. *Community resources may help patient develop potential, independence, and self-reliance.*

Evaluations for expected outcomes

• Family members acknowledge their feelings about the patient's illness.

• Family members spend adequate time with the patient and seek to participate in care.

• Family members establish a visiting routine beneficial to both patient and themselves.

• Family members display competence in caring for patient through return demonstration and provide adequate level of care to maintain patient's health.

• Family members make contact with support resources available in their community.

Documentation

• Family's response to illness
• Family's current understanding of patient's illness
• Observations about family's interaction with patient and acceptance of current situation
• Evaluations for expected outcomes

■ Coping, ineffective family: Compromised

related to inadequate or incorrect information held by primary caregiver

Definition
Behavior of family members that compromises patient's and family's capacities to adapt

Assessment
• Family status, including normal pattern of interaction among family members, family's understanding and knowledge of patient's present condition, support systems available (financial, social, and spiritual), family's response to past crises, and communication patterns used to express anger, affection, confrontation, and conflict
• Patient's illness, including progression and severity of illness, patient's perception of health problem, and problem-solving techniques used by patient to cope with life problems

Defining characteristics
• Concern about family's response to current health problem
• Attempt by family member to assist or support patient with unsatisfactory results
• Inadequate understanding or knowledge base of family member that interferes with effective assistive or supportive behaviors
• Protective behavior of family member that is disproportionate to patient's abilities or need for autonomy
• Preoccupation of family member with how to respond to patient's health problem
• Family member's withdrawal from or limited communication with patient at time of need

Associated medical diagnoses (selected)
Any disorder that results in long-term disability or incapacitation, such as Alzheimer's disease, amyotrophic lateral sclerosis, chronic renal failure, cystic fibrosis, Huntington's disease, myocardial infarction, and paralysis

Expected outcomes
• Family will discuss impact of patient's illness and feelings about it with health care professional.
• Family will designate a spokesperson to receive information regarding the patient's illness.
• Family will establish a visiting routine beneficial to both patient and family.
• Family will state understanding of patient's health status.
• Family will identify and use available support systems.

Interventions and rationales
• Identify the spokesperson for the family *to avoid creating communication conflicts within family.*
• Facilitate family conferences; help family members identify key issues and select support services, if needed. *Involving patient and family in care planning promotes open communication throughout illness.*
• Help patient and family establish a visiting routine that won't tax their resources. Each family member may be responsible for a day or period of time, if desired. Use patient's daily routine to aid in planning; for example, no visiting during treatments or periods of uninterrupted sleep. *This enhances family's sense of contributing to patient's overall care.*
• Encourage family to contact a community agency for continued support, if necessary. *This is an effective health-related coping skill.*

• Provide family with clear, concise information about patient's condition. Be aware of what family has already been told and help them interpret information. *This ensures clear, uncluttered communication between patient, family, and caregivers.*
• Ensure privacy during patient and family visits. *This demonstrates respect and fosters open communication between family members.*
• Help family support patient's independence. Encourage attendance at therapy sessions, and allow patient to demonstrate new skills and abilities *to help family members learn how they can help promote patient's independence and self-care.*
• Provide emotional support to family by being available to answer questions. *This demonstrates your willingness to help family seek health-related information.*

Evaluations for expected outcomes
• Family members express feelings about patient's illness and discuss its impact on family functioning.
• A family member is designated as spokesperson to receive and communicate information regarding the patient's illness.
• Family members agree to follow a consistent visiting routine.
• Family members accurately describe the patient's health status.
• Family contacts at least one support person or group.

Documentation
• Family's response to illness
• Family's current understanding of patient's illness
• Observations about family's interaction with patient and acceptance of current situation
• Evaluations for expected outcomes

■ Coping, ineffective family: Compromised

related to prolonged disease

Definition
Behavior of family members that compromises patient's and family's ability to adapt

Assessment
• Patient's illness, including course and severity and effect on family members
• Patient's health care resources, including hospital, community resources, health care providers such as therapists, and case manager (outpatient)
• Family process, including involvement with patient, quality of relationships, communication patterns, coping strategies, demands posed by patient's condition, family's understanding of patient's illness, family's feelings regarding patient's illness, willingness of family members to commit time to patient care, and family's ability to provide care

Defining characteristics
• Concern about family's response to current health problem
• Attempt by family member to assist or support patient with unsatisfactory results
• Inadequate understanding or knowledge base of family member that interferes with effective assistive or supportive behaviors
• Protective behavior of family member that is disproportionate to patient's abilities or need for autonomy
• Preoccupation of family member with how to respond to patient's health problem

• Family member's withdrawal from or limited communication with patient at time of need

Associated medical diagnoses (selected)

Any disease or illness that results in long-term disability or incapacitation, such as bronchiectasis, cerebrovascular accident, chronic obstructive pulmonary disease, chronic renal failure, cirrhosis, Crohn's disease, diabetes mellitus, Down syndrome, fractures, glomerulonephritis, hydrocephalus, hydronephrosis, hypoparathyroidism, hypothyroidism, liver transplantation, and Parkinson's disease

Expected outcomes

• Family members will express their concerns about coping with patient's illness.
• Family members will identify their needs.
• Family members will contact appropriate sources of support.
• Family and patient will achieve better cooperation.

Interventions and rationales

• Assess effects of patient's disease on family functioning *to plan interventions that enhance long-term well-being of family and patient.*
• Encourage family members to hold conferences. Help them identify topics appropriate for discussion. Examples of such topics include developing coping strategies for dealing with patient's disease or resolving conflicts between meeting personal needs and meeting patient's health care needs. *Family members may find a group problem-solving approach helpful in correcting dysfunctional behaviors.*
• Evaluate and rectify any knowledge deficit that family members have about patient's disease and treatment. *Experience doesn't guarantee correct*

knowledge. Lack of knowledge can exacerbate frustration and tension within the family.
• Encourage family members to participate in appropriate support groups *to help them obtain social support and information and to provide an opportunity to express feelings.*
• Encourage family members to contact and use appropriate community agencies *to help prevent burnout among family members after patient leaves the hospital.* Families may need encouragement to use support and respite care services if past efforts to use such services proved unsuccessful.

Evaluations for expected outcomes

• Family members discuss impact of patient's prolonged disease with nurse.
• Family members communicate their needs regarding the patient's prolonged care.
• Family is aware of available sources of support and uses them appropriately.
• Family and patient negotiate meeting patient's care needs to their mutual satisfaction.

Documentation

• Assessment of family functioning (including family's level of insight into their behavior)
• Content of family conferences
• Community resources used, their effectiveness, and recommendations for future use (indicate family's level of acceptance of nurse's recommendations)
• Evaluations for expected outcomes

■ Coping, ineffective family: Disabling

related to unresolved emotional conflict between patient and family members

Definition
Behavior of family members that undermines the patient's and family's ability to adapt

Assessment
• Patient's illness, including its course, severity, and effect on family members
• Patient's health care resources, including hospital, community resources, health care providers such as therapists, and case manager
• Demands on family imposed by patient's condition
• Family status, including involvement with patient, quality of relationships, communication patterns, coping strategies, family's understanding of patient's illness, family's feelings about patient's illness, willingness of family members to commit time to patient care, and family's ability to provide care

Defining characteristics
• Family member's intolerance of patient's physical ailments or psychological weaknesses; disregard for patient's basic human needs; distorted perception of patient's health problem, including extreme denial about its existence or severity; or refusal to participate in patient care
• Patient's development of helplessness and dependence, along with corresponding decrease in activity level; expression of abandonment, agitation, depression, aggression, rejection, or hostility toward a family member; or

report of poor relationships with family members

Associated medical diagnoses (selected)
Any disorder that results in long-term disability or incapacitation, such as degenerative and terminal disorders, and traumatic injuries

Expected outcomes
• To the extent possible, family members will participate in aspects of patient's care without evidence of increased conflict.
• Patient will express confidence in his ability to make decisions, despite pressure from family members.
• Patient will contact appropriate sources of support outside the family.
• Patient will take steps to ensure that care needs are met despite family's shortcomings.
• Patient will express greater understanding of emotional limitations of family members.

Interventions and rationales
• Assess effects of patient's disease on family functioning *to plan interventions.*
• As possible, encourage family members to participate in patient care. *Family members should have an opportunity to overcome dysfunctional behavior.*
• Maintain objectivity when dealing with family conflicts. Don't become embroiled in the dynamics of a dysfunctional family *to maintain your ability to intervene effectively.*
• If patient and family members appear incapable of taking steps to heal their relationships, focus on being a patient advocate. Reaffirm patient's right to make his own decisions without interference from family members. Provide necessary information to patient to facilitate decision mak-

ing. *Dysfunctional family coping patterns evolve over many years and are unlikely to change just because patient has a serious illness. Accepting your limitations when working with family members will help you to avoid burnout and better meet patient's needs.*

• Encourage patient to seek emotional support his family can't provide by participating in a support group. Help patient select support group that best meets his personal needs and outlook. Consider recommending Codependents Anonymous, a group for individuals who have difficulty maintaining healthy relationships as a result of being raised in a dysfunctional family. *Participation in a support group may improve patient's ability to cope as well as provide an opportunity to form meaningful relationships.*

• Refer patient to a home health care agency, homemaker service, Meals On Wheels, or other appropriate outside agencies for assistance and follow-up. *Use of various community services may help to make up for shortcomings in family's ability to provide care.*

• Listen openly to patient's expressions of pain over unresolved conflicts with family members. Patient may have to grieve over the fact that he will never have an "ideal" family, capable of fully meeting his emotional needs. *Therapeutic listening helps patient to understand himself and his family better and to understand how conflicts from past affect his behavior.*

Evaluations for expected outcomes

• Family members demonstrate improved willingness to cooperate in the patient's care.
• Patient expresses increased confidence in his ability to make decisions.

• Patient contacts at least one support group in an effort to form meaningful relationships outside the family.
• Patient takes steps to meet his own care needs.
• Patient indicates, either verbally or through behavior, a better understanding of family members and an increased ability to accept their emotional limitations.

Documentation

• Family's response to patient's illness
• Observations of patient's interactions with family members
• Referrals made to support groups and community services
• Patient's expressions of grief, anger, and disappointment over unresolved conflicts with family members
• Evaluations for expected outcomes

■ Coping, ineffective individual

related to situational crisis

Definition
Inability to use adaptive behaviors in response to such difficult life situations as loss of health, a loved one, or job

Assessment
• Current health status
• Diversional activities
• Financial resources
• Occupation
• Patient's perception of present health problem or crisis
• Problem-solving techniques usually employed to cope with life problems
• Support systems, including family, companion, friends, and clergy

Defining characteristics
• Change in communication patterns
• Decreased use of social support
• Destructive behavior toward self or others
• Difficulty asking for help
• Fatigue
• High illness rate
• Inability to meet basic needs and role expectations
• Lack of goal-directed behavior, such as inability to attend, difficulty organizing information, poor concentration, and poor problem-solving abilities
• Maladaptive coping behaviors
• Risk-taking behaviors
• Sleep disturbance
• Statements indicating inability to cope
• Substance abuse

Associated medical diagnoses (selected)
Adult respiratory distress syndrome, amyotrophic lateral sclerosis, asthma, brain tumors, breast cancer, cardiac arrhythmias, cor pulmonale, Cushing's syndrome, depression, diabetes mellitus, drug addiction or overdose, encephalitis, end-stage disease (renal or cardiac), Guillain-Barré syndrome, hyperparathyroidism, hyperpituitarism, hypoparathyroidism, hypothyroidism, incest, infertility, interstitial cystitis, liver transplantation, lung abscess, myocardial infarction, osteomyelitis, Parkinson's disease, premature labor, seizure disorders

Expected outcomes
• Patient will communicate feelings about the present situation.
• Patient will become involved in planning own care.
• Patient will express feeling of having greater control over present situation.
• Patient will use available support systems, such as family and friends, to aid in coping.
• Patient will identify and demonstrate ability to use at least two healthy coping behaviors.

Interventions and rationales
• If possible, assign primary nurse to patient *to provide continuity of care and promote development of therapeutic relationship.*
• Arrange to spend uninterrupted periods of time with patient. Encourage expression of feelings, and accept what patient says. Try to identify factors that cause or exacerbate patient's inability to cope such as fear of loss of health or job. *Devoting time to listening helps patient express emotions, grasp situation, and cope effectively.*
• Identify and reduce unnecessary stimuli in environment *to avoid subjecting patient to sensory or perceptual overload.*
• Initially, allow patient to depend partly on you for self-care. *Patient may regress to a lower developmental level during initial crisis phase.*
• Explain all treatments and procedures and answer patient's questions *to allay fear and allow patient to regain sense of control.*
• Encourage patient to make decisions about care *to increase sense of self-worth and mastery over current situation.*
• Have patient increase self-care performance levels gradually *to allow patient to progress at his own pace.*
• Praise patient for making decisions and performing activities *to reinforce coping behaviors.*
• Encourage patient to use support systems to assist with coping, *thereby helping restore psychological equilibrium and prevent crisis.*

• Help patient look at current situation and evaluate various coping behaviors *to encourage a realistic view of crisis.*
• Encourage patient to try coping behaviors. *A patient in crisis tends to accept interventions and develop new coping behaviors more easily than at other times.*
• Request feedback from patient about behaviors that seem to work *to encourage patient to evaluate effect of these behaviors.*
• Refer patient for professional psychological counseling. *If patient's maladaptive behavior has high crisis potential, formal counseling helps ease nurse's frustration, increases objectivity, and fosters collaborative approach to patient's care.*

Evaluations for expected outcomes
• Patient discusses recent stressful event and describes related emotions.
• Patient cooperates with nurse to plan care.
• Patient identifies problems, makes plans, and takes action.
• Patient requests assistance from family and friends.
• Patient identifies and uses at least two healthy coping behaviors such as relaxation techniques.

Documentation
• Patient's perception of present situation and what it means
• Patient's verbal expression of feelings indicating comfort or discomfort
• Observations of patient's behaviors
• Interventions to help patient cope
• Patient's responses to interventions
• Evaluations for expected outcomes

■ Death anxiety
related to terminal illness

Definition
Feelings of threat experienced by patient when death is inevitable

Assessment
• Age
• History of present illness
• Mental status, including level of consciousness, orientation, cognition, memory, and insight
• Self-care status, including ability to carry out activities of daily living
• Sleep pattern, including hours of sleep, energy level before and after sleep, rest and relaxation patterns, and difficulty falling asleep
• Pain assessment, including location, quality, intensity on a scale of 1 to 10, temporal factors, sources of provocation, and relief
• Psychological status, including reaction to illness and dying, and expressions of fear, anger, hope, and anxiety
• Spiritual status, including religious affiliation, current perception of faith, religious practices, changes in religious beliefs or practices brought on by illness, and evidence of unmet spiritual needs (meaning and purpose, love and relatedness, forgiveness)
• Family status, including marital status, family roles, family communications, family's ability to meet patient's physical and emotional needs, extent to which religion defines patient's and family's value system, and changes patient's illness and impending death will make in family functioning

Defining characteristics
• Worry about the impact of one's death on significant others

• Powerlessness over issues related to dying
• Fear of loss of physical and metal abilities when dying
• Anticipated pain related to dying
• Concerns about overworking the caregiver as terminal illness incapacitates self
• Concern about meeting one's creator or feeling doubtful about the existence of a god or higher being
• Total loss of control over aspects of one's own death
• Negative death images or unpleasant thoughts about any event related to death or dying
• Fear of delayed demise
• Fear of premature death because it prevents the accomplishment of important life goals
• Worry about being the cause of other's grief or suffering
• Fear of leaving family alone after death
• Fear of developing a terminal illness
• Denial of one's own mortality or impending death

Associated medical diagnoses (selected)
Acquired immunodeficiency syndrome, amyotrophic lateral sclerosis, aneurysm (abdominal, thoracic, or cerebral), cancer, cerebrovascular accident, heart failure, multiple sclerosis, myocardial infarction, Parkinson's disease, renal failure (acute or chronic), respiratory failure, trauma

Expected outcomes
• Patient will identify need for time with others and need for time alone.
• Patient will identify comfort measures that enhance feelings of well-being.
• Patient will communicate important thoughts and feelings to family members.

• Patient will obtain the level of spiritual support he requests.
• Patient will use available support systems to cope with dying.
• Patient will express feelings of comfort and peacefulness.
• Patient will experience dying with dignity, sensitivity, and love.

Interventions and rationales
• Assess how much help patient wants. *Patient may need a higher degree of independence than caregiver wants to allow.*
• Offer to spend time either reading to patient or sitting quietly beside him. *Commonly, patient approaching death desires the presence of another but is not interested in conversing.*
• If patient is confused, provide reassurance by telling him who's in the room. *This information may help to reduce anxiety.*
• Provide comfort measures — bathing, massage, regulation of environmental temperature, mouth care, administration of ice chips or wet washcloth — according to patient's preferences. *Some patients may prefer not to be bothered unless they specifically request comfort measures.*
• Help family members identify, discuss, and resolve issues related to patient's dying. *Patient needs the support of family members. Family members may need help removing emotional blocks that prevent them from providing full support to patient.*
• Demonstrate to patient your willingness to discuss spiritual aspects of death and dying *to foster open discussion.* Keep conversation focused on patient's spiritual values and the role they play in coping with dying *to ensure that your interaction with patient remains therapeutic.*
• Refer patient to a priest, minister, rabbi, or spiritual counselor, accord-

ing to his preference, *to show respect for patient's beliefs and provide expert spiritual care.*

• Ask patient or family members if there is a prayer or words of spiritual comfort that are especially meaningful to him. If patient seems comfortable with your request, recite this special prayer with him. *Doing so will demonstrate support for patient's spiritual needs and convey caring and acceptance.*

• Help patient cope by listening actively to him and by communicating acceptance of his thoughts and feelings. *Dying patients need the opportunity to express their feelings.*

• Provide simple physical gestures of support such as holding hands with patient. Encourage family members to do the same. Verify with patient that your actions aren't intrusive. *As patients begin to let go, they sometimes want to experience less touching.*

• Reassure patient that he won't be left alone; however, respect patient's requests to be alone. *For some patients, asking to be alone is part of the process of letting go.*

Evaluations for expected outcomes

• Patient reports feelings of anxiety.
• Patient describes anxiety-inducing situations.
• Patient engages in conversation and activities with family, caregivers, and other support people.
• Patient makes appropriate care-related decisions.
• Patient experiences fewer physical symptoms associated with anxiety.
• Patient performs stress-reduction techniques at least twice daily.

Documentation

• Behavioral manifestations of anxiety

• Patient's expressions of feelings related to death and dying
• Patient's requests for visitors or expression of desire for solitude
• Conferences with family members
• Patient's requests for comfort measures and their effectiveness
• Referrals to clergy, spiritual advisors, or others
• Patient's response to nursing interventions
• Evaluations for expected outcomes

■ Decisional conflict

related to health care options

Definition

State of uncertainty about health-related course of action when choice involves risk, potential loss, or challenge to personal life values

Assessment

• Age
• Sex
• Perception of health care options
• Developmental state
• Marital status
• Family system (nuclear, extended role, and sibling position)
• Sociocultural factors, including educational level, occupation, socioeconomic status, ethnic group, sexual preference, and religious beliefs
• Level of functioning (cognitive, emotional, and behavioral)
• Coping mechanisms
• Past experience with decision making
• Available support system

Defining characteristics

• Delayed decision making
• Focusing on self

• Lack of experience or interference with decision making
• Physical signs of distress or tension
• Questioning personal values and beliefs while attempting to make a decision
• Vacillation between alternative choices
• Verbal statements describing undesired consequences of alternative actions being considered
• Verbal expression of distress and uncertainty about making choices

Associated medical diagnoses (selected)
Breast cancer, conditions requiring amputation of an extremity, end-stage disease (cardiac or renal), melanoma

Expected outcomes
• Patient will state feelings about current situation.
• Patient will discuss benefits and drawbacks of treatment options.
• Patient will make minor decisions related to daily activities.
• Patient will accept assistance from family, friends, clergy, and other people.
• Patient will practice progressive muscle relaxation to decrease tension created by decisional conflict.
• Patient will report feeling comfortable about ability to make an appropriate, rational choice.

Interventions and rationales
• Listen to patient's concerns about making a decision. Use a nonjudgmental approach and encourage expression of feelings *to demonstrate acceptance of patient and respect for his culture, beliefs, and value system.*
• Help patient identify available options and their possible consequences *to encourage rational decision making.*

• Help patient make decisions about daily activities *to enhance his feelings of autonomy.*
• Encourage visits with family, friends, and clergy; provide privacy during visits *to foster emotional support.*
• Teach progressive muscle-relaxation techniques *to decrease physical and psychological signs of tension.*
• Help patient identify decision-making areas that require assistance from others, and provide appropriate referrals. *Providing referrals will ensure ongoing support. Putting patient in touch with appropriate community resources will help promote feeling that others are genuinely interested in his well-being.*

Evaluations for expected outcomes
• Patient expresses anxiety, tension, and other feelings related to difficult medical treatment decisions.
• Patient describes benefits and drawbacks of treatment options.
• Patient makes minor decisions related to daily activities.
• Patient accepts assistance from family, friends, clergy, and other people.
• Patient practices progressive muscle relaxation to decrease tension created by decisional conflict.
• Patient reports feeling at ease with ability to choose treatment option that is appropriate for him.

Documentation
• Patient's statements that provide insight into conflict regarding treatment option
• Cognitive, emotional, and behavioral functioning
• Interventions to assist patient with resolving decisional conflict
• Patient's response to nursing interventions
• Evaluations for expected outcomes

■ Denial

related to fear or anxiety

Definition
Conscious or unconscious attempt to disavow the knowledge or meaning of an event to reduce anxiety or fear to the detriment of health

Assessment
• Perception of present health state, including awareness of diagnosis, perception of personal relevance or impact on life pattern, and description of symptoms
• Mental status, including general appearance, affect, mood, memory, orientation, communication, thinking process, perception, abstract thinking, judgment, and insight
• Coping behaviors
• Problem-solving strategies
• Support systems, including family, friends, clergy, and financial resources
• Belief system, including values, norms, and religion
• Self-concept, including self-esteem and body image

Defining characteristics
• Delay in seeking or refusal of medical attention to detriment of health
• Displacement of fear of condition's impact
• Displacement of sources of symptoms to other organs
• Failure to perceive personal relevance or danger of symptoms
• Inability to admit impact of disease on life pattern
• Inappropriate affect
• Minimization of symptoms
• Refusal to admit fear of death or invalidism

• Use of dismissive gestures or comments when speaking of distressing events
• Use of self-treatment to relieve symptoms

Associated medical diagnoses (selected)
Acquired immunodeficiency syndrome, angina pectoris, anorexia nervosa, anxiety disorder, bipolar disorder (manic or depressive phase), bulimia nervosa, chronic obstructive pulmonary disease, chronic renal failure, depression, drug or alcohol addiction, end-stage renal disease, fractures, myocardial infarction, obsessive-compulsive disorder, placenta previa, renal calculi, rheumatoid arthritis, self-destructive behavior, suicidal behavior

Expected outcomes
• Patient will describe knowledge and perception of present health problem.
• Patient will describe life pattern and report any recent changes.
• Patient will express knowledge of stages of grief.
• Patient will demonstrate behavior associated with grief process.
• Patient will discuss present health problem with doctor, nurses, and family members.
• Patient will indicate by conversation or behavior an increased awareness of reality.

Interventions and rationales
• Provide for a specific amount of uninterrupted, non-care-related time with patient each day. *This allows patient to ventilate knowledge, feelings, and concerns.*
• Encourage patient to express feelings related to present problem, its severity, and its potential impact on life pattern. *This helps patient express doubts and resolve concerns.*

• Maintain frequent communication with doctor to assess what patient has been told about illness. *This fosters consistent, collaborative approach to patient's care.*
• Listen to patient with nonjudgmental acceptance *to demonstrate positive regard for patient as person worthy of respect.*
• Help patient learn the stages of anticipatory grieving *to increase understanding and ability to cope.*
• Encourage patient to communicate with others, asking questions and clarifying concerns based on readiness. *Patient fixated in denial may isolate and withdraw from others.*
• Visit more frequently as patient begins to accept reality; alleviate fears when necessary. *This helps reduce patient's fear of being alone and fosters accurate reality testing.*

Evaluations for expected outcomes
• Patient describes present health problem.
• Patient describes life pattern and reports any recent changes.
• Patient communicates understanding of stages of grief.
• Patient demonstrates behavior appropriate to present phase of grieving process.
• When ready, patient discusses health problem with doctor, nurses, and family members.
• Patient displays increasing awareness of reality, either verbally or through behavior.

Documentation
• Patient's perception of health problem
• Mental status (baseline and ongoing)
• Patient's knowledge of grief process
• Patient's behavioral responses

• Interventions implemented to assist patient
• Patient's response to nursing interventions
• Evaluations for expected outcomes

■ Diarrhea
related to malabsorption, inflammation, or irritation of bowel

---

Definition
Interruption of normal elimination pattern characterized by frequent, loose stools

Assessment
• History of bowel disorder or surgery
• GI status, including nausea and vomiting, usual bowel elimination habits, change in bowel elimination habits, stool characteristics (color, amount, size, and consistency), pain, inspection of abdomen, auscultation of bowel sounds, palpation for masses and tenderness, percussion for tympany and dullness, laxative and enema use, medications (especially antibiotics), and results of stool culture, upper GI series, and barium enema
• Nutritional status, including dietary intake, change from normal diet, appetite, current weight, change from normal weight, food irritants and contaminants, and serum albumin levels
• Fluid and electrolyte status, including intake and output, urine specific gravity, skin turgor, mucous membranes, serum potassium and sodium levels, and blood urea nitrogen
• Psychosocial status, including personality, stressors (such as finances, job, marital discord, and disease process), coping mechanisms, support systems, lifestyle, and recent travel

Defining characteristics
- Abdominal pain and cramping
- At least three loose, liquid stools per day
- Hyperactive bowel sounds
- Urgency

Associated medical diagnoses (selected)
Accidental radiation exposure, bone marrow transplantation, chemotherapy, colon and rectal cancer, Crohn's disease, diverticulitis, food poisoning, pseudomembranous colitis, radiation therapy, salmonella, sepsis

Expected outcomes
- Patient will control diarrhea with medication.
- Patient's elimination pattern will return to normal.
- Patient will regain and maintain fluid and electrolyte balance.
- Patient's skin will remain intact.
- Patient will discuss causative factors, preventive measures, and changed body image.
- Patient will practice stress-reduction techniques daily.
- Patient will demonstrate skill in using ostomy devices.
- Patient will seek out persons with similar conditions or join a support group.

Interventions and rationales
- Monitor frequency and characteristics of stool; auscultate bowel sounds and record results at least every shift *to monitor treatment effectiveness.*
- Tell patient to notify staff of each episode of diarrhea *to promote comfort and maintain communication.*
- Give antidiarrheal medications, as ordered, *to improve bodily function, promote comfort, and balance body fluids, salts, and acid-base levels.* Monitor and report efficacy.
- Monitor and record patient's intake and output, including number of stools. Report imbalances. *Monitoring ensures correct fluid replacement therapy.*
- Check skin daily *to detect and prevent breakdown.* Report decreased skin turgor or excoriation of perianal area.
- Weigh patient daily until diarrhea is controlled *to detect fluid loss or retention.*
- Teach patient about:
  – causative and preventive factors *to promote understanding of problem.*
  – cleaning of perianal area, including use of powders and lotions, *to promote comfort and skin integrity.*
  – dietary restriction to control diarrhea, such as a lactose-free diet, *which reduces residual waste and decreases intestinal irritation and spasms.*
- Teach stress-reduction techniques, and help patient perform them daily by providing time, privacy, and needed equipment. *This temporarily relieves emotional distress.*
- Prepare patient for surgery and provide preoperative instruction for abdominal surgery *to reassure patient and maintain trust.* Provide information about ileostomy or colostomy, if indicated, *to help patient understand procedure and avoid threat to health equilibrium.*
- Demonstrate use of ostomy equipment *to encourage understanding and compliance.*
- Provide support and assistance while patient develops skill in caring for stoma *to improve understanding and reduce anxiety.*
- Encourage expression of feelings and concerns about impact of changed body image *to allow patient to pinpoint specific fears and promote self-knowledge and growth.*

• Encourage use of support groups, such as ileostomy clubs, *to provide patient with additional support and health care resources.*

Evaluations for expected outcomes
• Patient doesn't experience diarrhea.
• Patient's elimination pattern returns to normal.
• Patient maintains weight and fluid and electrolyte balance.
• Skin breakdown doesn't occur.
• Patient explains cause of diarrhea and steps to prevent recurrence.
• Patient demonstrates successful use of stress-reduction techniques.
• Patient demonstrates successful use of ostomy devices.
• Patient attends a support group for individuals with a similar condition.

Documentation
• Patient's expressions of concern about diarrhea, causative factors, surgery, and adaptation to changes in body image
• Observations of effects of medications, intake and output, weight, stool characteristics, skin condition, and stoma appearance
• Evaluations for expected outcomes

■ Diarrhea

related to stress and anxiety

Definition
Interruption of normal bowel movements resulting in frequent, loose stools

Assessment
• History of bowel disorder or surgery
• GI status, including nausea and vomiting, usual bowel elimination habits, change in bowel elimination habits, stool characteristics (color, amount, size, and consistency), pain and discomfort, inspection of abdomen, auscultation of bowel sounds, palpation for masses and tenderness, and percussion for tympany and dullness
• Nutritional status, including dietary intake, change from normal diet, appetite, current weight, and change from normal weight
• Fluid and electrolyte status, including intake and output, urine specific gravity, skin turgor, mucous membranes, serum potassium and sodium levels, and blood urea nitrogen
• Psychosocial status, including personality, stressors (such as finances, job, and marital discord), coping mechanisms, support systems (family members and others), and lifestyle

Defining characteristics
• Abdominal pain and cramping
• At least three loose, liquid stools per day
• Hyperactive bowel sounds
• Urgency

Associated medical diagnoses (selected)
Anxiety disorder, colitis

Expected outcomes
• Patient's diarrheal episodes will decline or disappear.
• Patient will resume usual bowel pattern.
• Patient will maintain weight and will regain and maintain fluid and electrolyte balance.
• Patient will keep skin clean and free of irritation or ulcerations.
• Patient will explain causative factors and preventive measures.
• Patient will discuss relationship of stress and anxiety to episodes of diarrhea.
• Patient will state plans to use stress-reduction techniques (specify).

• Patient will demonstrate ability to use at least one stress-reduction technique.

Interventions and rationales
• Monitor and record frequency and characteristics of stool *to monitor treatment effectiveness.* Instruct patient to record diarrheal episodes and report them to staff *to promote comfort and maintain effective patient-staff communication.*
• Administer antidiarrheal medications, as ordered, *to improve bodily function, promote comfort, and balance body fluids, salts, and acid-base levels.* Monitor and report medications' effectiveness.
• Provide replacement fluids and electrolytes, as prescribed. Maintain accurate records *to ensure balanced fluid intake and output.*
• Monitor perianal skin for irritation and ulceration; treat according to established protocol *to promote comfort, skin integrity, and freedom from infection.*
• Identify stressors and help patient solve problems *to provide more realistic approach to care.*
• Encourage patient to ventilate stresses and anxiety; *release of pent-up emotions can temporarily relieve emotional distress.*
• Teach patient to:
– use relaxation techniques *to reduce muscle tension and nervousness.*
– recognize and reduce intake of diarrhea-producing foods or substances (such as dairy products and fruit) *to reduce residual waste matter and decrease intestinal irritation.*
• Spend at least 10 minutes with patient twice daily to discuss stress-reducing techniques; *this can help patient pinpoint specific fears.*
• Encourage and assist patient to practice relaxation techniques *to reduce*

tension and promote self-knowledge and growth.

Evaluations for expected outcomes
• Episodes of diarrhea decline by at least 50%.
• Patient resumes usual bowel elimination pattern.
• Patient maintains weight and fluid and electrolyte balance.
• Patient doesn't experience skin breakdown, irritation, or ulcerations.
• Patient identifies cause of diarrhea and discusses steps to prevent recurrence.
• Patient explains how stress may contribute to diarrhea.
• Patient explains plan to use stress-reduction techniques.
• Patient describes and demonstrates stress-reduction techniques.

Documentation
• Patient's expressions of concern and ability to manage diarrhea produced by stress and anxiety
• Observations of effects of relaxation and stress-reduction techniques and dietary management on diarrhea
• Patient's responses and skill level in carrying out stress-reduction techniques and dietary changes
• Evaluations for expected outcomes

Disuse syndrome, risk for

Definition
State of being at risk for deterioration of body systems as a result of prescribed or unavoidable inactivity

Assessment
• Condition leading to prolonged inactivity or immobility
• Age

• Neurologic status, including mental status, level of consciousness (LOC), and sensory and motor ability
• Cardiovascular status, including blood pressure, heart rate, temperature, peripheral pulses, capillary refill, clotting profile, skin temperature and color, presence of edema, and chest pain or discomfort
• Respiratory status, including rate and rhythm, depth of inspiration, chest symmetry, use of accessory muscles, cough and sputum, percussion of lung fields, auscultation of breath sounds, chest pain or discomfort, and arterial blood gas (ABG) levels
• GI status, including inspection of abdomen, auscultation of bowel sounds, palpation for tenderness and masses, percussion for areas of dullness, usual bowel habits, change in bowel habits, laxative use, pain or discomfort, and characteristics of stool (color, size, amount, and consistency)
• Nutritional status, including dietary intake, appetite, current weight, and change from normal weight
• Fluid status, including intake and output, urine specific gravity, mucous membranes, serum electrolyte levels, blood urea nitrogen, and creatinine level
• Genitourinary status, including voiding pattern, characteristics of urine (color, odor, sediment, and amount), history of urinary problems or infections, palpation of bladder, pain or discomfort, use of urinary assistive device, urinalysis, and urine cultures
• Musculoskeletal status, including range of motion; muscle size, strength, and tone; coordination; and functional mobility scale:
0 = completely independent

1 = requires use of equipment or device
2 = requires help, supervision, or teaching from another person
3 = requires help from another person and equipment or device
4 = dependent; doesn't participate in activity
• Integumentary status, including color, texture, turgor, temperature, elasticity, sensation, moisture, hygiene, and lesions
• Psychosocial factors, including family support, coping style, current understanding of prescribed inactivity, willingness to cooperate with treatment, mood, behavior, motivation, and stressors (such as inactivity, finances, job, and marital discord)

Risk factors
• Altered LOC
• Mechanical immobilization
• Paralysis
• Prescribed immobilization
• Severe pain

Associated medical diagnoses (selected)
Cerebrovascular accident; dermatomyositis and polymyositis; end-stage cardiac, pulmonary, or renal disease; fractures; head injury; neuromuscular trauma; rheumatoid arthritis; spinal cord injury

Expected outcomes
• Patient will display no evidence of altered mental, sensory, or motor ability.
• Patient will have no evidence of thrombus formation, venous stasis, or altered cardiovascular function.
• Patient will show no evidence of decreased chest movement, cough stimulus, or depth of ventilation.
• Patient will show no pooling of secretions or signs of infection.

• Patient will have no evidence of constipation and will maintain normal bowel elimination patterns.

• Patient will maintain adequate dietary intake, hydration, and weight.

• Patient will show no evidence of urine retention, infection, or renal calculi.

• Patient will maintain muscle strength and tone and joint range of motion.

• Patient will show no evidence of contractures.

• Patient will show no evidence of skin breakdown.

• Patient will maintain normal neurologic, cardiovascular, respiratory, GI, nutritional, genitourinary, musculoskeletal, and integumentary functioning during period of inactivity.

• Patient will express feelings about prolonged inactivity.

Interventions and rationales

• Provide frequent contact with staff, diversionary materials (magazines, radio, and television), and orienting mechanisms (clock and calendar). *Reality orientation fosters patient awareness of environment.*

• Avoid positions that put prolonged pressure on body parts and compress blood vessels. Patient should change positions at least every 2 hours within prescribed limits. *These measures enhance circulation and avoid tissue or skin breakdown.*

• Inspect skin every shift and protect areas subject to irritation. Follow facility policy for prevention of pressure ulcers *to prevent or mitigate skin breakdown.*

• Use pressure-reducing or pressure-equalizing equipment as indicated or ordered (flotation pad, air pressure mattress, sheepskin pads, or special bed). *This helps prevent skin breakdown by relieving pressure.*

• Apply antiembolism stockings; remove for 1 hour every 8 hours. *Stockings promote venous return to heart, prevent venous stasis, and decrease or prevent swelling of lower extremities.*

• Monitor clotting profile. Administer and monitor anticoagulant therapy, if ordered, and monitor for signs and symptoms of bleeding *because anticoagulant therapy may cause hemorrhage.*

• Monitor temperature, blood pressure, pulse, and respirations at least every 4 hours *to assess for indications of infection or other complications.*

• Teach and monitor deep breathing, coughing, and use of incentive spirometer. Maintain regimen every 2 hours. *These measures help clear airways, expand lungs, and prevent respiratory complications.*

• Encourage fluid intake of 2,500 to 3,500 ml daily, unless contraindicated, *to maintain urine output and aid bowel elimination.* Weigh daily and monitor hydration status (serum electrolytes, blood urea nitrogen, creatinine, and intake and output).

• Monitor breath sounds and respiratory rate, rhythm, and depth at least every 4 hours *to rule out respiratory complications.* Monitor ABG levels or pulse oximetry, if indicated, *to assess oxygenation, ventilation, and metabolic status.*

• Suction airway as needed and ordered *to clear airway and stimulate cough reflex;* note secretion characteristics.

• Establish baseline *to compare elimination patterns and habits.* Elevate head of bed and provide privacy *to allow comfortable elimination.*

• Instruct patient to avoid straining during bowel movements; administer stool softeners, suppositories, or laxatives as ordered, and monitor effec-

tiveness. *Straining during bowel movements may be hazardous to patients with cardiovascular disorders and increased intracranial pressure.*
• Provide small, frequent meals of favorite foods *to increase dietary intake.* Increase fiber content *to enhance bowel elimination.* Increase protein and vitamin C *to promote wound healing.* Limit calcium *to reduce risk of renal and bladder calculi.*
• Monitor urine characteristics and patient's subjective complaints typical of urinary tract infection (burning, frequency, and urgency). Obtain urine cultures as ordered. *These measures aid early detection of urinary tract infection.*
• Identify level of functioning *to provide baseline for future assessment,* and encourage appropriate participation in care *to prevent complications of immobility and increase patient's feelings of self-esteem.*
• Perform active or passive range-of-motion exercises at least once per shift. Teach and monitor appropriate isotonic and isometric exercises. *These measures prevent joint contractures, muscular atrophy, and other complications of prolonged inactivity.*
• Provide or help with daily hygiene; keep skin dry and lubricated *to prevent cracking and possible infection.*
• Encourage patient and family to ventilate frustration. Allow open expression of all feelings associated with prolonged inactivity. *Open expression of feelings helps patient and family cope with treatment.*

Evaluations for expected outcomes
• Patient doesn't exhibit altered LOC, mental status, sensory ability, or motor ability.

• Patient doesn't exhibit evidence of thrombus formation, venous stasis, or altered cardiovascular function.
• Patient shows no evidence of decreased chest movement, cough stimulus, or depth of ventilation.
• Patient maintains clear breath sounds bilaterally and doesn't show evidence of fever, chills, cough, purulent sputum, pooled secretions, or rapid, shallow respirations.
• Patient's bowel elimination pattern remains normal.
• Patient maintains adequate dietary intake, daily fluid intake, and weight.
• Patient doesn't exhibit evidence of distended bladder, fever, chills, frequent burning or painful urination, urgency, hematuria, flank pain, or urine retention.
• Patient's muscle strength and tone and joint range of motion remain stable.
• Patient doesn't exhibit evidence of joint contractures.
• Patient doesn't experience skin breakdown.
• Patient maintains neurologic, cardiovascular, respiratory, GI, nutritional, genitourinary, musculoskeletal, and integumentary functioning.
• Patient openly expresses frustration, anger, despondency, and other feelings associated with prolonged inactivity.

Documentation
• Patient's concerns or perceptions of circumstances necessitating inactivity; willingness to accept and participate in treatment
• Assessment of body systems at risk for deterioration
• Interventions to provide preventive or supportive care and prescribed treatment

• Treatment given to patient and patient's understanding and demonstrated ability to carry out instructions
• Patient's response to nursing interventions
• Evaluations for expected outcomes

■ Diversional activity deficit

related to lack of environmental stimulation

Definition
Restriction or decline in ability to use unoccupied time to patient's advantage or satisfaction

Assessment
• Physical status, including mobility and activity tolerance
• Cardiovascular status
• Respiratory status
• Neurologic status, including level of consciousness, orientation, mood, behavior, and memory
• Psychosocial status, including family or friends, hobbies, interests, favorite music, television, reading matter, and changes or adaptations needed to carry out activities

Defining characteristics
• Physical or environmental limitations affecting participation in usual activities
• Statements of boredom or wishing for something to do

Associated medical diagnoses (selected)
Blindness, depression, endocarditis, fractures, or any condition requiring isolation, intensive care, or prolonged hospitalization

Expected outcomes
• Patient will express interest in using leisure time meaningfully.
• Patient will express interest in activities provided.
• Patient will participate in chosen activity.
• Patient will watch selected television program or listen to radio program or selected music daily.
• Patient will report satisfaction with use of leisure time.
• Patient or caregiver will modify environment to provide maximum stimulation, such as by hanging posters or cards and moving bed next to a window.

Interventions and rationales
• Encourage discussion of previously enjoyed hobbies, interests, or skills *to direct planning of new activities.* Suggest performing an activity helpful to others or otherwise productive.
• Obtain radio or television (if desired) and allow patient to select programs. Communicate patient's desires to coworkers. Turn on television set at _____ (time) to _____ (channel). *Selective television or radio use can help pass time.*
• Ask volunteers (friends, family, or hospital volunteer) to read newspapers, books, or magazines to patient at specific times. *Personal contact helps alleviate boredom.*
• Engage patient in conversation while carrying out routine care. Discuss patient's favorite topics as much as possible. *Conversation conveys caring and recognition of patient's worth.*
• Provide supplies and set time to carry out hobby; for example, give crochet hook and yarn to patient daily at _____ (time). *Specifying time for activity indicates its value.*

• Avoid scheduling procedures during patient's leisure time, *which is integral to quality of life.*
• Provide talking books or records if available. *These provide low-effort sources of enjoyment for bedridden patient.*
• Obtain an adapter for television *to provide captions for hearing-impaired patient.*
• Encourage patient's family or caregiver to bring in personal articles (posters, cards, and pictures) to help make environment more stimulating. *Patient may respond better to objects with personal meaning.*
• Make referral to recreational, occupational, or physical therapist for consultation on adaptive equipment to carry out desired activity; arrange for therapy sessions. *Adaptive equipment allows patient to continue enjoying activities or may stimulate interest in new activities.*
• Provide plants for patient to tend. *Caring for live plants may stimulate interest.*
• Change scenery when possible; for example, place patient's bed in hall for short period or take patient outside in wheelchair *to help reduce boredom.*
• Identify type of music patient prefers; get help from family and hospital resources to provide selected music daily. *Music may relieve boredom.*

Evaluations for expected outcomes
• Patient expresses desire to participate in activities during leisure time.
• Patient discusses recent activity with staff members, family, or others.
• Patient engages in activity.
• Patient discusses content of television or radio program.
• Patient reports reduced feelings of boredom.

• Environment is modified to increase patient stimulation.

Documentation
• Patient's expression of boredom, frustration, and desire to carry out leisure activity
• Patient's interests and ability to carry out activity and necessary modifications required to accomplish activity
• Observations of patient's skill level and extent of participation in activity
• Patient's expression of satisfaction with use of unoccupied time
• Evaluations for expected outcomes

■ Diversional activity deficit

related to long-term hospitalization or frequent, lengthy treatments

Definition
Restriction or decrease in ability to use unoccupied time to one's advantage or satisfaction

Assessment
• Physical status, including mobility and activity tolerance
• Cardiovascular status
• Respiratory status
• Neurologic status, including level of consciousness, orientation, mood, behavior, and memory
• Psychosocial status, including family, hobbies, interests, favorite music, television, reading matter, and changes or adaptations needed to carry out activities

Defining characteristics
• Physical or environmental limitations affecting participation in usual activities

• Statements of boredom or wishing for something to do

Associated medical diagnoses (selected)

Burns, cystic fibrosis, long-term disability, peripheral vascular disease, spinal cord injury, or any condition requiring prolonged hospitalization

Expected outcomes

• Patient will express interest in using leisure time meaningfully.
• Patient will participate in chosen activity.
• Patient will state satisfaction with use of leisure time.
• Patient will express interest in activities provided.
• Patient will make decisions about timing and spacing of treatments.
• Patient will express satisfaction with established schedule of treatment routines.

Interventions and rationales

• Schedule time daily to pursue leisure activities; for example, have patient sit at desk daily in wheelchair to use paint-by-number kit. *Diversional activities improve patient's quality of life; scheduling activities indicates their value.*
• Encourage family members to bring in familiar objects. Provide space for favorite plants, cards, reading material, and hobby supplies. For bedridden patients, use ceiling for posters and other objects. *Maintaining personal contacts and involvement relieves boredom and stimulates interest.*
• Encourage patient to express enjoyment of past hobbies, interests, or skills. *This conveys a sense of worth and caring and helps patient to think of new activities.*
• Work with patient and family to find ways to carry out desired activities. Use imagination and creativity; for

example, a former carpenter may adapt to carving small objects rather than building large ones. *Adaptive equipment helps patient pursue previous activities within new limits.*
• Provide radio or television at patient's request *to help relieve boredom and increase enjoyment.*
• Engage patient in conversation while carrying out procedures, if desired by patient. Discuss favorite topics. *Conversation during treatments reduces discomfort by diverting attention; it also increases patient's sense of self-worth.*
• Encourage visitors to involve patient in favorite activities through discussion, reading, and attendance at programs, if appropriate, *to reduce boredom.*
• Keep patient informed of current events through discussion; encourage patient to read newspapers or books and watch television or listen to radio. *Keeping current helps reduce the isolation of long-term hospitalization.*
• Schedule treatments to allow adequate rest periods and pursuit of favorite activity; for example, no treatments between _____ and _____ (time), to allow time for watching television show. *This gives patient more control over environment.*
• Streamline treatments as much as possible. Have all equipment ready before starting; thoroughly instruct new personnel in routine and plan schedule for minimal interruptions. *Efficiency conveys respect for value of patient's time.*

Evaluations for expected outcomes

• Patient expresses desire to participate in activity during leisure hours.
• Patient engages in chosen activity.
• Patient reports decrease in feelings of boredom.

• Patient discusses recent activity with staff members, family, or others.
• Patient makes decisions about timing and spacing of treatments.
• Patient expresses a positive attitude about the treatment schedule.

Documentation
• Patient's expressions of boredom, desire to carry out leisure activity, and frustration at being restricted
• Patient's interests, skills, and abilities to carry out activity
• Observations of patient's skill level and extent of participation in activity
• Patient's expression of satisfaction with use of non-treatment-related time
• Evaluations for expected outcomes

■ Dysreflexia

related to spinal cord trauma

Definition
State in which a patient with spinal cord injury at T7 or above experiences or risks life-threatening, uninhibited sympathetic response to a noxious stimulus

Assessment
• History of spinal cord trauma, including level of injury or lesion, and previous episodes of dysreflexia
• Patient's description of symptoms, including headache, nasal congestion, blurred vision, chest pain, diaphoresis and flushing above level of lesion, chilling, paresthesia, cutis anserina ("goose flesh") above level of lesion, metallic taste, and nausea
• Neurologic status, including level of consciousness, orientation, pupillary response, sensory status, and motor status

• Cardiovascular status, including blood pressure, heart rate and rhythm, and skin temperature and color
• Genitourinary status, including urine output, palpation of bladder, signs of urinary tract infection, and examination of urinary assistive devices such as catheter
• GI status, including nausea and vomiting, usual bowel elimination pattern, last bowel movement, inspection of abdomen, auscultation of bowel sounds, palpation for masses, and percussion for areas of dullness
• Environmental conditions, including changes in temperature (for example, cold draft) and objects putting pressure on skin

Defining characteristics
• Paroxysmal hypertension (sudden periodic elevated blood pressure, systolic over 140 mm Hg and diastolic over 90 mm Hg); bradycardia or tachycardia (pulse under 60 or over 100 beats/minute); diaphoresis above injury; red splotches (vasodilation) on skin above injury; pallor below injury; or diffuse headache not confined to any nerve distribution area
• Chilling, conjunctival congestion, Horner's syndrome (contracted pupils, partial ptosis, enophthalmos, sometimes loss of sweating on affected side of face), paresthesia, pilomotor reflex, blurred vision, chest pain, metallic taste, or nasal congestion

Associated medical diagnoses (selected)
Spinal cord injury or tumor above T7 level

Expected outcomes
• Cause of dysreflexia will be identified and corrected.
• Patient will experience cardiovascular stability as evidenced by _____ sys-

tolic range, _____ diastolic range, and _____ heart rate range.

• Patient will avoid bladder distention and urinary tract infection.

• Patient will have no fecal impaction.

• Patient's environment will have no noxious stimuli.

• Patient will state relief from symptoms of dysreflexia.

• Patient will have few if any complications.

• Patient's bladder elimination pattern will remain normal.

• Patient's bowel elimination pattern will remain normal.

• Patient, family members, or caregiver will demonstrate knowledge and understanding of dysreflexia and will describe care measures.

• Patient will experience few if any dysreflexic episodes.

Interventions and rationales

• Assess for signs of dysreflexia (especially severe hypertension) *to detect condition promptly.*

• Place patient in sitting position or elevate head of bed *to aid venous drainage from brain, lower intracranial pressure, and temporarily reduce blood pressure.*

• Ascertain and correct probable cause of dysreflexia:

– Check for bladder distention and patency of catheter. If necessary, irrigate catheter with small amount of solution or insert a new catheter immediately. *A blocked urinary catheter can trigger dysreflexia.*

– Check for fecal mass in rectum. Apply dibucaine ointment (Nupercainal) or another product, as ordered, to anus and 1″ (2.5 cm) into rectum 10 to 15 minutes before removing impaction. *Failure to use ointment may aggravate autonomic response.*

– Check environment for cold drafts and objects putting pressure on pa-

tient's skin, *which could act as dysreflexia stimuli.*

– Send urine for culture if no other cause becomes apparent *to detect possible urinary tract infection.*

• If hypertension persists despite other measures, administer ganglionic blocking agent, vasodilator, or other medication as ordered. *Drugs may be required if hypertension persists or if noxious stimuli can't be removed.*

• Take vital signs frequently *to monitor effectiveness of prescribed medications.*

• Instruct patient, family members, or caregiver about dysreflexia, its causes, signs and symptoms, and care measures *to prepare them to handle possible dysreflexic emergencies.*

• Implement and maintain bowel and bladder elimination programs *to avoid stimuli that could trigger dysreflexia.*

Evaluations for expected outcomes

• Cause of dysreflexia is identified and corrected.

• Patient experiences cardiovascular stability as evidenced by ___ systolic range, _____ diastolic range, and ___ heart rate range.

• Palpation doesn't reveal a distended bladder or signs of urinary tract infection.

• Patient's bowel elimination program is successfully implemented and maintained. Fecal impaction is absent.

• Patient's environment remains free of noxious stimuli.

• Patient expresses relief from signs and symptoms of dysreflexia.

• Patient doesn't experience complications of dysreflexia, including contractures, venous stasis, thrombus formation, skin breakdown, and hypostatic pneumonia.

• Patient's bladder elimination program is successfully implemented and maintained, urinary catheter is patent and without kinking or blockage, and urine output remains within specified volume.

• Patient's bowel elimination pattern remains normal.

• Patient, family members, or caregiver expresses understanding of causes, signs and symptoms, and treatment of autonomic dysreflexia and demonstrate measures to implement if dysreflexia occurs.

• Because of successful maintenance of bladder and bowel elimination programs, preventive skin care measures, and patient and family teaching, patient experiences few or no dysreflexic episodes.

Documentation

• Objective assessment of dysreflexic episode

• Patient's description of dysreflexic episode

• Interventions to identify and eliminate causes of dysreflexia and patient's response to these

• Instructions given to patient, family, and caregiver

• Patient's expressions of understanding and demonstrated ability to prevent or manage dysreflexic episode

• Implementation, alteration, or continuation of bladder and bowel programs

• Evaluations for expected outcomes

Dysreflexia, risk for autonomic

Definition

Presence of risk factors, such as spinal cord trauma and spinal cord tumor, that can lead to uninhibited, *life-threatening response to a noxious stimulus*

Assessment

• History of spinal cord trauma or spinal cord tumor, including level of injury or lesion; previous episodes of dysreflexia

• Neurologic status, including level of consciousness, orientation, pupillary response, sensory status, and motor status

• Cardiovascular status, including blood pressure, heart rate and rhythm, and skin temperature and color

• Genitourinary status, including urine output, palpation of bladder, signs of urinary tract infection, and urinary assistive devices such as catheter

• GI status, including nausea and vomiting, usual bowel pattern, bowel habits, last bowel movement, inspection of abdomen, auscultation of bowel sounds, palpation for masses and tenderness, and percussion for areas of tympany and dullness

• Environmental conditions, including changes in temperature (for example, cold drafts) and objects putting pressure on skin

Risk factors

• Constipation or fecal impaction

• Noxious environmental stimuli, including changes in temperature or objects putting pressure on skin

• Spinal cord trauma or spinal cord tumor

• Urinary tract infection, bladder distention, or urinary catheter blockage

Associated medical diagnoses (selected)

Spinal cord injury or tumor above the T6 vertebra level

Expected outcomes
• Risk factors for dysreflexia will be identified and reduced.
• Patient will avoid bladder distention.
• Urinary tract infection will be absent.
• Patient will maintain normal urinary and bowel elimination patterns.
• Patient will be free from fecal impaction.
• Patient's environment will be free from noxious stimuli that may cause dysreflexia.
• Patient, family member, or caregiver will express understanding of the causes of dysreflexia.
• Patient, family member, or caregiver will demonstrate understanding of measures to prevent dysreflexia.

Interventions and rationales
• Assess for risk factors of dysreflexia, such as constipation, fecal impaction, distended bladder, and presence of noxious stimuli. *Identifying risk factors can prevent or minimize dysreflexic episodes.*
• Monitor and record intake and output accurately *to ensure adequate fluid replacement, thereby helping to prevent constipation.*
• Check for bladder distention and patency of catheter. *A blocked catheter can trigger dysreflexia.*
• Check for abdominal distention. Assess bowel sounds. Monitor and record characteristics and frequency of stool. *Fecal impaction may lead to dysreflexia.*
• Encourage fluid intake of 2.5 L (2½ qt) daily, unless contraindicated. *Adequate fluid intake helps maintain patency of catheter and aids bowel elimination.*
• Administer laxative, enema, or suppositories, as prescribed, *to promote elimination of solids and gases from GI tract.* Monitor effectiveness.

• Consult with dietitian about increasing fiber and bulk in diet to maximum prescribed by doctor *to improve intestinal muscle tone and promote comfortable elimination.*
• Implement and maintain bowel and bladder programs *to avoid stimuli that could trigger dysreflexia.*
• Monitor vital signs frequently *to ensure effectiveness of preventive measures. Severe hypertension may indicate dysreflexia.*
• Instruct patient, family member, or caregiver about risk factors, signs and symptoms, and care measures for dysreflexia *to help prevent a possible dysreflexic episode and help him respond appropriately should dysreflexia occur.*

Evaluations for expected outcomes
• Risk factors for dysreflexia are identified and reduced.
• Patient avoids bladder distention.
• Urinary tract infection is absent.
• Patient maintains normal urinary and bowel elimination patterns.
• Patient is free from fecal impaction.
• Patient's environment is free from noxious stimuli that may cause dysreflexia.
• Patient, family member, or caregiver expresses understanding of the causes of dysreflexia.
• Patient, family member, or caregiver demonstrates understanding of measures to prevent dysreflexia.

Documentation
• Presence of risk factors of dysreflexia
• Interventions to minimize risk of dysreflexia and patient's response
• Patient's, family members', or caregiver's expressions of concern about the risk for dysreflexia

• Instructions given to patient, family member, or caregiver regarding prevention of dysreflexic episodes
• Implementation or alteration of bowel and bladder program
• Evaluations for expected outcomes

■ Energy field disturbance

Definition
Disharmony in a person's inner sense of well-being that results in physical, emotional, or spiritual distress

Assessment
• Psychological status, including anxiety, fatigue, depression, somatic complaints, and recent lifestyle changes (death of loved one, conflict in a relationship, or loss of job)
• Health status, including presence of disorder that is life-threatening or requires surgery
• Sensory status, including pain and disorders that may affect senses
• Spiritual status, including religious beliefs and affiliation; support system; helplessness, hopelessness, anger, and withdrawal
• Caregiver's readiness to provide therapeutic healing, including education and training in therapeutic touch or similar treatment technique

Defining characteristics
• Disruption of field (vacant, hold, spike, bulge)
• Movement (wave, spike, tingling, dense, flowing)
• Sounds (tone, words)
• Temperature change (warmth, coolness)
• Visual changes (image, color)

Associated medical diagnoses (selected)
Amputation, cancer, infection, trauma, any illness that is life-threatening or requires surgery

Expected outcomes
• Patient will feel increasingly relaxed, as demonstrated by slower and deeper breathing, skin flushing in treated area, audible sighing, or reports of feeling more relaxed.
• Patient will visualize images that relax him.
• Patient will report feeling less tension or pain.
• Patient will use self-healing techniques, such as meditation, guided imagery, yoga, and prayer.
• Patient will express increased sense of well-being.

Interventions and rationales
• Implement measures to promote therapeutic healing. Place your hands 4″ to 6″ (10 to 15 cm) above patient's body. Pass your hands over entire skin surface. *This technique helps you become attuned to patient's energy field, which is the flow of energy that surrounds a person's being.* With experience and training in therapeutic touch or similar treatment, a practitioner can identify sensory cues to energy field disturbances, such as heat, cold, tingling, and an electric sensation.
• Try to gain patient's cooperation as you perform healing techniques such as therapeutic touch *to enhance effectiveness of healing techniques and foster participation in spiritual aspects of care.*
• Continue to treat patient using therapeutic healing techniques. *One treatment rarely restores a full sense of inner well-being.*
• Suggest that patient use self-healing techniques, such as meditation, guid-

ed imagery, yoga, and prayer, *to encourage patient to participate in his care.*

Evaluations for expected outcomes
• Patient shows evidence of relaxation, such as slower and deeper breathing.
• Patient reports experiencing relaxing visual images.
• Patient reports reduction in tension or pain.
• Patient uses self-healing techniques, such as meditation, guided imagery, yoga, and exercise.
• Patient reports an increased sense of well-being.

Documentation
• Summary of patient's psychosocial status
• Patient's progress in learning techniques that enhance relaxation
• Patient's perceptions of benefits of healing and self-healing techniques
• Evaluations for expected outcomes

■ Environmental interpretation syndrome, impaired

Definition
Consistent lack of orientation to person, place, time, or circumstances that lasts for more than 6 months and necessitates placement in a protective environment

Assessment
• Cultural status, including age, sex, level of education, occupation, living arrangements, nationality, race, ethnic group, religion, and personal habits
• Family status, including marital status, family composition, and family

members' ability to meet patient's needs
• Cardiovascular status, including vital signs; skin color (especially lips and nails); chest pain, fatigue on exertion, dyspnea, and dizziness; and electrocardiography or echocardiography results
• Neurologic status, including level of consciousness (LOC), motor activity, thought and speech, mood and affect, memory, attention span, judgment, orientation, comprehension, and perception; cerebellar function, cranial nerve function, sensation, reflexes, and pupillary response; and medications
• Psychological status, including changes in appearance, appetite, energy level, motivation, personal hygiene, self-image, self-esteem, sleep patterns, or LOC; alcohol and drug use; and life changes (recent divorce, separation, job loss, loss of a loved one, or relocation)
• Psychiatric history, including age at onset of illness, severity of symptoms, impact on functioning, and type of treatment and response
• Self-care status, including functional ability (muscle tone, size, and strength; range of motion; and coordination); daily activities (dressing, grooming, bathing, toileting, and hygiene); and use of adaptive equipment
• Social status, including interaction with others and ability to function in social or occupational roles
• Sensory status, including presence of visual or hearing deficits and use of hearing aid or eyeglasses

Defining characteristics
• Consistent disorientation to environment
• Chronic confusion

• Inability to reason, concentrate, or follow simple directions or instructions
• Loss of occupation or social function resulting from memory decline
• Slow response to questions

Associated medical diagnoses (selected)

Acquired immunodeficiency syndrome, Alzheimer's disease, angina, atherosclerosis, brain tumor, cerebral aneurysm, cerebrovascular accident, dementia, epilepsy, head trauma, human immunodeficiency virus infection, hypertension, multiple sclerosis, organic brain disorders, substance abuse, transient ischemic attacks

Expected outcomes

• Staff members will communicate clear, concise goals for coping with disorientation to patient and caregiver.
• Patient will acknowledge and respond to efforts by others to establish communication.
• Patient will remain oriented to environment to fullest extent possible.
• Family members will participate in efforts to help patient cope with disorientation.
• Patient will remain free from injury.
• Caregiver will describe measures for helping patient cope with disorientation.
• Caregiver will demonstrate reorientation techniques.
• Caregiver will describe ways to ensure that home is made safe for patient.
• Caregiver will describe plans to continue to help patient cope with disorientation in the least restrictive way possible.
• Caregiver, in cooperation with patient, will identify and contact appropriate support services.

Interventions and rationales

• Spend time with patient and caregiver *to establish a trusting relationship.*
• Be clear, concise, and direct in establishing goals and skills for coping with disorientation *so patient and caregiver can understand them.*
• Consider performing the following interventions:
– Assess patient's sight and hearing, and assist him with glasses or a hearing aid as necessary.
– Minimize distractions by turning off radios or television.
– When speaking to patient, face him, maintain eye contact, and smile.
– Speak slowly in clear, low tones, using simple, direct language. Repeat your remarks as needed.
– Be aware that patient may be sensitive to your unspoken feelings about him.
These measures will help foster communication with patient. Successful communication is necessary to implement interventions.
• Orient patient to reality as needed *to improve his awareness of himself and his environment:*
– Call him by name.
– Tell him your name.
– Provide background information (place, time, and date) frequently throughout the day. Reinforce this information verbally and by using a reality orientation board.
– Orient him to his environment.
• Place patient's photograph or name on room door *to aid memory and help him find his room.*
• Keep items in the same places. *A consistent, stable environment reduces confusion, decreases frustration, and aids successful completion of activities of daily living.*
• Ask family members to provide patient with photographs (labeled with

the name and relationship on the back) and favorite belongings. *Belongings may spark his memory and promote a sense of security.*
• Have someone accompany a patient who wanders *to prevent patient injury.*
• Place patient in a room close to nursing station, clear the area of as many hazards as possible, make sure he wears an identification bracelet, and provide hospital security with a recent photograph of him *to prevent patient from getting lost or being injured.*
• Encourage patient to interact with others *to increase social activity and ease isolation that may result from disorientation.*
• Provide reassurance, and praise patient for completing simple tasks *to increase patient's self-esteem.*
• Help patient and caregiver identify feelings associated with disorientation *to help improve their ability to cope.*
• Work with patient and caregiver to establish goals for coping with disorientation in the least restrictive way *to maximize independence and reduce feelings of loneliness.*
• Demonstrate reorientation techniques to caregiver and provide time for supervised return demonstrations *to prepare the caregiver to cope with patient when he returns home.*
• Instruct caregiver on how to maintain a safe home environment for patient. *Patient may be unable to consider his own safety needs.*
• Refer patient and caregiver to appropriate social service and mental health care agencies *to ensure continued care.*

Evaluations for expected outcomes
• Staff members communicate clear, concise goals for coping with disorientation to patient and caregiver.

• Patient acknowledges and responds to efforts by others to establish communication.
• Patient remains oriented to environment to fullest extent possible.
• Family members participate in efforts to help patient cope with disorientation.
• Patient remains free from injury.
• Caregiver describes measures for helping patient cope with disorientation.
• Caregiver demonstrates reorientation techniques.
• Caregiver describes measures to improve safety of home for patient.
• Caregiver describes plans to help patient cope with disorientation in least restrictive way possible.
• Caregiver identifies and contacts appropriate support services.

Documentation
• Assessment of patient's level of orientation
• Assessment of patient's response to various interventions
• Instructions to caregiver on how to reorient patient and how to maintain a safe home environment
• Referrals to community agencies
• Evaluations for expected outcomes

■ Family process alteration

related to situational crisis

Definition
Disruption in expected role functions within the family structure because of such situational crises as protracted physical or emotional illness

Assessment
• Family status, including normal patterns of interaction among family members, family members' and patient's understanding of present situation, and support systems available (financial, social, and spiritual)
• Family's past response to crises, including coping patterns and communication patterns to express anger, affection, and confrontation

Defining characteristics
Changes in the following:
• assigned tasks and effectiveness in completing those tasks
• availability for affective responsiveness and intimacy
• availability for emotional support
• communications patterns
• expressions of conflict with or isolation from community resources
• expressions of conflict within family
• mutual support
• participation in problem solving and decision making
• patterns and rituals
• power alliances
• satisfaction with family
• somatic complaints
• stress-reduction behaviors

Associated medical diagnoses (selected)
Any disease or illness that results in long-term disability or incapacitation, including acute renal failure, Alzheimer's disease, anorexia nervosa, bulimia nervosa, cerebrovascular accident, chronic renal failure, congenital heart disease, degenerative disease, dementia, Down syndrome, hemodialysis, hydrocephalus, incest, kidney transplantation, peritoneal dialysis, and polycystic kidney disease

Expected outcomes
• Family members will agree on who is the primary decision maker.

• Family members will develop adaptive responses by assuming duties carried out by the ill member; for example, meal preparation, transportation, shopping, laundry, cleaning, and providing emotional support to other family members.
• Family members will identify support systems to assist them and will participate in mobilizing those systems.
• Family members will contact a community agency or support group for continued assistance (depending on the type, severity, and prognosis of illness); for example, American Cancer Society, American Lung Association, Arthritis Foundation, Hospice, Myasthenia Gravis Foundation, Multiple Sclerosis Society, or National Kidney Foundation.
• Family members will share feelings about illness in the family.

Interventions and rationales
• Identify individual assuming role as head of family *to establish family hierarchy and functional ability.*
• Provide head of family with information necessary for decision making, such as updated information on patient's condition. *This avoids potential for misinterpretation and places responsibility for communication within family unit.*
• Help head of family decide which support systems need to be mobilized and used. *This allows opportunity to evaluate head of family's management ability and family's problem-solving ability.*
• Provide emotional support to head of family regarding altered role and additional responsibilities. *This encourages family member to ventilate feelings, ask questions, seek help, and make decisions.*

• Expedite communication within family *to allow members to express their feelings about present situation. This encourages supportive behavior to meet reciprocal needs in a crisis.*
• Arrange for and participate in family conferences, if appropriate.
– Whenever possible, ensure privacy to family members for their discussions or conferences.
– Include patient in family conferences and family interaction as often as possible.
These measures allow you to help family identify and work toward mutual goals and facilitate effective family coping.
• Make referrals to social services or community agencies, as appropriate, *to provide family with access to additional coping resources.*

Evaluations for expected outcomes
• Family members identify individual to take on responsibilities of head of family.
• Family members assume responsibilities formerly carried out by ill member.
• Family members identify and contact available resources as needed.
• Family members contact community support groups and associations and attend at least two meetings.
• Family members openly share feelings about present situation.

Documentation
• Observations of family's reactions to situation
• Interventions to assist family and family's responses to those interventions
• Referrals to outside agencies
• Evaluations for expected outcomes

Fatigue

Definition
Overwhelming sense of exhaustion and decreased capacity for physical and mental work, regardless of adequate sleep

Assessment
• History of underlying disease process
• Respiratory status, including dyspnea on exertion and respiratory rate and depth
• Cardiovascular status, including skin color, temperature, turgor, and blood pressure
• Age
• Sleep pattern, including hours slept at night and amount of time awake before becoming tired
• Nutritional status, including appetite, dietary intake, current weight, and change from normal weight
• Neurologic status, including headaches
• Activity status, including type and duration of exercise, occupation, and use of leisure time
• Psychosocial status, including personality stressors (finances, job, and marital discord), coping mechanisms, support systems (family members and others), and lifestyle
• Menstrual history, including length of periods and amount of menstrual flow

Defining characteristics
• Decreased libido
• Decreased performance
• Disinterest in surroundings
• Drowsiness
• Failure of sleep to restore energy
• Lack of energy
• Guilt for not meeting responsibilities

• Inability to maintain usual routines
• Impaired concentration
• Increased need for rest
• Increased physical complaints
• Lethargy or listlessness
• Perceived need for more energy for routine tasks
• Verbalization of overwhelming lack of energy

Associated medical diagnoses (selected)
Accidental radiation exposure, anemias, cerebrovascular accident, cervical cancer, chronic bronchitis, chronic fatigue syndrome, chronic obstructive pulmonary disease, cor pulmonale, depression, emphysema, esophageal cancer, Guillain-Barré syndrome, heart failure, Lyme disease, melanoma, mitral insufficiency, mitral stenosis, mitral valve prolapse, multiple myeloma, multiple sclerosis, myasthenia gravis, pleurisy, rheumatic fever, thoracic surgery, tuberculosis

Expected outcomes
• Patient will identify measures to prevent or modify fatigue.
• Patient will incorporate as part of daily activities those measures necessary to modify fatigue.
• Patient will explain relationship of fatigue to disease process and activity level.
• Patient will verbally express increased energy.
• Patient will articulate plan to resolve fatigue problems.
• Patient will employ measures to prevent and modify fatigue.

Interventions and rationales
• Prevent unnecessary fatigue; for example, avoid scheduling two energy-draining procedures on same day. *Using energy-conserving techniques avoids overexertion and potential for exhaustion.*

• Conserve energy through rest, planning, and setting priorities *to prevent or alleviate fatigue.*
• Alternate activities with periods of rest. Encourage activities that can be completed in short periods of time or divided into several segments; for example, read one chapter of a book at a time. *Scheduling regular rest periods helps decrease fatigue and increase stamina.*
• Discuss effect of fatigue on daily living and personal goals. Explore with patient the relationship between fatigue and the disease process *to help increase patient compliance with the schedule for activity and rest.*
• Reduce demands placed on patient; for example, ask one family member to call at specified times and relay messages to friends and other family members *to reduce physical and emotional stress.*
• Structure patient's environment; for example, set up daily schedule based on patient's needs and desires. *This encourages compliance with treatment regimen.*
• Encourage patient to eat foods rich in iron and minerals, unless contraindicated. *This helps avoid anemia and demineralization.*
• Postpone eating when patient is fatigued *to avoid aggravating the condition.*
• Provide small, frequent feedings *to conserve patient's energy and encourage increased dietary intake.*
• Establish a regular sleeping pattern. *Getting 8 to 10 hours of sleep nightly helps reduce fatigue.*
• Avoid highly emotional situations, *which aggravate patient's fatigue.*
• Encourage patient to explore feelings and emotions with a supportive counselor, clergy, or other professional *to help cope with illness.*

Evaluations for expected outcomes
• Patient describes at least three strategies to prevent or modify fatigue
• Patient incorporates at least three measures to modify fatigue into daily routine.
• Patient discusses the relationship of fatigue to disease process and activity level — for example, in heart disease, fatigue is a sign that the heart can't meet increased oxygen demands.
• Patient states that his fatigue level is reduced.
• Patient describes plan to resolve fatigue problems, including both physiologic and emotional remedies.
• Patient follows measures to prevent and modify fatigue.

Documentation
• Patient's ability to describe fatigue and its relationship to the disease process and condition
• Patient's ability to decrease fatigue by using various effective methods
• Patient's level of activity in relation to fatigue
• Patient's dietary intake
• Evaluations for expected outcomes

■ Fear

related to separation from support system

Definition
Feeling of physiologic or emotional disruption related to an identifiable source

Assessment
• History of experience with illness, hospitalization, and surgery
• Availability of support systems, including family members, friends, and clergy
• Financial resources
• History of coping with fear
• Physiologic manifestations of fear, including changes in pulse rate, respiratory rate, blood pressure, skin temperature, and quality and pitch of voice
• Psychological manifestations of fear, including changes in behavior, appetite, and sleep pattern

Defining characteristics
• Aggression
• Bedwetting
• Decreased self-assurance
• Feelings of alarm, apprehension, dread, horror, panic, and terror
• Focus of attention on "something out there"
• Identification of and concentration on object of fear
• Impulsive behavior
• Increased alertness
• Increased heart rate
• Increased tension, worrying, and wariness
• Jitteriness
• Wide-eyed appearance
• Withdrawal

Associated medical diagnoses (selected)
This nursing diagnosis may occur in any hospitalized patient separated from family or friends. In elderly patients, hospitalization often disrupts routines or rituals.

Expected outcomes
• Patient will identify source of fear.
• Patient will communicate feelings about separation from support systems.
• Patient will communicate feelings of comfort or satisfaction.
• Patient will use situational supports to reduce fear.
• Patient will integrate into daily behavior at least one fear-reducing cop-

ing mechanism, such as asking questions about treatment progress or making decisions about care.

Interventions and rationales

• Ask patient to identify source of fear; try to assess patient's understanding of situation. *Patient's perceptions may be erroneously based.*
• If patient has no visitors, spend an extra 15 minutes each shift in casual conversation; encourage other staff members to stop for brief visits *to help patient cope with separation.*
• Help patient maintain contact with family on a daily basis:
– Arrange for telephone calls.
– Help write letters.
– Promptly convey messages to patient from family and vice-versa.
– Encourage patient to have pictures of loved ones.
– Provide privacy for visits; take patient to day room or other quiet area. *These measures help patient reestablish and maintain social relationships.*
• Involve patient in planning care and setting goals *to renew confidence and give sense of control in a crisis situation.*
• Instruct patient in relaxation techniques, such as imagery and progressive muscle relaxation, *to reduce symptoms of sympathetic stimulation.*
• Administer antianxiety medications as ordered and monitor effectiveness. *Drug therapy may be needed to manage high anxiety levels or panic disorders.*
• Answer questions and help patient understand care *to reduce anxiety and correct misconceptions.*
• When feasible and where policies permit, relax visiting restrictions *to reduce patient's sense of isolation.*

• Allow a close family member or friend to participate in care *to provide an additional source of support.*
• Support family and friends in their efforts to understand patient's fear and to respond accordingly *to help them understand that patient's emotions are appropriate in context of situation.*

Evaluations for expected outcomes

• Patient states causes of fear.
• Patient expresses distress caused by separation from support systems.
• Patient reports feeling less fearful.
• Patient reaches out to others for support through phone calls, letters, or other means.
• Patient demonstrates use of at least one coping mechanism daily to reduce fear.

Documentation

• Patient's expressions of concern about illness, hospitalization, and separation from support system, and overt expressions of fear
• Observations of physiologic and behavioral manifestations of patient's fear
• Interventions performed to allay patient's fears and encourage healthy coping mechanisms
• Patient's response to interventions
• Evaluations for expected outcomes

■ Fear

related to unfamiliarity

Definition

Feelings of threat or danger to self arising from an identifiable source

Assessment
• History of experience with illness, hospitalization, and surgery
• Availability of support systems, including family members, friends, and clergy
• Financial resources
• History of coping with fear
• Neurologic status, including mental status, orientation, and sensory status
• Physiologic manifestations of fear, including changes in pulse rate, blood pressure, respiratory rate, skin temperature, and quality and pitch of voice
• Psychological manifestations of fear, including changes in behavior, appetite, and sleep pattern

Defining characteristics
• Aggression
• Bedwetting
• Decreased self-assurance
• Feelings of alarm, apprehension, dread, horror, panic, and terror
• Focus of attention on "something out there"
• Identification of and concentration on object of fear
• Impulsive behavior
• Increased alertness
• Increased heart rate
• Increased tension, worrying, and wariness
• Jitteriness
• Wide-eyed appearance
• Withdrawal

Associated medical diagnoses (selected)
Acute renal failure, acute respiratory failure, atelectasis, bladder cancer, blindness, brain tumors, breast cancer, cardiac arrhythmias, cervical cancer, chronic bronchitis, chronic obstructive pulmonary disease, Crohn's disease, deafness, disseminated intravascular coagulation, emphysema, endometrial cancer, epididymitis, esophageal cancer, head injury, hemothorax, liver transplantation, lung cancer, meningitis, metastatic disease, narcissistic personality disorder, ovarian cancer, panic disorder, phobic disorder, placenta previa, pneumothorax, pregnancy-induced hypertension, pulmonary edema, spinal cord injury, testicular cancer, thoracic surgery, tuberculosis

Expected outcomes
• Patient will identify source of fear.
• Patient will state understanding of procedures.
• Patient will verbally express comfort with surroundings.
• Patient will manifest no physical signs or symptoms of fear.
• Patient will use available support systems to assist in coping with fear.
• Patient will integrate into daily behavior at least one fear-reducing coping mechanism, such as asking questions about treatment progress and making decisions about care.

Interventions and rationales
• Encourage patient to identify source of fear. *Patient's perceptions may be erroneously based.*
• Explain all treatments and procedures, answering any questions patient might have. Present information at patient's level of understanding or acceptance *to reduce patient's anxiety and enhance cooperation.*
• Orient patient to surroundings. Make any adaptations to compensate for sensory deficits. *This enhances patient's ability to orient to time, place, person, and events.*
• Assign the same nurse to care for patient whenever possible *to provide consistency of care, enhance trust, and reduce threat often associated with multiple caregivers.*

• Spend time with patient each shift *to allow time for expression of feelings, provide emotional outlet, and promote feeling of acceptance.*
• Involve patient in planning and providing care *to give patient some control over situation and restore sense of self-esteem.*
• Orient family to patient's specific needs, allowing family members to participate in giving care. *This helps them provide effective support.*
• Request that family bring pictures and other small, personal objects to patient. *This helps alleviate patient's altered mental state by familiarizing the environment.*
• Arrange for family member or friend to stay with patient *to help patient cope with fears.*
• If a language barrier is the source of fear, use family and other resources in the hospital (such as an interpreter) *to help reduce patient's fear and aid effective communication.*

Evaluations for expected outcomes
• Patient identifies causes of fear.
• Patient demonstrates comprehension of procedures.
• Patient reports feeling comfortable in hospital.
• Patient's blood pressure, pulse rate, and respirations remain within set limits.
• Patient requests assistance from support systems to diminish fears (specify).
• Patient uses at least one effective fear-reducing behavior each day.

Documentation
• Patient's verbal expressions of fear
• Behavioral and physiologic manifestations of fear
• Interventions performed to reduce patient's fear
• Patient's response to interventions

• Family's involvement in patient care
• Patient's response to family involvement
• Evaluations for expected outcomes

■ Fluid volume deficit
related to active loss

Definition
Excessive loss of body fluid and electrolytes

Assessment
• History of fluid loss, such as vomiting, nasogastric tube drainage, diarrhea, or hemorrhage
• Pulse, blood pressure, respirations, and temperature
• Fluid and electrolyte status, including weight, intake and output, urine specific gravity, skin turgor, and mucous membranes
• Laboratory studies, including serum electrolyte levels, blood urea nitrogen, hemoglobin, hematocrit, and stool cultures

Defining characteristics
• Changes in mental status
• Decreased pulse volume and pressure
• Decreased urine output
• Decreased venous filling
• Dry skin and mucous membranes
• Increased body temperature
• Increased hematocrit
• Increased pulse rate
• Increased urine concentration
• Low blood pressure
• Poor turgor of skin or tongue
• Sudden weight loss
• Thirst
• Weakness

Associated medical diagnoses (selected)

Accidental radiation exposure, acute renal failure with hemodialysis or peritoneal dialysis, adult respiratory distress syndrome, anorexia nervosa, asthma, bulimia nervosa, burns, chemotherapy, cholecystitis, chronic obstructive pulmonary disease, cirrhosis, colitis, colon and rectal cancer, colostomy, diabetes insipidus, diabetic ketoacidosis, disseminated intravascular coagulation, diverticulitis, ectopic pregnancy, empyema, encephalitis, endometriosis, epididymitis, esophageal varices, fractures, hemorrhage, hemothorax, hepatic coma, hydatidiform mole, hyperemesis gravidarum, hyperosmolar hyperglycemic nonketotic syndrome, ileostomy, kidney transplantation, meningitis, metabolic alkalosis, multisystem trauma, pelvic inflammatory disease, pemphigus, peritonitis, pneumonia, pseudomembranous colitis, pulmonary embolus, radiation therapy, renal cancer, shock, thoracic surgery, uterine rupture, viral hepatitis

Expected outcomes

• Patient's vital signs will remain stable.
• Skin color evaluations will be normal.
• Electrolyte levels will stay within normal range.
• Fluid volume will remain adequate.
• Patient will produce adequate urine volume.
• Patient will have normal skin turgor and moist mucous membranes.
• Urine specific gravity will remain between 1.005 and 1.010.
• Fluid and blood volume will return to normal.
• Patient will express understanding of factors that caused fluid volume deficit.

Interventions and rationales

• Monitor and record vital signs every 2 hours or as often as necessary until stable. Then monitor and record vital signs every 4 hours. *Tachycardia, dyspnea, or hypotension may indicate fluid volume deficit or electrolyte imbalance.*
• Cover patient lightly. Avoid overheating *to prevent vasodilation, blood pooling in extremities, and reduced circulating blood volume.*
• Measure intake and output every 1 to 4 hours. Record and report significant changes. Include urine, stool, vomitus, wound drainage, nasogastric drainage, chest tube drainage, and any other output. *Low urine output and high specific gravity indicate hypovolemia.*
• Administer fluids, blood or blood products, or plasma expanders *to replace fluids and whole blood loss and facilitate fluid movement into intravascular space.* Monitor and record effectiveness and any adverse effects.
• Weigh patient daily at the same time *to give more accurate and consistent data. Weight is a good indicator of fluid status.*
• Assess skin turgor and oral mucous membranes every 8 hours *to check for dehydration.* Give meticulous mouth care every 4 hours *to avoid dehydrating mucous membranes.*
• Test urine specific gravity every 8 hours. *Elevated specific gravity may indicate dehydration.*
• Don't allow patient to sit or stand up quickly as long as circulation is compromised *to avoid orthostatic hypotension and possible syncope.*
• Measure abdominal girth every shift *to monitor for ascites and third-space shift.* Report changes.
• Administer and monitor medications *to prevent further fluid loss.*

• Explain reasons for fluid loss, and teach patient how to monitor fluid volume — for example, by recording daily weight and measuring intake and output. *This encourages patient involvement in personal care.*

Evaluations for expected outcomes
• Patient's pulse rate, blood pressure, respirations, and body temperature remain within set limits.
• Patient's skin color remains normal.
• Patient's electrolyte values remain within normal range.
• Patient's fluid volume remains adequate.
• Urine output remains at volume established for patient.
• Patient's skin turgor and mucous membranes remain normal.
• Patient's specific gravity remains between 1.005 and 1.010, unless specified otherwise.
• Patient's fluid volume returns to normal and remains normal, as evidenced by stable vital signs.
• Patient and caregiver demonstrate understanding of factors precipitating fluid volume deficit.

Documentation
• Patient's complaints of thirst, weakness, dizziness, and palpitations
• Observations of physical findings
• Intake and output (amount and type)
• Patient's weight and abdominal girth
• Interventions performed to control fluid loss
• Patient's response to interventions
• Evaluations for expected outcomes

■ Fluid volume deficit, risk for

related to excessive loss

Definition
Presence of risk factors that can lead to excessive fluid and electrolyte loss

Assessment
• History of problems that can cause fluid loss, such as vomiting, diarrhea, indwelling tubes, and hemorrhage
• Pulse, blood pressure, respirations, and temperature
• Fluid and electrolyte status, including weight, intake and output, urine specific gravity, skin turgor, and mucous membranes
• Laboratory studies, including serum electrolyte levels, blood urea nitrogen, hemoglobin, and hematocrit

Risk factors
• Conditions that influence fluid needs (such as a hypermetabolic state)
• Excessive loss of fluid from normal routes (such as from diarrhea)
• Extremes of age or weight
• Factors that affect intake of, absorption of, or access to fluids (such as immobility)
• Knowledge deficit related to fluid volume
• Loss of fluid through abnormal routes (such as a drainage tube)
• Medications that cause fluid loss

Associated medical diagnoses (selected)
Altered level of consciousness, bowel fistula, breast cancer with mastectomy, burns, cystic fibrosis, diabetes insipidus, diabetes mellitus, diarrhea-producing disorders (such as salmonellosis), draining pressure ulcer, esophageal fistula, esophageal varices (ruptured), intestinal obstruction,

open surgical wounds, organic brain syndrome, paralytic ileus

Expected outcomes
• Patient's vital signs will remain stable.
• Patient's skin color will remain normal.
• Patient will maintain urine output of at least ___ ml/hour.
• Patient's electrolyte values will remain within normal range.
• Patient will maintain intake at _____ ml/24 hours.
• Patient's intake will equal or exceed output.
• Patient will express understanding of need to maintain adequate fluid intake.
• Patient will demonstrate skill in weighing self accurately and recording weight.
• Patient will measure and record own intake and output.
• Patient will return to normal, appropriate diet.

Interventions and rationales
• Monitor and record vital signs every 4 hours. *Fever, tachycardia, dyspnea, or hypotension may indicate hypovolemia.*
• Maintain accurate record of intake and output *to aid estimation of patient's fluid balance.*
• Measure urine output every hour. Record and report an output of less than ____ ml/hour. *Decreased urine output may indicate reduced fluid volume.*
• Measure and record drainage from all tubes and catheters *to take such losses into account when replacing fluid.*
• When copious drainage appears on dressings, weigh dressings every 8 hours and record with other output sources. *Excessive wound drainage*

causes significant fluid imbalances (1 kg dressing equals about 1 L [1⅛ qt] of fluid).
• Test urine specific gravity each shift. Monitor laboratory values and report abnormal findings to doctor. *Increased urine specific gravity may indicate dehydration. Elevated hematocrit and hemoglobin also indicate dehydration.*
• Monitor serum electrolyte levels and report abnormalities. *Fluid loss may cause significant electrolyte imbalance.*
• Obtain and record patient's weight at the same time every day *to help ensure accurate data. Daily weighing helps estimate body fluid status.*
• Monitor skin turgor each shift *to check for dehydration;* report any decrease in turgor. *Poor skin turgor is a sign of dehydration.*
• Examine oral mucous membranes each shift. *Dry mucous membranes are a sign of dehydration.*
• Cover wounds *to minimize fluid loss and prevent skin excoriation.*
• Determine patient's fluid preferences *to enhance intake.*
• Keep oral fluids at bedside within patient's reach and encourage patient to drink. *This gives patient some control over fluid intake and supplements parenteral fluid intake.*
• Instruct patient in maintaining appropriate fluid intake, including recording daily weight, measuring intake and output, and recognizing signs of dehydration. *This encourages patient and caregiver participation and enhances patient's sense of control.*
• Force oral fluids when possible and indicated *to enhance replacement of lost fluids.* (Bowel sounds should be present and patient awake before giving oral fluids.)

• Administer parenteral fluids, as prescribed, *to replace fluid losses.* Maintain parenteral fluids or blood transfusions at prescribed rate *to prevent further fluid loss or overload.*
• Progress patient to appropriate diet, as prescribed, *to help achieve fluid and electrolyte balance.*

Evaluations for expected outcomes
• Patient's temperature, pulse rate, blood pressure, and respirations are within set limits (specify).
• Patient's skin color remains normal.
• Patient's urine output remains at specified volume.
• Patient's electrolyte values remain normal.
• Patient's daily fluid intake remains within established limits (specify).
• Patient's cumulative intake equals or exceeds cumulative output.
• Patient demonstrates understanding of importance of maintaining fluid balance.
• Patient weighs self with same scale at same time each day and records results.
• Patient measures fluid intake and output; records are reviewed to ensure accuracy.
• Patient returns to normal, appropriate diet.

Documentation
• Observations of physical findings
• Intake and output
• Drainage from indwelling tubes and catheters, including amount, color, and consistency
• Amount, color, and odor of drainage on dressings
• Patient teaching about fluid intake and diet
• Patient's response to interventions
• Evaluations for expected outcomes

■ Fluid volume excess
related to compromised regulatory mechanisms

Definition
Excess fluid resulting from compromised regulatory mechanisms (internal physiologic controls that help the body adapt to changing needs, such as renin-angiotensin, antidiuretic hormone, aldosterone, hydrogen-bicarbonate ion exchange)

Assessment
• Neurologic status, including level of consciousness, orientation, and mental status
• Cardiovascular status, including skin color, temperature, and turgor; central venous pressure and pulmonary artery pressure (if available); heart rate and rhythm; blood pressure; heart sounds, electrocardiogram (ECG) results; and hemoglobin (Hb) and hematocrit (HCT)
• Respiratory status, including rate, depth, pattern of respiration; breath sounds; chest X-ray; and arterial blood gas levels
• Renal status, including intake and output, urine specific gravity, weight, serum electrolyte and serum and urine osmolality levels, and blood urea nitrogen (BUN), creatinine, and serum protein levels
• Endocrine status, including general appearance, size and body proportions, skin color and condition, and distribution of body hair

Defining characteristics
• Altered mental status
• Altered respiratory pattern
• Anasarca
• Azotemia

• Changes in blood pressure, pulmonary artery pressure, urine specific gravity, and electrolyte levels
• Crackles
• Decreased Hb and HCT
• Dyspnea
• Edema
• Increased central venous pressure
• Intake greater than output
• Jugular vein distention
• Oliguria
• Orthopnea
• Pleural effusion
• Positive hepatojugular reflex
• Pulmonary congestion
• Rapid weight gain
• Restlessness and anxiety
• S_3 heart sound

Associated medical diagnoses (selected)
Acute renal failure, aortic aneurysm, cardiac arrhythmias, cardiogenic shock, chronic renal failure, Cushing's syndrome, endocarditis, endstage cardiac disease, glomerulonephritis, heart failure, hemodialysis, hypertension, meningitis, multiple myeloma, pregnancy-induced hypertension, pulmonary edema, pyelonephritis

Expected outcomes
• Blood pressure will remain no lower than ____ mm Hg and no higher than ____ mm Hg.
• Patient will demonstrate no signs of hyperkalemia on ECG.
• Patient will maintain fluid intake of no more than ____ ml and output of no less than ____ ml.
• Urine specific gravity will remain between ____ and ____.
• HCT will stay above ____ %.
• BUN, creatinine, sodium, and potassium will stay within acceptable levels for specific patient.
• Patient will plan 24-hour fluid intake, as prescribed.

• Patient will tolerate restricted intake with no physical or emotional discomfort.
• Patient's skin will remain intact and infection-free.
• Patient will assist with activities of daily living (ADLs) without undue fatigue.
• Patient will ambulate and carry out ADLs safely and comfortably.
• Patient will demonstrate skill in selecting permitted foods, such as those low in sodium and potassium.
• Patient will describe signs and symptoms that require medical treatment.

Interventions and rationales
• Monitor blood pressure, pulse rate, cardiac rhythm, temperature, and breath sounds at least every 4 hours; record and report changes. *Changed parameters may indicate altered fluid or electrolyte status.*
• Carefully monitor intake, output, and urine specific gravity at least every 4 hours. *Intake greater than output and elevated specific gravity may indicate fluid retention or overload.*
• Monitor BUN, creatinine, electrolytes, Hb, and HCT. *BUN and creatinine indicate renal function; electrolytes, Hb, and HCT help indicate fluid status.*
• Weigh patient daily before breakfast, as ordered, *to provide consistent readings.* Check for signs of fluid retention, such as dependent edema, sacral edema, and ascites.
• Give fluids as ordered. Monitor I.V. flow rate carefully *because excess I.V. fluids can worsen patient's condition.*
• If oral fluids are allowed, help patient make a schedule for fluid intake. *Patient involvement encourages compliance.*

• Explain the reasons for fluid and dietary restrictions *to enhance patient's understanding and compliance.*
• Learn patient's food preferences and plan accordingly within prescribed dietary restrictions *to enhance compliance.*
• Provide mouth care every 4 hours. Keep mucous membranes moist with water-soluble lubricant *to prevent them from dehydrating.*
• Provide sour hard candy *to decrease thirst and improve taste.*
• Support patient with positive feedback about adherence to restrictions *to encourage compliance.*
• Give skin care every 4 hours. Change patient's position at least every 2 hours. Elevate edematous extremities. *These measures enhance venous return, reduce edema, and prevent skin breakdown.*
• Examine skin daily for signs of bruising or other discoloration. *Edema may cause decreased tissue perfusion with skin changes.*
• Encourage patient to help in performing ADLs. *This boosts self-image and helps mobilize fluid from edematous areas.*
• Alternate periods of rest and activity *to avoid worsening fatigue caused by electrolyte imbalance.*
• Increase patient's activity level as tolerated; for example, ambulate and increase self-care measures performed by patient. *Gradually increasing activity helps body adjust to increased tissue oxygen demand and possible increased venous return.*
• Apply antiembolism stockings or intermittent pneumatic compression stockings *to increase venous return.* Remove for 1 hour and inspect skin every 8 hours or according to facility policy.
• Assess skin turgor *to monitor for dehydration.*

• Measure abdominal girth every shift and report changes *to monitor for ascites.*
• Have dietitian see patient *to teach or reinforce dietary restrictions.*
• Educate patient regarding:
– environmental safety measures
– fluid restriction and diet
– signs and symptoms requiring immediate medical treatment
– medications (name, dosage, frequency, therapeutic effects, and adverse effects)
– activity level
– ways to prevent infection.
These measures encourage patient and family members to participate more fully in care.

Evaluations for expected outcomes
• Patient's blood pressure remains within established limits.
• Signs of hyperkalemia (peaked or elevated T waves, prolonged PR intervals, widened QRS complexes, or depressed ST segments) don't appear on ECG.
• Patient's fluid intake and output remain within established limits.
• Patient's urine specific gravity remains within established limits.
• Patient's HCT remains above specified level.
• Patient's electrolyte levels remain within established limits.
• Patient plans 24-hour fluid intake.
• Patient doesn't indicate discomfort with restricted fluid intake, either verbally or through behavior.
• Patient's skin remains intact and free of infection.
• Patient assists caregiver with ADLs without undue fatigue.
• Patient ambulates and carries out ADLs comfortably and safely.
• Patient plans own menu and selects foods low in sodium and potassium.

Patient follows other dietary restrictions (specify).
• Patient and caregiver list signs and symptoms that require medical attention.

Documentation
• Expression of patient's needs, desires, or perceptions of the situation
• Specific changes in patient's physical status
• Observations about patient's response to treatment
• Observations about how patient appears to be coping with fluid and dietary restrictions
• Condition of skin and mucous membranes
• Interventions performed to alleviate or resolve diagnosis
• Evaluations for expected outcomes

■ Fluid volume excess

related to excess fluid intake or retention, or excess sodium intake or retention

Definition
Imbalance of water or sodium causing increased total body fluid or fluid volume shift from one compartment to another

Assessment
• Neurologic status, including level of consciousness, orientation, and mental status
• Cardiovascular status, including skin color, temperature, and turgor; jugular venous pressure; central venous pressure (CVP) and pulmonary artery pressure (if available); heart rate and rhythm; blood pressure; heart sounds; ECG results; hemoglobin (Hb); and hematocrit (HCT)

• Respiratory status, including breath sounds, chest X-ray, arterial blood gas levels, and rate, depth, and pattern of respiration
• Renal status, including intake and output, urine specific gravity, weight, serum electrolyte levels, serum and urine osmolality, blood urea nitrogen, urine and serum creatinine, and serum protein level

Defining characteristics
• Altered mental status
• Altered respiratory pattern
• Anascara
• Azotemia
• Changes in blood pressure, pulmonary artery pressure, urine specific gravity, and electrolyte levels
• Crackles
• Decreased Hb and HCT
• Dyspnea
• Edema
• Increased CVP
• Intake greater than output
• Jugular vein distention
• Oliguria
• Orthopnea
• Pleural effusion
• Positive hepatojugular reflex
• Pulmonary congestion
• Rapid weight gain
• Restlessness and anxiety
• S_3 heart sound

Associated medical diagnoses (selected)
Bone marrow transplantation, cor pulmonale, end-stage renal or cardiac disease, heart failure, peritoneal dialysis

Expected outcomes
• Patient will state ability to breathe comfortably.
• Patient will maintain fluid intake at ___ ml/day.
• Patient will return to baseline weight.

• Patient will maintain vital signs within normal limits (specify).
• Patient will exhibit urine specific gravity of 1.005 to 1.010.
• Patient will have normal skin turgor.
• Patient will show electrolytes within normal range (specify).
• Patient will avoid complications of excess fluid.
• Patient will state understanding of health problem.
• Patient will demonstrate skill in health-related behaviors.

Interventions and rationales
• Help patient into a position that aids breathing, such as Fowler's or semi-Fowler's, *to increase chest expansion and improve ventilation.*
• Administer oxygen, as ordered, *to enhance arterial blood oxygenation.*
• Restrict fluids to _____ ml per shift. *Excessive fluids will worsen patient's condition.*
• Monitor and record vital signs at least every 4 hours. *Changes may indicate fluid or electrolyte imbalances.*
• Measure and record intake and output. *Intake greater than output may indicate fluid retention and possible overload.*
• Weigh patient at same time each day *to obtain consistent readings.*
• Administer diuretics *to promote fluid excretion.* Record effects.
• Test urine specific gravity every 8 hours and record results. Monitor laboratory values and report significant changes to doctor. *High specific gravity indicates fluid retention. Fluid overload may alter electrolyte levels.*
• Assess patient daily for edema, including ascites and dependent or sacral edema. *Fluid overload or decreased osmotic pressure may result in edema, especially in dependent areas.*

• Maintain patient on sodium-restricted diet, as ordered, *to reduce excess fluid and prevent reaccumulation.*
• Reposition patient every 2 hours, inspect skin for redness with each turn, and institute measures as needed *to prevent skin breakdown.*
• Apply antiembolism stockings or intermittent pneumatic compression stockings *to increase venous return.* Remove for 1 hour every 8 hours or according to facility policy.
• Encourage patient to cough and deep-breathe every 2 to 4 hours *to prevent pulmonary complications.*
• Educate patient regarding maintenance of daily weight record, daily measuring and recording of intake and output, diuretic therapy, and dietary restrictions, especially sodium. *These measures encourage patient and caregivers to participate more fully.*

Evaluations for expected outcomes
• Patient indicates, verbally and through behavior, ability to breathe comfortably.
• Patient's fluid intake remains at established daily limit (specify).
• Patient's weight returns to baseline and remains stable.
• Patient's pulse and respiratory rates, blood pressure, and temperature remain within established limits.
• Patient's urine specific gravity remains between 1.005 and 1.010.
• Patient's skin turgor remains normal.
• Patient's electrolyte levels remain within established range.
• Complications of excess fluid don't occur.
• Patient expresses understanding of health problem.
• Patient demonstrates skill in health-related behaviors, such as maintaining

weight and monitoring intake and output.

Documentation
- Patient's perceptions of the situation
- Observations of physical findings
- Interventions to correct fluid volume excess
- Patient's responses to fluid and dietary restrictions
- Patient's demonstration of skills
- Evaluations for expected outcomes

■ Fluid volume imbalance, risk for

related to excessive loss, intake, or retention

Definition
Presence of risk factors that may lead to an excessive increase or decrease in fluids

Assessment
- Age
- Vital signs
- History of problems related to fluid imbalance, including vomiting, diarrhea, hemorrhage, oliguria, pulmonary congestion, weight gain, increased fluid or salt intake
- Fluid and electrolyte status, including weight gain or loss, increased or decreased urine output, increased or decreased fluid intake, urine specific gravity, skin turgor, mucous membranes, serum electrolyte levels, central venous pressure, pulmonary artery pressure, and heart sounds
- Patient's and caregiver's understanding of factors that may lead to fluid imbalance
- Willingness and ability of patient and caregiver to participate in care

Risk factors
- Altered intake
- Clinical evidence of fluid or blood loss through artificial orifices or lumens, wounds, or drainage tubes
- Increased fluid output
- Increased fluid intake
- Hypernatremia or hyponatremia
- Hyperkalemia or hypokalemia
- Hypervolemia or hypovolemia
- Fluid shift
- Lack of knowledge of factors that contribute to fluid imbalance

Associated medical diagnoses (selected)
Crohn's disease, cystic fibrosis, diabetes insipidus, diabetes mellitus, diarrhea, head injury, heart failure, intestinal obstruction, meningitis, renal failure

Expected outcomes
- Patient will maintain normal weight in relation to height and age.
- Patient's fluid intake and output will remain at appropriate levels for age and physical condition.
- Patient will exhibit urine specific gravity of 1.005 to 1.015.
- Patient will maintain vital signs within normal limits for age.
- Patient's mucous membranes will appear pink and moist.
- Patient will have normal skin turgor.
- Patient will maintain electrolyte levels within normal range.
- Patient will demonstrate an understanding of factors that will reduce fluid imbalance and the problems associated with it.

Interventions and rationales
- Weigh patient daily before breakfast *to help detect changes in fluid balance.*
- Measure fluid intake and urine output *to obtain fluid status. Decreased intake or increased output results in*

fluid deficit. Increased intake or decreased output results in fluid excess.
• Monitor urine specific gravity. *Elevated specific gravity indicates dehydration. Low specific gravity indicates excess fluid volume.*
• Examine oral mucous membranes each day. *Dry mucous membranes are an indication of dehydration.*
• Determine which fluids patient prefers and keep these fluids at the bedside, as prescribed, *to enhance intake.*
• Monitor serum electrolyte levels. *Changes in electrolyte value may herald the onset of fluid imbalance.* For example, a patient with hyperkalemia is at risk for fluid overload.
• Encourage patient to follow his prescribed diet, *to help achieve fluid and electrolyte balance.* For example, teach patient with hyperkalemia to eat foods low in potassium.
• Administer parenteral fluids, as prescribed, *to help maintain fluid balance.*
• Explain the nature of hypervolemia or hypovolemia and the relationship of fluid volume imbalance to patient's medical condition. Describe the prescribed treatment for fluid imbalance. Teach patient about medications, including dosage, frequency, and possible adverse effects. *The more the patient understands his condition, the more likely he is to comply with treatment, thereby minimizing the risk of complications.*
• Instruct patient and family members how to maintain appropriate fluid intake, including recording daily weight, measuring intake and output, and recognizing signs of fluid imbalance. *This encourages patient and caregivers to participate in care, thereby promoting a sense of control.*

Evaluations for expected outcomes
• Patient maintains normal weight in relation to height and age.
• Patient's fluid intake and output remain at appropriate levels for age and physical condition.
• Patient exhibits urine specific gravity of 1.005 to 1.015.
• Patient maintains vital signs within normal limits for age.
• Patient's mucous membranes appear pink and moist.
• Patient has normal skin turgor.
• Patient maintains electrolyte levels within normal range.
• Patient demonstrates an understanding of factors that will reduce fluid imbalance and the problems associated with it.

Documentation
• Observations of physical findings
• Factors contributing to risk of fluid imbalance
• Intake and output
• Patient teaching about fluid balance
• Patient's responses to interventions
• Evaluations for expected outcomes

■ Gas exchange impairment

related to altered oxygen-carrying capacity of the blood

Definition
Interference in cellular respiration resulting from inadequate exchange or transport of oxygen and carbon dioxide

Assessment
• Neurologic status, including level of consciousness, orientation, and mental status

• Respiratory status, including respiratory rate and depth, symmetry of chest expansion, accessory muscle use, cough, sputum, palpation for fremitus, percussion of lung fields, auscultation of breath sounds, arterial blood gas (ABG) levels, and pulmonary function studies
• Cardiovascular status, including skin color and temperature, heart rate and rhythm, blood pressure, hemoglobin (Hb) and hematocrit (HCT), red blood cell count, white blood cell count, platelet count, prothrombin time (PT), partial thromboplastin time (PTT), and serum iron
• Activity status, including such functional capabilities as range of motion and muscle strength, activities of daily living, and occupation

Defining characteristics
• Abnormal pH and ABG levels
• Abnormal respiratory rate, rhythm, and depth
• Confusion
• Cyanosis (in neonates)
• Diaphoresis
• Dyspnea
• Headache upon awakening
• Hypoxia and hypoxemia
• Increased or decreased carbon dioxide levels
• Irritability
• Nasal flaring
• Pale, dusky skin
• Restlessness or somnolence
• Tachycardia

Associated medical diagnoses (selected)
Cerebrovascular accident, chemotherapy, coronary artery disease, cystic fibrosis, hemophilia, leukemia, lung cancer, myasthenia gravis, polycythemia vera, sarcoidosis, shock, sickle cell anemia

Expected outcomes
• Patient will carry out activities of daily living (ADLs) without weakness or fatigue.
• Patient will have no signs of active bleeding.
• Hb and HCT will return to normal level (specify).
• Clotting profile will remain within normal limits (specify).
• Patient will maintain adequate ventilation.
• Patient will communicate understanding of precautions needed to prevent bleeding.

Interventions and rationales
• Encourage patient to alternate periods of rest and activity. *Activity increases tissue oxygen demand; rest enhances tissue oxygen perfusion.*
• If patient is on bed rest, help him into a comfortable position and raise side rails *to prevent falls.* Have patient turn, cough, and deep-breathe every 4 hours *to prevent atelectasis or fluid buildup in lungs and to enhance blood oxygen level.*
• Move patient slowly *to avoid orthostatic hypotension.* Assist patient when out of bed *in case of dizziness.* Avoid bumps and scratches, *which may cause trauma and tissue bleeding.*
• Plan patient's activities within level of tolerance *to avoid fatigue.*
• Provide gentle oral hygiene *to avoid injuring oral mucosa.*
• Check all urine and stools for blood *to detect internal bleeding.* Check for evidence of bleeding at least once every 8 hours. *Hemorrhage or bleeding may cause anemia.*
• Administer blood or blood products and monitor for adverse reactions *to restore fluid volume and prevent complications.*

• Consolidate laboratory work *to avoid multiple needle sticks and reduce chance of hematoma or hemorrhage in patients with altered clotting mechanisms.* Apply pressure for at least 1 minute after puncture *to promote clotting.*
• Auscultate lungs every 4 hours and report abnormalities *to detect decreased or adventitious breath sounds.*
• Monitor vital signs, cardiac rhythm, and ABG and Hb levels *to detect impaired gas exchange.* Report abnormalities.
• Teach patient about safety at home and work, including:
– use of soft toothbrush
– use of an electric razor for shaving
– careful use of sharp objects, such as knives, tweezers, and scissors
– monitoring of urine, stools, and sputum for blood and reporting results immediately if blood is present
– disadvantages and risks of smoking
– using medications (name, dosage, therapeutic effect, adverse effects, and precautions).
These measures encourage patient and caregivers to participate in care.

Evaluations for expected outcomes
• Patient carries out ADLs without fatigue or weakness.
• Patient doesn't exhibit signs of active bleeding, such as oozing from wounds or puncture site, bruising, petechiae, and occult blood in stool or urine.
• Patient's Hb and HCT remain within established limits.
• Patient's clotting profile, including platelet count, PTT, PT, fibrinogen, and fibrin split products, remains within normal limits.
• Patient maintains adequate ventilation.

• Patient communicates understanding of precautions needed to prevent bleeding.

Documentation
• Patient's expression of personal feelings
• Observations about physical findings
• Results of laboratory studies that significantly affect nursing care
• Patient's response to interventions
• Evaluations for expected outcomes

■ Gas exchange impairment
related to altered oxygen supply

Definition
Interference in cellular respiration resulting from inadequate exchange or transport of oxygen and carbon dioxide

Assessment
• Neurologic status, including level of consciousness, orientation, and mental status
• Respiratory status, including respiratory rate and depth, symmetry of chest expansion, use of accessory muscles, cough, sputum, palpation for fremitus, percussion of lung fields, auscultation of breath sounds, arterial blood gas (ABG) levels, and pulmonary function studies
• Cardiovascular status, including skin color and temperature, heart rate and rhythm, blood pressure, and complete blood count
• Activity status, including such functional capabilities as range of motion and muscle strength, activities of daily living (ADLs), and occupation

Defining characteristics
- Abnormal pH and ABG levels
- Abnormal respiratory rate, rhythm, and depth
- Confusion
- Cyanosis (in neonates)
- Diaphoresis
- Dyspnea
- Headache upon awakening
- Hypoxia and hypoxemia
- Increased or decreased carbon dioxide levels
- Irritability
- Nasal flaring
- Pale, dusky skin
- Restlessness or somnolence
- Tachycardia
- Visual disturbances

Associated medical diagnoses (selected)
Acute respiratory failure, adult respiratory distress syndrome, anemias, aortic aneurysm, asthma, atelectasis, bronchiectasis, cardiogenic shock, chronic obstructive pulmonary disease, cor pulmonale, disseminated intravascular coagulation, drug overdose or toxicity, empyema, head injury, heart failure, hemothorax, infant respiratory distress syndrome, lung abscess, pleurisy, pneumonia, pneumothorax, pulmonary edema, pulmonary embolus, pulmonary fibrosis, rheumatic fever, sarcoidosis, thoracic surgery, thrombophlebitis, tuberculosis

Expected outcomes
- Patient will maintain respiratory rate within ±5 of baseline.
- Patient will express feeling of comfort in maintaining air exchange.
- Patient will cough effectively.
- Patient will expectorate sputum.
- Patient will sustain sufficient fluid intake to prevent dehydration: ___ ml/ 24 hours.
- Patient will perform ADLs to level of tolerance.
- Patient will have normal breath sounds.
- Patient's ABG levels will return to baselines: ___ pH; ___ partial pressure of arterial oxygen (Pao_2); ___ partial pressure of arterial carbon dioxide ($Paco_2$).
- Patient will perform relaxation techniques every 4 hours.
- Patient will use correct bronchial hygiene.

Interventions and rationales
- Assess and record pulmonary status every 4 hours or more frequently if patient's condition is unstable. *Poor pulmonary status may result in hypoxemia.*
- Monitor vital signs and cardiac rhythm at least every 4 hours *to detect tachycardia and tachypnea, which could indicate hypoxemia.*
- Place patient in position that best facilitates chest expansion *to enhance gas exchange.*
- Change patient's position at least every 2 hours *to mobilize secretions and allow aeration of all lung fields.*
- Perform bronchial hygiene as ordered, including coughing, percussion, postural drainage, and suctioning. *These measures promote drainage and keep airways clear.*
- Give medications, as ordered, *to improve oxygenation.* Monitor and record efficacy and adverse reactions *to guide treatment.*
- Monitor oxygen therapy, *which increases alveolar oxygen concentration and enhances arterial blood oxygenation.*
- Record intake and output *to monitor patient's fluid status.*
- Report signs of dehydration or fluid overload immediately. *Dehydration may hinder tissue perfusion and secretion mobilization; fluid overload may cause pulmonary edema.*

• Assist patient with ADLs *to decrease tissue oxygen demand.*
• Include periods of rest in plan of care *to reduce patient's tissue oxygen demand.*
• Monitor ABG levels and notify doctor immediately if Pao_2 or arterial oxygen saturation drops or $Paco_2$ rises. Administer endotracheal intubation and mechanical ventilation if needed. *This helps increase ventilation and gas exchange.*
• Teach patient relaxation techniques *to reduce tissue oxygen demand.*
• Have patient perform relaxation techniques every 4 hours *to establish the routine and reduce oxygen demand.*

Evaluations for expected outcomes
• Patient's respiratory rate remains within established limits.
• Patient doesn't experience dyspnea.
• Patient demonstrates ability to cough and produce sputum.
• Patient expectorates sputum produced by coughing and deep breathing.
• Patient's fluid intake remains sufficient to prevent dehydration.
• Patient performs ADLs without exhibiting dyspnea or other signs of abnormal ABG levels.
• Patient has normal breath sounds.
• Patient's pH, Pao_2, and $Paco_2$ return to and remain within established limits.
• Patient performs relaxation techniques every 4 hours.
• Patient uses correct bronchial hygiene.

Documentation
• Patient's complaints of dyspnea, headache, and restlessness
• Patient's expression of well-being
• Observations of physical findings
• Effectiveness of medications
• Other treatments performed by nurse
• Evaluations for expected outcomes

■ Grieving, anticipatory
related to perceived potential loss of significant object (such as person, job, possessions)

Definition
Intellectual and emotional responses through which an individual attempts to adjust self-concept based upon a perceived personal loss. The concept of anticipatory grieving can be applied to families and communities as well.

Assessment
• Type of loss expected
• Feelings about control of situation
• Usual patterns of coping with loss
• Ability of patient and family to grieve over loss
• Greatest fear about loss
• Behavioral manifestations of grieving
• Somatic problems associated with grieving process, including appetite, sleep patterns, activity, and libido
• Support systems, including family members, friends, and clergy

Defining characteristics
• Altered activity level
• Altered communication pattern
• Altered libido
• Anger
• Changes in eating habits
• Changes in sleep patterns or dream patterns
• Denial of significance of potential loss
• Difficulty taking on new or different roles

• Expression of distress at potential loss
• Expression of guilt or bargaining with a higher power
• Resolution of grief before the occurrence of loss
• Sorrow

Associated medical diagnoses (selected)

Acquired immunodeficiency syndrome, Alzheimer's disease, amyotrophic lateral sclerosis, breast cancer, burns, cataracts, cystic fibrosis, diabetes mellitus, endometrial cancer, glaucoma, juvenile rheumatoid arthritis, laryngeal cancer, limb amputation, ovarian cancer, urinary diversion

Expected outcomes

• Patient will identify the perceived potential loss.
• Patient will express feelings about potential loss.
• Patient will communicate understanding of grieving process and willingness to experience the process.
• Patient will exercise control by making decisions about care.
• Patient will use healthy coping mechanisms to deal with potential loss.
• Patient will seek support groups.
• Patient will make plans for future.

Interventions and rationales

• Help patient identify the potential loss *because patient may be unable to pinpoint cause of anxiety.*
• Plan time each shift to sit and listen to patient. If patient isn't ready to talk, spend the time in silence. *This demonstrates concern, understanding, and support for patient.*
• Encourage patient to express feelings about the potential loss and its impact on well-being and lifestyle. *This reinforces reality and helps alle-*

viate guilt through self-assurance that effort was made to prevent loss.
• Help patient understand grieving process and accept feelings being experienced as normal under the present circumstances. *This enhances patient's understanding and ability to cope.*
• Encourage patient to make simple decisions related to care issues *to give patient a sense of functional ability and control.*
• Emphasize patient's identified strengths. Provide positive reinforcement as patient demonstrates effective coping behavior. *This helps patient reestablish positive self-image and gain confidence.*
• Encourage patient to use family, friends, or other support systems *to bolster coping ability.*
• Inform patient about existing support groups in the facility and the community *to encourage patient to seek help from available resources.*
• Help make a specific plan for coping after discharge *to enable patient to integrate the loss and adjust to lifestyle.*
• Recognize that patients from different cultures may express grief differently:
– African Americans may cry loudly, pray, and read from scripture and rely on the support of family and friends. Provide privacy.
– Asian Americans may express grief less publicly and more quietly with the support of family.
– Hispanic Americans may come together as a family and grieve openly. Provide privacy.
Understanding how different cultures express grief allows you to help patient and family express grief within cultural norms.

Evaluations for expected outcomes
• Patient identifies potential loss.
• Patient expresses feelings about potential loss.
• Patient communicates understanding of stages of grief and accepts feelings and behavior brought on by potential loss.
• Patient plans own daily plan of care, such as deciding best time for bathing, resting, and receiving visitors.
• Patient uses healthy coping mechanisms to deal with potential loss.
• Patient contacts support groups for help in coping with potential loss.
• Patient discusses future plans for coping with potential loss.

Documentation
• Patient's verbal expressions
• Patient's eating, sleeping, activity patterns
• Observation of emotional responses, such as crying, anger, and withdrawal
• Patient's attempt to gain control, such as making decisions and using support systems
• Interventions performed to assist patient
• Patient's response to intervention
• Evaluations for expected outcomes

■ Grieving, dysfunctional

related to actual object loss

Definition
Extended, unsuccessful intellectual and emotional responses on the part of an individual attempting to work through the grief process. The concept of dysfunctional grieving can also be applied to families and communities.

Assessment
• History of recent loss
• Patient's usual patterns of coping with loss, including cultural, intellectual, and emotional responses
• Verbal expressions of feelings of control over the situation
• Behavioral manifestations of grieving, including presence and intensity of specific behaviors
• Somatic problems associated with grieving process, including appetite, sleep patterns, activity level, and libido
• Support systems, including family members, friends, and clergy

Defining characteristics
• Alterations in eating habits, sleep patterns, dream patterns, activity level, libido, concentration, or desire to pursue activities
• Anger
• Crying
• Denial of loss
• Developmental regression
• Difficulty in expressing loss
• Expressions of guilt
• Expressions of unresolved issues
• Idealization of lost object
• Prolonged interference with life functioning
• Labile affect
• Loss of health, family member, friend, job, or anything of importance to patient
• Reliving of past experiences with little or no reduction of intensity of grief
• Repetitive use of ineffective behaviors as part of effort to reinvest in lost relationship
• Sadness
• Verbal expression of distress at loss

Associated medical diagnoses (selected)
Abruptio placentae, breast cancer, Cushing's syndrome, infertility, spinal

cord injury (partial or total paralysis), spontaneous or therapeutic abortion

Expected outcomes
• Patient will identify the loss.
• Patient will express feelings about the loss.
• Patient will allow others to help in coping.
• Patient will begin using healthy coping mechanisms.
• Patient will communicate understanding that it's normal to grieve.
• Patient will seek out available support systems.
• Patient will allow self to experience grieving process alone and with family.
• Patient will begin planning for future.

Interventions and rationales
• Encourage patient to use expressions of feeling that are most comfortable; for example, crying, talking, writing, and drawing. *Dysfunctional grieving may result from inability to express feelings freely.*
• Spend at least 15 minutes each shift with patient. Allow this time for expression of feelings. Place limits on destructive or exaggerated behaviors. *Inability to identify anger as normal response to loss may cause patient to behave aggressively toward self or others.*
• Help patient focus realistically on changes the loss has brought about. *This is an initial step in planning for future and helps patient find new patterns of rewarding interactions.*
• Encourage patient's help in self-care activities *to reduce intensity of patient's mourning and enhance sense of functional ability.*
• Encourage patient to use available support systems *to provide emotional strength.*

• Encourage patient and family to reminisce. *Helping them engage in "life review" often creates peaceful atmosphere in which loss acquires purpose and meaning.*
• Inform patient and family about existing support groups in the agency and in the community *to help prevent or reduce maladaptive emotional responses to loss.*
• Help patient formulate goals for discharge and the future. *This helps patient to place loss in perspective and to move on to new situations and relationships.*
• Refer patient to an appropriate mental health professional. *Delayed grief reaction may indicate depression, which requires psychiatric intervention.*

Evaluations for expected outcomes
• Patient identifies recent loss.
• Patient discusses feelings about recent loss.
• Patient allows others to help cope with loss.
• Patient uses coping mechanisms, including discussing loss with others.
• Patient communicates understanding that grieving is an appropriate response to loss and comes to terms with own grief response.
• Patient actively participates in discussions about loss with support groups or seeks help from mental health professional.
• Patient allows himself to experience grief alone and with family members.
• Patient describes future plans for coping with loss and getting on with life.

Documentation
• Patient's verbal expressions of grieving
• Patient's observable behaviors, such as attempts at coping and interactions with family and staff

• Description of nursing interventions and patient's responses
• Evaluations for expected outcomes

■ Growth and development alteration

related to effects of physical disability

Definition
State in which an individual deviates from norms for age

Assessment
• Age (chronologic and developmental stage)
• Sex
• Nature of physical disability
• Past experience with hospitalization
• Family system (nuclear, extended, and sibling position)
• Communication skills (verbal and nonverbal)
• Motor skills
• Socialization pattern
• Knowledge, including educational background and understanding of physical disability
• Mental status, including orientation, cognitive and perceptual ability, memory, affect, and mood behavior

Defining characteristics
• Altered physical growth
• Delay or difficulty in performing skills typical of age-group (motor, social, expressive)
• Flat affect, listlessness, and decreased verbal or nonverbal response
• Inability to perform self-care or self-control activities appropriate for age

Associated medical diagnoses (selected)
Asphyxia, cerebrovascular accident, Down syndrome, hydrocephalus, orthopedic injuries, spinal cord injuries

Expected outcomes
• Patient will express concerns about physical disability.
• Patient will identify changes in usual communication, motor, and socialization skills.
• Patient will state a desire to regain age-appropriate skills and behaviors to the extent possible.
• Patient will demonstrate age-appropriate skills and behaviors to the extent possible.
• Patient and family members will agree to seek help from peer support groups or professional counselors to increase adaptive coping behaviors.

Interventions and rationales
• Spend specified amount of uninterrupted non-care-related time, perhaps 10 minutes twice daily, using active listening to encourage patient to express concerns. *Active listening, which includes attentive involvement and openness to patient's concerns without interpretation, allows patient to reveal concerns at own pace.*
• Urge patient to identify normal skills and behaviors and then describe how they could be altered in light of current disability. *Self-monitoring helps patient identify normal behaviors and relate behavioral changes to specific variables.*
• Instruct patient on age-appropriate skills and behaviors (chronologic and developmental) and request feedback on possible ways for patient to regain as many as possible. *This helps patient to recognize regressive behavior and noncompliance and to adjust accordingly.*
• Give patient positive reinforcement for demonstrating appropriate skills and behaviors *to promote similar behavior in future.*
• Tell patient and family members about social and professional support available, and advise about benefits of

using services after discharge. *This encourages patient to seek help from available resources.*

Evaluations for expected outcomes
• Patient expresses concerns about physical disability.
• Patient provides information about usual abilities and behaviors and reports changes seen as result of current situation (specify).
• Patient expresses a desire to regain appropriate skills and behaviors (specify).
• As much as possible, patient demonstrates age-appropriate skills and behavior.
• Patient and caregiver describe plans for participating in support groups after discharge.

Documentation
• Assessment of observed deviations from norm for patient's age-group
• Patient's report of concern about disability
• Interventions performed to assist patient in regaining age-appropriate skills and behaviors
• Patient's response to nursing interventions
• Evaluations for expected outcomes

■ Health maintenance alteration

related to lack of motor skills

Definition
Inability to maintain a healthy state

Assessment
• Neuromuscular status, including muscle strength and mass, gross and fine motor skills, joint mobility, and electromyelogram and electroencephalogram
• Abilities and limitations, including turning, transferring, ambulating, wheelchair use, driving, and activities of daily living
• Knowledge of health practices, including body maintenance, preventive health needs, health team follow-up, and safety measures
• Psychosocial support, including lifestyle, communication status (verbal, nonverbal, phone, and written), family members, and finances

Defining characteristics
• History of lack of health-seeking behaviors
• Impaired personal support systems
• Inability to take responsibility for meeting basic health needs
• Interest in improving health behaviors
• Lack of adaptive behaviors to internal or external changes
• Lack of knowledge regarding basic health practices
• Lack of necessary equipment or financial and other resources

Associated medical diagnoses (selected)
Amyotrophic lateral sclerosis, cerebrovascular accident, multiple sclerosis, muscular dystrophy, paralysis, spinal cord injury

Expected outcomes
• Patient will identify necessary health maintenance activities.
• Patient will make decisions about daily schedule.
• Patient will perform health maintenance activities according to level of ability (specify).
• Patient will communicate understanding of necessity for continuous self-monitoring of body functions.
• Patient will maintain muscle strength and joint mobility.

• Patient will demonstrate specific motor skills such as brushing teeth.
• Family members will demonstrate skill in carrying out activities patient can't perform.
• Patient will identify community and social resources available to help with health maintenance.

Interventions and rationales
• Discuss health maintenance needs with patient while carrying out routine activities *to reinforce their importance.*
• Involve patient in decision making by allowing choices in determining where, when, and how activities are to be carried out. Ask, for example, "Would you like a bath or shower in the morning or evening?" *Participation in decision making increases feelings of independence.*
• Help patient perform health maintenance activities, such as daily skin inspection and weekly catheterization for residual urine. *Encouraging skill development in patient promotes continued use of those skills after discharge.*
• Instruct patient in specific skills needed in monitoring health status *to prompt participation in self-care.* Allow patient to carry out skills *to encourage independence.*
• Perform or help patient perform passive and active range-of-motion exercises *to help maintain joint mobility and muscle strength.*
• Identify level of mobility (independent in feeding and bathing; needs assistance to brush teeth; dependent in use of wheelchair) and communicate skill level to all personnel *to provide continuity and preserve level of independence.*
• Educate family members in skills that patient can't perform unassisted, such as bathing, maintaining hygiene,

driving to appointments, transferring, or using walker. *This allows patient and family members to take active role in care.*
• Consult with social services or other health team members to identify health resources (for example, Meals On Wheels or homemaker services), and help patient contact and arrange for follow-up. *These resources can help patient maintain independence after discharge.*

Evaluations for expected outcomes
• Patient identifies health maintenance activities.
• Patient plans daily schedule.
• Patient's functional level is appropriate to capability level.
• Patient communicates understanding of importance of monitoring body functions, such as blood glucose levels, blood pressure, and pulse rate.
• Patient maintains muscle strength and joint mobility.
• Patient demonstrates motor skills correctly without prompting.
• Family members demonstrate skill in carrying out activities patient can't perform.
• Patient identifies and contacts community resources to assist with health maintenance, if needed.

Documentation
• Patient's identified health needs and perceptions and limitations in achieving them
• Patient's willingness to make decisions and participate in health maintenance activities
• Observations of motor abilities, level of skill performance, and health status
• Patient's response to nursing interventions
• Evaluations for expected outcomes

■ Health maintenance alteration

related to perceptual or cognitive impairment

Definition
Inability to maintain a healthy state

Assessment
• Age
• Current health status
• History of neurologic, sensory, or psychological impairment
• Neurologic status, including level of consciousness, orientation, cognition (memory, insight, and judgment), sensory ability, and motor ability
• Personal habits, such as smoking and alcohol consumption
• Psychosocial status, including support systems, personality, coping mechanisms, drug use, and communication status (verbal, nonverbal, phone, or written)

Defining characteristics
• History of lack of health-seeking behaviors
• Impaired personal support systems
• Inability to take responsibility for meeting basic health needs
• Interest in improving health behaviors
• Lack of adaptive behaviors to internal or external changes
• Lack of knowledge regarding basic health practices
• Lack of necessary equipment or financial and other resources

Associated medical diagnoses (selected)
Alzheimer's disease, bipolar disease (depressive phase), cataracts, chronic obstructive pulmonary disease, drug addiction, Huntington's disease, hypochondriasis, schizophrenia

Expected outcomes
• Patient will maintain current health status.
• Patient will sustain no harm or injury.
• Patient and family members will verbalize feelings and concerns.
• Patient and family members will explain health maintenance program.
• Patient and family members will demonstrate health maintenance program.
• Patient and family members will identify health resources available.
• Patient and family members will demonstrate appropriate coping skills.

Interventions and rationales
• Determine patient's capability to maintain health, degree of support available from family or others, degree of motivation, and level of dependence. Report any changes. *Comprehensive assessment provides a basis for evaluating future functional changes.*
• Perform prescribed treatment for condition causing perceptual or cognitive impairment. Monitor progress and report favorable and adverse responses. *Evaluating patient's responses to treatment and collaborating with doctor foster appropriate care planning.*
• Help patient and family members identify strengths and weaknesses in maintaining health (such as self-care deficits) *to provide focus for interventions.* Also help family members communicate with patient and understand what patient's behaviors mean. *This reduces patient's feelings of helplessness and gives a sense of control over situation.*
• Plan a health maintenance program with patient and family members, addressing current disabilities.

– Reorient patient as often as necessary *to enhance reality testing and mental status.* Adapt environment to appear somewhat familiar to patient. Display such personal objects as pictures and clocks from patient's home.

– Provide a structured care program in writing *to give patient sense of security.*

– Have same person provide care on an ongoing basis *to provide stability.*

– Fully describe all aspects of care to patient and family members *to elicit patient's cooperation.*

– When discussing care, give short, simple explanations geared to patient's level of understanding *to enhance cooperation.*

– If possible, prepare patient for any unexpected change *to minimize disruption.*

– Provide ample time for patient to perform health maintenance tasks *to reduce frustration and encourage success.*

• Instruct family members to carry out health maintenance practices. Demonstrate such necessary skills as bathing, feeding, and reality orientation; then have family members perform them under supervision. *Involving family members allows them to solve problems with supervision and support.*

• Instruct family members on how to maintain a safe environment *to reduce risk of patient injury.*

• Encourage patient and family members to verbalize feelings and concerns related to health maintenance *to help them develop greater understanding and better manage their health.*

• Help family members develop coping skills necessary to deal with patient. *If patient's illness is prolonged, family members could develop maladaptive coping strategies.*

• Help family members identify available social and community resources, such as stroke support group and Alzheimer's family support group. *This helps them gain social support and factual information and allows them to express feelings associated with patient's disorder.*

• Make referrals, as appropriate, to psychiatric liaison nurse and social services *to help prevent burnout among family members.*

Evaluations for expected outcomes
• Patient maintains health.
• Patient doesn't show signs of injury.
• Patient discusses impact of illness and self-care needs on others' lives. Family members voice feelings about patient's illness.
• Patient and family members state at least three health maintenance strategies.
• Patient performs health maintenance practices to extent possible. Family members assist patient as needed.
• Patient and family members identify and contact sources of support.
• Patient copes with current situation without experiencing severe emotional upset. Family members also display effective coping.

Documentation
• Expressions of concern by patient and family members about patient's inability to maintain health
• Observations of patient's impaired ability to perform self-care and response to treatment
• Patient's response to nursing interventions
• Instructions given to patient and family members, their level of understanding, and demonstrated skill in carrying out health maintenance program

• Referrals made for patient and family members
• Evaluations for expected outcomes

■ Health-seeking behaviors

related to absence of aerobic exercise as a risk factor for coronary artery disease

Definition
State in which a patient in stable health actively seeks ways to alter personal health habits or the environment in order to move toward optimal health

Assessment
• Risk factor analysis, including age, sex, cholesterol level, personal or family history of diabetes, ratio of high-density lipoprotein to low-density lipoprotein, blood pressure, weight, level of exercise, history of smoking, and stressors
• Current health status
• Psychosocial status, including lifestyle and motivation
• Recognition and realization of potential growth, health, and autonomy
• Understanding of risk modification

Defining characteristics
• Desire for increased control of health practice
• Desire to seek higher level of wellness
• Expressed concern about effect of environmental conditions on health status
• Lack of knowledge about behaviors that promote health
• Unfamiliarity with wellness community resources

Associated medical diagnoses (selected)
This diagnosis may coincide with any medical diagnosis, depending on patient and reasons for health visit.

Expected outcomes
• Patient will communicate understanding of benefits of aerobic exercise program.
• Patient will state guidelines for aerobic exercise.
• Patient will develop exercise routine.
• Patient will state proper target heart rate to achieve during exercise (60% to 80% of 220, minus patient's age).
• Patient will demonstrate ability to take pulse accurately.

Interventions and rationales
• Discuss benefits of regular exercise on cardiovascular and respiratory systems and on mental health status *to introduce patient to various benefits of exercise program.*
• Review basic components of aerobic exercise routine, including:
– frequency (minimum of three times weekly)
– duration (minimum of 20 minutes, not including 5 to 10 minutes of warm-up and cool-down)
– intensity (workload should progress only according to perceived exertion and target heart rate).
This informs patient of minimum requirements needed to get aerobic benefit from exercise program.
• Discuss aerobic activities, such as walking, jogging, swimming, cycling, and rowing. *Patient must build individualized program around enjoyable activity that meets aerobic criteria.*
• Recommend that patient consult with doctor before starting exercise program *so patient can have exercise stress test, if necessary, and receive*

medical clearance for exercise program.
• Recommend either a supervised or unsupervised exercise program, depending on patient's motivation to continue program. *Supervised program may help less motivated patients.*
• Review warm-up and cool-down techniques, *which prevent abrupt changes in heart rate,* and stretching muscles *to avoid injuries and an overworked heart.*
• Teach patient how to take his own pulse, and monitor accuracy. *Patient must know how to take pulse to maintain correct heart rate range.*
• Instruct patient to notify doctor of any adverse symptoms experienced while exercising *to detect any adverse effects early.*
• Provide patient with literature on exercise guidelines and community exercise programs *to reinforce teaching and provide references following discharge.*

Evaluations for expected outcomes
• Patient lists several benefits of aerobic exercise program.
• Patient outlines basic aerobic exercise program.
• Patient provides example of individualized exercise routine.
• Patient states personal target heart rate range.
• Patient demonstrates accurate pulse-taking techniques.

Documentation
• Patient's expression of concern about promoting a higher level of wellness
• Patient's response to nursing interventions
• Instructions given and patient's understanding of instructions

• Patient's plan of exercise after discharge from hospital
• Patient's ability to take and record pulse
• Literature provided and referrals made to resources in the community
• Evaluations for expected outcomes

■ Health-seeking behaviors

related to elevated serum cholesterol level as a risk factor for coronary artery disease

Definition
State in which a patient in stable health actively seeks ways to alter personal health habits or the environment in order to move toward optimal health

Assessment
• Risk factor analysis, including age, sex, cholesterol level, personal or family history of diabetes, ratio of high-density lipoprotein (HDL) to low-density lipoprotein (LDL), blood pressure, weight, level of exercise, history of smoking, and stressors
• Current health status
• Psychosocial status, including lifestyle and motivation
• Recognition and realization of potential growth, health, and autonomy
• Understanding of risk modification

Defining characteristics
• Desire for increased control over health practices
• Desire to seek higher level of wellness
• Expressed concern about effect of environmental conditions on health status

• Lack of knowledge about behaviors that promote health
• Unfamiliarity with wellness community resources

Associated medical diagnoses (selected)

This diagnosis may coincide with any medical diagnosis, depending on patient and reasons for health visit.

Expected outcomes

• Patient will state personal cholesterol level.
• Patient will report that elevated cholesterol level is risk factor for coronary artery disease.
• Patient will state appropriate dietary intake of fat and cholesterol to reduce cholesterol level.
• Patient will identify ways to decrease cholesterol level.
• Patient's cholesterol level will decline to desired level.
• Patient will not develop illness, or signs and symptoms of disease will be controlled.

Interventions and rationales

• Discuss patient's cholesterol level and HDL-LDL ratio *to inform patient of desirable results.*
• Discuss patient's understanding of cholesterol and its sources *to increase understanding of intrinsic and extrinsic sources and connection between high levels and coronary disease.*
• Discuss ways to lower cholesterol level *to encourage compliance with postdischarge diet plan.*
• Provide literature on cholesterol *to reinforce teaching after discharge.*
• Have patient meet with dietitian *to correct any dietary imbalances and reinforce healthy eating habits.*
• Review outside resources available to patient *to provide follow-up and reinforcement after discharge.*

• Review patient's dietary habits, foods high in cholesterol and saturated fats, and importance of adhering to a low-cholesterol, low-fat diet *to reinforce dietary teaching and healthy eating habits.*

Evaluations for expected outcomes

• Patient states cholesterol level.
• Patient states that elevated cholesterol level is risk factor for coronary artery disease.
• Patient communicates understanding of how diet affects cholesterol level.
• Patient describes other factors such as exercise that can decrease cholesterol level.
• Follow-up laboratory tests reveal reduction in patient's serum cholesterol level.
• Patient doesn't exhibit signs or symptoms of disease associated with elevated cholesterol level.

Documentation

• Patient's expression of concern about promoting a higher level of wellness
• Patient's response to nursing interventions
• Instructions provided and patient's understanding of instructions
• Literature recommended or provided to patient
• Evaluations for expected outcomes

■ Health-seeking behaviors

related to hypertension as a risk factor for coronary artery disease

Definition

State in which a patient in stable health actively seeks ways to alter

personal health habits or the environment in order to move toward optimal health

Assessment
• Risk factor analysis, including age, sex, cholesterol level, personal or family history of diabetes, ratio of high-density lipoprotein to low-density lipoprotein, blood pressure, weight, level of exercise, history of smoking, and stressors
• Current health status
• Psychosocial status, including lifestyle and motivation
• Recognition and realization of potential growth, health, and autonomy
• Understanding of risk modification

Defining characteristics
• Desire for increased control over health practices
• Desire to seek higher level of wellness
• Expressed concern about effect of environmental conditions on health status
• Lack of knowledge about behaviors that promote health
• Unfamiliarity with wellness community resources

Associated medical diagnoses (selected)
This diagnosis may coincide with any medical diagnosis, depending on patient and reasons for health visit.

Expected outcomes
• Patient will express interest in learning new behaviors to help reduce blood pressure.
• Patient will state that hypertension is a risk factor for coronary artery disease.
• Patient will identify and demonstrate appropriate interventions for lowering blood pressure.
• Patient will state own blood pressure range.
• Patient will express and demonstrate appropriate dietary measures used to reduce high blood pressure.
• Patient will maintain blood pressure within desired limits.
• Patient will not develop illness, or signs and symptoms of disease will be controlled.

Interventions and rationales
• Discuss patient's understanding of hypertension and how it affects the body. Clarify any misconceptions. *This increases patient's awareness of hypertension's dangers.*
• Inform patient of blood pressure reading each time it's taken *to reinforce acceptable range and give patient responsibility for maintaining it.*
• Provide patient with pamphlets on hypertension *for reinforcement and easy reference after discharge.*
• Encourage patient to continue prescribed antihypertensives, as ordered, *to control blood pressure.*
• Teach patient how to monitor own blood pressure *to help maintain normal pressure.*
• Instruct patient on methods to lower blood pressure *using simple exercise and dietary guidelines.*
• Have patient meet with dietitian *to discuss low-sodium diet, assess eating habits, and make appropriate modifications.*

Evaluations for expected outcomes
• Patient expresses desire to control blood pressure.
• Patient communicates that hypertension is a risk factor for coronary artery disease.
• Patient reports at least three methods to help control blood pressure.
• Patient states blood pressure range.

• Patient demonstrates use of appropriate dietary measures to reduce high blood pressure.
• Patient's blood pressure remains within desired limits.
• Patient doesn't exhibit signs or symptoms of disease associated with hypertension.

Documentation
• Patient's expression of concern about promoting a higher level of wellness
• Patient's response to nursing interventions
• Instructions provided and patient's understanding of instructions
• Literature recommended or provided to patient
• Referrals made to community resources
• Evaluations for expected outcomes

■ Health-seeking behaviors

related to smoking as a risk factor for coronary artery disease

Definition
State in which a patient in stable health actively seeks ways to alter personal health habits or the environment in order to move toward optimal health

Assessment
• Risk factor analysis, including age, sex, cholesterol level, ratio of high-density lipoprotein to low-density lipoprotein, blood pressure, weight, level of exercise, history of smoking, and stressors
• Current health status
• Psychosocial status, including lifestyle and motivation

• Recognition and realization of potential growth, health, and autonomy
• Understanding of risk modification

Defining characteristics
• Desire for increased control over health practices
• Desire to seek higher level of wellness
• Expressed concern about effect of environmental conditions on health status
• Lack of knowledge about behaviors that promote health
• Unfamiliarity with wellness community resources

Associated medical diagnoses (selected)
This diagnosis may coincide with any medical diagnosis, depending on patient and reasons for health visit.

Expected outcomes
• Patient will state need to stop or decrease smoking.
• Patient will state hazards of smoking and how it affects body.
• Patient will understand ways to stop or decrease smoking.
• Patient will choose which smoking cessation alternative to implement.
• Patient will stop smoking or enter a program to stop smoking.
• Patient will not develop illness, or signs and symptoms of disease will be controlled.

Interventions and rationales
• Determine patient's capability and motivation to promote a higher level of wellness. *Patient can't be forced to change; he must have inherent desire.*
• Discuss with patient hazards of smoking *to emphasize nicotine's long-term detriment to body.* Support behavior change.
• Assess patient's understanding of how smoking affects the body (blood

pressure, cholesterol, clotting, and heart rate). Clarify any misconceptions. *This reinforces patient's desire to change behavior.*
• Emphasize benefits of stopping smoking *to reinforce behavior changes.*
• Review with patient past methods used to decrease or stop smoking (successful or not) *to discover most effective methods for patient.*
• Suggest ways for patient to decrease or stop smoking:
– List reasons to stop.
– Set dates to stop.
– Get support.
– Switch brands.
– Cut down on number smoked.
– Perform alternative activities.
– Ask doctor about pharmacologic interventions such as nicotine patch. *These suggestions provide patient with practical measures he can implement.*
• Provide literature on smoking cessation *to reinforce teaching and provide easy reference after discharge.*
• Discuss resources available *to support patient's attempts to stop smoking after discharge.*

Evaluations for expected outcomes
• Patient voices desire to stop or decrease smoking.
• Patient lists several hazards associated with smoking.
• Patient lists several options for assistance with efforts to stop smoking (such as self-help group, smoking cessation class, and hypnosis).
• Patient chooses method to stop smoking and signs a self-contract (including rewards for smoking cessation) to commit to program.
• Patient implements chosen option to stop smoking.

• Patient is free of signs and symptoms of disorders associated with smoking.

Documentation
• Patient's expression of concern about promoting a higher level of wellness
• Patient's response to nursing interventions
• Instructions provided and patient's understanding of instructions
• Referrals made to smoking cessation programs available in hospital and community
• Evaluations for expected outcomes

■ Health-seeking behaviors

related to stress as a risk factor for coronary artery disease

Definition
State in which a patient in stable health actively seeks ways to alter personal health habits or the environment in order to move toward optimal health

Assessment
• Risk factor analysis, including age, sex, cholesterol level, ratio of high-density lipoprotein to low-density lipoprotein, blood pressure, weight, level of exercise, history of smoking, and stressors
• Current health status
• Psychosocial status, including lifestyle and motivation
• Recognition and realization of potential growth, health, and autonomy
• Understanding of risk modification

Defining characteristics
- Desire for increased control over health practices
- Desire to seek higher level of wellness
- Expressed concern about effect of environmental conditions on health status
- Lack of knowledge about behaviors that promote health
- Unfamiliarity with wellness community resources

Associated medical diagnoses (selected)
This diagnosis may coincide with any medical diagnosis, depending on patient and the circumstances of hospitalization.

Expected outcomes
- Patient will state that stress is a risk factor for coronary artery disease.
- Patient will identify and list factors that create stress in life.
- Patient will voice understanding of how stress affects body.
- Patient will state ways to maximize positive aspects and minimize negative aspects of stress.

Interventions and rationales
- Inform patient that stress is a risk factor for many major health problems, including coronary artery disease. *Patient may not know that stress can contribute to disease and death.*
- Review stressors in patient's personal and professional life and mechanisms used to cope with them. *This increases patient's awareness of stressors and provides baseline for stress management tools.*
- Discuss how stress affects patient's body and how decreasing stress changes these effects. *This encourages patient to manage stress as a way to improve quality of life.*

- Discuss difference between type A and type B personalities. *Type A and B behaviors define personality type and provide framework for dealing with stress.*
- Discuss with patient stress management techniques, including:
  – perceiving situation differently
  – managing time
  – taking a mental health day or evening periodically
  – practicing relaxation techniques
  – being assertive when faced with unreasonable demands
  – improving self-image and self-esteem
  – exercising
  – facing problems and discussing alternatives with family or friends
  – setting realistic goals
  – relaxing standards of living.
  These measures provide tools to manage stress.
- Review available community resources for stress management and provide literature *to reinforce teaching after discharge.*

Evaluations for expected outcomes
- Patient states that stress contributes to coronary artery disease.
- Patient identifies habits and situations that create stress.
- Patient identifies physiologic responses to stress.
- Patient states methods to minimize harmful stressors and ways to cope better with daily stress.

Documentation
- Patient's expression of concern about promoting a higher level of wellness
- Patient's response to nursing interventions
- Instructions provided and patient's understanding of instructions

• Referrals made and literature provided about stress management courses available in community
• Evaluations for expected outcomes

■ Home maintenance management impairment

related to inadequate support system

Definition
Insufficient resources available to meet self-care needs adequately and safely in patient's home

Assessment
• Psychosocial status
• Support systems, including family in the home, close friends, and organizations with which patient is affiliated; if patient lives alone, access to family, friends, and pets
• Financial resources
• Home environment
• Patient's and family members' knowledge of disease and self-care requirements

Defining characteristics
• Household disrepair, marked by excessive clutter, unwashed clothing and cooking equipment, offensive odors, presence of rodents and insects, accumulation of dirt and food wastes, and inappropriate temperature
• Outstanding debts or financial crisis
• Difficulty in maintaining a comfortable home
• Request for assistance with home maintenance
• Lack of necessary equipment or aids
• Overtaxed family members

Associated medical diagnoses (selected)
This diagnosis may coincide with any medical diagnosis and frequently occurs in geriatric or impoverished patients.

Expected outcomes
• Patient and family members will express need to make adjustments in home to help manage patient's condition.
• Patient and family members will identify individuals or organizations that may provide assistance.

Interventions and rationales
• Help patient and family members explore available resources *to help identify discharge problems and ease transition from hospital to home.*
• Provide sufficient information to patient and family members *to ensure knowledge necessary for them to make appropriate decisions.*
• Refer patient to social service department, *which can assist with follow-up care after discharge.*
• Suggest referral to home health agency, homemaker service, Meals On Wheels, or other appropriate outside agencies for assistance and follow-up. *Patient may need a range of community services to meet various needs.*

Evaluations for expected outcomes
• Patient and family members describe changes needed to promote maximum health and safety at home.
• Patient and family members list agencies that can assist with home care.

Documentation
• Patient's and family members' perception of problem
• Observations regarding problem's magnitude

• Interventions performed to alleviate problem
• Responses of others asked to assist with problem
• Evaluations for expected outcomes

■ Home maintenance management impairment

related to impaired cognitive or emotional functioning

Definition
Inability to meet self-care needs adequately because of cognitive or emotional dysfunction of patient or family member

Assessment
• Home environment
• Financial resources
• Patient's and family's knowledge of self-care requirements
• Patient's and family's psychological status, including perception of reality, communication patterns, assignment of responsibilities, degree of awareness and concern, and history of psychiatric illness
• Drug or alcohol abuse
• Support systems, including close friends, organizations with which patient is affiliated, and community resources

Defining characteristics
• Household disrepair, marked by excessive clutter, unwashed clothing and cooking equipment, offensive odors, presence of rodents and insects, accumulation of dirt and food wastes, and inappropriate temperature
• Outstanding debts or financial crisis
• Difficulty in maintaining a comfortable home

• Request for assistance with home maintenance
• Lack of necessary equipment or aids
• Overtaxed family members

Associated medical diagnoses (selected)
Alzheimer's disease, antisocial personality disorder, anxiety disorder, bipolar disorder (manic phase), cerebrovascular accident, chronic obstructive pulmonary disease, delusional disorder, depression, dissociative disorder, heart failure, multiple personality disorder, obsessive-compulsive disorder, schizophrenia

Expected outcomes
• Patient and family members will express concern about poor home maintenance.
• Patient and family members will verbalize plan to correct health and safety hazards in home.
• Patient and family members will identify community resources available to help maintain home.

Interventions and rationales
• Discuss obstacles to effective home maintenance management with patient and family *to develop understanding of potential and actual health and safety hazards.*
• Help family members assign responsibilities for household care and establish appropriate expectations *to aid communication and help set realistic goals.*
• Help family members establish daily and weekly home maintenance activities and assignments *to impose structure on family's routine and set standards for measuring progress.*
• Encourage weekly discussions about progress in maintaining home maintenance schedule *to develop family unity and allow members to address*

problems before they become over-whelming.

• Help family members contact community resources that can assist them in their efforts to improve home maintenance management, such as self-help groups, cleaning services, and exterminators. *Community resources can lessen family's burden while members learn to function independently.*

Evaluations for expected outcomes

• Patient and family members establish and follow daily and weekly schedule for home management.
• With the help of appropriate community resources as needed, patient and family members clear home of clutter, debris, and waste.
• Patient and family members contact community resources.

Documentation

• Patient's and family members' expressions of difficulty in maintaining household
• Patient's and family members' mental status
• Presence of health hazards, such as filth, rodents, and waste matter
• Presence of safety hazards such as faulty wiring
• Presence of offensive odors
• Patient's and family members' understanding of home maintenance management and resources
• Interventions to improve home maintenance skills
• Patient's and family members' responses to nursing interventions
• Evaluations for expected outcomes

■ Hopelessness

related to chronic illness

Definition

Subjective state in which an individual sees few or no available alternatives or personal choices and can't mobilize energy on own behalf

Assessment

• Nature of chronic illness
• Patient's and family members' knowledge of illness
• Mental status, including cognitive functioning, affect, mood, and stage in grieving process
• Communication, including verbal (speech content, quality, and quantity), nonverbal (body positioning, eye contact, and facial expression), and quality of interactions with others
• Nutritional status, including alteration in appetite or body weight
• Motivation level, including personal hygiene, therapies (physical and occupational), use of diversional activities, and sense of control over current life situation
• Developmental stage, including age and role in family
• Disruption in usual roles and activities and losses (real and perceived)
• Actual or perceived self-care deficits (specify)
• Number and types of stressors
• Coping mechanisms and decision-making ability
• Support systems, including clergy, family, and friends
• Spiritual values or religious beliefs

Defining characteristics

• Decreased affect
• Decreased appetite
• Decreased response to stimuli
• Decreased verbalization

- Increased or decreased sleep
- Lack of involvement in self-care
- Nonverbal cues, such closing eyes, shrugging in response to questions, and turning away from speaker
- Passivity and lack of initiative
- Verbal cues, including sighing and despondent comments such as "I can't"

Associated medical diagnoses (selected)

Affective disorders, Alzheimer's disease, bipolar disorder (depressive phase), chronic bronchitis, chronic fatigue syndrome, chronic obstructive pulmonary disease, chronic pain, cor pulmonale, Cushing's syndrome, depression, diabetes mellitus, emphysema, heart failure, long-term disability, lupus erythematosus, paralysis, Parkinson's disease, schizophrenia, spinal cord injury

Expected outcomes

- Patient will express feelings of hopelessness.
- Patient will recognize and accept limitations of chronic illness.
- Patient will work through stages of grief.
- Patient will develop coping mechanisms to deal with feelings of hopelessness.
- Patient will recognize benefit of positive social interactions.
- Patient will participate in self-care activities and in decisions regarding care planning.
- Patient will resume and maintain as many former roles as possible.
- Patient will regain and maintain self-esteem.
- Patient will begin to develop feelings of hope.

Interventions and rationales

- Assess for evidence of self-destructive behavior. *Assessment for suicide*

potential in a depressed patient is a nursing care priority.
- If possible, assign a primary nurse to patient *to encourage establishment of a therapeutic relationship between patient and nurse.*
- Allow for specific amount of uninterrupted, non-care-related time each shift to talk with patient. Encourage verbal response with open-ended statements and questions. If patient chooses not to talk, spend time in silence. *This establishes rapport with depressed patient even if patient talks little.*
- Provide for appropriate physical outlets for expression of feelings (punching bag, walking) *to help patient release hostilities, thereby decreasing tension and anxiety.*
- Convey belief in patient's ability to develop and use coping skills *to increase patient's self-esteem and reduce feelings of dependence.*
- Acknowledge patient's pain. Encourage patient to express feelings of depression, anger, guilt, and sadness. Convey to patient that all these feelings are appropriate. *This will help patient work through stages of coming to terms with chronic illness.*
- Identify patient's strengths and encourage putting strengths to use *to maintain optimal functioning.*
- Encourage patient's participation in self-care to fullest extent possible *to reduce feelings of helplessness.*
- Help patient to participate in usual activities as strength, energy, and time permit. *Patient needs to maintain a sense of being connected to others.*
- Encourage patient to identify enjoyable diversions and to participate in them *to decrease negative thinking and enhance self-esteem.*
- Encourage positive thinking. Convey a sense of confidence in patient's

ability to cope with illness *to promote an optimistic outlook.*
• Provide positive reinforcement for patient's efforts to participate in self-care activities *to encourage patient to participate in self-care.* Encourage patient to establish self-care schedule *to enhance feelings of usefulness and control.*
• Assist patient with hygiene and grooming needs *to help enhance patient's self-esteem.*
• Offer patient and family a realistic assessment of situation, and communicate hope for immediate future. *This facilitates acceptance, helps promote patient safety and security, and allows planning of future health care.*
• Encourage patient to identify spiritual needs and facilitate fulfillment of those needs *to help patient come to terms with chronic illness and its limitations.*
• Involve patient and family members in care planning, and allow patient to choose degree of self-involvement on a continuing basis. Begin by offering patient a choice between two alternatives. Increase alternatives as initiative improves. *Cognitive disturbances associated with anxiety or depression often prevent patient from making healthy decisions.*
• Teach patient and family members how to manage illness, prevent complications, and control factors in the environment that affect patient's health. *Education enables family members to become resources in patient's care.*
• Refer patient and family members to other caregivers (such as dietitian, social worker, clergyman, and mental health clinical nurse specialist) or support groups as necessary. *Referrals to outside specialists ensure continuity of care. Support groups give*

patient chance to discuss illness with others similarly affected.

Evaluations for expected outcomes
• Patient talks about negative feelings instead of acting on them.
• Patient expresses understanding of lifestyle changes imposed by chronic illness.
• Patient discusses impact of illness and sees the future realistically.
• Patient demonstrates at least ___(specify) coping mechanisms.
• Patient interacts with others and regains involvement in life experiences.
• Patient demonstrates understanding that involvement in self-care is necessary to maintain optimal functioning.
• Patient demonstrates involvement in as many former roles as possible.
• Patient acknowledges a belief in self and demonstrates increased energy and will to live.
• Patient states that feelings of hopelessness are less frequent and expresses feelings of hope.

Documentation
• Patient's perception of chronic illness
• Patient's responses to treatment regimen
• Patient's mental and emotional status (baseline and ongoing)
• Patient education, counseling, and precautions taken to maintain or enhance patient's level of functioning
• Interventions to help patient deal with daily stressors
• Interventions to protect patient from harming self
• Patient's response to nursing interventions
• Evaluations for expected outcomes

■ Hopelessness

related to failing or deteriorating physiologic condition

Definition
Subjective state in which an individual sees few or no available alternatives or personal choices and can't mobilize energy on own behalf

Assessment
• Nature of current medical diagnosis
• Patient's and family members' knowledge of diagnosis and prognosis
• Actual or perceived self-care deficits (specify)
• Mental status, including cognitive functioning, affect, and mood
• Communication, including verbal (speech content, quality, and quantity) and nonverbal (body positioning, eye contact, and facial expression)
• Available support systems, including clergy, family, and friends
• Past experience with loss, including body part or function, death, residence, and employment
• Coping mechanisms and decision-making ability
• Nutritional status, including alteration in appetite or body weight
• Sleep pattern
• Motivation level for personal hygiene, therapies (physical and occupational therapy), and diversional activities
• Developmental stage (Erikson's model), including age and role in family

Defining characteristics
• Decreased affect
• Decreased appetite
• Decreased response to stimuli
• Decreased verbalization
• Increased or decreased sleep
• Lack of involvement in self-care
• Nonverbal cues, such closing eyes, shrugging in response to questions, and turning away from speaker
• Passivity and lack of initiative
• Verbal cues, including sighing and despondent comments such as "I can't"

Associated medical diagnoses (selected)
Acquired immunodeficiency syndrome, amyotrophic lateral sclerosis, cerebrovascular accident, degenerative disease, diabetes insipidus, end-stage disease (cardiac or renal), hyperparathyroidism, leukemia, lymphomas, muscular dystrophy

Expected outcomes
• Patient will identify feelings of hopelessness regarding current situation.
• Patient will demonstrate more effective communication skills, including direct verbal responses to questions and increased eye contact.
• Patient will resume appropriate rest and activity pattern.
• Patient will participate in self-care activities and in decisions regarding care planning.
• Patient will use diversional activities (specify).
• Patient will identify factors that make him feel more hopeful.
• Patient will identify social and community resources for continued assistance.

Interventions and rationales
• Follow medical regimen *to manage patient's physiologic condition and increase potential for patient's physiologic recovery.*
• Allow specific amount of uninterrupted, non-care-related time each shift to talk with patient. If patient

chooses not to talk, spend time in silence. *This time together establishes rapport with depressed patient even if patient talks little.*
• Encourage patient to talk about personal assets and accomplishments and about improvements in condition, no matter how small. Give positive feedback. *Conversation helps you evaluate patient's self-concept and adaptive abilities; positive feedback reinforces patient's healthy perceptions.*
• Direct patient's focus beyond current state. For example, "Your nasogastric tube will come out tomorrow and you'll feel more comfortable." *This helps instill hope in a depressed patient with no time perspective.*
• Encourage patient to identify enjoyable diversions and to participate in them. *Pleasurable activity decreases potential hazard of crisis situation.*
• Keep patient informed of what to expect and when to expect it. *Accurate information reduces patient's anxiety.*
• Involve patient and family members in care planning, and allow patient to choose degree of self-involvement. Begin by offering patient a choice between two alternatives. Increase alternatives as initiative improves. *Cognitive disturbances associated with anxiety or depression often prevent patient from making healthy decisions.*
• Use comfort measures (give back rub, dim room light, reduce noise level, and minimize procedures) in addition to prescribed sleep medication *to help induce sleep.*
• Refer patient and family members to other disciplines (such as dietitian, social worker, clergy, and mental health clinical nurse specialist) or support groups (such as I Can Cope, Ostomy Support Group, and Reach For Recovery) as necessary. *These groups give patient chance to discuss illness with others similarly afflicted.*
• Help patient mobilize resources before discharge, including contacting family and scheduling follow-up appointments with referral groups. *This helps give patient a sense of future direction.*
• If not contraindicated medically, allow patient to use therapies practiced in his culture in conjunction with normal treatment *to increase his sense of control.*

Evaluations for expected outcomes
• Patient voices feelings of hopelessness.
• Patient responds to questions and, at least once each day, participates in a conversation.
• Patient sleeps at least 6 hours per night and remains awake during day, except for two rest periods.
• Patient performs self-care measures and makes decisions related to care.
• Patient engages in diversional activity (specify) at least twice daily.
• Patient identifies factors that make him feel more hopeful (specify).
• Patient seeks out help from social support groups and professional agencies.

Documentation
• Patient's and family's knowledge of current condition
• Patient's mental status
• Patient's verbal and nonverbal behaviors
• Interventions to increase patient's feelings of hope, self-worth, and initiative in self-care
• Patient's and family's responses to nursing interventions
• Evaluations for expected outcomes

■ Hopelessness

related to prolonged activity restriction, creating isolation

Definition

Subjective state in which an individual sees few or no available alternatives or personal choices and can't mobilize energy on own behalf

Assessment

• Nature of illness or injury
• Activity or rest pattern before illness or injury
• Past experience with prolonged inactivity
• Actual or perceived self-care deficit (specify)
• Mental status, including affect, cognitive functioning, and mood
• Communication, including verbal (speech content, quality, and quantity) and nonverbal (body positioning, eye contact, and facial expression)

Defining characteristics

• Decreased affect
• Decreased appetite
• Decreased response to stimuli
• Decreased verbalization
• Increased or decreased sleep
• Lack of involvement in self-care
• Nonverbal cues, such as closing eyes, shrugging in response to questions, and turning away from speaker
• Passivity and lack of initiative
• Verbal cues, including sighing and despondent comments such as "I can't"

Associated medical diagnoses (selected)

Cardiovascular disease, long-term disability, orthopedic injuries requiring skeletal traction, prolonged hospitalization, pulmonary disease requiring ventilatory support, vertebral fracture requiring prolonged bed rest

Expected outcomes

• Patient will identify feelings of hopelessness regarding current situation.
• Patient will demonstrate more effective communication.
• Patient will initiate self-involvement in care.
• Patient will describe persons, events, and interventions that instill hope.
• Patient will join in diversional activities.
• Patient will resume appropriate sleep pattern and dietary intake.
• Patient will mobilize support systems as necessary.
• Patient will begin to make plans regarding activity after discharge.

Interventions and rationales

• Follow medical regimen *to manage patient's physiologic condition and increase potential for patient's physiologic recovery.*
• Visit frequently, allowing for specific amount of uninterrupted, non-care-related time each shift to talk with patient. Encourage verbal response with open-ended statements and questions. *This time together establishes rapport with depressed patient even if patient talks little.*
• Provide structured schedule of daily routine, including morning care, meals, therapies, and rest periods; post schedule within patient's range of vision. *A structured environment helps patient move beyond emotional self-absorption and focus on external factors.*
• Encourage patient's participation in self-care to extent possible *to reduce patient's feeling of helplessness.*

• Ask patient to identify support systems and enjoyable diversions, and encourage their use. *Supportive persons and pleasurable diversions decrease potential hazard of a crisis situation.*
• Ask family member to bring patient a few personal belongings from home, such as a radio, family photographs, clock, and pillow. *Familiar environment reduces patient's stress.*
• Assist patient with plans for resuming activity after discharge. *As feelings of hopelessness subside, patient will be more willing to discuss future plans.*

Evaluations for expected outcomes
• Patient voices feelings of hopelessness.
• Patient responds to questions and engages in conversation at least once daily.
• Patient performs self-care measures without prompting.
• Patient identifies factors that make him feel more hopeful (specify).
• Patient engages in diversional activity (specify) at least once daily.
• Patient sleeps at least 6 hours per night and maintains caloric intake appropriate for age and sex.
• Patient seeks out support persons or agencies for assistance.
• Patient discusses plans for resuming activity after discharge.

Documentation
• Patient's perception of current situation
• Patient's previous rest or activity pattern
• Patient's mental status
• Patient's verbal and nonverbal behavior
• Interventions to increase patient's hope, initiative, and involvement in self-care and diversional activities

• Patient's response to nursing interventions
• Evaluations for expected outcomes

■ Hyperthermia
related to dehydration

Definition
Elevation of body temperature above normal range

Assessment
• History of pathologic conditions known to cause dehydration, such as anorexia nervosa and infection
• Medications (diuretics, for example)
• Physiologic manifestations of fever, including pulse, respiration, and blood pressure
• Skin temperature, color, and turgor
• Fluid and electrolyte status, including blood urea nitrogen level, creatinine level, intake and output, mucous membranes, serum electrolyte levels, and urine specific gravity
• Neurologic status, including level of consciousness (LOC), mental status, and orientation
• Nutritional status, including current weight, dietary pattern, and normal weight
• Psychosocial status, including change in financial status, coping skills, and recent traumatic event

Defining characteristics
• Fever
• Flushed, warm skin
• Increased heart and respiratory rate
• Seizures

Associated medical diagnoses (selected)
Anorexia nervosa, bulimia nervosa, diabetes mellitus (uncontrolled), drug

overdose or toxicity, hyperthermia, pleural effusion

Expected outcomes
• Temperature will remain normal.
• Fluid balance will remain stable (intake approximately equals output).
• Patient will state increased comfort.
• Patient will not develop such complications as seizures.
• Patient will identify risk factors that exacerbate the problem.
• Patient will state measures to prevent dehydration.

Interventions and rationales
• Monitor body temperature every 4 hours or more often if indicated *to evaluate effectiveness of interventions.* Identify and record route *to ensure accurate data comparison.*
• Administer antipyretic medication as ordered *to reduce fever.* Record effectiveness.
• Employ measures to reduce excessive fever, such as removing blankets and placing loincloth over patient, applying ice bags to axilla and groin, sponging with tepid water, and using hypothermia blanket if temperature rises above 103° F (39.4° C). *These measures promote patient comfort and lower body temperature.*
• Monitor and record heart rate and rhythm, central venous pressure (CVP), blood pressure, respiratory rate, level of responsiveness, and skin temperature at least every 4 hours. *Increased heart rate, decreased CVP, and decreased blood pressure may indicate hypovolemia, which leads to decreased tissue perfusion. Cool and blanched or mottled skin may also indicate decreased tissue perfusion. Increased respiratory rate compensates for tissue hypoxia.*
• Observe patient for confusion or disorientation. Report changes to doc-

tor. *Changed LOC may result from tissue hypoxia.*
• Determine patient's preference for liquids (specify). *Offering patient liquids he prefers promotes adequate hydration.*
• Keep liquids at bedside and within reach *to allow patient easy access.*
• Treat patient for dehydration:
– Monitor and record intake and output accurately.
– Administer I.V. fluids as ordered. *These measures prevent excessive loss of water, sodium chloride, and potassium.*
• Discuss precipitating factors with patient, if known, *to develop recommendations for keeping cool and avoiding heat-related illnesses.*
• Encourage adherence to other aspects of health care management, including dietary habits *to help reduce fever.* Patient should drink plenty of fluids, such as water, fruit or vegetable juices, and decaffeinated beverages *to replace losses from sweating.*

Evaluations for expected outcomes
• Patient's temperature remains within normal range.
• Patient's fluid intake approximately equals output.
• Patient indicates increased comfort, through either verbal reports or behavior.
• Patient doesn't develop complications of hyperthermia.
• Patient lists risk factors that exacerbate hyperthermia.
• Patient identifies measures to prevent dehydration associated with hyperthermia.

Documentation
• Physical findings
• Nursing interventions carried out
• Effectiveness of medications

• Patient's response to nursing actions (behavioral, cognitive, and physiologic)
• Evaluations for expected outcomes

■ Hyperthermia

related to infection

Definition
Elevation of body temperature above normal range

Assessment
• History of present illness
• History of exposure to communicable disease
• Health history, including chronic disease or disability, pathologic conditions known to cause dehydration, recent traumatic event, exposure to sources of infection, exposure to communicable diseases, and other related events
• Medications
• Physiologic manifestations of fever, including vital signs and skin temperature and color
• Fluid and electrolyte status, including skin turgor, intake and output, mucous membranes, serum electrolyte levels, and urine specific gravity
• Laboratory studies, including white blood cell count and culture and sensitivity findings
• Neurologic status, including level of consciousness (LOC) and orientation
• Skin integrity, including open lesions and rashes

Defining characteristics
• Fever
• Flushed, warm skin
• Increased heart and respiratory rate
• Seizures

Associated medical diagnoses (selected)
Abnormal rupture of membranes, burns, encephalitis, food poisoning, hyperthermia, Lyme disease, meningitis, rheumatic fever, rubella, salmonella, scarlet fever, sepsis, streptococcal throat

Expected outcomes
• Patient will remain afebrile.
• Patient will maintain adequate hydration:
– Intake and output will be balanced and within normal limits.
– Urine specific gravity will range from 1.005 to 1.015.
• Patient will exhibit moist mucous membranes.
• Patient will exhibit good skin turgor.
• Patient will remain alert and responsive.

Interventions and rationales
• Take temperature every 1 to 4 hours *to obtain an accurate core temperature.* Identify route and record measurements.
• Administer antipyretic medication, as prescribed, and record effectiveness. *Antipyretics act on hypothalamus to regulate temperature.*
• Use nonpharmacologic measures to reduce excessive fever, such as removing sheets, blankets, and most clothing; placing ice bags on axillae and groin; and sponging with tepid water. Explain these measures to patient. *Nonpharmacologic measures lower body temperature and promote comfort. Sponging reduces body temperature by increasing evaporation from skin. Tepid water is used because cold water increases shivering, thereby increasing metabolic rate and causing temperature to rise.*
• Use hypothermia blanket if patient's temperature rises above 103° F (39.4° C). Monitor vital signs every 15 min-

utes for 1 hour and then as indicated. Turn off blanket if shivering occurs. *Shivering increases metabolic rate, increasing temperature.*

• Monitor heart rate and rhythm, blood pressure, respiratory rate, LOC and level of responsiveness, and capillary refill time every 1 to 4 hours *to evaluate effectiveness of interventions and monitor for complications.*

• Determine patient's preferences for oral fluids, and encourage patient to drink as much as possible, unless contraindicated. Monitor and record intake and output, and administer I.V. fluids if indicated. *Because insensible fluid loss increases by 10% for every 1° C increase in temperature, patient must increase fluid intake to prevent dehydration.*

Evaluations for expected outcomes

• Patient remains afebrile.
• Patient maintains adequate hydration:
– Intake and output are balanced and within normal limit for age.
– Urine specific gravity ranges from 1.005 to 1.015.
• Patient exhibits moist mucous membranes.
• Patient exhibits good skin turgor.
• Patient remains alert and responsive.

Documentation

• Observations of physical findings
• Nursing interventions, including administration of medications
• Patient's response to interventions, including antipyretics
• Evaluations for expected outcomes

■ Hypothermia

related to exposure to cold or cold environment

Definition

State in which body temperature is reduced below normal range

Assessment

• History of present illness
• Circumstances surrounding development of hypothermia
• Age
• Medication history
• Neurologic status, including level of consciousness, mental status, motor status, and sensory status
• Cardiovascular status, including blood pressure, capillary refill time, electrocardiogram (ECG), heart rate and rhythm, pulses (apical, peripheral), and temperature
• Respiratory status, including arterial blood gas analysis, breath sounds, and rate, depth, and character of respirations
• Integumentary status, including color, temperature, and turgor
• Nutritional status, including current weight and dietary pattern
• Fluid and electrolyte status, including blood urea nitrogen level, intake and output, serum electrolyte levels, and urine specific gravity
• Psychosocial status, including behavior, financial resources, mood, and occupation

Defining characteristics

• Body temperature below normal range
• Cool, pale skin
• Cyanotic nail beds
• Increased capillary refill time
• Increased blood pressure and heart rate

• Piloerection
• Shivering

Associated medical diagnoses (selected)
Adrenal insufficiency, asphyxia, burns, drug overdose or toxicity, hypothermia, intoxication

Expected outcomes
• Body temperature will remain within normal range.
• Skin will feel warm and dry.
• Heart rate and blood pressure will remain within normal range.
• Patient won't shiver.
• Patient will express feelings of comfort.
• Patient will show no complications associated with hypothermia, such as soft-tissue injury, fracture, dehydration, and hypovolemic shock if warmed too quickly.
• Patient will understand how to prevent further episodes of hypothermia.

Interventions and rationales
• Monitor body temperature at least every 4 hours or more frequently, if indicated, *to evaluate effectiveness of interventions.* Record temperature and route *to allow accurate data comparison. Baseline temperatures vary, depending on route used.* If temperature drops below 95° F (35° C), use a low-reading thermometer *to obtain accurate reading.*
• Monitor and record neurologic status at least every 4 hours. *Falling body temperature and metabolic rate reduce pulse rate and blood pressure, which reduces blood perfusion to brain, resulting in disorientation, confusion, and unconsciousness.*
• Monitor and record heart rate and rhythm, blood pressure, and respiratory rate at least every 4 hours. *Blood pressure and pulse decrease in hypothermia. During rewarming, pa-*

tient may develop hypovolemic shock. During warming, ventricular fibrillation and cardiac arrest may occur, possibly signaled by irregular pulse.
• Provide supportive measures, such as placing patient in warm bed and covering with warm blankets, removing all wet or constrictive clothing, and covering all metal or plastic surfaces that contact patient's body. *These measures protect patient from heat loss.*
• Follow prescribed treatment regimen for hypothermia:
– As ordered, administer medications to prevent shivering *to avoid overheating.* Monitor effectiveness and record.
– As ordered, administer analgesic *to relieve pain associated with warming.* Monitor effectiveness and record.
– Use hyperthermia blanket *to warm patient* if temperature drops below 95° F (35° C). Warm patient to 97° F (36.1° C).
– As appropriate, administer fluids during rewarming *to prevent hypovolemic shock.* If administering large volumes of I.V. fluids, consider using a fluid warmer *to avoid heat loss.*
• Discuss precipitating factors with patient, if indicated. *The patient may require community outreach assistance with certain precipitating factors, including inadequate living conditions, insufficient finances, and abuse of medications (such as sedatives and alcohol).*
• Instruct patient in precautionary measures to avoid hypothermia, such as dressing warmly even when indoors, eating proper diet, and remaining as active as possible. *Precautions help to prevent accidental hypothermia.*

Evaluations for expected outcomes
• Patient's temperature remains within normal range.
• Patient's skin is warm and dry.
• Patient's heart rate and blood pressure remain within normal range.
• Patient doesn't shiver.
• Patient voices feelings of comfort.
• Patient doesn't develop complications associated with hypothermia.
• Patient describes measures to prevent further episodes of hypothermia.

Documentation
• Patient's shivering and complaints of coldness
• Observations of physical findings
• Interventions carried out to resolve nursing diagnosis
• Patient's response to interventions, including physiologic, behavioral, and cognitive
• Evaluations for expected outcomes

■ Incontinence, bowel

related to neuromuscular involvement

Definition
Involuntary passage of stool

Assessment
• History of neuromuscular disorder
• GI status, including usual bowel elimination pattern, history of bowel disorder, laxative or enema use, incontinence characteristics (frequency, awareness of need to defecate, and precipitating factors), presence or absence of anal sphincter reflex, and bowel sounds
• Fluid and electrolyte status, including intake and output, urine specific gravity, skin turgor, and mucous membranes
• Nutritional status, including usual dietary pattern, appetite, tolerance or intolerance for foods, current weight, and change from normal weight
• Activity status, including type of exercise, frequency, and duration

Defining characteristics
• Constant dribbling of soft stool
• Fecal odor
• Fecal staining of clothing or bedding
• Feeling of rectal fullness
• Ignoring of urge to defecate
• Inability to delay defecation
• Inability to feel rectal fullness or urge to defecate
• Red perianal skin
• Urgency

Associated medical diagnoses (selected)
Amyotrophic lateral sclerosis, cerebrovascular accident, Guillain-Barré syndrome, head injury, multiple sclerosis, myasthenia gravis, paralysis, Parkinson's disease, spinal cord injury or tumor

Expected outcomes
• Patient will establish and maintain a regular pattern of bowel care.
• Patient will state understanding of bowel care routine.
• Patient or caregiver will demonstrate skill in carrying out bowel care routine with help from nurse.
• Patient or caregiver will demonstrate increasing skill in performing bowel care routine independently.
• Patient will participate in social activities.

Interventions and rationales
• For upper motor neuron lesion (anal reflex intact):
– Establish regular pattern for bowel care; for example, after breakfast every other day, maintain patient in

upright position after inserting suppository and allow half an hour for suppository to melt and maximum reflex response to occur. *Regular pattern encourages adaptation and routine physiologic function.*
– Discuss bowel care routine with patient and family *to promote feelings of safety, adequacy, and comfort.*
– Demonstrate bowel care to patient and caregivers *to reduce anxiety from lack of knowledge or involvement in care.*
– Observe return demonstration of bowel care routine by patient and caregivers *to check skills and establish a therapeutic relationship.*
– Establish a date when patient or caregivers will carry out bowel routine independently, with supportive assistance, *to reassure patient of dependable care.*
– Instruct patient and family on need to regulate foods and fluids that cause diarrhea or constipation *to encourage good nutritional habits.*
– Maintain dietary intake diary *to identify irritating foods*; instruct patient to avoid foods that are spicy, rich, or produce gas *to prevent painful flatulence.*
– Obtain order allowing modified bowel preparations for tests and procedures *to avoid interrupting routine and to encourage regular bowel function.*
– Encourage patient to use protective padding under clothing, changing it as necessary *to prevent odor, skin breakdown, or embarrassment and to promote positive self-image.*
• For lower motor neuron lesion (flaccid sphincter):
– Establish regular pattern for bowel care; for example, after breakfast every other day, turn patient on left side, put waterproof pads under buttocks, administer prescribed enema,

and allow him to remain in place 2 to 5 minutes. Then perform digital removal of stool, clean perianal area, and remove soiled pads. *These procedures encourage regular physiologic function, stimulate peristalsis, minimize infection, and promote comfort and elimination.*
– Follow rest of interventions for upper motor neuron lesion.

Evaluations for expected outcomes
• Patient establishes and maintains regular pattern of bowel care.
• Patient states understanding of bowel care routine.
• Patient or caregiver demonstrates competence in performing bowel care routine with assistance from nurse.
• Patient or caregiver carries out bowel routine independently.
• Patient attends social events without experiencing bowel incontinence.

Documentation
• Patient's feelings about problem and bowel routine
• Bowel care routine and administration of suppositories and enemas
• Description of incontinent episodes, including known precipitating factors, time of day, and other relevant details
• Patient's and caregivers' skills in bowel care
• Evaluations for expected outcomes

■ Incontinence, bowel

related to perceptual or cognitive impairment

Definition
Involuntary passage of stool

Assessment
- History of neurologic or psychiatric disorder
- Fluid and electrolyte status, including intake and output, skin turgor, urine specific gravity, and mucous membranes
- GI status, including usual bowel elimination habits, change in bowel habits, stool characteristics (color, amount, size, and consistency), pain or discomfort, inspection of abdomen, auscultation of bowel sounds, palpation for masses and tenderness, percussion for tympany and dullness, and laxative and enema use
- Characteristics of incontinence, including frequency, time of day, before or after meals, relationship to activity, and behavior pattern (restlessness)
- Neurologic status, including orientation, level of consciousness, memory, and cognitive ability

Defining characteristics
- Constant dribbling of soft stool
- Fecal odor
- Fecal staining of clothing or bedding
- Feeling of rectal fullness
- Ignoring of urge to defecate
- Inability to delay defecation
- Inability to feel rectal fullness or urge to defecate
- Red perianal skin
- Urgency

Associated medical diagnoses (selected)
Alzheimer's disease, brain tumor, cerebrovascular accident, head injury, Huntington's disease, meningitis

Expected outcomes
- Patient will experience bowel movement every ___ day(s) when placed on commode or toilet at ___ a.m./p.m.
- Patient's skin will remain clean and intact.
- Patient will improve control of incontinent episodes.
- Caregiver will state understanding of bowel routine.
- Caregiver will demonstrate skill in placing patient on commode.
- Caregiver will demonstrate skill in use of suppository, if indicated.
- Caregiver will understand and explain relationship of food and fluid regulation to promotion of continence.
- Patient will maintain self-respect and dignity through participation and acceptance within group.

Interventions and rationales
- Establish a regular pattern for bowel care; for example, after breakfast every other day, place patient on commode chair 1 hour after inserting suppository and allow patient to remain upright for 30 minutes for maximum response; then clean anal area. *Procedure encourages adaptation and routine physiologic function.*
- Monitor and record incontinent episodes; keep baseline record for 3 to 7 days *to track effectiveness of toileting routine.*
- Discuss bowel care routine with family or caregiver *to foster compliance.*
- Demonstrate bowel care routine to family or caregiver *to reduce anxiety from lack of knowledge or involvement in care.*
- Arrange for return demonstration of bowel care routine *to help establish therapeutic relationship with patient and family or caregiver.*
- Establish a date when family or caregiver will carry out bowel care routine with supportive assistance; *this will ensure that patient receives dependable care.*

• Instruct family or caregiver on need to regulate foods and fluids that cause diarrhea or constipation *to encourage helpful nutritional habits.*
• Maintain diet log *to identify irritating foods,* and then eliminate them from patient's diet.
• Clean and dry perianal area after each incontinent episode *to prevent infection and promote comfort.*
• Maintain patient's dignity by using protective padding under clothing, by removing patient from group activity after incontinent episode, and by cleaning and returning patient to group without undue attention. *These measures prevent odor, skin breakdown, and embarrassment and promote patient's positive self-image.*

Evaluations for expected outcomes
• Patient has one soft bowel movement every _____ day(s).
• Patient's skin remains clean, dry, and intact.
• Episodes of incontinence decrease by 50%.
• Caregiver can explain bowel routine.
• Caregiver successfully demonstrates placing patient on commode.
• Caregiver successfully demonstrates insertion of suppositories.
• Caregiver explains the relationship between the food and fluid intake and the regulation of continence and plans appropriate diet for patient.
• Patient expresses positive self-image.

Documentation
• Patient's level of awareness, response to incontinent episodes, and acceptance of bowel care routine
• Family's or caregiver's response to incontinence and to establishment and implementation of a bowel care routine

• Observation of effects of bowel care routine, episodes of incontinence, stool characteristics, and condition of skin
• Family's or caregiver's skill in carrying out bowel care routine and modifying diet
• Evaluations for expected outcomes

■ Incontinence, functional
related to cognitive deficits

Definition
Involuntary and unpredictable passage of urine in socially unacceptable situations, where patient usually doesn't recognize warning signs of bladder fullness

Assessment
• History of mental illness
• Age
• Sex
• Vital signs
• Genitourinary status, including frequency and voiding pattern
• Fluid and electrolyte status, including blood urea nitrogen level, creatinine level, intake and output, mucous membranes, serum electrolyte levels, and skin turgor
• Neuromuscular status, including daily living activities, mental status, mobility, and sensory ability to perceive bladder fullness
• Psychosocial status, including behavior before and after voiding, support from family members, impact of incontinence on self and others, and stressors (family, job, and change in environment)

Defining characteristics
• Ability to empty bladder completely
• Inability to sense need to void

• Loss of urine before reaching toilet
• Occurrence only in early morning (in some patients)

Associated medical diagnoses (selected)

Alzheimer's disease, anxiety disorder, cerebrovascular accident, dementia, depression, drug overdose, hypothyroidism, schizophrenia, urinary incontinence

Expected outcomes

• Patient will void at appropriate intervals.
• Patient will not void in unacceptable situations.
• Patient will have minimal, if any, complications.
• Patient and family members will demonstrate skill in managing incontinence.
• Patient will discuss impact of incontinence on self and family members.
• Patient and family members will identify resources to assist with care following discharge.

Interventions and rationales

• Monitor and record patient's voiding patterns *to ensure correct fluid replacement therapy.*
• Assist with specific bladder elimination procedures, such as:
– bladder training. Place patient on commode or toilet every 2 hours while awake and once during night. *Successful bladder training revolves around adequate fluid intake, muscle-strengthening exercises, and carefully scheduled voiding times.*
– rigid toilet regimen. Place patient on toilet at specific intervals (every 2 hours or after meals). Note whether patient was wet or dry and whether voiding occurred at each interval. *This helps patient adapt to routine physiologic function.*

– behavior modification. Reward continence or voiding in lavatory. Don't punish unwanted behavior such as voiding in the wrong place. Reinforce behavior consistently, using social or material rewards. *This helps patient learn alternatives to maladaptive behaviors.*
– use of external catheter. Apply according to established procedure and maintain patency. Observe condition of perineal skin and clean with soap and water at least twice daily. *This ensures effective therapy and prevents infection and skin breakdown.*
– application of protective pads and garments. Use only when interventions have failed *to prevent infection and skin breakdown and promote social acceptance.* Allow at least 4 to 6 weeks for trial period. *Establishing continence requires prolonged effort.*
• Maintain continence based on patient's voiding patterns and limitations.
– Use reminders. *Reminders help limit amount of information patient must retain in his memory.*
– Orient patient to toileting environment: time, place, and activity. *A structured environment offers security and helps patient with elimination problems.*
– Stimulate patient's voiding reflexes (give patient drink of water while on toilet; stroke area over bladder; or pour water over perineum). *External stimulation triggers bladder's spastic reflex.*
– Provide hyperactive patient with distraction, such as magazine, to occupy attention while on toilet. *This reduces anxiety and eases voiding.*
– Provide privacy and adequate time to void *to allow patient to void easily without anxiety.*

– Praise successful performance *to give patient a sense of control and to encourage compliance.*

– Change wet clothes *to accustom patient to dry clothes.*

– Teach family members and support personnel to assist, *thus reducing anxiety that results from noninvolvement and increasing chances for successful treatment.*

– Respond to patient's call light promptly *to avoid delays in voiding routine.*

– Choose patient's clothing to promote easy dressing and undressing. (For example, use Velcro fasteners and gowns instead of pajamas.) *This reduces patient's frustration with voiding routine.*

• Schedule patient's fluid intake to encourage voiding at convenient times. Maintain adequate hydration up to 3,000 ml daily, unless contraindicated. *Scheduling fluid intake promotes regular bladder distention and optimal time intervals between voidings.* Limit fluid intake to 150 ml after dinner *to reduce need to void at night.*

• Instruct patient and family members on continence techniques to use at home *to increase chances of successful bladder retraining.*

• Encourage patient and family members to share feelings related to incontinence. *This allows specific problems to be identified and resolved. Attentive listening conveys recognition and respect.*

• Refer patient and family members to psychiatric liaison nurse, home health care agency, or support group *to provide access to additional community resources.*

Evaluations for expected outcomes

• Record of voiding pattern indicates that patient voids at appropriate intervals, with minimal episodes of incontinence.

• Patient recognizes urge to void, undresses without assistance, and uses toilet.

• Patient doesn't experience urinary tract infection, skin breakdown, or other complications related to incontinence.

• Patient and family members demonstrate proper procedures for managing incontinence.

• Patient expresses feelings about condition and its effect on family. Patient and family members are neither overwhelmed nor excessively optimistic about patient's condition.

• Patient and family members contact support group or home health care agency, if needed.

Documentation

• Observations of incontinence and response to treatment regimen
• Interventions to provide supportive care and patient's response to supportive care
• Instructions given to patient and family members; return demonstration of knowledge and skills needed to carry out continence management techniques
• Patient's expression of concern about incontinence and motivation to participate in self-care
• Evaluations for expected outcomes

■ Incontinence, functional

related to sensory or mobility deficits

Definition

Involuntary and unpredictable passage of urine in socially unacceptable situations, where patient usually doesn't recognize warning signs of bladder fullness

Assessment

• History of mental retardation, trauma, and alcohol abuse
• Medication history
• Age
• Sex
• Vital signs
• Genitourinary status, including extent of clothing wetness due to urine, frequency, palpation of bladder, urine leakage when standing or sitting, and voiding pattern
• Fluid and electrolyte status, including blood urea nitrogen level, creatinine level, intake and output, mucous membranes, serum electrolyte levels, skin turgor, and urine specific gravity
• Neuromuscular status, including manual dexterity, mental status, mobility, motor ability to start and stop urine stream, rectal examination (muscle tone, prostate size, and fecal impaction), and sensory ability to perceive bladder fullness
• Psychosocial status, including behavior before and after voiding, coping skills, support from family members, perception of health problem, self-concept, and stressors (such as finances, job, and change in environment)

Defining characteristics

• Ability to empty bladder completely
• Inability to sense need to void
• Loss of urine before reaching toilet
• Occurrence only in early morning (in some patients)

Associated medical diagnoses (selected)

Alcohol addiction, cerebrovascular accident, dementia, drug overdose or toxicity

Expected outcomes

• Patient will void in appropriate situation using suitable receptacle.
• Patient will void at specific times.
• Patient will have no wet episodes.
• Patient will maintain fluid balance, with intake approximately equaling output.
• Patient will have minimal, if any, complications.
• Patient and family members will demonstrate skill in managing incontinence.
• Patient will discuss impact of incontinence on self and family members.
• Patient and family members will identify resources to assist with care following discharge.

Interventions and rationales

• Monitor patient's voiding pattern; document and report intake and output *to ensure correct fluid replacement therapy.*
• Assist with specific bladder elimination procedures, such as:
– bladder training. Place patient on commode or toilet every 2 hours while awake and once during the night. *Successful bladder training revolves around adequate fluid intake, muscle-strengthening exercises, and carefully scheduled voiding times.*
– rigid toilet regimen. Place patient on toilet at specific intervals (every 2 hours or after meals). Note whether patient was wet or dry and whether voiding occurred at each interval. *This helps patient adapt to routine physiologic function.*
– use of external catheter. Apply according to established procedure and maintain patency. Observe condition of perineal skin and clean with soap and water at least twice daily. *This ensures effective therapy and prevents infection and skin breakdown.*

– application of protective pads and garments. Use only after incontinence management procedures have failed *to prevent infection and skin breakdown and promote social acceptance.* Allow at least 4 to 6 weeks for trial period. *Establishing continence requires prolonged effort.*

• Maintain continence based on patient's voiding patterns and limitations.

– Use reminders.

– Orient patient to toileting environment: time, place, and activity. *A structured environment offers security and helps patient with elimination problems.*

– Stimulate voiding reflexes. Give patient a drink of water while on the toilet; stroke the area over the bladder; or pour water over the perineum. *External stimulation triggers bladder's spastic reflex.*

– For hyperactive patients, provide distraction, such as a magazine, to occupy attention while on the toilet. *This reduces anxiety and eases voiding.*

– Provide privacy and adequate time to void *to allow patient to void easily without anxiety.*

– Praise successful performance *to give patient a sense of control and encourage compliance.*

– Change wet clothes *to accustom patient to dry clothes.*

– Teach family members and support personnel to assist, *thus reducing anxiety that results from noninvolvement and increasing chances for successful treatment.*

– Respond quickly to patient's call light *to avoid delays in voiding routine.*

– Choose patient's clothing to promote ease in dressing and undressing. (For example, use Velcro fasteners and gowns instead of pajamas.) *This*

reduces patient's frustration with voiding routine.

• Keep skin as clean and dry as possible. Use mild soap and water *to clean urea burns and prevent skin breakdown.*

• Schedule patient's fluid intake to encourage voiding at convenient times. Maintain adequate hydration up to 3,000 ml daily, unless contraindicated. *Scheduling fluid intake promotes regular bladder distention and optimal time intervals between voidings.* Limit fluid intake to 150 ml after dinner *to reduce need to void at night.*

• Decrease patient's use of alcohol *to reduce sensory or mobility deficits.*

• Instruct patient and family members on continence techniques to use at home. Have patient and family members return demonstrations. *This will increase chances for successful bladder retraining.*

• Encourage patient and family members to share feelings related to incontinence. *This allows specific problems to be identified and resolved. Attentive listening conveys recognition and respect.*

• Refer patient and family members to psychiatric liaison nurse, home health care agency, support group, and similar resources when appropriate *to provide access to additional community resources.*

Evaluations for expected outcomes

• Patient voids in appropriate situation using suitable receptacle.

• Record of voiding pattern indicates that patient voids at appropriate intervals, with minimal episodes of incontinence.

• Patient has no wet episodes.

• Patient maintains fluid balance with intake approximately equal to output.

• Patient doesn't experience urinary tract infection, skin breakdown, or

other complications related to incontinence.
• Patient and family members demonstrate the proper procedures for managing incontinence.
• Patient expresses feelings about condition and its effect on family. Patient and family members are neither overwhelmed nor excessively optimistic about patient's condition.
• Patient and family members contact support group or home health care agency, if needed.

Documentation
• Observations of incontinence and response to treatment regimen
• Interventions to provide supportive care and patient's response
• Instructions given to patient and family members; return demonstration of knowledge and skills needed to carry out continence management techniques
• Patient's expression of concern about incontinence problem and motivation to participate in self-care
• Evaluations for expected outcomes

■ Incontinence, reflex

related to sensory or neuromuscular impairment

Definition
Involuntary loss of urine, controlled by spinal cord reflex, occurring at somewhat predictable intervals when a specific bladder volume is reached

Assessment
• History of sensory or neuromuscular impairment
• History of urinary tract disease, trauma, surgery, or infection
• Genitourinary status, including bladder palpation, residual urine volume after voiding, urinalysis, urine characteristics, urine culture and sensitivity, and voiding patterns
• Neuromuscular status, including anal sphincter tone, motor ability to start and stop urine stream, neuromuscular function, sensory ability to perceive bladder fullness and voiding, and involuntary voiding after stimulation of skin on abdomen, thighs, or genitals
• Fluid and electrolyte status, including blood urea nitrogen level, creatinine level, intake and output, medication history, mucous membranes, serum electrolyte levels, skin turgor, and urine specific gravity
• Sexuality status, including capability, concerns, and habits
• Psychosocial status, including coping skills, self-concept, and perception of problem by patient and family members

Defining characteristics
• Complete emptying (with lesion above pontine micturition center) or incomplete emptying (with lesion above sacral micturition center) of bladder
• Either inability to sense full bladder, urge to void, or voiding, or ability to sense urge to void without ability to voluntarily inhibit bladder contraction
• Inability to voluntarily inhibit or initiate voiding
• Predictable pattern of voiding
• Sensations associated with full bladder (sweating, restlessness, and abdominal discomfort)

Associated medical diagnoses (selected)
Paralysis, prolapsed intervertebral disk, spinal cord injury, spinal tumor, urinary incontinence

Expected outcomes

• Patient will maintain fluid balance, with intake approximately equaling output.
• Patient will have minimal, if any, complications.
• Patient will achieve urinary continence.
• Patient and family members will demonstrate skill in managing urinary incontinence.
• Patient will discuss impact of incontinence on self and family.
• Patient and family members will identify resources to assist with care following discharge.

Interventions and rationales

• Monitor intake and output *to ensure correct fluid replacement therapy.* Report output greater than intake.
• Implement and monitor effectiveness of specific bladder elimination procedure, such as:
– stimulating reflex arc. Patient who voids at somewhat predictable intervals may be able to regulate voiding by reflex arc stimulation. Trigger voiding at regular intervals (for example, every 2 hours) by stimulating skin of abdomen, thighs, or genitals to initiate bladder contractions. Avoid stimulation at nonvoiding times. Stimulate primitive voiding reflexes by giving patient water to drink while he sits on the toilet or pouring water over the perineum. *External stimulation triggers bladder's spastic reflex.*
– applying external catheter according to established procedure and maintaining patency. Observe condition of perineal skin and clean with soap and water at least twice daily. *Cleanliness prevents skin breakdown and infection. External catheter protects surrounding skin, promotes accurate output measurement, and keeps patient dry. Applying foam strip*

in spiral fashion increases adhesive surface and cuts risk of impaired circulation.
– inserting indwelling catheter. Monitor patency and keep tubing free of kinks *to avoid drainage pooling and ensure accurate therapy.* Keep drainage bag below level of bladder *to avoid urine reflux into bladder.* Perform catheter care according to established procedure. Maintain closed drainage system *to prevent bacteriuria.* Secure catheter to leg (female) or abdomen (male) *to avoid tension on bladder and sphincter.*
– applying suprapubic catheter. Change dressing according to established procedure *to avoid skin breakdown.* Monitor patency and keep tubing free of kinks *to avoid drainage pooling in loops of catheter.* Keep drainage bag below bladder level *to avoid urine reflux into bladder.* Maintain closed drainage system *to prevent bacteriuria.*
– changing wet clothes *to prevent patient from becoming accustomed to wet clothes.*
• Encourage high fluid intake (3,000 ml daily, unless contraindicated) *to stimulate micturition reflex.* Limit fluid intake after 7 p.m. *to prevent nocturia.*
• Instruct patient and family members on continence techniques to use at home. Have patient and family members return demonstrations until they can perform procedure well. *Patient education begins with assessment and depends on nurse's therapeutic relationship with patient and family.*
• Encourage patient and family members to share feelings and concerns regarding incontinence. *A trusting environment allows nurse to make specific recommendations to resolve patient's problems.*

• Refer patient and family members to psychiatric liaison nurse, home health care agency, support group, or other resources as appropriate. *Community resources often provide health care not available from other health agencies.*

Evaluations for expected outcomes
• Records indicate that fluid intake equals output. Patient maintains fluid balance.
• Patient avoids complications associated with incontinence, such as infections, swelling of penis (because of external catheter), skin breakdown, catheter obstruction, and urine odor. Results of urinalysis are normal.
• Patient achieves urinary continence.
• Patient and family members successfully demonstrate chosen technique for bladder control.
• Patient expresses both positive and negative feelings about condition. Patient can cope with dependence brought on by condition.
• Patient and family members initiate contact with support group or visiting nurse.

Documentation
• Observations of urologic condition and response to treatment regimen
• Interventions to provide supportive care and patient's response
• Instructions given to patient and family members; return demonstration of knowledge and skills needed to carry out continence management techniques
• Patient's expression of concern about incontinence and its impact on body image and lifestyle; patient's motivation to participate in self-care
• Evaluations for expected outcomes

■ Incontinence, stress
related to weak pelvic musculature

Definition
Loss of urine (less than 50 ml) resulting from increased abdominal pressure

Assessment
• History of long-term use of tranquilizers, multiple pregnancies, prolonged or difficult labor, surgery, trauma, and vaginal infections
• Age
• Sex
• Vital signs
• Genitourinary status, including inspection of abdomen for scars from previous surgeries, rectal examination, vaginal examination, voiding pattern, and leakage of urine during sneezing, laughing, vomiting, coughing, defecating, physical exertion, or change from prone to upright position
• Fluid and electrolyte status, including creatinine level, blood urea nitrogen level, estrogen levels, intake and output, mucous membranes, serum electrolyte levels, and skin turgor
• Nutritional status, including appetite, dietary habits, and present weight
• Neuromuscular status, including degree of neuromuscular function, motor ability to start or stop urine stream, and sensory ability to perceive fullness
• Sexuality status, including capability, concerns, habits, and patterns
• Psychosocial status, including coping skills, self-concept, stressors (such as finances, family, and job), and perception of problem by family members

Defining characteristics
• Dribbling with increased abdominal pressure
• Frequency
• Urgency

Associated medical diagnoses (selected)
Atrophic senile vaginitis, fractures, multiple births, obesity, urinary incontinence, urinary tract infection, uterine prolapse

Expected outcomes
• Patient will maintain continence.
• Patient will state increased comfort.
• Patient will state understanding of treatment.
• Patient will state understanding of surgical procedure.
• Patient and family members will demonstrate skill in managing urinary elimination problems.
• Patient and family members will identify resources to assist with care following discharge.

Interventions and rationales
• Observe patient's voiding patterns, time of voiding, amount voided, and whether voiding is provoked by stimuli. *Accurate, thorough assessment forms basis of an effective treatment plan.*
• Provide appropriate care for patient's urologic condition, monitor progress, and report patient's responses to treatment. *Patient expects to receive adequate care and to participate in decisions regarding care.*
• Help patient to strengthen pelvic floor muscles by Kegel exercises for sphincter control. *Exercises increase muscle tone and restore cortical control.*
• Promote patient's awareness of condition through education *to help patient understand illness as well as treatment.*

• Help patient reduce intra-abdominal pressure by:
– losing weight
– avoiding heavy lifting
– avoiding chairs or beds that are too high or too low.
These measures reduce intra-abdominal pressure and bladder pressure.
• Provide supportive measures:
– Respond to call light quickly, assign patient to bed next to bathroom, put night light in bathroom, and have patient wear easily removable clothing (gown rather than pajamas and Velcro fasteners rather than buttons or zippers). *Early recognition of problems promotes continence; easily removed clothing reduces patient frustration and helps achieve continence.*
– Provide privacy during toileting *to reduce anxiety and promote elimination.*
– Have patient empty bladder before meals, at bedtime, and before leaving accessible bathroom area *to promote elimination, avoid accidents, and help relieve intra-abdominal pressure.*
– Limit fluids to 150 ml after dinner *to reduce need to void at night.*
– Encourage high fluid intake, unless contraindicated, *to moisten mucous membranes and maintain hydration.*
– Suggest patient eat increased amount of salty food before going on a long trip (unless contraindicated). *Increased sodium decreases urine production.*
– Make protective pads available for patient's undergarments, if needed, *to absorb urine, protect skin, and control odors.*
• If surgery is scheduled, give attentive, appropriate preoperative and postoperative instructions and care *to reduce patient's anxiety and build trust in caregivers.*
• Encourage patient to ventilate feelings and concerns related to urologic

problems. *This helps patient focus on specific problem.*
• Refer patient and family members to psychiatric liaison nurse, support group, or other resources, as appropriate. *Community resources often provide health care not available from other health agencies.*
• Alert patient and family members to need for toilet schedule. Prepare for discharge according to individual needs *to ensure that patient will receive proper care.*

Evaluations for expected outcomes
• Patient maintains continence.
• Patient expresses satisfaction with progress in overcoming stress incontinence.
• Patient expresses understanding of techniques to reduce intra-abdominal pressure and other supportive measures.
• Patient explains surgical procedure, including risks and expected outcome.
• Patient and family members demonstrate all procedures and supportive measures to enable patient to remain continent. They also make arrangements for home care, such as providing bedroom near bathroom and purchasing easily removable clothing.
• Patient and family members contact appropriate community resources.

Documentation
• Observations of urologic condition and patient's response to treatment regimen
• Interventions to provide supportive care and patient's response to interventions
• Instructions given to patient and family members on patient's urologic problem, their response to instructions, and demonstrated ability to carry out self-care management

• Patient's expression of concern about urologic problem and its impact on body image and lifestyle
• Patient's motivation to participate in self-care
• Evaluations for expected outcomes

■ Incontinence, total
related to neurologic dysfunction

Definition
Continuous and unpredictable passage of urine

Assessment
• History of trauma, sensory or neuromuscular impairment, surgery, and congenital anomalies
• Vital signs
• Age
• Sex
• Genitourinary status, including palpation of bladder, previous bladder elimination procedures, urinalysis, urine characteristics, use of urinary assistive devices, and voiding pattern
• Fluid and electrolyte status, including blood urea nitrogen level, creatinine level, intake and output, mucous membranes, skin turgor, and serum electrolyte levels
• Neuromuscular status, including degree of neuromuscular function, motor ability to start or stop urine stream, and sensory ability to perceive bladder fullness
• Sexuality status, including capability, concerns, and sexual partner
• Psychosocial status, including patient's perception of health problem, coping skills, family, and self-concept

Defining characteristics
• Constant flow of urine that occurs at unpredictable times without disten-

tion or uninhibited bladder contractions or spasms
• Incontinence refractory to treatments
• Lack of awareness of incontinence, perineal fullness, or bladder filling
• Nocturia

Associated medical diagnoses (selected)
Cerebrovascular accident, diabetes mellitus, head injury, labor, multiple sclerosis, neuromuscular trauma, spinal cord injury or tumor, urinary incontinence

Expected outcomes
• Patient will maintain fluid balance, with intake approximately equaling output.
• Patient will state increased comfort.
• Patient will have minimal, if any, complications.
• Patient will maintain continence with assistive devices.
• Patient and family members will demonstrate skill in managing incontinence.
• Patient and family members will discuss impact of incontinence on their lives.
• Patient and family members will identify resources to assist with care following discharge.

Interventions and rationales
• Monitor patient's voiding pattern; document and report intake and output *to ensure correct fluid replacement therapy.*
• Assist with specific bladder elimination devices, such as:
– external catheter. Apply according to established procedure and maintain patency. Avoid constriction. Observe condition of perineal area and clean with soap and water at least twice daily. Reusable penile sheaths are available for long-term use. *Cleanliness prevents skin breakdown or infection. External catheter protects surrounding skin, promotes accurate output measurement, and keeps patient dry. Applying foam strip in spiral fashion increases adhesive surface and cuts risk of impaired circulation.*
– indwelling catheter. Monitor patency and keep tubing free of kinks *to avoid drainage pooling and ensure accurate therapy.* Keep drainage bag below level of bladder *to avoid urine reflux into bladder.* Clean urinary meatus according to established procedure *to reduce risk of infection.* Maintain closed drainage system *to prevent bacteriuria.* Secure catheter to leg (female) or abdomen (male) *to avoid tension on bladder and sphincter.*
– suprapubic catheter. Monitor patency, change dressing, and clean catheter site according to established policy *to avoid skin breakdown.* Keep tubing free of kinks; keep drainage bag below level of bladder *to prevent urine reflux into bladder.* Maintain closed drainage system *to prevent bacteriuria.*
– body-worn appliances. These body-worn "urinals" fit over the penis and have a drainage bag and waist and leg straps for body attachment *to protect skin and keep patient dry.* Selection depends on patient's self-help skills. Appliances need regular, careful washing *to protect skin and keep patient dry.*
– incontinence aids. As needed, provide patient with absorbent pad and pants with protective waterproof shield, a drip collector (an absorbent pouch that fits over penis), and absorbent pad that protects patient's bed. *These aids trap urine to keep it away from patient's skin.*

• Disguise urinary bag by placing it in shopping bag or tote bag *to enhance patient's self-image.*
• Provide supportive measures:
– Regulate fluid intake on a specific schedule *to encourage voiding at convenient times.* Maintain adequate hydration up to 3,000 ml daily, unless contraindicated. Limit fluid intake to 150 ml after dinner *to reduce need to void at night.*
– Clothe patient to promote ease in dressing and undressing and to accommodate appliance. (For example, use Velcro fasteners and gowns rather than pajamas.) *Unwieldy clothing increases patient frustration with voiding routine.*
– Keep skin as clean and dry as possible *to promote skin integrity.* Treat urea burns by cleaning with mild soap and water.
• Instruct patient and family members on continence techniques for home use. Provide for return demonstrations. *Patient education begins with assessment and depends on nurse's establishing therapeutic relationship with patient and family.*
• Encourage patient and family members to share feelings and concerns related to incontinence. *A trusting environment allows nurse to make specific recommendations to resolve patient's problems.*
• Refer patient and family members to psychiatric liaison nurse, home health care agency, support group, or other resources, as appropriate. *Community resources often provide health care not available from other health agencies.*

Evaluations for expected outcomes
• Patient takes in enough fluid to void approximately eight times each day.
• Patient remains dry, maintains usual lifestyle, and doesn't experience skin breakdown or infection. Patient expresses increased comfort.
• Patient has minimal, if any, complications.
• Patient maintains continence, using assistive devices.
• Before discharge, patient and family members demonstrate skill in managing incontinence.
• Patient and family members discuss impact of incontinence on their lives.
• Patient and family members identify two resources in community to assist with care following discharge.

Documentation
• Observations of incontinence and response to treatment regimen
• Interventions to provide supportive care and patient's response to interventions
• Instructions given to patient and family members, their understanding of information, and their demonstrated ability to carry out continence management techniques
• Patient's expressions of concern about incontinence and motivation to participate in self-care
• Evaluations for expected outcomes

■ Incontinence, urge
related to decreased bladder capacity

Definition
Involuntary passage of urine occurring shortly after a strong sense of urgency to void

Assessment
• History of cerebrovascular accident, urinary tract disease, spinal cord injury, surgery, or infection
• Medication history

• Vital signs
• Genitourinary status, including cystometrogram, pain or discomfort, urinalysis, urine specific gravity, use of urinary assistive devices, and voiding pattern
• Fluid and electrolyte status, including blood urea nitrogen level, creatinine level, intake and output, mucous membranes, postvoiding residual volume, skin turgor, and serum electrolyte levels
• Neuromuscular status, including ambulation ability, degree of neuromuscular function, dexterity, and sensory ability to perceive fullness
• Sexuality status, including capability, concerns, habits, and sexual partner
• Psychosocial status, including coping skills, self-concept, stressors (such as finances, family, and job), and perception of health problem by patient and family members

Defining characteristics
• Bladder contraction or spasm
• Frequency
• Inability to reach toilet in time
• Increased or decreased volume
• Nocturia
• Urgency

Associated medical diagnoses (selected)
Bladder cancer, cystitis, gonorrhea, urinary tract infection

Expected outcomes
• Patient will have fewer episodes of incontinence.
• Patient will state increased comfort.
• Patient will state understanding of treatment.
• Patient will have minimal, if any, complications.
• Patient will discuss impact of urologic disorder on self and family members.

• Patient and family members will demonstrate skill in managing incontinence.

Interventions and rationales
• Observe voiding pattern; document intake and output. *This ensures correct fluid replacement therapy and provides information about patient's ability to void adequately.*
• Provide appropriate care for patient's urologic condition, monitor progress, and report patient's responses to treatment. *Patient should receive adequate care and take part in decisions about care as much as possible.*
• Provide supportive measures:
– Administer pain medication and monitor effectiveness. *Patient's knowledge that pain can be alleviated reduces tension and anxiety.*
– Prepare pleasant toilet environment that's warm, clean, and free of odors *to promote continence.*
– Place commode next to bed, or assign patient bed next to bathroom. *A bedside commode or convenient bathroom requires less energy expenditure than bedpan.*
– Keep bed and commode at same level *to facilitate patient's movements.*
– Provide good lighting from bed to bathroom *to reduce sensory misinterpretation.*
– Remove all obstacles between bed and bathroom *to reduce chance of falling.*
– Provide clock *to help patient maintain voiding schedule through self-monitoring.*
– Unless contraindicated, maintain fluids to 3,000 ml daily *to moisten mucous membranes and ensure hydration*; limit patient to 150 ml after dinner *to reduce need to void at night.*
– Have patient wear easily removable clothes (gown instead of pajamas and

Velcro fasteners instead of buttons or zippers) *to reduce frustration and delay in voiding routine.*
– If patient loses control on way to bathroom, instruct patient to stop and take a deep breath. *Anxiety and rushing may strengthen bladder contractions.*
• Assist with specific bladder elimination procedures, such as:
– bladder training. Place patient on commode every 2 hours while awake and once during the night. Provide privacy. Gradually increase intervals between toileting. *These measures aim to restore a regular voiding pattern.*
– rigid toilet regimen. Place patient on toilet at specific times (for example, every 2 hours). *This aids adaptation to routine physiologic function.* Keep baseline micturition record for 3 to 7 days *to monitor toileting effectiveness.*
• Encourage patient to ventilate feelings and concerns related to his urologic problem *to identify patient's fears.*
• Explain urologic condition to patient and family members; include instructions on preventive measures and established bladder schedule. *Patient education begins with educational assessment and depends on establishing a therapeutic relationship with patient and family.* Prepare patient for discharge according to individual needs *to allow patient to practice under supervision.*
• Instruct patient and family members on continence techniques for home use. *This reduces fear and anxiety resulting from lack of knowledge of patient's condition and reassures patient of continuing care.*
• Refer patient and family members to psychiatric liaison nurse, support group, or other resources, as appropri-

ate. *Community resources often provide health care not available from other health agencies.*

Evaluations for expected outcomes
• Patient maintains continence.
• Patient expresses increased comfort and reduces requests for pain medication.
• Patient expresses understanding of treatment.
• Patient doesn't experience nighttime incontinence or other complications.
• Patient expresses feelings about condition.
• Patient and family members discuss treatment of urologic condition and home bladder schedule. They also demonstrate necessary skills.

Documentation
• Observations of urologic condition and patient's response to treatment regimen
• Interventions to provide supportive care
• Patient's response to nursing interventions
• Instructions given to patient and family members on urologic problem, their response to instructions, and their demonstrated ability to carry out self-care management
• Patient's expression of concern about urologic problem and its impact on body image and lifestyle; patient's motivation to participate in self-care
• Evaluations for expected outcomes

■ Infection, risk for
related to external factors

Definition
Presence of internal or external hazards that threaten physical well-being

Assessment

- Health history, including accidents, allergies, falls, hyperthermia, hypothermia, poisoning, seizures, trauma, and exposure to pollutants
- Sensory or perceptual changes (auditory, gustatory, kinesthetic, olfactory, tactile, and visual)
- Circumstances of present situation that could lead to infection
- Neurologic status, including level of consciousness, mental status, and orientation
- Laboratory studies, including clotting factors, hemoglobin and hematocrit, platelet count, serum albumin, white blood cell (WBC) count, and cultures of blood, body fluid, sputum, urine, and wound drainage

Risk factors

- Altered immune function
- Amniotic membrane rupture
- Chronic illness
- Drug use
- Environmental exposure to pathogens
- Invasive procedures
- Lack of knowledge about causes of infection
- Lack of primary (such as skin) or secondary (such as inflammatory response) defenses
- Malnutrition
- Tissue destruction
- Trauma

Associated medical diagnoses (selected)

Although any patient can develop a nosocomial infection, debilitated, elderly, and postoperative patients (especially transplantation patients) are at greatest risk. Associated medical diagnoses include accidental radiation exposure, acquired immunodeficiency syndrome, acute renal failure, acute respiratory failure, adrenal insufficiency, adult respiratory distress syndrome, anemias, asthma, bone marrow transplantation, breast engorgement, bronchiectasis, burns, chemotherapy, chlamydia, cholecystitis, chronic bronchitis, chronic obstructive pulmonary disease, chronic renal failure, congenital heart disease, cor pulmonale, diabetes mellitus, Down syndrome, emphysema, empyema, encephalitis, endometriosis, esophageal cancer, genital herpes, glomerulonephritis, gonorrhea, hemodialysis, hepatic coma, Hodgkin's disease, hydrocephalus, hydronephrosis, hyperosmolar hyperglycemic nonketotic syndrome, ileostomy, lesions, leukemia, lupus erythematosus, lymphomas, meningitis, metastatic disease, multiple myeloma, multiple sclerosis, multisystem trauma, nutritional deficiencies, open wounds, peripheral vascular disease, peritoneal dialysis, pleural effusion, polycystic kidney disease, pressure ulcer, prostatectomy, pyelonephritis, renal calculi, rheumatic fever, rubella, salmonella, scarlet fever, shock, spinal cord injury, streptococcal throat, syphilis, thoracic surgery, urinary calculi, urinary tract infection (UTI), and viral hepatitis.

Expected outcomes

- Patient's temperature will stay within normal range.
- Patient's WBC count and differential will stay within normal range.
- No pathogens will appear in cultures.
- Patient will maintain good personal and oral hygiene.
- Patient's respiratory secretions will be clear and odorless.
- Patient's urine will remain clear, yellow, odorless, and free of sediment.
- Patient will show no evidence of diarrhea.

• Patient's wounds and incisions will appear clean, pink, and free of purulent drainage.
• Patient's I.V. sites will show no signs of inflammation.
• Patient will show no evidence of skin breakdown.
• Patient will take ___ ml of fluid and ___ g of protein daily.
• Patient will state infection risk factors.
• Patient will identify signs and symptoms of infection.
• Patient will remain free of all signs and symptoms of infection.

Interventions and rationales
• Minimize patient's risk of infection by:
– washing hands before and after providing care. *Hand washing is the single best way to avoid spreading pathogens.*
– wearing gloves to maintain asepsis when providing direct care. *Gloves offer protection when handling wound dressings or carrying out various treatments.*
• Monitor temperature at least every 4 hours and record on graph paper. Report elevations immediately. *Sustained temperature elevation after surgery may signal onset of pulmonary complications, wound infection or dehiscence, UTI, or thrombophlebitis.*
• Monitor WBC count as ordered. Report elevations or depressions. *Elevated total WBC count indicates infection. Markedly decreased WBC count may indicate decreased production resulting from extreme debilitation or severe lack of vitamins and amino acids. Any damage to bone marrow may suppress WBC formation.*
• Culture urine, respiratory secretions, wound drainage, or blood according to facility policy and doctor's order.

This identifies pathogens and guides antibiotic therapy.
• Help patient wash hands before and after meals and after using bathroom, bedpan, or urinal. *Hand washing prevents spread of pathogens to other objects and food.*
• Assist patient when necessary to ensure that perianal area is clean after elimination. *Cleaning perineal area by wiping from area of least contamination (urinary meatus) to area of most contamination (anus) helps prevent genitourinary infections.*
• Instruct patient to report incidents of loose stools or diarrhea. Inform doctor immediately. *Diarrhea or loose stools may indicate need to discontinue or change antibiotic therapy. It may also indicate need to test for* Clostridium difficile.
• Offer oral hygiene to patient every 4 hours *to prevent colonization of bacteria and reduce risk of descending infection. Disease and malnutrition may reduce moisture in mucous membranes of mouth and lips.*
• Use strict aseptic technique when suctioning lower airway, inserting indwelling urinary catheters, inserting I.V. catheters, and providing wound care *to avoid spreading pathogens.*
• Change I.V. tubing and give site care every 24 to 48 hours or as facility policy dictates *to help keep pathogens from entering the body.*
• Rotate I.V. sites every 48 to 72 hours or as facility policy dictates *to reduce chances of infection at individual sites.*
• Have patient cough and deep-breathe every 4 hours after surgery *to help remove secretions and prevent pulmonary complications.*
• Provide tissues and disposal bags for expectorated sputum. *Convenient disposal encourages expectoration;*

sanitary disposal reduces spread of infection.
• Help patient turn every 2 hours. Provide skin care, particularly over bony prominences, *to help prevent venous stasis and skin breakdown.*
• Use sterile water for humidification or nebulization of oxygen. *This prevents drying and irritation of respiratory mucosa, impaired ciliary action, and thickening of secretions within respiratory tract.*
• Encourage fluid intake of 3,000 to 4,000 ml daily, unless contraindicated, *to help thin mucous secretions.*
• Ensure adequate nutritional intake. Offer high-protein supplements unless contraindicated. *This helps stabilize weight, improves muscle tone and mass, and aids wound healing.*
• Arrange for protective isolation if patient has compromised immune system. Monitor flow and number of visitors. *These measures protect patient from pathogens in environment.*
• Teach patient about:
– good hand-washing technique
– factors that increase infection risk
– infection signs and symptoms.
These measures allow patient to participate in care and help patient modify lifestyle to maintain optimum health level.

Evaluations for expected outcomes
• Patient's temperature remains within normal range.
• Patient's WBC count and differential remain within normal range.
• Cultures don't exhibit pathogen growth.
• Patient demonstrates appropriate personal and oral hygiene.
• Patient's respiratory secretions remain clear and odorless.
• Patient's urine remains clear, yellow, odorless, and free of sediment.

• Patient's bowel patterns remain normal.
• Patient's incisions or wounds remain clear, pink, and free of purulent drainage.
• Patient's I.V. sites don't show signs of inflammation.
• Patient's skin doesn't exhibit signs of breakdown.
• Patient's fluid and protein intake remains at specified levels.
• Patient lists risk factors for infection.
• Patient lists signs and symptoms of infection.
• Patient remains free of signs and symptoms of infection.

Documentation
• Temperature
• Dates, times, and sites of all cultures
• Dates, times, and sites of all catheter insertions
• Appearance of all invasive catheter sites, tube sites, and wounds
• Interventions performed to reduce infection risk
• Patient's response to nursing interventions
• Evaluations for expected outcomes

■ Infection, risk for
related to surgical incision

Definition
Accentuated risk of invasion of a surgical wound by a pathogenic organism (bacteria, virus, fungus, protozoa, or parasite) from either endogenous or environmental sources

Assessment
• Age
• Sex
• Weight

- Reason for surgery
- Type of surgery
- Current health status, including vital signs, nutritional status, and integumentary status
- Laboratory studies, including hematocrit and hemoglobin, complete blood count, electrolytes, urinalysis, blood cultures, blood coagulation studies, immunologic and serologic tests, and liver function tests
- Presence of infection (urinary, respiratory, or oral)
- Health history, including drug allergies, recent infection, substance abuse, and chronic metabolic or systemic disease (diabetes mellitus; cardiovascular, hepatic, or renal disease; coagulation disorders; and splenic or bone marrow disorders)
- Mobility status
- Anticipated length of surgery
- Current medical treatments, including radiation therapy, chemotherapy, antibiotic or antifungal therapy, steroid treatment, anticoagulant or thrombolytic therapy, and immunosuppressive therapy
- Presence of invasive devices, including indwelling urinary catheter, endotracheal tube, tracheostomy tube, I.V. lines, central venous and arterial lines, drains, and gastric feeding tubes
- Wound classification (clean, clean-contaminated, contaminated, or dirty)

Risk factors
- Altered immune function
- Amniotic membrane rupture
- Chronic illness
- Drug use
- Environmental exposure to pathogens
- Invasive procedures
- Lack of knowledge about causes of infection
- Lack of primary (such as skin) or secondary (such as inflammatory response) defenses
- Malnutrition
- Tissue destruction
- Trauma

Associated medical diagnoses (selected)
Appendectomy, bowel resection, craniotomy, joint replacement, kidney or liver transplantation, open heart surgery, urinary diversion

Expected outcomes
- Patient's vital signs and laboratory values will remain within normal limits.
- Incision site will remain free of signs and symptoms of infection.
- Dehiscence will not occur.

Interventions and rationales
- Document and report results of preoperative nursing assessment. Identify risk factors predisposing patient to infection. *A complete nursing assessment allows development of an individualized plan of care.*
- Make sure all surgical team members wear appropriate operating room attire. *The human body is a major source of microbial contamination.*
- Inspect operating room for cleanliness before opening supplies and instruments *to provide a safe environment.*
- Perform a surgical hand scrub. Put on sterile gown and gloves. Place sterile drapes on patient, furniture, and equipment. *Surgical hand scrub minimizes number of microorganisms on skin. Sterile gown and gloves protect against contamination. Sterile drapes create sterile field.*
- Check package integrity, chemical indicator, and, if appropriate, expiration date on all sterile items before dispensing them onto sterile field. *All*

items used within field must be sterile or field will become contaminated.
• Closely monitor sterile field and initiate corrective measures when a break in technique occurs. *Contamination of sterile field may lead to wound contamination and subsequent infection.*
• Use proper technique when opening items onto sterile field *to avoid contamination.*
• Perform preoperative skin preparation of surgical site. *Skin preparation reduces resident microbial count to subpathogenic amounts and inhibits rapid rebound growth of microbes.*
• Keep operating room doors closed at all times and minimize traffic in and out. *Air turbulence caused by movement and mixing of corridor air with room air can sharply increase bacterial counts in operating room.*
• Maintain room temperature of 68° to 75° F (20° to 23.9° C) and relative humidity at 50% + 10, unless contraindicated. *Cooler air temperature and lower humidity inhibit microbial growth.*
• Classify surgical wound according to degree of contamination of wound and surrounding tissue. *Classification helps to assess risk of wound infection from an endogenous source and determine need for antibiotic therapy.*
• Wash hands following contact with patient or any object contaminated with blood or body fluids. *Hand washing is the most effective means for preventing microbial transmission.*
• Administer antibiotics as ordered. *Intraoperative administration of antibiotics can decrease incidence of wound infection and lessen its severity.*
• Disinfect and sterilize all instruments and equipment before and immediately after surgical procedure.

All instruments and equipment used during surgery must be free of microorganisms. Sterilizing instruments and equipment after use prevents growth and spread of microorganisms during storage.
• Promptly clean areas outside sterile field that become contaminated by blood, tissue, or body fluids with an approved disinfectant *to prevent distribution of microbes into environment.*
• Apply sterile dressing to surgical wound before removing surgical drapes *to avoid wound contamination and subsequent infection.*

Evaluations for expected outcomes
• Patient's oral temperature remains below 100° F (37.8° C). Postoperative vital signs and laboratory values (especially white blood cell count) are consistent with preoperative values.
• Patient's incision site remains free of erythema, edema, undue tenderness, warmth, induration, foul odor, purulent drainage, and other signs and symptoms of infection.
• Wound edges are approximated, and evidence of dehiscence is absent.

Documentation
• Results of preoperative nursing assessment
• Operative procedure
• Type of anesthesia
• Surgical times (time patient entered operating room, time incision was made, time incision was closed, and time patient left operating room)
• Wound classification
• Intraoperative administration of antibiotics
• Presence of packing, drains, indwelling urinary catheter, or other invasive devices
• Intraoperative insertion of permanent or temporary implants

- Type of wound closure method
- Type of dressing applied
- Estimated intraoperative blood loss
- Evaluations for expected outcomes

■ Injury, risk for

related to lack of awareness of environmental hazards

Definition
Accentuated risk of physical harm caused by lack of awareness of dangers in the environment

Assessment
- Age
- Health history, including accidents, falls, and exposure to environmental hazards
- Environmental factors, including household layout, electrical wiring, lighting, utilities, fire precautions, presence of toxic or noxious substances, medications, special safety needs, and childproofing
- Mental status, including mood, affect, thought processes, thought content, orientation, judgment, and ability to perform activities of daily living
- Knowledge, including understanding of household safety precautions and automobile safety
- Participation in recreational activities, such as swimming, diving, motorcycling, bicycling, and contact sports

Risk factors
- Abnormal blood profile
- Altered mobility
- Confusion
- Disorientation
- Exposure to biological or chemical hazards
- Malnutrition

- Skin breakdown

Associated medical diagnoses (selected)
Alzheimer's disease, blindness, brain abscess, burns, cataracts, dementia, depression, diabetes mellitus, Down syndrome, hemophilia, Huntington's disease, inhalation injuries, joint replacement, osteomyelitis, osteoporosis, poisoning, syphilis

Expected outcomes
- Patient and family will acknowledge presence of environmental hazards in their everyday surroundings.
- Patient and family will practice safety and take safety precautions in home.
- Adults in household will instruct children in safety habits.
- Adults in household will childproof house to ensure safety of young children and cognitively impaired adults.

Interventions and rationales
- Help patient identify situations and hazards that can cause accidents *to increase patient's awareness of potential dangers.*
- Encourage patient to make repairs and remove potential safety hazards from environment *to decrease possibility of injury.*
- Encourage adults to discuss safety rules with children. For example:
  – Don't play with matches.
  – Use electrical equipment carefully.
  – Know location of fire escape route.
  – Don't speak to strangers.
  – Dial 911 in an emergency.
  Teaching by parents fosters household safety.
- Arrange environment of patient with dementia to minimize risk of injury:
  – Place furniture against walls.
  – Don't use throw rugs.

– Maintain lighting so that patient can find his way around room and to bathroom. *Arranging patient's environment helps prevent injury.*
• Refer patient to appropriate community resources for more information about identifying and removing safety hazards. *This enables patient and family to alter environment to achieve optimal safety level.*

Evaluations for expected outcomes
• Patient and family identify and eliminate safety hazards in their surroundings.
• Patient and family members demonstrate prevention and safety measures.
• Children describe safety measures they have learned.
• Patient and family point out evidence of childproofing measures in the home.

Documentation
• Patient's statements about situations that cause accidents and injuries
• Patient's lack of awareness of, or disregard for, safety hazards
• Patient's cognitive deficits that inhibit learning or attention to safety hazards
• Interventions to help patient recognize and eliminate safety hazards
• Patient's or family's response to nursing interventions
• Evaluations for expected outcomes

■ Injury, risk for

related to sensory or motor deficits

Definition
Accentuated risk of physical harm caused by sensory or motor deficits

Assessment
• Age
• Nature of sensory or motor deficit
• Health history, including cerebral function, mobility, sensory function, and use of adaptive devices
• Psychological status, including substance abuse, familiarity with surroundings, mental status, coping skills, and self-concept
• Medication history and use, including understanding of medications, compliance with prescribed regimen, use of over-the-counter medications, and interactions
• Knowledge, including understanding of safety precautions
• Pain or fatigue
• Laboratory studies, complete blood count and differential, and coagulation studies
• Diagnostic tests, including chest X-ray and brain scan
• Sensory status, including hearing, vision, touch, and taste

Risk factors
• Abnormal blood profile
• Altered mobility
• Confusion
• Disorientation
• Exposure to biological or chemical hazards
• Malnutrition
• Skin breakdown

Associated medical diagnoses (selected)
Amputation, brain tumors, cerebral aneurysm, cerebrovascular accident, deafness, detached retina, fractures, glaucoma, head injury, heart failure, hepatic coma, metabolic acidosis, metabolic alkalosis

Expected outcomes
• Patient will identify factors that increase potential for injury.

• Patient will help identify and apply safety measures to prevent injury.
• Patient and family members will develop strategy to maintain safety.
• Patient will optimize activities of daily living within sensorimotor limitations.

Interventions and rationales

• Observe for factors that may cause or contribute to injury *to increase awareness of patient, family members, and caregivers.*
• Improve environmental safety as needed:
– Orient patient to environment. Assess patient's ability to use call bell, side rails, and bed positioning controls. Keep bed at lowest level, and conduct close night watch. *These measures will help patient cope with unfamiliar surroundings.*
– Teach patient and family about need for safe illumination. Advise patient to wear sunglasses to reduce glare. Advise using contrasting colors in household furnishings. *These measures will enhance visual discrimination.*
– Test heating pads and bath water before using; assess extremities daily for injury *to assist patient with decreased tactile sensitivity.*
– For patient with hearing loss, encourage use of hearing aid *to minimize deficit.*
– Teach patient with unstable gait correct use of adaptive devices *to decrease potential for injury.*
• Provide additional patient teaching as needed. Possible topics may include household, automobile, and pedestrian safety. Refer patient to appropriate resources (police, fire, and home health care agency) for more information. *Health education can help patient take steps to prevent injury.*

Evaluations for expected outcomes

• Patient identifies two factors that increase risk of injury.
• Patient applies safety measures.
• Patient and family members describe and demonstrate preventive measures to minimize potential for injury.
• Patient increases self-care activities within limits posed by sensorimotor limitations.

Documentation

• Statements by patient and family members about potential for injury due to sensory or motor deficits
• Manifestations of deficit
• Observation or knowledge of unsafe practices
• Interventions to decrease risk of injury to patient
• Patient's responses to nursing interventions
• Evaluations for expected outcomes

■ Intracranial adaptive capacity, decreased

Definition

A state in which physiologic mechanisms that normally compensate for increased intracranial volumes are compromised, resulting in disproportionate increases in intracranial pressure (ICP) in response to stimuli

Assessment

• Cardiovascular status, including vital signs, skin color and temperature, carotid and apical pulses, heart sounds, jugular vein distention, electrocardiography, and history of hypertension
• GI status, including bowel elimination patterns, dietary intake, and ab-

dominal inspection, palpation, and auscultation
• Musculoskeletal status, including range of motion (ROM); joint and muscle symmetry; muscle size, strength, and tone; functional mobility; contractures, subluxation, dislocation, and atrophy; previous trauma; and degenerative joint diseases
• Neurologic status, including mental status; cranial nerve function; cerebellar function; reflexes (deep tendon, superficial, and pathologic [Babinski's reflex]); peripheral sensory system (pain, position, and vibration); pupillary size and reactivity; use of anticonvulsant, neuroleptic, antidepressant, antimanic, analgesic, or illicit drugs; history of head injury; alcohol abuse; history of lethargy, restlessness, stupor, headaches, seizures, tremors, paresthesia, paresis, incoordination, ticks, fasciculation, pain, psychiatric disorders, or abnormal posturing (decorticate or decerebrate); and tests such as computed tomography scan, magnetic resonance imaging, cerebral arteriography, electroencephalography, evoked potential studies, and Glasgow Coma Scale
• Respiratory status, including chest expansion; rate, depth, and pattern of respirations; tracheal position; fremitus; auscultation of lung fields; arterial blood gas (ABG) analysis, pulse oximetry, and mixed venous oxygen saturation; history of lung disease; tobacco use; and use of bronchodilators, antibiotics, or diuretics
• Sensory status, including visual and auditory acuity, use of hearing aid or glasses, tactile sensitivity eye disorders, and hearing loss

Defining characteristics
• Baseline ICP equal to or greater than 10 mm Hg; wide amplitude ICP waveform

• Disproportionate increase in ICP following single nursing maneuver
• Elevated P2 ICP waveform
• Repeated increases in ICP exceeding 10 mm Hg for more than 5 minutes following external stimuli
• Volume pressure response test variation (volume-pressure ratio greater than 2, pressure-volume index less than 10)

Associated medical diagnoses (selected)
Brain abscess, brain tumors, cerebral aneurysm, cerebrovascular accident, craniotomy, head injury, Reye's syndrome

Expected outcomes
• Patient will maintain patent airway, effective breathing patterns, and normal ABG levels.
• Patient will show no evidence of fever.
• Patient's position will promote venous drainage from the brain.
• Patient will not experience sustained rise in ICP in response to stimulation.
• Patient's environment will be modified to reduce noxious stimuli.
• Patient will maintain regular bowel function.
• Patient will maintain skin integrity.
• Patient will remain free of signs and symptoms of infection.
• Patient will show no evidence of neurologic compromise.
• Patient and family members will express feelings about treatment and recovery.

Interventions and rationales
• Perform thorough nursing history and head-to-toe assessment and document *to establish baseline of patient's condition for future comparison and to ensure continuity and consistency of care among nursing staff.*

• Monitor neurologic status, including level of consciousness, pupillary size and reactivity, eye movement, selected reflexes, and motor and sensory function *to identify changes that indicate increased ICP.*

• Monitor vital signs and hemodynamic parameters (mean arterial blood pressure and pulmonary artery pressure) *to assess hemodynamic stability and to note trends.*

• Maintain ICP monitoring systems, if used. Use aseptic technique for dressing changes. Maintain closed system. *Aseptic technique prevents contamination of equipment and subsequent infections.*

• Monitor ICP waveforms for trends over time (A waves, B waves, C waves). Assess intracranial pulse waves (P1 percussion waves, P2 tidal waves, P3 dicrotic waves). Monitor for damped waveforms, absent waveforms, or abnormally high or low readings. *Waveforms provide information about cerebral compliance. Cerebral compliance is the body's attempt to cope with changes in intracranial content (brain tissue, blood volume, and cerebral spinal fluid). Compliance is expressed as a mathematic ratio between volume and pressure changes within the skull.*

• Assess cerebral perfusion pressure. *Adequate cerebral perfusion pressure is critical to prevent cerebral ischemia. Cerebral perfusion pressure is calculated by taking the mean arterial pressure and subtracting ICP.*

• Assess temperature every 2 hours. *Fever increases cerebral metabolic demands, cerebral blood flow, and ICP.*

• Maintain patent airway. Assess rate, depth, and rhythm of respirations *to monitor lung expansion and presence of abnormal sounds.*

• Suction patient only if needed. Limit suctioning to 10 to 15 seconds per pass of the catheter. *Suctioning stimulates coughing and Valsalva's maneuver; Valsalva's maneuver increases intrathoracic pressure, decreases cerebral venous drainage, and increases cerebral blood volume, resulting in increased ICP.*

• Administer 100% oxygen for 1 minute before and after suctioning. *Hypercapnia results in cerebral vasodilation, increased cerebral blood volume, and increased ICP. Giving supplemental oxygen helps avoid hypoxemia and tissue ischemia.*

• Administer lidocaine, if prescribed, I.V. or into endotracheal (ET) tube before suctioning. *Lidocaine suppresses cough reflex, thereby preventing increases in ICP.*

• Monitor ABG levels. Observe for signs and symptoms of respiratory distress. *Hypercapnia results in vasodilation, increased cerebral blood volume, and increased ICP. Hypoxia may contribute to tissue ischemia.*

• Elevate head of bed 15 to 30 degrees or as ordered. Keep patient's head and neck straight. Use sandbags, rolled towels, or small pillows to keep head in neutral position. Avoid hip flexion of 90 degrees or more. *Neutral head position promotes venous drainage from head. Some positions cause increased intra-abdominal and intrathoracic pressure that can interfere with venous drainage from head.*

• When performing neurologic assessment, use the minimal amount of stimuli required to obtain a response. *Unpleasant or painful stimuli increase ICP.*

• Limit environmental noise as much as possible. *Auditory stimuli can contribute to increased ICP.*

• Monitor for seizure activity. Maintain seizure precautions. Administer anticonvulsant drugs as prescribed. *Tonic-clonic seizures increase intrathoracic pressure, decrease cerebral venous outflow, and increase cerebral blood volume, thereby raising ICP.*

• Maintain intake and output. Maintain fluid restriction, if ordered. *Fluid restriction helps decrease extracellular fluid, thereby decreasing ICP.*

• Administer osmotic diuretics, if prescribed. Monitor for signs and symptoms of dehydration (increased sodium, serum osmolality, and decreased urine output). *Osmotic diuretics pull fluid from nonedematous areas of brain, thereby decreasing ICP.*

• Administer loop diuretics, if prescribed, *to decrease water in injured brain tissue and to decrease overall body water, thereby reducing cerebral edema and lowering ICP.* Monitor for signs of dehydration and hypokalemia, *which are adverse effects of diuretics.*

• Turn and reposition patient every 2 hours and as needed *to prevent pressure ulcer formation.*

• While turning, keep patient's head in neutral position *to promote venous drainage from head.*

• Use a draw sheet to reposition patient. Instruct patient to exhale, if conscious, when turning or moving in bed *to avoid Valsalva's maneuver, which can increase ICP by increasing intrathoracic and intra-abdominal pressures.*

• Monitor and record bowel movements. Administer stool softeners, as prescribed. Instruct patient not to hold his breath or strain on defecation. *Straining associated with constipation can cause Valsalva's maneuver, increasing ICP.*

• Instruct patient, if he can follow simple commands, to avoid pushing against footboard or digging heels into mattress when moving up in bed.

Remove footboard if possible, especially if patient has decerebrate or abnormal posturing. *Isometric muscle contraction can increase ICP.*

• Perform passive ROM exercises *to maintain muscle tone and prevent atrophy and contractures.*

• Maintain normothermia. Administer antipyretics if ordered. Apply hypothermia blanket. Assess rectal temperature every 30 minutes while patient is on blanket. Control shivering. Administer chlorpromazine if prescribed. *Shivering causes isometric muscle contraction, which can increase ICP.*

• Continue frequent neurologic assessment. Compare results with previous findings. *Frequent assessment allows detection of subtle changes in neurologic signs that indicate improvement or deterioration in patient's status.*

• Try to limit painful procedures, if possible. Avoid unnecessary tension or pulling on tubes (such as ET tube or indwelling urinary catheter). *Unpleasant or painful stimuli increase ICP.*

• Involve family members in gentle stroking of patient's face, hand, or arm. *Recent studies have shown touch provided by family members may lower ICP in some patients.*

• Speak in a low, soft voice. Provide nursing care in calm, reassuring manner. Explain all procedures before touching patient. *Explanations can help prevent emotional upsets that may increase ICP.*

• Avoid discussion of upsetting topics near patient's bedside. Patient may be upset by discussion of his prognosis, treatment procedures, or his level of pain. Instruct patient's family members not to discuss upsetting topics within patient's hearing range. *Emotional upsets may increase ICP.*

• Ask family members to bring in audiotapes of familiar voices and patient's favorite music. Play audiotapes through earphones, if appropriate. *Family members' voices and preferred music have been shown to decrease ICP in some patients.*
• Provide uninterrupted rest periods as much as possible. Avoid awakening patient during rapid eye movement (REM) sleep. *Cerebral blood flow increases during REM sleep.* Don't carry out nursing activities known to increase ICP during that time. *Nursing procedures performed during REM sleep may cause additional elevations in patient's ICP.*
• Schedule sufficient time, at least 10 minutes, between nursing care activities (such as bathing, turning, and suctioning) *to allow patient to rest and to avoid cumulative effects of continuous activity on ICP. Close spacing of activities has been known to cause sustained increases of ICP.*
• Encourage patient and family to ventilate feelings associated with diagnosis, treatment, and recovery. *Expression of feelings helps patient and family cope with treatment.*
• Refer patient and family to appropriate support groups *to assist them in dealing with the injury, diagnosis, or recovery.*

Evaluations for expected outcomes
• Patient maintains effective breathing patterns, patent airway, and normal ABG levels.
• Patient shows no evidence of fever.
• Patient maintains proper positioning to promote venous drainage from brain.
• Patient shows no evidence of sustained increase in ICP in response to stimulation.

• Patient's environment contains fewer noxious stimuli as a result of modifications.
• Patient is free from constipation.
• Patient has intact skin.
• Patient has no signs or symptoms of infection.
• Patient shows no evidence of neurologic compromise.
• Patient and family members openly express fear, anxiety, anger, and other feelings associated with treatment and recovery.

Documentation
• Results of initial nursing assessment
• Monitoring procedures and results
• Nursing interventions and patient's response
• Instructions to patient, family, or caregiver and their demonstrated understanding of those instructions
• Evaluations for expected outcomes

■ Knowledge deficit
related to cognitive impairment

Definition
Inadequate understanding of information or inability to perform skills needed to practice health-related behaviors

Assessment
• Psychosocial status, including age, learning ability (affective, cognitive, and psychomotor domains), decision-making ability, developmental stage, financial resources, interest in learning, knowledge and skills related to current health problem, obstacles to learning, support systems (willingness and capability of others to help patient), and usual coping pattern

• Neurologic status, including level of consciousness, memory, mental status, and orientation

Defining characteristics
• Inability to follow through with instruction
• Inability to perform well on test
• Inappropriate or exaggerated behaviors (hysteria, hostility, agitation, apathy)
• Verbalization of problem

Associated medical diagnoses (selected)
Alzheimer's disease, cerebrovascular accident, Down syndrome, Huntington's disease, metabolic acidosis

Expected outcomes
• Patient will demonstrate ability to perform simple self-care measures, such as feeding, maintaining hygiene, dressing, and toileting.
• Family members will communicate understanding of patient's cognitive impairment.
• Family members will express willingness to help patient maintain maximum independence.
• Family members will demonstrate method being used to teach patient.

Interventions and rationales
• Provide all equipment needed for each self-care measure patient must learn. *This reduces frustration, aids learning, and minimizes dependence by promoting self-care.*
• When teaching self-care measures, go slowly and repeat frequently. Offer small amounts of information and present it in various ways. *By building cognition, patient will be better able to complete self-care measures.*
• Have patient practice each task. Provide positive reinforcement each time patient performs task correctly. *This encourages desired behavior.*

• Discuss patient's limitations with family members. *Communication promotes working relationship and reduces fear and anxiety.*
• Demonstrate to family members how each self-care measure is broken down into simple tasks *to enhance patient's success and foster sense of control.*
• Encourage family members to participate in patient's learning process *to help create an encouraging, therapeutic climate after discharge.*
• Have family members give return demonstration of patient's methods of performing self-care measures. *This provides hands-on experience with equipment, builds confidence, and encourages compliance.*
• Refer family members to outside agencies, such as a home health care organization, for assistance after patient's discharge. *This ensures continuity of care and assistance with follow-up after discharge.*

Evaluations for expected outcomes
• Patient practices simple self-care measures and demonstrates ability to perform activities of daily living.
• Family members describe cause of patient's cognitive impairment.
• Family members demonstrate willingness to help patient learn to perform self-care measures.
• Family members provide return demonstration of patient's methods of performing self-care measures.

Documentation
• Patient's abilities and limitations in performing self-care measures
• Progress made by patient in learning each specific task
• Information given to family members concerning patient's limitations and progress in learning tasks

• Family members' participation in learning process
• Referrals to outside agencies
• Evaluations for expected outcomes

■ Knowledge deficit
related to lack of exposure

Definition
Inadequate understanding of information or inability to perform skills needed to practice health-related behaviors

Assessment
• Psychosocial status, including age, learning ability (affective, cognitive, and psychomotor domains), decision-making ability, developmental stage, financial resources, health beliefs and attitudes, interest in learning, knowledge and skill regarding current health problem, obstacles to learning, support systems (willingness and capability of others to help patient), and usual coping pattern
• Neurologic status, including level of consciousness, memory, mental status, and orientation

Defining characteristics
• Inability to follow through with instruction
• Inability to perform well on test
• Inappropriate or exaggerated behaviors (hysteria, hostility, agitation, apathy)
• Verbalization of problem

Associated medical diagnoses (selected)
This nursing diagnosis can be associated with any medical diagnosis. Examples include alcohol addiction, aortic insufficiency, aortic stenosis, cardiac arrhythmias, cellulitis, child abuse, chronic renal failure, coronary artery disease, dermatomyositis and polymyositis, diabetes mellitus, endocarditis, endometriosis, glaucoma, gout, head injury, heart failure, hemodialysis, hemorrhoids, hypertension, hyperthermia, hypothermia, infertility, interstitial cystitis, kidney transplantation, lesions, mitral insufficiency, mitral stenosis, open wounds, osteoarthritis, panic disorder, Parkinson's disease, peritoneal dialysis, pregnancy-induced hypertension, rheumatic fever, rheumatoid arthritis, syphilis, and trigeminal neuralgia.

Expected outcomes
• Patient will communicate need to know.
• Patient will state or demonstrate understanding of what has been taught.
• Patient will demonstrate ability to perform new health-related behaviors as they are taught and will list specific skills and realistic target dates for each.
• Patient will set realistic learning goals.
• Patient will state intention to make needed changes in lifestyle, including seeking help from health professional when needed.

Interventions and rationales
• Establish environment of mutual trust and respect to enhance learning. *Comfort with growing self-awareness, ability to share this awareness with others, receptiveness to new experiences, and consistency between actions and words form basis of trusting relationship.*
• Negotiate with patient to develop goals for learning. *Involving patient in planning meaningful goals encourages follow-through.*
• Select teaching strategies (such as discussion, demonstration, role-play-

ing, and visual materials) appropriate for patient's individual learning style (specify) *to enhance teaching effectiveness.*
• Teach skills that patient must incorporate into daily lifestyle. Have patient give return demonstration of each new skill *to help gain confidence.*
• Have patient incorporate learned skills into daily routine during hospitalization (specify skills). *This allows patient to practice new skills and receive feedback.*
• Provide patient with names and telephone numbers of resource people or organizations *to provide continuity of care and follow-up after discharge.*
• As needed, arrange for interpreter. *Patient who doesn't speak English may understand health-related behaviors but may need interpreter to express them.*

Evaluations for expected outcomes
• Patient expresses desire to overcome lack of knowledge.
• Patient states understanding of what he has learned.
• Patient demonstrates newly learned health-related behaviors.
• Patient develops realistic learning goals and performs new skills by target date.
• Patient identifies specific changes in lifestyle needed to promote optimal health.

Documentation
• Patient's statements of information and skills he knows and doesn't know
• Expressions of need to know and motivation to learn
• Learning objectives
• Methods used to teach patient
• Information imparted
• Skills demonstrated
• Patient's responses to teaching

• Evaluations for expected outcomes

■ Knowledge deficit
related to lack of motivation

Definition
Inadequate understanding of information or inability to perform skills needed to practice health-related behaviors

Assessment
• Psychosocial status, including age, learning ability (affective, cognitive, and psychomotor domains), decision-making ability, developmental stage, financial resources, interest in learning, knowledge and skills related to current health problem, obstacles to learning, support systems (willingness and capability of others to help patient), and usual coping pattern
• Neurologic status, including level of consciousness, memory, mental status, and orientation

Defining characteristics
• Inability to follow through with instruction
• Inability to perform well on test
• Inappropriate or exaggerated behaviors (hysteria, hostility, agitation, apathy)
• Verbalization of problem

Associated medical diagnoses (selected)
Chronic bronchitis, chronic obstructive pulmonary disease, emphysema, hypertension, polycystic kidney disease

Expected outcomes
• Patient will express interest in learning new behaviors.

• Patient will gradually set realistic learning objectives (specify).
• Patient will strive to meet each objective by target date.
• Patient will practice new health-related behaviors during hospitalization (for example, selecting appropriate diet, self-medicating, weighing self daily, and monitoring intake and output).
• Patient will develop realistic plan for maintaining new skills at home.

Interventions and rationales
• Provide uninterrupted time for patient to state reasons for not wanting to learn or practice new health-related behaviors. *Attentive listening conveys caring attitude, encouraging patient to talk.*
• Avoid nonconstructive criticism. Rather, encourage expression of feelings. *Nonjudgmental approach encourages patient to express feelings more freely.*
• Ascertain what patient already knows *to determine what patient needs to know. Building on known information leads to successful learning.*
• Explore with patient impact of behavior on self and family members. *Learning is more effective if patient recognizes need to know.*
• Urge patient to ask questions *to help clarify information and evaluate patient's comprehension.*
• Determine whether patient enjoys learning through such media as videotapes, audiotapes, books, and discussions *to discover most effective teaching tools.*
• Begin negotiating learning objectives with patient. *Involving patient in defining goals increases understanding and encourages compliance.*

• Be patient; offer praise when patient attempts new behaviors *to motivate patient to learn more.*
• Provide emotional support as patient attempts distasteful or anxiety-producing behaviors. *Support will help patient perform tasks successfully.*
• Suggest that patient discuss situation with someone who has developed skill in managing a similar health problem *to encourage patient to air feelings and concerns.*
• Help patient plan realistically for continuing new behaviors; include teaching family members as needed. *Setting realistic goals increases probability of compliance. Involving others adds support after discharge.*

Evaluations for expected outcomes
• Patient expresses desire to change behavior.
• Patient participates in developing educational goals.
• Patient displays motivation to attain each goal by target date.
• Patient practices new health-related behaviors.
• Patient states plans for inclusion of new activities into daily routine after discharge.

Documentation
• Statements of motivation or lack of interest in learning
• Observations that indicate readiness or lack of readiness to learn
• Goals set by patient
• Methods used to teach patient
• Information imparted
• Skills demonstrated
• Patient's responses to trying new behaviors
• Evaluations for expected outcomes

■ Latex allergy response

Definition
A systemic or local allergic response to contact with latex products

Assessment
• Age
• Sex
• Weight
• Occupation
• Health history, including past episodes of latex allergy; food, pollen, or drug allergy; multiple surgical history; spina bifida; and asthma
• Current health status, including temperature, blood pressure, respiratory status, and other vital signs
• Integumentary status, including color, elasticity, hygiene, lesions, moisture, sensation, texture, and turgor
• Reports of contact with latex products, including when, where, and what
• Laboratory studies, including arterial blood gas levels, complete blood count, immunoglobulin E level, radioallergosorbent test, and scratch test

Defining characteristics
• Local reaction, such as edema, erythema, itching, open or weeping wounds, pain, skin cracking or breakdown, and urticaria
• Systemic reaction, such as chest tightness, cough (sometimes productive), facial edema (especially around eyes), increased respiratory rate, rhinitis (with secretions from clear to yellow-green), shortness of breath, use of accessory muscles, and wheezing

Associated medical diagnoses (selected)
Asthma, atopy (from food, pollen, or drugs), spina bifida

Expected outcomes
• Vital signs, respiratory status, and laboratory values will return to normal.
• Skin will be clear, moist, and free from erythema, edema, itching, urticaria, and breakdown.
• Patient will express awareness of allergic response to latex-containing products.
• Patient will state intention to avoid contact with latex-containing products.

Interventions and rationales
• If the patient exhibits compromised respiratory status, implement treatment immediately and document findings. *Airway maintenance is a primary health consideration and must be attended to immediately.*
• Conduct nursing assessment and document results *to allow for development of an individualized plan of care.*
• Monitor respiratory status and document findings *to detect changes in status and respond appropriately. Accurate documentation is necessary to maintain continuity of care among staff.*
• Administer prescribed drugs and treatments in a timely fashion. *Wheezing and shortness of breath can quickly deteriorate to respiratory distress and failure. Skin with urticaria and itching is uncomfortable and unsightly, so patients appreciate timely treatment.*
• Become familiar with potential adverse effects of administered drugs. *Bronchodilators, antihistamines, and corticosteroids may cause systemic adverse effects; becoming familiar with these effects and ways to respond to them may help prevent serious reactions.*

• When latex allergy is confirmed, document on the patient record and label the record clearly *to prevent future contact with the allergen.*
• Remove all latex products from immediate proximity of the patient and the staff treating the patient. *If latex products are nearby, they may be inadvertently used by the staff or patient, increasing risk of contact and allergic reaction.*
• Educate the patient and family about allergic reaction to latex products *to prevent future contact and allergic reactions.*
• Give the patient and family a list of household items containing latex and emphasize the importance of avoiding these. Tell them about nonlatex product substitutes. *Prevention is the foundation of treatment for latex allergy.*
• Educate the patient and family members about the importance of quickly seeking medical treatment for allergic reaction *to foster timely intervention.*
• Emphasize the need to inform all health care providers — including emergency medical rescuers — about the patient's latex sensitivity. Stress the importance of wearing a medical identification bracelet that specifies latex sensitivity *to prevent future contact and allergic reactions.*
• Provide documentation of latex allergy for the patient to take to his employer. With the patient's permission, communicate with the employee health department and discuss the patient's need to avoid contact with latex products *to help prevent the patient's further contact with latex products and avoid latex allergy reaction.*

Evaluations for expected outcomes
• Vital signs, respiratory status, and laboratory values return to normal levels.

• Skin is clear, moist, and free from erythema, edema, itching, urticaria, and breakdown.
• Patient expresses awareness of allergic response to latex-containing products.
• Patient expresses intention to avoid contact with latex-containing products.

Documentation
• Results of nursing assessment
• Diagnosis of latex allergy
• Treatment for allergic reaction, including drugs administered
• Respiratory status throughout episode of allergic reaction
• Integumentary status throughout episode of allergic reaction
• Evidence of refrain from latex product use during patient's care and of removal of latex products from immediate patient area; explanation of latex product substitutes
• Evidence of patient and family education regarding latex allergy and avoidance of latex products
• Evaluations for expected outcomes

■ Latex allergy response, risk for

Definition
Accentuated risk of allergic reaction, either systemic or local, due to contact with latex products

Assessment
• Age
• Sex
• Weight
• Occupation
• Current health status, including vital signs, respiratory status, and integumentary status

• Health history, including drug, food, or pollen allergies; surgical history; chronic disease such as spina bifida; and previous local or systemic allergic reactions
• Laboratory studies, such as immunoglobulin E level, complete blood count, radioallergosorbent test, and scratch tests

Risk factors
• Diagnosis of spina bifida
• Frequent medical or occupational exposure to latex
• History of atopy
• History of food allergies, such as allergy to bananas, kiwi, avocados, chestnuts, or pineapples
• History of latex allergy
• History of multiple surgeries, especially genitourinary surgery
• Lack of knowledge about latex allergy
• Unexplained anaphylaxis with a previous medical or dental exposure, especially if latex products were used

Associated medical diagnoses (selected)
Asthma, atopy, spina bifida

Expected outcomes
• Vital signs, especially respirations, will remain within patient's normal limits.
• Skin will remain free from erythema, edema, urticaria, and breakdown.
• Nasal passages and laryngeal area will remain clear and free from edema and secretions.
• Patient and family members will express understanding of risk of latex allergy.
• Patient and family members will state intention to take precautions to avoid contact with latex products.

Interventions and rationales
• Conduct nursing assessment and document results *to allow for development of an individualized plan of care.*
• Remove all latex-containing products from the patient's room *to reduce risk of allergic reaction.*
• Use only nonlatex products when caring for the patient *to reduce risk of latex allergy reaction in the patient.*
• Make sure all personnel are aware of risk of latex allergy and refrain from using latex products during diagnostic procedures. *Communication with other health care personnel allows for continuity of care and reduces the risk of latex allergy reaction.*
• Educate the patient and family about the risk of latex allergy *to prevent allergic reaction due to contact with latex products.*
• Explain that although some reactions to latex are relatively minor (such as sneezing and runny nose), others are life-threatening. *This will foster awareness of serious nature of risk.*
• Educate the patient and family regarding the symptoms of allergic reaction and the need for quick treatment if symptoms appear. *Rapid response to allergic reaction may help prevent complications, such as skin infection (with local reaction) and respiratory failure (with systemic reaction).*
• Give the patient and family a list of household items containing latex and emphasize the importance of avoiding these. Tell them about nonlatex product substitutes. *Prevention is the foundation of treatment for latex allergy.*
• Emphasize the need to inform all health care providers — including emergency medical rescuers — about the patient's latex sensitivity. Stress

the importance of wearing a medical identification bracelet that specifies latex sensitivity *to prevent future contact and allergic reactions.*
• Provide emotional support to help the patient cope with stress. *Fear of latex exposure can cause a high level of stress in a latex-sensitive patient. Some patients are afraid to seek medical help for fear of latex exposure.*

Evaluations for expected outcomes
• Vital signs, especially respirations, remain within patient's normal limits.
• Skin remains free from erythema, edema, urticaria, and breakdown.
• Nasal passages and laryngeal area remain clear and free from edema and secretions.
• Patient and family members express understanding of risk of latex allergy.
• Patient and family members state intention to take precautions to avoid contact with latex products.

Documentation
• Results of nursing assessment
• Presence of risk factors
• Communication of risk factors to health care personnel involved in care or diagnostic studies of patient
• Teaching provided to patient and family members about risk factors and symptoms of allergic reactions
• Patient's and family members' statements indicating understanding of risk factors and symptoms of allergic reactions
• Evaluations for expected outcomes

■ Loneliness, risk for

Definition
A subjective state in which an individual is at risk for experiencing vague dysphoria associated with feelings of isolation from others

Assessment
• Family status, including family composition, presence of a spouse, ability of family to meet patient's physical and emotional needs, conflicts between patient's needs and family's ability to meet them, and family members' feelings of self-worth
• Psychological status, including changes in appetite, behavior, energy level, mood, motivation, self-image, self-esteem, or sleep patterns; alcohol and drug consumption; recent death, job loss, loss of loved one, or relocation; and psychiatric history
• Social status, including interpersonal skills, size of social network, quality of relationships, degree of trust in others, level of self-esteem, and ability to function in social and occupational roles
• Health history, including medical illness, disabilities, and deformities
• Spiritual status, including religious or church affiliation, description of faith and religious practices, and support network (family, clergy, and friends)

Risk factors
• Deprivation of physical or emotional energy
• Deprivation of affection
• Physical isolation
• Social isolation

Associated medical diagnoses (selected)
Acquired immunodeficiency syndrome, affective disorders, anxiety disorders, blindness, depression, eating disorders, genital herpes, Parkinson's disease, personality disorders, posttraumatic stress disorder, tuberculosis

Expected outcomes
• Patient will identify feelings of loneliness and will desire to socialize more.
• Patient will identify behaviors that lead to loneliness.
• Patient will identify people who will likely support and accept him.
• Patient will spend time with others.
• Patient will be comfortable in social settings, will interact with peers, and will receive support from others
• Patient will make specific plans to continue involvement with others such as through recreational activities or social interaction groups.

Interventions and rationales
• Spend sufficient time with patient to allow him to express his feelings of loneliness *to establish trusting relationship.*
• Inform patient that you will help him express feelings of loneliness and identify ways to increase social activity *to bring issue into open and help patient understand that you want to help him.*
• Work with patient to identify factors and behaviors that have contributed to loneliness *to begin changing behaviors that may alienate others.*
• Help patient identify feelings associated with loneliness *to lessen their impact and mobilize energy to counteract them.*
• Help patient curb feelings of loneliness by encouraging one-on-one interaction with others who are likely to accept him — for example, church members or patients with similar health problems — *to promote feelings of acceptance and support.*
• Encourage patient to address needs assertively. *By being assertive, patient assumes responsibility for meeting his needs, without anger or guilt.*

• As patient's comfort level improves, encourage him to attend group activities and social functions *to promote use of social skills.*
• Help patient identify social activities he can initiate, such as becoming active in a support group or volunteer organization, *to foster feelings of control and increase social contacts.*
• Help patient accept that other people may view him differently because of his illness, and explore ways of coping with their reactions. *Patient must learn to cope with stigma associated with illness.*
• Work with patient to establish goals for reducing feelings of loneliness after he leaves health care setting *to focus energy on specific objectives.*
• Refer patient and family to social service agencies, mental health center, and appropriate support groups *to ensure continued care and maintain social involvement.*

Evaluations for expected outcomes
• Patient expresses feelings of loneliness.
• Patient describes behaviors that lead to loneliness.
• Patient lists at least __ (specify) people who will likely support and accept him.
• Patient initiates conversations with peers.
• Patient participates in group activities.
• Patient describes plans to continue involvement with others.

Documentation
• Patient's statements of loneliness
• Observations of patient's behaviors and problems associated with loneliness
• Patient's choice of activities to end isolation
• Teaching of new coping methods

- Goals established by patient
- Evidence of efforts to use new coping mechanisms
- Referral
- Evaluations for expected outcomes

■ Management of therapeutic regimen, ineffective: family

related to family conflict, complex therapy, economic difficulties, or difficulty coping with the health care system

Definition
Difficulty integrating measures to cope with illness into a family's daily routine

Assessment
- Family status, including marital status, family composition, communication patterns, coping skills, drug or alcohol abuse, psychiatric history, and beliefs and attitudes about health and illness
- Health status, including chronic or terminal illness and severely disabling physical conditions
- Socioeconomic factors, including financial status, insurance, accessibility of health care, availability of health care providers, and transportation system
- Social status, including communication skills, size of social network, degree of trust in others, self-esteem, and ability to function in social and occupational roles
- Spiritual status, including religious or church affiliation and description of faith and religious practices

Defining characteristics
- Acceleration of signs and symptoms of illness of family member
- Expressed inability to reduce risk factors for progression of illness
- Expressed desire to manage treatment
- Expressed difficulty with regulating or integrating treatment
- Inappropriate family activities for meeting goals of treatment or prevention
- Inattention to illness or its sequelae

Associated medical diagnoses (selected)
Acquired immunodeficiency syndrome, drug or alcohol addiction, eating disorders, prolonged hospitalization

Expected outcomes
- Family members will identify behaviors that lead to conflict.
- Family members will participate in family therapy sessions and openly express feelings about illness of family member.
- Family members will express desire to have help in resolving conflicts.
- Family members will describe coping mechanisms that help reduce conflicts.
- Family members will cooperate in finding ways to incorporate therapeutic regimen into their lifestyle.
- Family members will express desire to carry out therapeutic regimen.
- Family members will plan for future course of illness.

Interventions and rationales
- Spend time with family, get to know each family member individually, and establish trusting relationship with each family member *to help identify measures that will increase family cohesiveness.*

• Encourage family members to attend and participate in family therapy sessions *to strengthen family unit and promote resolution of conflict.*

• Help family members describe feelings associated with illness of their relative *to bring family conflict into open. Unresolved family conflicts may prevent family members from fully implementing therapeutic regimen.*

• Elicit family members' personal beliefs about illness and review relevant information *to establish their support for improving management of therapeutic regimen.*

• Educate family members about pathophysiology of illness, and explain relationship between pathophysiology and therapeutic regimen. *If family members know reasons for specific behaviors, they may be more willing to adjust their lifestyle.*

• Work with family members to identify behaviors that have contributed to family conflict, and help them identify alternative behaviors *to promote resolution of the conflict.*

• Encourage family members to address individual needs assertively *to promote healthy interactions within family.*

• Help family members clarify values associated with their lifestyle *to enhance understanding of conflicts between their lifestyle and demands of therapeutic regimen.*

• Work with family members to develop daily routine for managing therapeutic regimen that fits with their lifestyle. *Collaboration with family members makes it possible to incorporate lifestyle factors, such as culture, family dynamics, and finances, into plan for managing illness.*

• Assist family members in modifying factors (such as lack of supportive behaviors among family members) that interfere with treatment management *to enhance level of care.*

• Work with family in establishing goals for coping with conflicts *to focus their energy on achievable objectives and to foster hope.*

• Refer family members to appropriate agencies, if needed. *This can ensure continued family support and help reduce conflicts.*

• Help family members plan for future course of illness. *Planning enhances family members' abilities to develop appropriate strategy to manage therapeutic regimen.*

Evaluations for expected outcomes

• Family members identify unresolved conflicts.

• Family members attend and participate in family therapy sessions.

• Family members express a desire to resolve conflicts.

• Family members describe coping mechanisms that can reduce conflicts.

• Family members successfully incorporate components of therapeutic regimen into daily activities.

• Family members carry out therapeutic regimen.

• Family members establish a plan for coping with future course of illness.

Documentation

• Description of each family member's understanding of patient's illness

• Family members' expressions of feelings regarding patient's illness

• Compliance with participation in family therapy sessions

• Evaluations for expected outcomes

■ Management of therapeutic regimen, effective: individual

Definition
An effective pattern of regulating and integrating into daily life a program for treating illness and its sequelae

Assessment
• Family status, including marital status and family composition
• Psychological status, including changes in appetite, behavior, energy level, mood, motivation, self-image, and sleep; alcohol and drug use; life changes; psychiatric history; and blood and urine toxicology
• Self-care status, including ability to carry out voluntary activities, use of adaptive devices, and neurologic, sensory, and psychological impairment
• Social status, including communication skills, size of social network, quality of relationships, degree of trust in others, and ability to function in social and occupational roles
• Spiritual status, including religious or church affiliation, religious practices, and support network (family, clergy, and friends)

Defining characteristics
• Expressed desire to manage treatment and prevent sequelae
• Expressed desire to take action to reduce risk factors for progression of illness
• Symptoms within expectations

Associated medical diagnoses (selected)
This diagnosis may coincide with any medical diagnosis. It's appropriate for any patient who is successful in managing his illness or condition.

Expected outcomes
• Patient will recognize potential problems and identify needs.
• Patient will work toward establishing objectives to meet needs.
• Patient will make plans to ensure meeting future needs.

Interventions and rationales
• Help patient identify needs, potential problems, and sources of stress *to maintain highest level of well-being.*
• Help patient identify resources necessary to meet needs and develop strategies for using these resources *to solve problems.*
• Assist patient in identifying major stressors in his life and what needs demand immediate attention. Help to establish priorities for addressing problems *to focus energy on important issues.*
• Encourage patient to contact appropriate agencies *so that they can give preventive care, reduce stress, and enhance patient's well-being.*
• Continue to monitor patient's progress in identifying needs, problems, and stressors *to reinforce patient's efforts to obtain maximum well-being.*
• Support patient's plans for meeting future needs *to foster independence.*

Evaluations for expected outcomes
• Patient describes potential problems and establishes plan to meet therapeutic needs.
• Patient includes specific actions in plan.
• Patient makes changes to plan that allow him to meet needs and solve problems after discharge.

Documentation
• Patient's description of problems and needs

• Patient's plan to resolve current issues, including resources required, priorities, and strategies
• Patient's progress toward meeting goals
• Evaluations for expected outcomes

■ Management of therapeutic regimen, ineffective: individual

related to health beliefs

Definition
Failure to integrate program for treating illness into daily living

Assessment
• Medical history
• Physical examination
• Prescriptions for treatment, including medications, activity, diet, and other treatments
• Current medication schedule, including medications used at home (prescribed and over-the-counter)
• Activities of daily living and exercise pattern
• Nutrition pattern, including 3-day diet history or 1-day diet recall
• Weight
• Patient's and family members' health-related goals
• Self-care abilities and resources, including presence of family members or others
• Health beliefs, including perception of susceptibility to illness, seriousness of illness, effectiveness of treatment, and barriers to managing regimen
• Other influences on health-related behavior, including age, sex, knowledge, and social pressures

Defining characteristics
• Acceleration of signs and symptoms of illness
• Expressed desire to manage treatment and reduce risk factors for progression of illness
• Expressed difficulty with following treatment regimen and including it in daily routine
• Expressed inability to take action to reduce risk factors for progression of illness
• Inappropriate daily living choices for meeting goals of treatment or prevention program

Associated medical diagnoses (selected)
Any illness has potential to be managed ineffectively by patient. Common examples include acquired immunodeficiency syndrome, asthma, chronic fatigue syndrome, diabetes mellitus, hypertension, multiple sclerosis, Parkinson's disease, rheumatoid arthritis, and spinal cord injury.

Expected outcomes
• Patient will express personal beliefs about illness and its management.
• Patient and family members will develop plan for integrating components of therapeutic regimen, such as medications, activity, and diet, into pattern of daily living.
• Patient will select daily activities to meet goals of treatment or prevention program.
• Patient will express intent to reduce risk factors for progression of illness.
• Patient and family members will use available support services.

Interventions and rationales
• Discuss patient's personal beliefs about illness and review relevant information *to establish common understanding for developing plan to*

improve management of therapeutic regimen.

• Educate patient about pathophysiology of illness, and explain relationship between pathophysiology and therapeutic regimen. *A patient who knows reasons for specific behaviors may be more willing to adjust lifestyle.*

• Help patient and family members clarify values associated with lifestyle *to enhance understanding of conflicts between lifestyle and demands of therapeutic regimen.*

• Work with patient and family members to develop daily routine for managing therapeutic regimen that fits with lifestyle. *Collaboration with patient and family members makes it possible to combine scientific knowledge of illness with lifestyle factors such as culture, family dynamics, and finances.*

• Correct patient's misconceptions about susceptibility to and seriousness of illness. *Misconceptions may undermine treatment.*

• Assist patient and family members in modifying factors (such as social pressures, lack of family support, and previous behavior patterns) that interfere with treatment management *to enhance level of care.*

• Provide verbal reminders to reinforce health-promoting behaviors. For example, remind patient with heart disease to stop smoking. *Verbal cues may stimulate patient to take action; if not immediately, then at a later time.*

• Provide clearly written literature about treatment regimen *to reinforce patient's knowledge.*

• Assist patient and family members in selecting appropriate options for managing therapeutic regimen *to help patient and family members integrate potentially complicated and disrup-*

tive therapeutic interventions into their lifestyle.

• Refer patient or family members to support groups or self-help organizations *to empower patient and family members to continue effective management of therapeutic regimen.*

• Help patient and family members plan for future course of illness. For example, patient or family members may need to make structural changes at home to accommodate wheelchair or hospital bed. *Planning enhances patient's and family members' abilities to develop appropriate management strategies.*

Evaluations for expected outcomes

• Patient expresses personal beliefs about illness and therapeutic regimen.

• Patient and family members successfully incorporate components of therapeutic regimen into daily activities.

• Patient describes daily activities that will help him achieve goals of treatment or prevention program and carries out therapeutic regimen.

• Patient states intent to reduce risk factors for illness.

• Patient and family members contact appropriate support services.

Documentation

• Patient's knowledge and beliefs about illness and therapeutic regimen

• Patient's explanation of values and lifestyle

• Information provided to clarify misconceptions

• Actions taken to modify patient's environment or behavior

• Written materials given to patient

• Referrals to support services

• Evaluations for expected outcomes

■ Memory impairment

related to neurologic disturbance

Definition
Inability to remember or recall fragments of information or behavioral skills

Assessment
• Age, sex, level of education, occupation, and living arrangements
• Cardiovascular status, including vital signs, apical pulse, pulse rate and rhythm, and heart sounds; color of skin, lips, and nails; fatigue on exertion, dyspnea, and dizziness; history of hypertension, chest pain, or anoxia; and complete blood count and differential, thyroid studies, electrocardiography, and echocardiography
• Family status, including household composition and marital status (presence of a spouse, length of marriage, divorce, or death of spouse)
• Neurologic status, including mental status (abstract thinking, insight about present situation, judgment, long-term and short-term memory, cognition, and orientation to person, place, and time); level of consciousness; sensory ability; fine and gross motor functioning; history of neurologic disorder, head injury, or psychiatric illness; medication use; and computed tomography scan, magnetic resonance imaging, cerebral angiography, electroencephalography, toxicology studies, thyroid function, and serotonin levels
• Psychological status, including changes in appetite, behavior, energy level, mood, motivation, self-image, self-esteem, and sleep patterns; alcohol and drug consumption; recent divorce, separation, death, job loss, loss of loved one, relocation, or physical or emotional trauma; and psychiatric history
• Self-care status, including ability to carry out voluntary activities and use of adaptive equipment

Associated medical diagnoses (selected)
Acquired immunodeficiency syndrome, Alzheimer's disease, cerebrovascular accident, dementia, head injury, multiple sclerosis, seizure disorders, transient ischemic attacks

Defining characteristics
• Inability to determine whether a behavior was performed
• Inability to learn new skills or information or to perform previously learned skills
• Inability to recall factual information and recent or past events
• Incidences of forgetting, including forgetting to perform a behavior at a scheduled time

Expected outcomes
• Patient will express feelings about memory impairment.
• Patient will acknowledge need to take measures to cope with memory impairment.
• Patient will identify coping skills to deal with memory impairment.
• Patient and family members will state specific plans to modify lifestyle.
• Patient and family members will establish realistic goals to deal with further loss of memory.

Interventions and rationales
• Observe patient's thought processes during every shift. Document and report any changes. *Changes may indicate progressive improvement or a decline in patient's underlying condition.*

• Implement appropriate safety measures to protect patient from injury. *He may be unable to provide for his own safety needs.*
• Call patient by name and tell him your name. Provide background information (place, time, and date) frequently throughout the day *to provide reality orientation.* Use a reality orientation board *to visually reinforce reality orientation.*
• Spend sufficient time with patient to allow him to become comfortable discussing memory loss *to establish trusting relationship.*
• Inform patient that you are aware of his memory loss and that you will help him cope with his condition *to bring issue into the open and help patient understand that your goal is to help him.*
• Be clear, concise, and direct in establishing goals *so that patient can maximize use of his remaining cognitive skills.*
• Offer short, simple explanations to patient each time you carry out any medical or nursing procedure *to avoid confusion.*
• Label patient's personal possessions and photos, keeping them in same place as much as possible, *to reduce confusion and create a secure environment.*
• Encourage patient to develop a consistent routine for performing activities of daily living *to enhance his self-esteem and increase his self-awareness and awareness of environment.*
• Teach patient ways to cope with memory loss — for example, using a beeper to remind him when to eat or take medications, using a pillbox organized by days of the week, keeping lists in notebooks or a pocket calendar, and having family members or friends remind him of important tasks. *Reminders help to limit amount of information patient must maintain in his memory.*
• Encourage patient to interact with others *to increase social involvement, which may decline with memory loss.*
• Encourage patient to express feelings associated with impaired memory *to reduce impact of memory impairment on patient's self-image and to lessen anxiety.*
• Help patient and family members establish goals for coping with memory loss. Discuss with family members need to maintain least restrictive environment possible. Instruct them on how to maintain a safe home environment for patient. *This helps ensure that patient's needs are met and promotes his independence.*
• Demonstrate reorientation techniques to family members and provide time for supervised return demonstrations *to prepare them to cope with patient with memory impairment.*
• Help family members identify appropriate community support groups, mental health services, and social service agencies *to assist in coping with effects of patient's illness or injury.*

Evaluations for expected outcomes
• Patient expresses feelings about memory impairment.
• Patient acknowledges need to take measures to cope with memory impairment.
• Patient describes mechanisms for coping with memory loss.
• Patient and family members describe plans to modify lifestyle.
• Patient and family members set realistic goals to cope with further memory loss.

Documentation
• Description of patient's mental status, including documentation of changes from shift to shift
• Outline of goals for helping patient cope with memory loss
• Response of family members to techniques for keeping patient functioning at maximal level
• Referrals to community support groups
• Evaluations for expected outcomes

■ Mobility impairment, physical

related to neuromuscular impairment

Definition
Limitation of physical movement

Assessment
• History of neuromuscular disorder or dysfunction
• Musculoskeletal status, including coordination, gait, muscle size and strength, muscle tone, range of motion (ROM), and functional mobility scale:
0 = completely independent
1 = requires use of equipment or device
2 = requires help, supervision, or teaching from another person
3 = requires help from another person and equipment or device
4 = dependent; doesn't participate in activity
• Neurologic status, including level of consciousness, motor ability, and sensory ability

Defining characteristics
• Difficulty turning

• Substitution of other behaviors for impaired mobility (for instance, increased attention to other's activity and controlling behavior)
• Gait changes (for instance, shuffling gait and exaggerated lateral postural sway)
• Limited fine and gross motor skills
• Limited range of motion
• Movement-induced tremor
• Postural instability when performing routine activities of daily living
• Slowed movement
• Shortness of breath
• Slowed reaction time
• Uncoordinated or jerky movements

Associated medical diagnoses (selected)
Brain abscess, cerebral aneurysm, cerebrovascular accident, craniotomy, dermatomyositis and polymyositis, Guillain-Barré syndrome, head injury, Huntington's disease, multiple sclerosis, muscular dystrophy, myasthenia gravis, paralysis, Parkinson's disease, prolapsed intervertebral disk, Reye's syndrome, spinal cord injury or tumor

Expected outcomes
• Patient will maintain muscle strength and joint ROM.
• Patient will show no evidence of complications, such as contractures, venous stasis, thrombus formation, skin breakdown, and hypostatic pneumonia.
• Patient will achieve highest level of mobility (will transfer independently, will be wheelchair-independent, or will ambulate with such assistive devices as walker, cane, and braces).
• Patient or family member will carry out mobility regimen.
• Patient or family member will make plans to use resources to help maintain level of functioning.

Interventions and rationales

• Perform ROM exercises to joints, unless contraindicated, at least once every shift. Progress from passive to active, as tolerated. *This prevents joint contractures and muscular atrophy.*

• Turn and position patient every 2 hours. Establish turning schedule for dependent patients; post at bedside and monitor frequency of turning. *This prevents skin breakdown by relieving pressure.*

• Place joints in functional position, use trochanter roll along thigh, abduct thighs, use high-top sneakers, and put small pillow under head. *These measures maintain joints in functional position and prevent musculoskeletal deformities.*

• Identify level of functioning using a functional mobility scale (see Assessment). Communicate patient's skill level to all staff members *to provide continuity and preserve identified level of independence.*

• Encourage independence in mobility by helping patient to use trapeze and side rails, to use unaffected leg to move affected leg, and to perform such self-care activities as combing hair, feeding, and dressing. *This increases muscle tone and patient's self-esteem.*

• Place items within reach of unaffected arm if patient has one-sided weakness or paralysis *to promote patient's independence.*

• Monitor and record daily any evidence of immobility complications (such as contractures, venous stasis, thrombus, pneumonia, and urinary tract infection). *Patients with history of neuromuscular disorders or dysfunction may be more prone to develop complications.*

• Carry out medical regimen to manage or prevent complications; for example, administer prophylactic heparin for venous thrombosis. *This promotes patient's health and well-being.*

• Provide progressive mobilization to limits of patient's condition (bed mobility to chair mobility to ambulation) *to maintain muscle tone and prevent complications of immobility.*

• Refer to physical therapist for development of mobility regimen *to help rehabilitate musculoskeletal deficits.*

• Encourage attendance at physical therapy sessions, and support activities on unit by using same equipment and technique. Request written mobility plans and use as reference. *All members of health care team should reinforce learned skills in same manner.*

• Instruct patient and family members in ROM exercises, transfers, skin inspection, and mobility regimen *to help prepare patient for discharge.*

• Demonstrate mobility regimen, and note date. Have patient and family members return mobility regimen demonstration, and note date. *This ensures continuity of care and use of proper technique.*

• Assist in identifying resources to carry out mobility regimen, such as American Heart Association and National Multiple Sclerosis Society. *These resources help provide comprehensive approach to rehabilitation.*

Evaluations for expected outcomes

• Patient maintains muscle strength and joint ROM.

• Patient shows no evidence of contractures, venous stasis, thrombus formation, skin breakdown, hypostatic pneumonia, or other complications.

• Patient achieves highest mobility level possible identified by health care team (specify).

• Patient or family member carries out mobility regimen.

• Patient or family member identifies and contacts at least one resource person or group to help maintain level of functioning.

Documentation
• Patient's expression of concern about loss of mobility, current status of functional abilities, and goals set for self
• Observations of patient's mobility status, presence of complications, and response to mobility regimen
• Instruction and demonstration of skills in carrying out mobility regimen
• Patient's response to nursing interventions
• Evaluations for expected outcomes

■ Mobility impairment, physical
related to pain or discomfort

Definition
Limitation of physical movement

Assessment
• History of recent surgery, injury, or disorder causing pain or discomfort
• Medication history
• Musculoskeletal status, including coordination, gait, muscle size and strength, muscle tone, range of motion (ROM), and functional mobility scale:
0 = completely independent
1 = requires use of equipment or device
2 = requires help, supervision, or teaching from another person
3 = requires help from another person and equipment or device
4 = dependent; doesn't participate in activity

• Pain, including environmental and cultural influences, intensity, location, quality, and temporal factors
• Psychosocial status, including coping mechanisms, family members, lifestyle, personality, and stressors (disease process, finances, job, and marital discord)

Defining characteristics
• Difficulty turning
• Substitution of other behaviors for impaired mobility (such as focusing on one's pre-illness activities or on another person's activities)
• Gait changes (for instance, shuffling gait and exaggerated lateral postural sway)
• Limited fine and gross motor skills
• Limited ROM
• Movement-induced tremor
• Postural instability when performing routine activities of daily living
• Slowed movement
• Shortness of breath
• Slowed reaction time
• Uncoordinated or jerky movements

Associated medical diagnoses (selected)
Acute renal failure, atelectasis, bone sarcomas, bronchiectasis, burns, bursitis, carpal tunnel syndrome, cellulitis, chemotherapy, encephalitis, food poisoning, fractures, gout, Hodgkin's disease, joint replacement, juvenile rheumatoid arthritis, lupus erythematosus, metastatic disease, orthopedic injuries, osteoarthritis, osteomyelitis, peripheral vascular disease, pneumonia, pressure ulcers, pyelonephritis, radiation therapy, Reiter's syndrome, rheumatic fever, rheumatoid arthritis, sickle cell anemia, tendinitis

Expected outcomes

• Patient will state relief from pain.
• Patient will display increased mobility.
• Patient will show no evidence of such complications as contractures, venous stasis, thrombus formation, skin breakdown, and hypostatic pneumonia.
• Patient will attain highest degree of mobility possible within confines of disease.
• Patient or family member will demonstrate mobility regimen.
• Patient will begin to accept limitations imposed by immobility and accompanying lifestyle changes.
• Patient will express willingness to participate in care.

Interventions and rationales

• Observe patient's functional ability daily; document and report any changes using functional mobility scale (see Assessment). *Changes may indicate progressive decline or improvement in underlying disorder.*
• Encourage patient to verbalize pain and discomfort. Observe for nonverbal cues of pain, including favoring a body part and grimacing. *This aids assessment of location, quality, and intensity of pain.*
• Perform prescribed treatment regimen for underlying condition producing pain or discomfort. Monitor progress and report favorable and adverse responses to treatment *to assess effectiveness of treatment.*
• Administer pain medication and assess nonverbal cues, verbal reports, and vital signs *to monitor effectiveness.*
• Ensure patient comfort by padding extremities prone to skin breakdown (such as heels and elbows), ensuring correct measurement of crutches, and using convoluted foam mattress on bed. *These measures prevent skin breakdown.*
• Encourage patient's active movement by using assistive devices *to increase muscle tone and increase patient's feelings of self-esteem;* promote joint rest between activities.
• Implement ROM exercises every shift after pain medication, unless medically contraindicated; progress from passive to active, as tolerated. *This prevents joint contracture and muscle atrophy.*
• Reposition patient every 2 hours and provide meticulous skin care *to prevent skin breakdown.*
• Promote progressive mobilization to maximum, within limits of patient's tolerance for pain (bed mobility to chair mobility to ambulation). *This maintains muscle tone and prevents complications of immobility.*
• Discuss use of distraction and other nonpharmacologic pain-relief methods with patient. Instruct patient and family members on preferred method and monitor effectiveness. Encourage patient to choose an alternative if method is ineffective. Document response. *In addition to providing pain relief, nonpharmacologic techniques may help patient achieve sense of control. Documentation helps ensure continuity of care.*
• Explain necessity of movement even during painful periods, unless contraindicated, to prevent greater pain such as occurs in arthritic conditions and after surgery. Let patient know when to expect to move; provide pain-relief measures before moving patient. *Movement alleviates effects of immobility. Medication alleviates pain and maintains patient's functional activity level.*
• Instruct patient and family members in ROM exercises, transfers, skin inspection, and mobility regimen. Have

patient and family members return mobility demonstration under supervision. *Education will enable patient and family members to prevent complications of immobility.*
• Encourage patient to discuss feelings and concerns about altered state of mobility *to reduce anxiety and promote compliance.*
• Encourage adherence to other aspects of health care management *to control or minimize effects on mobility. This promotes health and wellbeing by alleviating pain and preventing complications.*
• Refer to psychiatric liaison nurse, social service agency, support group, or other resources as appropriate *to provide patient with alternative approaches to care.*

Evaluations for expected outcomes
• Patient expresses relief from pain.
• Patient demonstrates increased mobility.
• Patient shows no evidence of contractures, venous stasis, thrombus formation, skin breakdown, hypostatic pneumonia, or other complications.
• Patient attains highest mobility level possible as determined by health care team (specify).
• Patient or family member carries out mobility regimen.
• Patient begins to accept limitations imposed by immobility and accompanying lifestyle changes.
• Patient expresses willingness to participate in care.

Documentation
• Patient's expression of feelings and concerns about immobility, impact on lifestyle, and willingness to participate in care
• Observations of patient's impaired mobility, pain, and response to treatment

• Interventions to provide supportive care
• Instructions to patient and family members, their understanding of instructions, and demonstrated skill in carrying out prescribed mobility and pain-relief program
• Patient's response to nursing interventions
• Evaluations for expected outcomes

■ Mobility impairment, physical

related to perceptual or cognitive impairment

Definition
Limitation of physical movement

Assessment
• History of neurologic, sensory, or psychological disorder with impaired movement
• Musculoskeletal status, including coordination, gait, muscle size and strength, muscle tone, range of motion (ROM), and functional mobility scale:
0 = completely independent
1 = requires use of equipment or device
2 = requires help, supervision, or teaching from another person
3 = requires help from another person and equipment or device
4 = independent; doesn't participate in activity
• Neurologic status, including cognition, communication skills, insight and judgment, level of consciousness, memory, motor ability, orientation, and sensory ability
• Psychosocial status, including coping mechanisms, family members, lifestyle, personality, and stressors

(disease process, finances, job, and marital discord)

Defining characteristics
- Difficulty turning
- Substitution of other behaviors for impaired mobility (for instance, increased attention to other's activity and controlling behavior)
- Gait changes (for instance, shuffling gait and exaggerated lateral postural sway)
- Limited fine and gross motor skills
- Limited ROM
- Movement-induced tremor
- Postural instability when performing routine activities of daily living
- Slowed movement
- Shortness of breath
- Slowed reaction time
- Uncoordinated or jerky movements

Associated medical diagnoses (selected)
Alcohol addiction, amyotrophic lateral sclerosis, bipolar disease (manic phase), blindness, cataracts, lupus erythematosus, Ménière's disease

Expected outcomes
- Patient will maintain functional mobility.
- Patient will have minimal, if any, complications.
- Patient will state feelings about impairment.
- Family members will communicate understanding of mobility regimen.
- Family members will demonstrate skill in carrying out mobility regimen.
- Family members will obtain support necessary to continue care.

Interventions and rationales
- Observe patient's functional ability daily; document and report any changes using functional mobility scale (see Assessment). *Changes may*

indicate progressive decline or improvement in underlying disorder.
- Determine patient's degree of perceptual or cognitive impairment and ability to follow directions *to determine presence of deficits.* Modify interventions accordingly.
- Perform prescribed treatment regimen for underlying condition producing pain or discomfort. Monitor progress, reporting favorable and adverse response to treatment, *to assess effectiveness of treatment.*
- Allow patient and family members to ventilate frustration and other negative feelings regarding difficulty in performing mobility tasks. *Expressing feelings helps patient and family members cope with impaired mobility.*
- Ask patient to perform one task at a time; offer encouragement and provide simple, direct instructions ("walk to the bathroom") to avoid confusion. *Limiting new skills to small, critical units enhances learning.*
- Provide patient with ample time to perform each new mobility-related task. *Patient may need extensive supervision and repetition to master new tasks.*
- Provide supportive measures as indicated:
  – Perform ROM exercises to joints (unless medically contraindicated) every shift; progress from passive to active, as tolerated, and monitor progress. *This prevents joint contracture and muscle atrophy.*
  – Turn and position patient every 2 hours; establish a turning schedule for dependent patients. Post at bedside and monitor effectiveness. *Regular turning and positioning prevents skin breakdown.*
  – Place joints in functional position (for example, trochanter roll along thigh) on an alternating schedule.

This prevents musculoskeletal deformities.
– Encourage active movement by helping patient to use trapeze and side rails, to use his unaffected leg to move his affected leg, and to perform self-care activities. Provide frequent reinforcement and demonstrations. *This increases muscle tone and feelings of self-esteem and reinforces learning.*
– Walk patient with one or two assistants on regular schedule, if possible. *This preserves muscle tone, has positive psychological effect on patient and family, and prevents complications of immobility.*
• Teach patient (if capable) and family members how to perform ROM exercises, transfers, skin inspection and mobility regimen; provide time for return demonstrations with supervision. *Informed patient and family members will be better prepared to prevent complications of immobility.*
• Encourage adherence to other aspects of health care management *to control or minimize effects on mobility. This promotes health and well-being by alleviating pain and preventing complications.*
• Refer to psychiatric liaison nurse, social service agency, support group, or other resources as appropriate *to provide patient with alternative approaches to care.*

Evaluations for expected outcomes
• Patient maintains functional mobility.
• Patient shows no evidence of skin breakdown, contractures, venous stasis, thrombus formation, hypostatic pneumonia, or other complications.
• Patient begins to accept limitations imposed by mobility impairment and impact on lifestyle.

• Family members communicate understanding of purpose and principles of mobility regimen.
• Family members successfully demonstrate ROM exercises, transfers, skin inspection, and other aspects of mobility regimen.
• Family members identify and contact at least two sources for support.

Documentation
• Observations of patient's impaired mobility, perceptual or cognitive status, and response to treatment
• Interventions to provide supportive care
• Instructions to patient and family members, their understanding of instructions, and demonstrated skill in carrying out prescribed mobility program
• Patient's response to nursing interventions
• Patient's and family members' expressions of feelings and concern about immobility, impact on lifestyle, and capacity for participating in care
• Evaluations for expected outcomes

■ Nausea

related to irritation to the GI system

Definition
An unpleasant, wavelike sensation in the back of the throat, epigastrium, or throughout the abdomen that may or may not lead to vomiting

Assessment
• Health history, including illnesses, pregnancy, and medication use
• Nutritional status, including height, weight, fluctuations in weight, food preferences, and usual dietary patterns

• Psychosocial status, including ethnic background, family dynamics, lifestyle, perception of self, recent stressful events, and coping skills

Defining characteristics
• Cold, clammy skin
• Increased salivation
• Tachycardia
• Gastric stasis
• Diarrhea
• Reports "nausea" or "sick to stomach"

Associated medical diagnoses (selected)
Acute pancreatitis, chemotherapy, Crohn's disease, food poisoning, hepatitis, infections, labyrinthitis, Ménière's disease, motion sickness, peritonitis, psychiatric disorders, radiation therapy, volvulus

Expected outcomes
• Patient will state reasons for nausea and vomiting.
• Patient will take steps to manage episodes of nausea and vomiting.
• Patient will ingest sufficient nutrients to maintain health.
• Patient will take steps to ensure adequate nutrition when nausea abates.
• Patient will maintain weight within specified range.

Interventions and rationales
• Ask patient the reasons for nausea or inability to eat and document his explanation in his own words *to plan interventions.*
• Observe the patient's fluid and food intake and document findings *to assess nutrient consumption and need for supplements.*
• Encourage patient to eat dry, bland foods (such as dry toast or crackers) during periods of nausea *to make it possible for him to eat.*

• Suggest that the patient avoid offensive foods and food odors, shorten food preparation time, and eat and drink slowly. *These measures may help to prevent nausea from getting worse.*
• Administer antinausea medications, as prescribed, *to provide relief from nausea and allow the patient to eat.*
• Teach relaxation techniques and help the patient to use such techniques during mealtime *to reduce stress and divert attention from nausea, thereby helping the patient to eat and drink.*
• Encourage the patient to make a list of best-tolerated and least-tolerated foods *to help him choose foods wisely once nausea abates.*
• When nausea abates, encourage the patient to eat larger amounts of food *to help the patient consume adequate nutrients over time.*

Evaluations for expected outcomes
• Patient states reasons for nausea and vomiting.
• Patient takes steps to manage episodes of nausea and vomiting.
• Patient ingests sufficient nutrients to maintain health.
• Patient takes steps to ensure adequate nutrition when nausea abates.
• Patient maintains weight within specified range.

Documentation
• Patient's statements regarding nausea and its causes
• Episodes of nausea or vomiting
• Intake and output measurements
• Types of food and fluids ingested and patient's tolerance
• Nursing interventions, including teaching provided to patient
• Patient's response to nursing interventions
• Evaluations for expected outcomes

■ Neglect, unilateral

related to neurologic illness or trauma

Definition

Lack of awareness of a body part

Assessment

• History of neurologic impairment
• Age
• Neurologic status, including awareness of body parts, cognition, level of consciousness, mental status, memory, sensory function, orientation, position sense, visual acuity, visual fields, ability to communicate (verbally and nonverbally), and bowel and bladder control
• Musculoskeletal status, including coordination, muscle size and strength, muscle tone, range of motion (ROM), and functional mobility scale:
0 = completely independent
1 = requires use of equipment or device
2 = requires help, supervision, or teaching from another person
3 = requires help from another person and equipment or device
4 = dependent; doesn't participate in activity
• Integumentary status, including color, texture, turgor, temperature, elasticity, sensation, moisture, hygiene, and lesions
• Psychosocial status, including coping mechanisms, support systems (family and others), lifestyle, and understanding of physical condition
• Self-care abilities, including preparation of equipment and supplies, technical or mechanical skills, and use of assistive devices

Defining characteristics

• Failure to eat food on plate on affected side
• Failure to look toward or respond to stimuli on affected side
• Inadequate self-care
• Need for positioning and safety precautions to protect affected side

Associated medical diagnoses (selected)

Bell's palsy, body image agnosia, cerebrovascular accident, head injury, hemianopsia, neoplastic brain disease

Expected outcomes

• Patient will avoid injury to affected body part.
• Patient will avoid skin breakdown.
• Patient will avoid contractures.
• Patient will recognize neglected body part.
• Patient and family members will demonstrate exercises for affected body part.
• Patient and family members will demonstrate measures and arrange environment to protect affected body part.
• Patient and family members will express feelings about altered state of health and neurologic deficits.
• Patient and family members will identify community resources and support groups to help cope with the effects of illness.

Interventions and rationales

• Place sling on affected arm *to prevent dangling or injury.* Support affected leg and foot while in bed, place foot strap on wheelchair, and perform other measures as appropriate *to keep limbs in functional position and avoid contractures.* Use drawsheet to move patient up in bed *to avoid skin abrasions.*
• Touch and rub affected limb. Describe it in conversation with patient

to remind patient of neglected body part.

• Direct patient to perform activities that require use of affected limb. *A patient who uses paretic or paralyzed limb will more easily integrate affected limb into his body image.*

• Encourage patient to check position of affected body part with each repositioning or transfer *to reestablish awareness of body part.*

• Establish and follow a regular turning schedule *to maintain skin integrity.*

• Request consultations with occupational and physical therapists about adaptive equipment, exercise program, and other recommendations *to increase patient's awareness of affected limb.*

• Use safety belts or protective devices according to facility policy. *Safety devices remind patient of limitations and help prevent falls.*

• Remove splints and other devices at least every 2 hours. Inspect skin for pressure areas. Reapply splint. *Proper use of splints and other devices prevents deformities and maintains skin integrity.*

• Perform ROM exercises on affected side at least once every shift, unless medically contraindicated, *to maintain joint flexibility and prevent contractures.*

• Instruct family and nursing personnel to observe position of affected body part frequently. Remove food or drainage from face if unnoticed by patient. Place arm or leg in proper position as often as necessary *to prevent injury.*

• Arrange environment for maximum functioning; for example, place water, television controls, and call light within reach. *These measures enhance orientation and encourage independence.*

• Assist with activities of daily living (ADLs) or provide supervision as appropriate *to protect patient's affected side.*

• Encourage patient and family members to express feelings regarding patient's condition and level of functioning *to release tension and enhance coping.*

• Refer patient and family members to appropriate support groups and other community resources *to assist patient and family in adjusting to altered state of health.*

Evaluations for expected outcomes

• Patient doesn't experience injury.
• Patient's skin doesn't show signs of breakdown.
• Patient doesn't show evidence of contractures.
• Patient recognizes and protects neglected body part when carrying out ADLs.
• Patient and family members demonstrate exercise routine and program for protecting affected body part.
• Patient's environment is arranged for maximum functioning.
• Patient and family members openly express fear and other feelings associated with patient's neurologic deficits and altered level of functioning.
• Patient and family members identify and contact appropriate community resources and support groups.

Documentation

• Patient's expressions of feelings about neglected side of body
• Safety measures taken to prevent injury
• Patient's ability to perform ADLs and nursing measures taken to overcome deficits
• Observations of patient's and family's coping skills

• Patient's response to nursing interventions, including verbal expressions or behavior that indicates increased awareness of affected limb
• Evaluations for expected outcomes

■ Noncompliance

related to patient's value system

Definition

Unwillingness to practice prescribed health-related behaviors

Assessment

• Age
• Health beliefs
• Patient's perceptions of health problem, treatment regimen, and importance of complying with treatment regimen
• Patient's ability to learn and perform prescribed treatment (activity, diet, and medications)
• Financial resources
• Cultural and ethnic influences
• Religious influences
• Educational and language background

Defining characteristics

• Complications or exacerbation of signs and symptoms
• Failure to keep appointments and adhere to treatment regimen
• Objective indications (such as physiologic tests) of failure to progress

Associated medical diagnoses (selected)

This nursing diagnosis can be associated with any medical diagnosis and depends upon patient's value system. Examples include chronic bronchitis, chronic obstructive pulmonary disease, cystitis, diabetes mellitus, emphysema, and hypertension.

Expected outcomes

• Patient will identify factors that influence noncompliance.
• Patient will demonstrate level of compliance that doesn't interfere with physiologic safety.
• Patient will contract with nurse to perform ____ (specify behavior and frequency).
• Patient will use support systems to modify noncompliant behavior.

Interventions and rationales

• Listen to patient's reasons for noncompliance. *Active listening may reveal concerns not clearly stated in words and helps individualize teaching process.*
• Approach patient in nonjudgmental manner. *This demonstrates unconditional positive regard for patient.*
• Identify specific areas of patient's noncompliant behavior *to help develop appropriate interventions.*
• Attempt to identify influencing factors associated with noncompliant behaviors, such as lack of understanding, unrealistic expectations, and cultural differences. *Reasons for noncompliance may range widely and include lack of knowledge, forgetting, feeling better or worse, and getting contradictory advice from family, friends, and health care providers.*
• Emphasize positive aspects of compliance. *Understanding that compliance can reduce risk factors, prevent complications, and help manage certain chronic diseases may encourage patient to comply.*
• Help patient clarify his values *to allow him to explore both intellectual and emotional components of values, which form basis for his behavior.*
• Acknowledge patient's right to choose against carrying out prescribed regimen. *Patient's autonomy must be respected; control over pa-*

tient's action is legitimate only if needed to prevent harm to patient, to others, or to yourself.
• Contract with patient to practice only nonthreatening behaviors. *This involves both patient and caregiver in formal commitment and gives patient sense of personal control.*
• Use support systems to enforce or reinforce negotiated behaviors. *Support from patient's family helps foster compliance.*
• Give positive reinforcement for compliant behavior *to encourage patient to continue such behavior.*
• As medically appropriate, support patient who chooses to follow Eastern therapies instead of traditional Western medical practices. *Such support demonstrates your respect for patient's beliefs.*
• Determine whether patient's perceived noncompliance actually stems from lack of financial resources. Contact appropriate agencies to help patient meet costs of medical treatment and supplies and other financial needs. *Helping patient meet financial requirements of treatment improves compliance.*

Evaluations for expected outcomes
• Patient describes factors that influence noncompliance with health care regimen.
• Patient performs daily self-care in compliance with health care regimen.
• Patient performs behaviors agreed upon in contract with nurse.
• Patient uses available support resources as needed.

Documentation
• Patient's statements that indicate noncompliant behavior
• Direct observation of noncompliant behavior

• Statements by patient that provide insight into causes of noncompliant behavior
• Terms agreed upon by patient in performing negotiated behaviors
• Patient's daily progress in complying with treatment regimen
• Evaluations for expected outcomes

■ Nutrition alteration: Less than body requirements

related to inability to digest or absorb nutrients because of biological factors

Definition
Change in normal eating pattern that results in decreased body weight

Assessment
• GI assessment, including antibiotic therapy, auscultation of bowel sounds, change in bowel habits, stool characteristics (color, amount, size, and consistency), history of disorder or surgery, inspection of abdomen, pain or discomfort, usual bowel elimination pattern, palpation for masses and tenderness, percussion for tympany and dullness, and nausea and vomiting
• Nutritional status, including change in type of food tolerated, financial resources, height and weight, meal preparation, serum albumin level, sociocultural influences, usual dietary pattern, and weight fluctuations over past 10 years
• Change in intrapersonal or interpersonal factors, including internal or external cues that trigger desire to eat, rate of food consumption, and stated food preference
• Psychosocial status
• Activity level

• Coping behaviors
• Body image, including perception of observer and self-perception

Defining characteristics
• Abdominal pain or cramping, with or without pathology
• Altered taste sensation
• Aversion to or lack of interest in eating
• Body weight 20% or more under ideal weight
• Diarrhea and steatorrhea
• Evidence of lack of food
• Excessive hair loss
• Fragile capillaries
• Hyperactive bowel sounds
• Inadequate food intake (less than recommended daily allowances)
• Lack of information or misinformation about nutrition
• Loss of body weight despite adequate food intake
• Pale conjunctivae and mucous membranes
• Perceived inability to ingest food
• Poor muscle tone
• Satiety immediately after eating
• Sore, inflamed buccal cavity
• Weakness of muscles required for chewing or swallowing

Associated medical diagnoses (selected)
Bone marrow transplantation, burns, cholecystitis, chronic obstructive pulmonary disease, cirrhosis, colitis, colostomy, Crohn's disease, diverticulitis, duodenal ulcer, emphysema, esophageal varices, gastric ulcer, glomerulonephritis, hepatic coma, hyperemesis gravidarum, hypoparathyroidism, ileostomy, lupus erythematosus, multiple sclerosis, peritoneal dialysis, pressure ulcers, sepsis

Expected outcomes
• Patient will show no further evidence of weight loss.

• Patient will tolerate oral, tube, or I.V. feedings without adverse effects.
• Patient will take in ____ calories daily.
• Patient will gain ____ lb weekly.
• Patient and family members will communicate understanding of preoperative instructions.
• Patient and family members will communicate understanding of special dietary needs.
• Patient and family members will demonstrate ability to plan diet after discharge.

Interventions and rationales
• Obtain and record patient's weight at same time every day *to obtain accurate readings.*
• Monitor fluid intake and output *because body weight may decrease as a result of fluid loss.*
• Maintain parenteral fluids, as ordered, *to provide patient with needed fluids and electrolytes.*
• Provide diet prescribed for patient's specific condition *to improve patient's nutritional status and increase weight.*
• Determine food preferences and provide them within limitations of patient's prescribed diet. *This enhances compliance with diet regimen.*
• Monitor electrolyte levels and report abnormal values. *Poor nutritional status may cause electrolyte imbalances.*
• If patient vomits, record amount, color, and consistency. Keep a record of all stools. *Vomitus and stool characteristics indicate status of nutrient absorption.*
• Refer to dietitian or nutritional support team for dietary management (possible regimens include yogurt feedings and low-bulk diet). *Dietitian or nutritional support team can help patient and health care team individ-*

ualize patient's diet within prescribed restrictions.

• If patient is receiving tube feeding:

– Add food coloring if patient has altered state of consciousness or diminished gag reflex *to help detect aspiration.*

– If possible, use continuous infusion pump for tube feeding *to avoid diarrhea.*

– Begin tube feeding regimen with small amount and diluted concentration *to decrease diarrhea and improve absorption.* Increase volume and concentration as tolerated.

– Keep head of bed elevated during tube feeding *to reduce risk of aspiration.*

– Check feeding tube placement each shift *to verify placement in GI tract rather than in lungs.*

• If patient receives total parenteral nutrition:

– Ensure delivery as prescribed. *Electrolytes, amino acids, and other nutrients must be tailored to patient's needs.*

– Monitor blood glucose levels and urine specific gravity at least once each shift. *Because glucose is main component of total parenteral nutrition, patient may become hyperglycemic if not carefully monitored.*

• Monitor bowel sounds once a shift. *Normal active bowel sounds may indicate readiness for enteral feedings; hyperactive sounds may indicate poor absorption and may be accompanied by diarrhea.*

• Reinforce medical regimen by explaining to patient and family members reasons for present regimen. *Collaborative practice enhances patient's overall care.*

• Teach principles of good nutrition for patient's specific condition. *This encourages patient and family members to participate in patient's care.*

• Provide or assist with oral hygiene *to help keep patient comfortable.*

• Provide preoperative teaching, if needed, *to reduce patient's fear and anxiety and promote understanding.*

• Involve family members in meal planning *to encourage them to help patient comply with diet regimen after discharge.*

Evaluations for expected outcomes

• Patient remains at or above specified weight.

• Patient doesn't develop adverse reactions from feedings, such as aspiration of food particles into lungs, diarrhea, and hyperglycemia.

• Patient consumes specified number of calories daily.

• Patient's weight increases by specified amount weekly.

• Patient and family communicate understanding of preoperative instructions, either verbally or through behavior.

• Patient and family communicate understanding of special dietary needs, either verbally or through behavior.

• Patient and family plan appropriate diet for patient to follow after discharge.

Documentation

• Daily weight
• Mouth care
• Maintenance of nasogastric tube
• Intake and output
• Bowel sounds
• Blood glucose levels
• Urine specific gravity
• Patient's ability to eat
• Incidence of vomiting or diarrhea
• Presence of other complications
• Patient's statements of understanding of dietary education
• Evaluations for expected outcomes

■ Nutrition alteration: Less than body requirements

related to inability to ingest foods

Definition
Change in normal eating pattern that results in decreased body weight

Assessment
• GI assessment, including auscultation of bowel sounds, change in bowel habits, characteristics of stool (color, amount, size, and consistency), history of GI disorder or surgery, inspection of abdomen, pain or discomfort, palpation for masses and tenderness, percussion for tympany and dullness, nausea and vomiting, and usual bowel pattern
• Nutritional status, including financial resources, height, meal preparation, serum albumin level, sociocultural influences, usual dietary pattern, weight, and weight fluctuations over past 10 years
• Intrapersonal and interpersonal factors, including internal and external cues that trigger desire to eat, rate of food consumption, and stated food preference
• Psychosocial status
• Activity level
• Coping behaviors
• Body image, including perception of observer and self-perception

Defining characteristics
• Abdominal pain or cramping, with or without pathology
• Altered taste sensation
• Aversion to or lack of interest in eating
• Body weight 20% or more under ideal weight
• Diarrhea and steatorrhea
• Evidence of lack of food

• Excessive hair loss
• Fragile capillaries
• Hyperactive bowel sounds
• Inadequate food intake (less than recommended daily allowances)
• Lack of information or misinformation about nutrition
• Loss of body weight despite adequate food intake
• Pale conjunctivae and mucous membranes
• Perceived inability to ingest food
• Poor muscle tone
• Satiety immediately after eating
• Sore, inflamed buccal cavity
• Weakness of muscles required for chewing or swallowing

Associated medical diagnoses (selected)
Achalasia, acoustic neuroma, adult respiratory distress syndrome, Alzheimer's disease, appendicitis, bronchiectasis, cerebrovascular accident, chemotherapy, endocarditis, esophageal cancer, esophageal varices, gastric cancer, head injury, Hodgkin's disease, hydrocephalus, hyperparathyroidism, intestinal obstruction, leukemia, lung cancer, metastatic disease, multiple myeloma, nutritional deficiencies, ovarian cancer, Parkinson's disease, pemphigus, pneumonia, radiation therapy, tracheostomy, trigeminal neuralgia, viral hepatitis

Expected outcomes
• Patient will show no further evidence of weight loss.
• Patient will tolerate ___ ml of nasogastric (NG) or gastrostomy tube feedings.
• Patient will avoid aspiration, diarrhea, and hyperglycemia.
• Patient will gain ___ lb weekly.
• Patient will consume ___ calories daily.

• Patient will avoid skin breakdown and infection around tube site.
• Patient and family members will communicate understanding of special dietary needs.
• Patient and family members will demonstrate correct tube feeding procedures.

Interventions and rationales
• Obtain and record patient's weight at same time every day *to obtain accurate readings.*
• Monitor fluid intake and output *because body weight may increase as result of fluid retention.*
• Administer prescribed amount of food *to provide patient with needed nutrition.*
– Begin regimen with small amount and diluted concentration *to decrease diarrhea and improve absorption.* Increase volume and concentration as tolerated.
– Elevate head of bed during tube feeding *to reduce risk of aspiration.*
– Check feeding tube placement at least once every shift *to verify placement in GI tract rather than in lungs.*
– Give water and juices, as needed, *to maintain adequate hydration.*
– If possible, use continuous infusion pump *to prevent diarrhea.*
– Put food coloring in the food *to monitor for aspiration.*
• Provide nares care every 4 hours *to prevent ulceration and skin breakdown.* Tape NG tube *to prevent visual obstruction.* Use hypoallergenic tape *to minimize skin reactions.*
• Change gastrostomy dressing daily or according to facility protocol *to prevent infection.*
• Ensure proper temperature of feeding (room temperature); change feeding tube bags and tubing according to facility protocol *to maximize tolerance and minimize infection.*

• Assess and record bowel sounds once a shift *to monitor for increase or decrease.*
• Auscultate and record breath sounds every 4 hours *to monitor for aspiration.* Report wheezes, rhonchi, crackles, or decreased breath sounds. If aspiration is suspected, stop tube feeding. Keep suction apparatus at bedside and suction as needed. Turn patient on side *to avoid further aspiration.*
• Instruct patient and family members in tube feeding procedures. Supervise return demonstrations until competency is achieved. *This encourages patient and family members to participate in patient's care.*

Evaluations for expected outcomes
• Patient shows no further evidence of weight loss.
• Patient tolerates NG or gastrostomy tube feedings without adverse effects.
• Patient doesn't exhibit signs of aspiration, diarrhea, or hyperglycemia.
• Patient gains specified amount of weight weekly.
• Patient consumes specified amount of calories daily.
• Patient avoids skin breakdown and infection around tube site.
• Patient and family members communicate understanding of special dietary needs and plan appropriate diet.
• Patient and family members demonstrate correct tube feeding procedures.

Documentation
• Daily weight
• Intake and output
• Tolerance of tube feeding
• Incidents of vomiting, aspiration, and diarrhea
• Bowel sounds
• Breath sounds
• Response to instructions

• Demonstration of feeding procedures
• Evaluations for expected outcomes

■ Nutrition alteration: Less than body requirements

related to psychological factors

Definition
Change in normal eating pattern that results in decreased body weight

Assessment
• History of eating disorders
• Nutritional history, including financial resources, height and weight, hereditary influences, meal preparation, sociocultural influences, usual dietary pattern, and weight fluctuations over past 10 years
• Change in intrapersonal or interpersonal factors, including internal and external cues that trigger desire to eat, rate of food consumption, and stated food preference
• Activity level
• Coping behaviors
• Body image, including perception of observer and self-perception

Defining characteristics
• Abdominal pain or cramping, with or without pathology
• Altered taste sensation
• Aversion to or lack of interest in eating
• Body weight 20% or more under ideal weight
• Diarrhea and steatorrhea
• Evidence of lack of food
• Excessive hair loss
• Fragile capillaries
• Hyperactive bowel sounds
• Inadequate food intake (less than recommended daily allowances)

• Lack of information or misinformation about nutrition
• Loss of body weight despite adequate food intake
• Pale conjunctivae and mucous membranes
• Perceived inability to ingest food
• Poor muscle tone
• Satiety immediately after eating
• Sore, inflamed buccal cavity
• Weakness of muscles required for chewing or swallowing

Associated medical diagnoses (selected)
Anorexia nervosa, bipolar disease (depressive phase), bulimia nervosa, depression

Expected outcomes
• Patient will consume at least _____ calories daily.
• Patient will gain _____ lb weekly.
• Patient will eat independently, without being prodded.
• Patient will identify emotional and psychological factors that interfere with eating.
• Patient will develop plan to monitor and maintain target weight at discharge.
• Patient will plan to use mental health resources to help resolve psychological problems.

Interventions and rationales
• Provide opportunities for patient to discuss reasons for not eating *to help assess causes of eating disorder.*
• Observe and record patient's intake (both liquid and solid) *to assess what nutrients patient consumes and what supplements she needs.*
• Determine patient's food preferences and attempt to obtain these foods. Offer foods that appeal to olfactory, visual, and tactile senses *to enhance patient's appetite.*

• Offer high-protein, high-calorie supplements, such as milk shakes, custard, and ice cream. *Such foods prevent body protein breakdown and provide caloric energy.*
• Serve foods that require little cutting or chewing *to help prevent malingering at meals.*
• Provide pleasant environment at mealtime *to enhance patient's appetite.*
• Keep snacks at bedside *to give patient some control over eating time.*
• With some patients, begin with nutritious liquids and gradually introduce solids. *Severely malnourished patient may not be able to chew solid foods immediately.*
• Avoid asking whether patient is hungry or wants to eat. Be positive in offering food. *A positive, undemanding attitude avoids confrontation with patient.*
• Whenever possible, sit with patient for predetermined length of time during meal. *This inhibits patient from dawdling during meal and from hiding or hoarding food.*
• Monitor and record elimination patterns. *Patient may be taking laxatives or diuretics to keep weight low in spite of eating.*
• Weigh patient at same time every day. Reinforce weight gain with privileges or rewards. *This yields accurate data and gives patient some control over foods eaten and privileges or rewards gained.*
• Set target weight and have patient record daily weight *to involve patient in treatment.*
• Refer patient and family members to appropriate mental health professional. *Most eating disorders are psychological. Patient and family members require treatment and follow-up to prevent recurrence.*

Evaluations for expected outcomes

• Patient consumes specified number of calories daily.
• Patient gains specified amount of weight weekly.
• Patient eats independently without constant encouragement.
• Patient lists emotional and psychological factors that interfere with eating.
• Patient states plan to monitor and maintain specific target weight after discharge.
• Patient contacts support groups and mental health resources as needed.

Documentation

• Patient's expressed attitudes toward food and eating at present time
• Patient's expressed feelings about weight, body image, and emotional status
• Patient's daily intake (liquid and solid) and output (urine, stool, and vomitus)
• Daily weight and progression of weight gain
• Interventions to feed patient adequately
• Emotional support provided
• Patient's response to nursing interventions
• Evaluations for expected outcomes

■ Nutrition alteration: More than body requirements

related to excessive intake

Definition

Change in normal eating pattern that results in increased body weight

Assessment
• Nutritional history, including financial resources, height and weight, hereditary influences, history of obesity, meal preparation, sociocultural influences, usual dietary pattern, and weight fluctuations over past 10 years
• Change in intrapersonal or interpersonal factors, including internal and external cues that trigger desire to eat, motivation to lose weight, rate of food consumption, and stated food preference
• Psychosocial status
• Activity level
• Coping patterns
• Body image, including perception of observer and self-perception

Defining characteristics
• Body weight 20% or more over ideal weight
• Dysfunctional eating patterns, such as concentrating food intake at end of day, eating in response to internal cue other than hunger (such as anxiety), eating in response to external cues (such as social situations), and pairing food with other activities
• Sedentary lifestyle
• Triceps skin fold greater than 15 mm in men and 25 mm in women

Associated medical diagnoses (selected)
Anxiety disorder, cerebrovascular accident, coronary artery disease, Cushing's syndrome, depression, diabetes mellitus, gout, hypertension, myocardial infarction, obesity

Expected outcomes
• Patient will voice feelings about present weight.
• Patient will identify internal and external cues that increase food consumption.
• Patient will state need to lose weight.
• Patient will set a weight-loss goal of _____ lb weekly.
• Patient will plan menus appropriate to prescribed diet.
• Patient will adhere to prescribed diet.
• Patient will lose at least ___ lb weekly.
• Patient will set target weight before discharge.
• Patient will state plan to monitor and maintain target weight.
• Patient will participate in selected exercise program _____ times weekly.

Interventions and rationales
• Help patient identify problem, feelings associated with eating, and circumstances in which patient turns to food. *Permanent weight loss starts with examination of factors contributing to weight gain.*
• Discuss patient's normal food preferences *to evaluate eating habits and include preferred foods in patient's diet.*
• Have dietitian calculate caloric intake patient will require to reach desirable weight *to allow planning of appropriate diet.*
• Have dietitian discuss meal planning with patient during hospitalization *to help patient plan nutritious, satisfying meals.*
• If resource is available, refer patient to mental health professional for behavior modification *to help patient change poor eating habits and ensure permanent weight loss.*
• Teach patient about low-calorie, nutritious foods. *This encourages patient to eat foods that provide energy without causing weight gain.*
• Help patient set realistic goals for losing weight. *This aids positive reinforcement and reduces frustration.*
• Give patient emotional support and positive feedback for adhering to pre-

scribed dietary regimen *to promote compliance.* Encourage nondietary rewards, such as purchase of new accessory or book, *to promote continuation of dietary plan and help patient avoid using food as reward.*
• Weigh patient weekly or as prescribed *to monitor effectiveness of diet plan.*
• Set target weight with patient and have patient record weight. *This involves patient in plan and provides positive reinforcement.*
• Explore feasibility of having patient participate after discharge in Weight Watchers, Overeaters Anonymous, or other group or individual diet therapies. *Such resources provide reinforcement and information.*
• Help patient select an exercise program (such as walking, jogging, aerobics, and swimming) appropriate to age and physical condition. *Besides aiding weight loss, such activities offer an alternative to eating to alleviate stress.*

Evaluations for expected outcomes
• Patient expresses feelings about present weight.
• Patient identifies cues that increase food consumption.
• Patient expresses desire to lose weight.
• Patient and health care professional establish weekly weight loss goal.
• Patient and family plan menus within parameters of prescribed diet.
• Patient adheres to prescribed diet.
• Patient loses specified amount of weight weekly.
• Patient and health care professional set target weight before discharge.
• Patient summarizes plan to monitor and maintain specified target weight.
• Patient participates in specified number of selected exercise activities weekly.

Documentation
• Patient's expressions of feelings about weight, eating, food, and dieting
• Goals set by patient
• Record of weight
• Foods consumed by patient
• Behaviors that promote or impede weight reduction
• Evaluations for expected outcomes

■ Nutrition alteration, risk for: More than body requirements
related to excessive intake

Definition
Accentuated risk of change in normal eating pattern that results in increased body weight

Assessment
• Nutritional history, including financial resources, height and weight, hereditary influences, history of obesity, meal preparation, sociocultural influences, usual dietary pattern, and weight fluctuations over past year
• Eating patterns, including internal and external cues that trigger desire to eat, rate of food consumption, and stated food preferences
• Psychosocial status, including behavior, mood, stressors (finances, job, and marital discord), coping mechanisms, sources of support (family, friends, and others), lifestyle, knowledge level, hobbies, and interests
• Activity levels
• Body image, including perception of observer and self-perception
• Additional circumstances that may lead to excessive intake

Risk factors

• Consumption of solid food as major food source before age 5 months
• Dysfunctional eating patterns, such as concentrating food intake at end of day, using food as reward or comfort measure, eating in response to internal cues other than hunger (such as anxiety), and eating in response to external cues (such as social situations)
• High baseline weight at beginning of each pregnancy
• Obesity in one or both parents
• Rapid movement across growth percentiles (in infant or child)

Associated medical diagnoses (selected)

Anxiety disorder, depression, diabetes mellitus

Expected outcomes

• Patient will express need to maintain or stabilize weight within 5 to 10 lb (2.3 to 4.5 kg) of target weight.
• Patient will plan to monitor weight and sustain target weight.
• Patient will express feelings regarding dietary regimen and current weight.
• Patient will identify internal and external cues that lead to increased food consumption.
• Patient will plan menus appropriate for prescribed diet.
• Patient will adhere to prescribed diet.
• Patient will participate in selected exercise program every week (specify).
• Patient will achieve weight goal.

Interventions and rationales

• Weigh patient weekly or as prescribed *to monitor effectiveness of diet.*
• Work with patient to establish realistic target weight. Instruct patient how to record weight. *Involvement in nursing plan of care improves compliance.*
• Instruct patient to keep food diary. *This helps patient confront actual intake, break through denial, and achieve more objective view of eating habits.*
• Monitor fluid intake and output and assess for edema. *Fluid retention may increase body weight.*
• Encourage patient to express feelings about dietary restrictions *to assess his perception of problem.* Help patient identify emotions associated with food and situations that trigger eating episodes. *Permanent weight maintenance requires an understanding of risk factors that contribute to weight gain.*
• Determine patient's food likes and dislikes *to evaluate eating habits and to include preferred foods in patient's diet.*
• Encourage consumption of foods low in calories and fat and high in complex carbohydrates and fiber. Have patient meet with dietitian to discuss meal planning. *These steps will help patient plan nutritious, well-balanced meals.*
• Refer patient to appropriate resource for behavior modification and cognitive therapy *to prevent relapse into high-risk eating behaviors.*
• Give patient emotional support and positive feedback for adhering to prescribed diet. *This will foster compliance and help ensure adherence to regimen.*
• Recommend patient explore group diet therapies, such as Weight Watchers and Overeaters Anonymous, *to provide additional sources of information and encouragement.*
• Discuss importance of incorporating exercise into lifestyle. Help patient select program with variety of activities (such as swimming, walking, aer-

obics, and biking) appropriate for age and physical condition. *Exercise burns calories, offers alternative to eating to alleviate stress, and fosters sense of accomplishment.*

Evaluations for expected outcomes
• Patient expresses need to maintain or stabilize weight.
• Patient states plan to maintain food diary, weighs self weekly, and expresses motivation to sustain current weight.
• Patient expresses feelings regarding dietary regimen and current weight.
• Patient identifies at least three internal and three external cues that lead to increased food consumption.
• When filling out menus, patient selects low-fat, high-fiber foods that are high in complex carbohydrates.
• Patient adheres to prescribed diet, as evidenced by selection of well-balanced meals and low-calorie snacks.
• Patient selects at least two activities for exercise program.
• Patient achieves weight goal.

Documentation
• Patient's expression of feelings about weight, eating, and dietary regimen
• Patient's weight
• Ability of patient to maintain target weight
• Foods consumed by patient
• Behaviors that promote or impede weight maintenance
• Evaluations for expected outcomes

■ Oral mucous membrane alteration

related to dehydration

Definition
Altered mouth integrity

Assessment
• History of pathologic conditions known to cause dehydration such as diabetes mellitus
• Medications, such as diuretics and antihistamines
• Vital signs
• Fluid and electrolyte status, including blood urea nitrogen level, creatinine level, intake and output, mucous membranes, serum electrolyte levels, skin turgor, and urine specific gravity
• Oral status, including inspection of oral cavity (gums and tongue), pain or discomfort, and salivation
• Nutritional status, including current weight, change from normal weight, and dietary pattern
• Psychosocial status, including change in financial status, coping skills, habits (smoking and alcohol intake), patient's perception of health problem, and recent traumatic event

Defining characteristics
• Bleeding
• Coated tongue
• Desquamation
• Difficulty eating, speaking, or swallowing
• Diminished, absent, or bad taste
• Dry mouth
• Edema
• Enlarged tonsils
• Fissures and chelitis
• Gingival hyperplasia or recession (pockets deeper than 4 mm)
• Gingival or mucosal pallor
• Halitosis

• Mucosal denudation
• Oral lesions, ulcers, pain, or discomfort
• Purulent drainage or exudate; presence of pathogens
• Smooth, atrophic, sensitive tongue
• Spongy patches or white, curdlike exudate
• Stomatitis
• Vesicles, nodules, or papules
• White patches and plaque

Associated medical diagnoses (selected)

Asthma, chronic obstructive pulmonary disease, diabetes insipidus, diabetes mellitus (uncontrolled), fractures, hemorrhage, hyperthermia, metabolic acidosis, metabolic alkalosis, shock

Expected outcomes

• Patient will maintain fluid balance (intake equals output).
• Patient will state increased comfort.
• Patient will have pink, moist oral mucous membranes.
• Patient will have minimal, if any, complications.
• Patient will correlate precipitating factors with appropriate oral care.
• Patient will demonstrate oral hygiene practices.

Interventions and rationales

• Inspect patient's oral cavity every shift. Describe and document condition; report any change in status. *Regular assessments can anticipate or alleviate problems.*
• Perform prescribed treatment regimen, including administering I.V. or oral fluids, *to improve condition of patient's mucous membranes.* Monitor progress, reporting favorable and adverse responses to treatment regimen.
• Provide supportive measures as indicated:

– Assist with oral hygiene before and after meals *to promote feeling of comfort and well-being.*
– Use toothbrush with suction if patient can't spit out water *to minimize risk of aspiration.*
– Provide mouthwash or gargles, as ordered, *to increase patient comfort and maintain moisture in mouth.*
– Lubricate patient's lips frequently with water-based lubricant *to prevent cracked, irritated skin.*
• Instruct patient in oral hygiene practices, if necessary. Have patient return demonstration of oral care routine.
– Use soft-bristled toothbrush.
– Brush with circular motion downward from gums.
– Include tongue when brushing.
– Review need for routine visits to dentist (annually for adults).
These measures increase patient's awareness of oral hygiene practices and reduce discomfort, resulting in increased nutrition and hydration.
• Tell patient to chew gum or suck on sugarless hard candy *to stimulate salivation.*
• Discuss precipitating factors, if known, and work to prevent future episodes. For example, encourage patient to avoid exercising in heat and to report effects of medication. *Patient's increased awareness of causative factors will help prevent recurrence.*
• Encourage adherence to other aspects of health care management (controlling diabetes, changing dietary habits, and avoiding alcoholic beverages) *to control or minimize effects on mucous membranes.*

Evaluations for expected outcomes

• Patient's total daily fluid intake equals total output.
• Patient chews and swallows without discomfort.

• Patient's mucous membranes remain moist, pink, and free of cuts and abrasions.
• Patient doesn't develop complications related to extended dehydration of mucous membranes.
• Patient discusses possible causes of alteration in oral mucous membranes, such as heat exhaustion and reactions to medication.
• Patient discusses and demonstrates preventive measures such as regular oral hygiene.

Documentation
• Observations of condition, healing, and response to treatment
• Interventions to provide supportive care and patient's response to supportive care
• Instructions given, patient's understanding of instructions, and patient's demonstrated skill in carrying out prescribed oral care measures
• Evaluations for expected outcomes

■ Oral mucous membrane alteration

related to mechanical trauma

Definition
Altered mouth integrity

Assessment
• History of oral surgery, dentures, braces, or dental problems
• Medications, such as diuretics and antihistamines
• Vital signs
• Fluid and electrolyte status, including blood urea nitrogen level, creatinine level, intake and output, mucous membranes, serum electrolyte levels, skin turgor, and urine specific gravity

• Oral status, including inspection of oral cavity (with gums and tongue), pain or discomfort, and salivation
• Nutritional status, including current weight, change from normal weight, and dietary pattern
• Psychosocial status, including coping skills, patient's perception of health problem, and recent traumatic event

Defining characteristics
• Bleeding
• Coated tongue
• Desquamation
• Difficulty eating, speaking, or swallowing
• Diminished, absent, or bad taste
• Dry mouth
• Edema
• Enlarged tonsils
• Fissures and chelitis
• Gingival hyperplasia or recession (pockets deeper than 4 mm)
• Gingival or mucosal pallor
• Halitosis
• Mucosal denudation
• Oral lesions, ulcers, pain, or discomfort
• Purulent drainage or exudate; presence of pathogens
• Smooth, atrophic, sensitive tongue
• Spongy patches or white, curdlike exudate
• Stomatitis
• Vesicles, nodules, or papules
• White patches and plaque

Associated medical diagnoses (selected)
Abscessed tooth, facial fracture, hemorrhagic gingivitis, impacted wisdom teeth, jaw fracture, other conditions requiring oral surgery

Expected outcomes
• Patient will maintain fluid balance (intake equals output).

• Patient will have pink, moist oral mucous membranes.
• Patient will state increased comfort.
• Patient will have minimal, if any, complications.
• Patient will correlate precipitating factors with appropriate oral care.
• Patient will demonstrate correct oral hygiene practices.

Interventions and rationales
• Inspect patient's oral cavity every shift. Describe and document condition and report any status change. *Ill-fitting dentures, jagged teeth, braces, oral surgery, and insertion of endotracheal tube may cause mechanical trauma. Regular assessments can anticipate or alleviate problems.*
• Establish and follow routine oral hygiene schedule. For example, soak dentures every evening, clean with denture cream, rinse, and keep in properly labeled container at patient's bedside. *Routine oral hygiene can improve condition of mucous membranes.*
• Provide supportive measures, as indicated:
– Assist with oral hygiene before and after meals *to promote feeling of comfort and well-being.*
– Use toothbrush with suction if patient can't spit out water *to minimize risk of aspiration.*
– Provide mouthwash or gargles, as ordered, *to increase patient comfort.*
– Lubricate patient's lips frequently with water-based lubricant. *Fluid and food intake increases when patient is more comfortable.*
• Instruct patient in oral hygiene practices, if necessary. Have patient return demonstration of oral care routine. Tell patient to stimulate saliva by chewing gum or sucking on sugarless hard candy. *These measures increase patient's awareness of oral hygiene*

practices and reduce discomfort, resulting in increased nutrition and hydration.
• Discuss precipitating factors, if known, and work to prevent future episodes (for example, weight loss may change contours of oral cavity). *Patient's increased awareness of causative factors will help prevent recurrence.*
• Encourage adherence to other aspects of health care management *to control or minimize effects on mucous membranes.* For example, encourage patients with braces to avoid popcorn, chewing gum, and caramels. *These measures reduce risk of trauma to oral mucous membrane.*
• Refer patient to dentist, dental hygienist, or other appropriate resource to correct ill-fitting dentures, modify braces, and adjust jaw wires as needed. *Regularly scheduled dental follow-up reduces risk of trauma to oral mucous membranes.*

Evaluations for expected outcomes
• Patient's total daily fluid intake equals output.
• Patient's mucous membranes remain moist, pink, and free of cuts and abrasions.
• Patient chews and drinks without discomfort.
• Patient doesn't exhibit complications related to trauma to oral mucous membranes.
• Patient discusses possible causes of alteration in oral mucous membrane, such as ill-fitting dentures or braces.
• Patient discusses preventive measures such as regular oral hygiene, including cleaning of dentures, and demonstrates prescribed oral hygiene measures.

Documentation
• Observations of condition, healing, and response to treatment
• Interventions to provide supportive care and patient's response to supportive care
• Instructions given, patient's understanding of instructions, and demonstrated skill in carrying out prescribed oral care measures
• Evaluations for expected outcomes

■ Oral mucous membrane alteration

related to pathologic condition

Definition
Altered mouth integrity

Assessment
• History of oral cavity disorder or surgery
• Medication history
• Oral status, including condition of teeth, inspection of oral cavity (including gums and tongue), oral hygiene routine, pain or discomfort, palpation of buccal mucosa, and salivation
• Nutritional status, including current weight, change from normal weight, dietary pattern, and vitamin intake
• Psychosocial status, including coping skills, family members' habits (smoking and alcohol intake), patient's perception of health problem, self-concept, and stressors (finances, family, and job)

Defining characteristics
• Bleeding
• Coated tongue
• Desquamation
• Difficulty eating, speaking, or swallowing
• Diminished, absent, or bad taste
• Dry mouth
• Edema
• Enlarged tonsils
• Fissures and chelitis
• Gingival hyperplasia or recession (pockets deeper than 4 mm)
• Gingival or mucosal pallor
• Halitosis
• Mucosal denudation
• Oral lesions, ulcers, pain, or discomfort
• Purulent drainage or exudate; presence of pathogens
• Smooth, atrophic, sensitive tongue
• Spongy patches or white, curdlike exudate
• Stomatitis
• Vesicles, nodules, or papules
• White patches and plaque

Associated medical diagnoses (selected)
Bone marrow transplantation, chemotherapy, head and neck cancer, leukemia, melanoma, pemphigus, radiation therapy, scarlet fever, Sjögren's syndrome, streptococcal throat

Expected outcomes
• Patient's lesions or wounds will show improvement or heal.
• Patient will have minimal, if any, complications.
• Patient will voice increased comfort.
• Patient will demonstrate understanding of surgical measures.
• Patient will voice feelings about condition.
• Patient will explain oral care routine.
• Patient will demonstrate oral hygiene practices.

Interventions and rationales
• Inspect patient's oral cavity every shift. Describe and document condition, reporting any status change.

Regular assessment prevents recurrence or exacerbation of problems.
• Perform prescribed treatment regimen for underlying pathologic condition. Report favorable and adverse responses to treatment regimen. *Treating underlying condition improves condition of oral mucous membranes.*
• Encourage patient to state feelings and concerns about oral condition and its impact on body image *to help him accept changes in body image.*
• Provide supportive measures as indicated:
– Assist with oral hygiene before and after meals. Use soft-bristled toothbrush or cotton applicator and nonalcoholic mouthwash *to minimize trauma to damaged tissues.*
– Lubricate patient's lips frequently *to prevent cracking and irritation.*
– Use artificial saliva solution if mouth remains dry *to restore normal moisture.*
– Avoid serving hot, cold, spicy, fried, or citrus foods *to avoid irritating damaged tissue.*
– Suction oral cavity *to prevent drooling and aspiration of accumulated secretions. Aspiration may lead to pneumonia or coughing and further trauma.*
– Give soft or pureed foods, which don't irritate tissues, *to reduce pain.*
• If oral surgery is scheduled, give appropriate preoperative and postoperative instruction and care. Document response. *Instruction enhances compliance with therapy.*
• Instruct patient in oral hygiene practices and have patient give return demonstration. Suggest referral to dentist or dental hygienist. *This increases patient's awareness of oral hygiene and reduces discomfort, resulting in increased nutrition and hydration.*

• Encourage patient to stop smoking. *Smoking has been linked to mucous membrane breakdown and cancer.*
• Refer to psychiatric liaison nurse or support group *to help patient cope with altered body image.*

Evaluations for expected outcomes
• Patient has no lesions or wounds, or they cause patient less discomfort.
• Patient doesn't exhibit complications related to trauma to oral mucous membranes.
• Patient chews and swallows without discomfort.
• Patient discusses impending surgical procedures.
• Patient discusses fear of oral surgery and outcome.
• Patient discusses postoperative oral care routine.
• Patient demonstrates oral hygiene practices, including treatments and medications.

Documentation
• Patient's expression of concern about oral condition and its impact on body image
• Patient's willingness to join in own care
• Observations of condition, healing, and response to treatment
• Interventions to provide supportive care and patient's response to supportive care
• Instructions given, patient's understanding of instructions, and demonstrated skill in carrying out prescribed oral care measures
• Evaluations for expected outcomes

■ Pain

related to physical, biological, or chemical agents

Definition

An unpleasant sensory and emotional experience arising from actual or potential tissue damage or described in terms of such damage; pain may be of sudden or slow onset, vary in intensity from mild to severe, and be constant or recurring; pain lasts less than 6 months; and period of pain has an anticipated or predictable end

Assessment

• Descriptive characteristics of pain, including location, quality, intensity on a scale of 1 to 10, temporal factors, and sources of relief
• Physiologic variables, such as age and pain tolerance
• Psychological variables, such as body image, personality, previous experience with pain, anxiety, and secondary gain
• Sociocultural variables, including cognitive style, culture or ethnicity, attitude and values, sex, and birth order
• Environmental variables, such as setting and time

Defining characteristics

• Alteration in muscle tone (may range from listless to rigid)
• Autonomic responses (diaphoresis; blood pressure, pulse rate, and respiratory rate changes; and dilated pupils)
• Changes in appetite and eating
• Communication (verbal or coded) of pain
• Distracting behavior (such as pacing, seeking out other people, and performing repetitive activities)
• Expressions of pain (such as moaning and crying)
• Facial mask of pain (grimacing)
• Guarding or protective behavior
• Narrowed focus (including altered time perception, withdrawal from social contact, and impaired thought process)
• Self-focusing
• Sleep disturbance

Associated medical diagnoses (selected)

Acoustic neuroma, adrenal insufficiency, amputation, angina pectoris, aortic aneurysm, appendicitis, arterial occlusion, bladder cancer, bone sarcomas, brain abscess, breast cancer, breast engorgement, burns, carpal tunnel syndrome, cellulitis, cervical cancer, cholecystitis, chronic fatigue syndrome, colitis, colon and rectal cancer, coronary artery disease, craniotomy, Crohn's disease, cystitis, detached retina, diverticulitis, duodenal ulcer, ectopic pregnancy, encephalitis, endometrial cancer, epididymitis, esophageal cancer, fractures, gastric ulcer, glaucoma, gout, Guillain-Barré syndrome, head or neck cancer, heart failure, hemophilia, hemorrhoids, hemothorax, hydrocephalus, hyperemesis gravidarum, hyperparathyroidism, hyperpituitarism, interstitial cystitis, intestinal obstruction, joint replacement, leukemia, lung abscess, Lyme disease, maternal nipple anomaly, meningitis, metastatic disease, multiple myeloma, multiple sclerosis, myocardial infarction, osteoarthritis, osteomyelitis, pelvic inflammatory disease, pemphigus, pericarditis, peripheral vascular disease, peritonitis, pleurisy, pneumothorax, polycystic kidney disease, polycythemia vera, prolapsed intervertebral disk, prostate cancer, pulmonary embolus, pyelonephritis, radiation therapy, Reiter's syndrome, renal calculi, renal cancer, rheumatic fever, rheumatoid arthritis, sarcoidosis, scarlet fever, sickle cell anemia, Sjögren's syndrome, testicular cancer, thrombophlebitis, trigeminal neuralgia, urinary calculi, urinary diversion, urinary tract infection, uterine rupture

Expected outcomes
• Patient will identify pain characteristics.
• Patient will articulate factors that intensify pain and will modify behavior accordingly.
• Patient will state and carry out appropriate interventions for pain relief.
• Patient will report more than 4 hours of sleep nightly.
• Patient will decrease amount and frequency of pain medication needed.
• Patient will express feeling of comfort and relief from pain.

Interventions and rationales
• Assess patient's signs and symptoms of pain and administer pain medication as prescribed. Monitor and record medication's effectiveness and adverse effects. *Assessment allows for plan of care modification as needed.*
• Perform comfort measures to promote relaxation, such as massage, bathing, repositioning, and relaxation techniques. *These measures reduce muscle tension or spasm, redistribute pressure on body parts, and help patient focus on non-pain-related subjects.*
• Plan activities with patient to provide distraction, such as reading, crafts, television, and visits, *to help patient focus on non-pain-related matters.*
• Provide patient with information to help increase pain tolerance; for example, reasons for pain and length of time it will last. *This educates patient*

and encourages compliance in trying alternative pain relief measures.
• Manipulate environment to promote periods of uninterrupted rest. *This promotes health, well-being, and increased energy level important to pain relief.*
• Apply heat or cold as ordered (specify) *to minimize or relieve pain.*
• Help patient into comfortable position and use pillows to splint or support painful areas, as appropriate, *to reduce muscle tension or spasm and to redistribute pressure on body parts.*
• Collaborate with patient in administering prescribed analgesics when alternative methods of pain control are inadequate. *Gaining patient's trust and involvement helps ensure compliance and may reduce medication intake.*
• When possible, allow patient to use alternative pain treatments from his culture (such as acupuncture) as a substitute for or complement to Western treatments *to promote nonpharmacologic pain management.*

Evaluations for expected outcomes
• Patient's pain rating is documented (using a scale of 1 to 10) before administering medication and 30 to 45 minutes afterward.
• Patient articulates factors that intensify pain and modifies behavior accordingly.
• Patient carries out alternative pain control measures such as heat or cold applications.
• Patient reports more than 4 hours sleep nightly (reports of less than 4 hours require further assessment).
• Patient decreases amount and frequency of pain medication within 72 hours.
• Patient expresses feeling of comfort.

Documentation
• Patient's description of physical pain, pain relief, and feelings about pain
• Observations of patient's physical, psychological, and sociocultural responses to pain
• Comfort measures and medications provided to reduce pain and effectiveness of interventions
• Information provided to patient about pain and pain relief
• Other interventions performed to assist patient with pain control
• Evaluations for expected outcomes

■ Pain

related to psychological factors

Definition
An unpleasant sensory and emotional experience arising from actual or potential tissue damage or described in terms of such damage; pain may be of sudden or slow onset, vary in intensity from mild to severe, and be constant or recurring; pain lasts less than 6 months; and period of pain has an anticipated or predictable end

Assessment
• History of exposure to physical, biological, or chemical agents as a cause of pain
• Descriptive characteristics of pain, including location, quality, intensity on a scale of 1 to 10, temporal factors, and sources of provocation or relief
• Physiologic variables, such as age and pain tolerance
• Psychological variables, such as body image, personality, previous experience with pain, anxiety, and secondary gain
• Sociocultural variables, including cognitive style, culture and ethnicity, attitude and values, sex, and birth order
• Environmental variables, such as time and setting

Defining characteristics
• Alteration in muscle tone (may range from listless to rigid)
• Autonomic responses (diaphoresis; blood pressure, pulse rate, and respiratory rate changes; and dilated pupils)
• Changes in appetite and eating
• Communication (verbal or coded) of pain
• Distracting behavior (such as pacing, seeking out other people, and performing repetitive activities)
• Expressions of pain (such as moaning and crying)
• Facial mask of pain (grimacing)
• Guarding or protective behavior
• Narrowed focus (including altered time perception, withdrawal from social contact, and impaired thought process)
• Self-focusing
• Sleep disturbance

Associated medical diagnoses (selected)
Depending on the variables present in assessment, such psychological factors as stress, depression, and ineffective coping mechanisms may intensify pain caused by physical, biological, or chemical agents. An example of psychological pain is the phantom pain often experienced following limb amputation.

Expected outcomes
• Patient will identify specific characteristics of pain.
• Patient will express relief from pain within a reasonable time after taking prescribed medication.

• Patient will help develop a plan for pain control.
• Patient will articulate possibility of physical pain being associated with emotional stressors.
• Patient will require less pain medication (specify).
• Patient will state satisfaction with pain management regimen.
• Patient will use available resources to understand pain phenomenon and will cooperate with treatment plan.

Interventions and rationales

• Assess physical symptoms that require pain medication, and administer medication as prescribed. *Continuous reassessment documents patient's subjective complaints and behavior with organic pathology.*
• Return to patient in 30 minutes to check medication's effectiveness. *This establishes trusting-caring relationship that encourages accurate communication.*
• Discuss with patient possible association between exacerbation of pain and patient's identified stressors. *This helps patient explore exacerbating emotional or environmental factors that may affect pain.*
• Ask patient to help establish goals and develop plan for pain control. *This gives patient sense of control.*
• Provide patient with positive feedback about progress toward reaching goals *to improve motivation and encourage compliance.*
• Spend at least 15 minutes per shift allowing patient to express feelings, *which will help give patient a sense of control.*
• Consider services of psychiatric mental health professional to help patient and staff members establish realistic plan to resolve problem. *Patients who remain helpless, unmotivated, uncooperative, and manipulative are*

self-destructive. Underlying causes should be explored.
• Plan activities to distract patient, such as reading, television, and family visits, *to help keep patient from focusing on pain.*

Evaluations for expected outcomes

• Patient discusses characteristics of pain, including location, duration, and frequency.
• Patient reports achieving pain relief with analgesia or other measures.
• Patient participates in development of health care plan and discusses modifications.
• Patient acknowledges that pain may be related to emotional factors and lists stressors that may exacerbate pain.
• Patient achieves reduction in use of pain medication.
• Patient states satisfaction with pain management regimen.
• Patient displays motivation by seeking out resources to explain pain phenomenon and cooperating with treatment plan.

Documentation

• Patient's expressions of physical pain and well-being and emotional pain and well-being
• Observations of patient's physical well-being
• Interventions performed to help patient control pain
• Results of interventions
• Evaluations for expected outcomes

■ Pain, chronic

related to physical disability

Definition

An unpleasant sensory and emotional experience arising from actual or potential tissue damage or described in terms of such damage; pain may be of sudden or slow onset, vary in intensity from mild to severe, and be constant or recurring; pain lasts more than 6 months; and period of pain doesn't have an anticipated or predictable end

Assessment

• Descriptive characteristics of pain, including location, quality, intensity on a scale of 1 to 10, temporal factors, duration, precipitating factors (food, alcohol, activity, and stress), and comfort factors
• Physiologic variables, such as general health state, length of pain, organ system involvement, pain tolerance, disability (work, family, or social), and pain interventions (such as injection, traction, ice, physical therapy, and transcutaneous electrical nerve stimulation)
• Psychological variables, such as age, self-esteem, self-worth, role (worker, husband, breadwinner), coping behavior (appropriate or inappropriate), secondary gains (disability insurance, workmen's compensation, litigation), suffering (emotional component), manipulative behavior, dependence on others or on system, and previous hospital experience
• Sociocultural variables, including educational level, motivation, culture or ethnicity, sex, values and beliefs, pain behaviors, financial distress, and religion
• Environmental variables, such as setting and time
• Pharmacologic variables, including type of drugs, amount used in one day, use of illicit drugs, and use of alcohol

Defining characteristics

• Altered ability to continue previous activities
• Atrophy of involved muscle group
• Changes in sleep pattern
• Depression
• Facial mask
• Fatigue
• Fear of reinjury
• Irritability
• Protective or guarding behavior
• Reduced social interaction
• Restlessness
• Self-focusing
• Sympathetic-mediated responses (such as change in temperature and hypersensitivity)
• Weight gain or loss

Associated medical diagnoses (selected)

Cervical pain, chronic low back pain, diabetic neuropathy, intermittent or chronic headaches, phantom limb, postherpetic neuralgia, postsurgical pain, reflex sympathetic dystrophy, spinal cord injury

Expected outcomes

• Patient will identify characteristics of pain and pain behaviors.
• Patient will develop pain management program that includes activity and rest schedule, exercise program, and medication regimen that isn't pain-contingent.
• Patient will carry out resocialization behavior and activities.
• Patient will state relationship of increasing pain to stress, activity, and fatigue.

• Patient will state importance of self-care behavior or activities.

Interventions and rationales
• Assess patient's physical symptoms of pain, physical complaints, and daily activities. Administer pain medication as prescribed. Monitor and record effectiveness and adverse effects of medication. (Keep in mind that pain behavior and pain talk may be inconsistent.) *Correlating patient's pain behavior with activities, time of day, and visits may be useful in modifying tasks.*
• Develop behavior-oriented plan of care; for instance, set up plan to follow activity schedule. *Behavioral-cognitive measures can help patient modify learned pain behaviors.*
• Teach patient how to use relaxation techniques, guided imagery, massage, or music therapy to relieve pain. *These methods work as adjunct to medications, increase self-help, and foster independence.*
• Teach patient and family members such techniques as massage, application of ice, and exercise *to relieve pain and foster independence.*
• Work closely with staff and patient's family *to achieve pain management goals and maximize patient's cooperation.*
• Use behavior modification; for example, spend time with patient only if discussion includes no pain talk. Use contingency rewards for decreasing pain talk and pain behavior. *Reducing pain talk helps patient refocus on other, more important matters.*
• Encourage self-care activities. Develop a schedule. *This helps patient gain sense of control and reduces dependence on caregivers and society.*
• Establish specific time to talk with patient about pain and its psychological and emotional effects *to establish trusting, supportive relationship that encompasses patient's physiologic, emotional, social, sexual, and financial concerns.*

Evaluations for expected outcomes
• Patient maintains activity diary and pain level chart that rates severity of pain on a scale of 1 to 10.
• Patient maintains pain management program that includes activity and rest schedule, exercise program, and medication regimen.
• Patient documents increased activity in daily activity diary.
• Patient states that stress, activity, and fatigue may increase pain.
• Patient states that self-care activities are important.

Documentation
• Patient's description of physical pain, pain relief, and feelings about pain
• Pain talk and pain behavior and affect
• Relationship of reports of pain to activities
• Treatments and pain talk
• Time out of bed
• Comfort measures initiated by nurse, patient, or family members
• Response to interventions
• Response to pharmacologic agents
• Interaction with staff
• Evaluations for expected outcomes

■ Perioperative positioning injury, risk for

Definition
Accentuated risk of tissue injury, neuromuscular impairment, vascular compromise, or impaired gas exchange during surgery

Assessment

- Reason for surgery
- Type of surgery and its expected length
- Health status, including age, weight, vital signs, nutritional status, integumentary status, musculoskeletal status, hydration status, temperature, peripheral vascular status, neurologic status, and smoking history
- Laboratory studies, including hematocrit and hemoglobin, complete blood count, electrolyte levels, urinalysis, blood coagulation studies, and liver function tests
- Mobility status, including range of motion (ROM), presence of prosthesis, and limb abnormality, impairment, or injury
- Current medical treatments, including radiation therapy, chemotherapy, and steroid therapy

Risk factors

- Disorientation
- Edema
- Emaciation
- Immobilization
- Muscle weakness
- Obesity
- Sensory-perceptual disturbances from anesthesia

Associated medical diagnoses (selected)

Any disease that may require surgery.

Supine position: Abdominal aortic aneurysm resection, appendectomy, arthroscopy, arthrotomy, bowel resection, bronchoscopy, cholecystectomy, colostomy, coronary artery bypass grafting, cystectomy, exploratory laparotomy, gastrectomy, hernia repair, ileal conduit, mediastinoscopy, splenectomy, total abdominal hysterectomy, pacemaker insertion, rotator cuff repair

Prone position: Achilles tendon repair, anal fissurectomy or fistulectomy, hemorrhoidectomy, laminectomy, pilonidal cyst excision, posterior cervical fusion, spinal fusion with Harrington rods

Lateral position: Descending thoracic aortic aneurysm resection, nephrectomy, nephrolithotomy, thoracotomy, total hip arthroplasty

Lithotomy position: Anterior or posterior vaginal repair, conization of the cervix, dilatation and curettage, hemorrhoidectomy and other rectal procedures, laparoscopy, perineal condyloma, low anterior bowel resection, rectovaginal or vesicovaginal fistulectomy, total vaginal hysterectomy, uterine or bladder suspension

Expected outcomes

- Patient will maintain effective breathing patterns.
- Patient will maintain adequate cardiac output.
- Surgical positioning will facilitate gas exchange.
- Patient will show no evidence of neurologic, musculoskeletal, or vascular compromise.
- Patient will maintain tissue integrity.

Interventions and rationales

- Document and report results of preoperative nursing assessment. Identify factors predisposing patient to tissue injury. *This information guides interventions.*
- Use appropriate mode of patient transportation (stretcher, patient bed, wheelchair, or crib) *to ensure patient safety.*
- Make sure adequate number of staff members assist with transferring patient — at least two for moving patient onto operating room bed and at least four for moving anesthetized patient off operating room bed. *Adequate staffing enhances safety.*

• Check operating room bed before surgery for proper functioning. *Intraoperative bed malfunction can result in increased anesthesia time and more difficult surgical approach.*

• Ensure proper positioning.

Supine position:

– Check neck and spine for proper alignment *to avoid trauma.*

– Check that legs are straight and ankles uncrossed. *Crossed ankles cause pressure on tissue, vessels, and nerves.*

– Place safety strap 2″ (5 cm) above knees, tight enough to restrain without compromising superficial venous return. *Applied too tightly, safety strap may cause venous thrombosis or compression of tibial, peroneal, or sciatic nerves.*

– Secure arms at sides with drawsheet, with palms down, making sure no part of arm or hand extends over mattress. Alternatively, secure arms on padded arm boards at less than 90-degree angle from body, with palms supinated. *Hyperextension can cause injury to brachial plexus. Supination of palms minimizes pressure.*

– Apply eye pads if eyelids won't remain closed or if surgery is being performed on head, neck, or chest. *If allowed to remain open, eye may dry out and become infected. Corneal abrasions may result from drapes and other foreign material rubbing against eye.*

– If surgery is expected to last more than 2 hours or if patient is predisposed to pressure injury, place padding under occiput, scapulae, olecranon, sacrum, coccyx, and calcaneus *to protect potential pressure points.* Apply padded footboard *to support feet, avoid plantar flexion, and prevent stretching of tibial nerve and subsequent footdrop.*

– Unless contraindicated, place foam doughnut or small pillow under head *to prevent stretching of neck muscles. Prone position:*

– Make sure at least four staff members assist when turning patient *to ensure safety.*

– Place foam doughnut or small pillow under head. Check lower eye and ear for excessive pressure. Apply eye pads. *Head support helps maintain cervical and thoracic spine alignment. Checking dependent ear and eye lowers risk of pressure injury. Pads protect eyes.*

– Place arms on arm boards extended in front beside head with elbows slightly flexed and palms pronated *to prevent strain on shoulder, elbows, and wrist joints.*

– Check for proper alignment of neck and spine *to avoid trauma.*

– Check female patient's breasts and male patient's genitalia for excessive pressure from chest rolls or laminectomy brace *to avoid soft-tissue and nerve injury.*

– Check bilateral pulses of upper and lower extremities. *Top and bottom edges of chest rolls or laminectomy brace may compress radial and femoral arteries.*

– Place padding under knees *to avoid injury to soft tissue and knee joint.*

– Place pillow under ankles *to avoid putting pressure on toes and feet, stretching tibial nerve, or causing plantar flexion.*

– Place safety strap 2″ (5 cm) above knees, securely but not too tightly, *to restrain patient without compromising superficial venous return.*

– If surgery is expected to last more than 2 hours or if patient is predisposed to pressure injury, place padding under acromion process, olecranon, and anterior iliac spine *to protect pressure points.*

Lateral position:
– Make sure at least four staff members assist when turning patient *to ensure safety.*
– Check neck and spine for proper alignment *to avoid trauma.*
– Place foam doughnut or small pillow under patient's head. Check dependent eye and ear for excessive pressure. Apply eye pads. *Head supports help maintain cervical and thoracic spine alignment. Checking dependent ear and eye lowers risk of pressure injury. Pads protect patient's eyes.*
– Place small roll under dependent lower axilla *to relieve pressure on chest and axilla, allow for adequate chest expansion, and prevent compression of brachial plexus by humeral head.*
– Place lower arm on arm board at less than 90-degree angle from body, palm supinated. Place upper arm on elevated padded support at less than 90-degree angle from body, with palm pronated, and apply restraints *to avoid injury to brachial plexus.*
– Place bottom leg flexed at hip and knee and top leg straight. *Flexing bottom leg provides greater stability for torso, decreases pressure on lateral aspect of lower leg, and prevents bony areas of knees and ankles from pressing against each other.*
– Place pillows between knees and ankles *to support top leg, prevent strain on top hip, and pad pressure points on medial aspects of both legs.*
– Place padding under lateral aspects of bottom knee and ankle *to reduce risk of tissue injury to area over lateral malleolus of ankle and peroneal nerve damage (footdrop).*
– Place safety strap across upper thighs or wide tape over hips. Attach strap or tape to bed *to ensure safety.*

– If surgery is expected to last more than 2 hours or if patient is predisposed to pressure injury, place padding under acromion process, ilium, and greater trochanter *to protect pressure points.*
Lithotomy position:
– Secure arms on arm boards or at sides. If arms are placed at sides, position fingers away from break in table *to prevent fingers from becoming compressed in bed mechanism.*
– Check neck and spine for proper alignment *to avoid trauma.*
– Position stirrups at equal height and attach them to bed securely *to prevent accidental movement. Uneven leg flexion and hip abduction can cause strain on lumbar and sacral areas.*
– Place loop straps of post stirrup behind ankle and under foot. Pad post portion of stirrup if it could come in contact with leg. *Loop straps support and secure legs.*
– Pad popliteal knee support stirrups *to prevent possible thrombosis of superficial vessels and pressure injury to femoral and obturator nerves.*
– If surgery is expected to last more than 2 hours or if patient is predisposed to pressure injury, place padding under occiput, scapulae, olecranon, and sacrum *to protect potential pressure points.*
– With help of coworker, raise and lower patient's legs simultaneously and slowly *to prevent ankle and knee injury and hip dislocation. Lowering legs too quickly may cause sudden hypotension.*
• Assess patient position following each positional change *to ensure proper body alignment and adequate padding and support.*
• Apply restraints after positioning patient *to prevent falls and injury.*

Evaluations for expected outcomes

• Patient maintains effective breathing patterns. Patient's position doesn't restrict ventilation. Patient has adequate chest expansion.

• Patient maintains adequate cardiac output. Patient doesn't experience any significant episodes of hypertension or hypotension.

• Positioning allows for adequate gas exchange, as evidenced by patient's ventilation-perfusion ratio and oxygen saturation.

• Patient shows no evidence of neurologic, musculoskeletal, or vascular compromise. Patient's mobility status and ROM remain at preoperative levels. Patient doesn't experience pain, numbness, tingling, or weakness in positioned body parts.

• Patient's tissue integrity remains intact; skin doesn't become reddened, discolored, ulcerated, edematous, or excoriated.

Documentation

• Results of preoperative nursing assessment

• Operative procedure, type of anesthesia, and surgical positioning

• Surgical times, including time patient entered operating room, time incision was made, time incision was closed, and time patient left operating room

• Method of patient transport and transfer

• Estimated intraoperative blood loss

• Types and placement of padding, restraints, and positional devices

• Intraoperative repositioning of patient

• Intraoperative insertion of permanent or temporary implants

• Peripheral pulses

• Evaluations for expected outcomes

■ Peripheral neurovascular dysfunction, risk for

Definition

Accentuated risk of disruption in circulation or sensation in or motion of an extremity

Assessment

• History of trauma or vascular injuries

• Inspection of extremities, including signs of soft-tissue injury, such as abrasions, lacerations, and contusions

• Pain sensation, including characteristics (sharp, dull, constant, or intermittent) of pain, precipitating factors, and reaction to passive stretching of affected muscles

• Tactile sensation in areas innervated by major nerves of upper extremities, including deltoid, radial side of forearm, palmar surface of thumb, fingers, palmar surface of little finger, and webbed space between thumb and index finger

• Tactile sensation in lower extremities, including medial side of foot and leg, medial side of thigh, sole of foot, and lateral aspect of leg below the knee

• Motor nerve function of upper extremities, including arm abduction at shoulder, arm flexion at elbow, thumb and little finger opposition, abduction and adduction of fingers, and extension of wrist and fingers

• Motor nerve function of lower extremities, including knee extension, thigh adduction, plantar flexion and dorsiflexion of ankle, and flexion and extension of toes

• Pulses in upper and lower extremities, including radial, ulnar, brachial, femoral, popliteal, posterior tibial, and dorsalis pedis. Perform bilateral comparison and rank quality using following scale:

0 = absent
1 = very weak, barely palpable
2 = weak, reduced
3 = slightly weak, easily located
4 = normal, easily located

• Vascular status, including capillary refill time, blanching, skin temperature, and skin color
• Point tenderness, especially over bony prominences
• Edema
• Increased intracompartmental pressure
• Cranial nerves (if patient has halo cast)

Risk factors
• Burns
• Fractures
• Immobilization
• Mechanical compression (such as tourniquet, cast, brace, dressing, and restraint)
• Orthopedic surgery
• Trauma
• Vascular obstruction

Associated medical diagnoses (selected)
Carpal tunnel syndrome, compartment syndrome, ganglion cyst, fractures, neurovascular compression, peripheral circulatory failure, peripheral nerve entrapment syndrome, peripheral vascular disease, spinal cord injury, vascular insufficiency, vascular occlusion

Expected outcomes
• Patient won't experience disability related to peripheral neurovascular dysfunction after injury or treatment.
• Patient will maintain circulation in extremities.
• Patient will feel and move each toe or finger after application of cast, brace, or splint.

• Patient will demonstrate correct body positioning techniques.
• Patient and family members will express understanding of risk for altered neurovascular status and need to report symptoms of impaired circulation.
• If appropriate, patient will enroll in smoking cessation program.
• Symptoms of neurovascular compromise will be absent.

Interventions and rationales
• Note if patient is to undergo surgery or procedure that increases his risk of peripheral neurovascular dysfunction *to anticipate complications.*
• Immobilize joints directly above and below suspected fracture site, leaving room for pulse assessment *to facilitate monitoring of circulatory status.*
• As appropriate, assess circulation before application of cast, brace, or splint. After application of cast, brace, or splint, have patient move fingers and toes every 4 hours until discharge *to detect signs of impaired circulation.*
• Remove clothing around suspected fracture site, clean site, apply sterile dressings to open wounds, and carefully apply cast, brace, or splint *to avoid further infection and trauma.*
• Follow facility guidelines for application of such devices as tourniquets, restraints, and tape *to ensure adequate circulation in affected extremity.*
• If you suspect nerve compression, assess position of extremity that has cast, brace, or splint. *Positioning of extremity may affect circulation.*
• Elevate limb above heart level after surgery or trauma *to reduce risk of edema.* If increased intracompartmental pressure is evident, maintain affected limb at heart level *to reduce pressure.*

• If edema appears in affected extremity, split, bivalve, slit, or cut a window in cast and padding according to facility protocol *to avoid neurovascular impairment.*

• Inject prescribed neurotoxic agents (such as penicillin G, hydrocortisone, tetanus toxoid, and diazepam) away from affected extremity and major nerves *to avoid injury.*

• Avoid flexing affected extremity. *Flexion may reduce venous circulation, increasing risk of neurovascular complications.*

• If patient smokes, encourage him to enroll in a smoking cessation program. *Quitting smoking may enhance oxygenation, decreasing risk of peripheral neurovascular dysfunction.*

• Take steps to ease patient's anxiety. *Stress may lead to vasoconstriction.*

• Administer and monitor effectiveness of vasodilators, as ordered, *to control vasospasm.*

• If patient requires fasciotomy to restore circulation, provide educational material that explains this emergency procedure *to reduce patient anxiety.*

• Instruct patient and family members in proper positioning when lying in bed and when sitting and in methods of obtaining pressure relief *to avoid pooling of blood and pressure ulcers.*

• If appropriate, discuss cause of injury and safety precautions *to avoid further injury.* Injuries to upper extremities usually result from industrial accidents; injuries to lower extremities, from automobile accidents.

• Instruct patient and family members in recognizing symptoms of peripheral neurovascular dysfunction, including numbness, pain, and tingling. Emphasize need to report symptoms to doctor *to prevent onset of neurovascular damage after discharge.*

Evaluations for expected outcomes

• Patient doesn't experience disability related to peripheral neurovascular dysfunction.

• Patient maintains circulation in extremities.

• Patient demonstrates ability to move each toe or finger after application of cast, brace, or splint.

• Patient demonstrates correct body positioning techniques.

• Patient and family members express understanding of risk for altered neurovascular status.

• Patient enrolls in smoking cessation program.

• Patient has no symptoms of neurovascular compromise.

Documentation

• Results of neurovascular assessment (baseline and ongoing)

• Nature of injury or treatment

• History of illnesses and surgeries

• Symptoms of neurovascular dysfunction reported by patient and family members

• Patient's turning schedule

• Instructions provided to patient and family members at discharge

• Evaluations for expected outcomes

■ Poisoning, risk for

related to external factors

Definition

Accentuated risk of accidental exposure to or ingestion of drugs or dangerous products in doses sufficient to cause poisoning

Assessment

• Health history, including accidents, allergies, exposure to pollutants, falls, hyperthermia, hypothermia, poison-

ing, sensory or perceptual changes (auditory, gustatory, kinesthetic, olfactory, tactile, and visual), and trauma
• Circumstances surrounding present situation that might lead to injury
• Neurologic status, including level of consciousness (LOC), mental status, and orientation
• Psychosocial history, including age, habits (drug or alcohol use), occupation, and personality
• Laboratory studies, including clotting factors, hemoglobin and hematocrit, platelet count, white blood cell count, and toxicology screening

Risk factors
• Atmospheric pollutants
• Chemical contamination of food or water
• Dangerous products or drugs stored within reach of children or confused people
• Use of illegal drugs contaminated with poisonous additives
• Flaking or peeling paint or plaster in presence of young children
• Storing of large amounts of drugs in home
• Poisonous plants
• Unprotected contact with heavy metals or chemicals
• Use of paint, lacquer, or similar materials in poorly ventilated area or without effective protection

Associated medical diagnoses (selected)
Alcohol addiction, Alzheimer's disease, cerebrovascular accident, diabetes mellitus, self-destructive behavior, suicidal behavior

Expected outcomes
• Patient won't ingest or be exposed to dangerous substances.
• Patient will communicate an understanding of need for self-protection.
• Patient and family members will state method for safekeeping of potentially dangerous products.

Interventions and rationales
• Observe, record, and report falls, seizures, and unsafe practices *to ensure implementation of appropriate interventions. Overdose of certain medications (such as phenothiazines) can cause such neurologic problems as seizures.*
• Monitor and record respiratory status *because certain poisons can cause respiratory depression.*
• Monitor and record neurologic status *because excessive toxic exposure can cause coma.* Patient may have pinpoint or dilated pupils, depending on type of drug ingested and length of time patient has been hypoxic.
• Monitor vital signs, intake and output, and LOC. Record and report any changes. *Severe hypotension may develop following overdose. It may be related to central nervous system defect, direct myocardial depression, or vasodilation. Marked hyperthermia can occur with salicylate overdose, which affects metabolic rate. Dehydration may develop in some patients from increased respiratory rate, sweating, vomiting, and urine losses.*
• Remove all dangerous or potentially dangerous products from environment *to avoid injury.*
• Check settings on oxygen flow meters every hour on all patients known to retain carbon dioxide (for example, some patients with chronic obstructive pulmonary disease). *This avoids carbon dioxide narcosis from excessive oxygen therapy in poorly ventilated patients; if unchecked, patient may stop breathing.*
• Provide patient and family members with information about such specific products as medications, oxygen, and

total parenteral nutrition. Tailor instructions to specific product and patient's capability for learning self-care. *This enables patient and family members to identify and alter environmental or lifestyle factors to achieve optimum health level.*

Evaluations for expected outcomes
• Patient doesn't report or exhibit signs or symptoms resulting from exposure to or ingestion of dangerous substances.
• Patient requests information on protection from dangerous products.
• Patient and family members describe method for safekeeping of potentially dangerous products.

Documentation
• Patient's statements that indicate potential for injury
• Physical findings
• Observations or knowledge of unsafe practices
• Interventions performed to prevent injury
• Patient's response to nursing interventions
• Evaluations for expected outcomes

■ Poisoning, risk for

related to internal factors (biological, psychological, developmental)

Definition
Accentuated risk of accidental exposure to or ingestion of drugs or dangerous products in doses sufficient to cause poisoning

Assessment
• Health history, including accidents, allergies, exposure to pollutants, falls, hyperthermia, hypothermia, poisoning, seizures, trauma, and sensory-perceptual changes (auditory, gustatory, kinesthetic, olfactory, tactile, and visual)
• Circumstances of present situation that might lead to injury
• Neurologic status, including level of consciousness (LOC), mental status, and orientation
• Psychosocial history, including age, habits (drug or alcohol use), occupation, and personality
• Laboratory studies, including clotting factors, hemoglobin and hematocrit, platelet count, white blood cell count, and toxicology screening

Risk factors
• Cognitive or emotional difficulties
• Insufficient resources
• Lack of drug education
• Lack of safety precautions
• Occupational setting without adequate safeguards
• Reduced vision

Associated medical diagnoses (selected)
Alzheimer's disease, brain tumor, cerebrovascular accident, depression, head injury, schizophrenia, self-destructive behavior, suicidal behavior

Expected outcomes
• Patient won't ingest or be exposed to dangerous products.
• Patient will communicate understanding of need for self-protection.
• Patient and family members will explain method for safekeeping of dangerous products.

Interventions and rationales
• Observe, record, and report falls, seizures, and unsafe practices *to ensure implementation of appropriate interventions. Overdose of certain*

medications can cause such neurologic problems as seizures.

• Monitor and record respiratory status *because certain poisons can cause respiratory depression.*

• Monitor and record neurologic status *because excessive toxic exposure can cause coma.* Patient may have pinpoint or dilated pupils, depending on type of drug ingested and length of time patient has been hypoxic.

• Remove dangerous or potentially dangerous products from environment *to avoid injury.*

• Monitor vital signs, intake and output, and LOC. Record and report any changes. *Severe hypotension may develop following overdose. It may be related to central nervous system defect, direct myocardial depression, or vasodilation. Marked hyperthermia can occur with salicylate overdose, which affects metabolic rate. Dehydration may develop in some patients from increased respiratory rate, sweating, vomiting, and urine losses.*

• Provide patient and family members with information about such specific products as medications, oxygen, and total parenteral nutrition. Tailor instructions to specific product and patient's capability for learning self-care. *This enables patient and family members to identify and alter environmental or lifestyle factors to achieve optimum health level.*

Evaluations for expected outcomes

• Patient doesn't report or exhibit signs or symptoms related to exposure to or ingestion of dangerous products.

• Patient requests information on self-protection from dangerous products.

• Patient and family members state method for safekeeping of potentially dangerous products.

Documentation

• Patient's statements about situation that indicate potential for injury

• Physical findings

• Record of falls, seizures, and unsafe practices

• Interventions that reduce risk of injury

• Patient's response to nursing interventions

• Evaluations for expected outcomes

■ Posttrauma syndrome

related to accidental injury

Definition

Sustained painful response to an unexpected life event

Assessment

• History and circumstances of accident

• Physical injuries sustained, including cardiopulmonary, musculoskeletal, genitourinary, and integumentary

• Neurologic status

• Emotional reactions, including grief reaction, self-concept, and sleep pattern

• Cognitive reactions, including concentration, memory, and orientation

• Behavioral reactions, including available support systems, clergy, coping patterns, family members, problem-solving ability, and social interactions

Defining characteristics

• Aggression, anxiety, anger, rage

• Avoidance, alienation, altered moods

• Compulsive behavior

• Denial, grief, fear, depression

• Detachment

• Exaggerated startle response, flashbacks
• Guilt
• Headaches
• Hypervigilance
• Intrusive dreams, nightmares, or thoughts; difficulty in concentrating
• Irritability
• Numbness
• Panic attacks
• Psychogenic amnesia
• Repression
• Shame
• Substance abuse

Associated medical diagnoses (selected)
This nursing diagnosis can occur in any patient seriously injured by sudden, unexpected trauma, such as a gunshot wound, motor vehicle accident, airplane crash, train derailment, and fall. Examples of medical diagnoses include head injury, neuromuscular trauma, posttraumatic stress disorder, and spinal cord injury.

Expected outcomes
• Patient will recover or be rehabilitated from physical injuries to extent possible.
• Patient will state feelings and fears related to traumatic event.
• Patient will express feelings of safety.
• Patient will use available support systems.
• Patient will use effective coping mechanisms to reduce fear.
• Patient will maintain or reestablish adaptive social interactions with family members.

Interventions and rationales
• Follow medical regimen to manage physical injuries. *Attention to physical needs remains primary, according to Maslow's hierarchy.*
• Provide emotional support:

– Visit patient frequently *to reduce fear of being alone.*
– Be available to listen *to respond empathetically to patient's feelings.*
– Accept and encourage statement of patient's feelings *to reassure patient that feelings are appropriate and valid.*
– Assure patient of safety, and take measures needed to ensure it. *Frequent nightmares or flashbacks may cause patient to question safety of environment.*
– Avoid care-related activities or environmental stimuli that may intensify symptoms associated with trauma (loud noises, bright lights, abrupt entrances to patient's room, or painful procedures or treatment). *Environmental stimuli can easily intensify flashbacks to traumatic event.*
– Reorient patient to surroundings and reality as frequently as necessary. *Posttrauma psychic numbing impairs orientation, memory, and reality perception.*
– Instruct patient in at least one fear-reducing behavior such as seeking support from others when frightened. *As patient learns to reduce fears, coping skills will increase.*
• Support patient's family members:
– Provide time for them to express feelings.
– Help them understand patient's reactions.
This reduces their anxiety and gives them chance to help patient.
• Offer referrals to other support persons or groups, including clergy, mental health professionals, and trauma support groups. *Referrals help patient to regain sense of universality, reduce isolation, share fears, and deal constructively with feelings.*
• Recognize that patient's culture may affect his response to trauma; remain supportive and nonjudgmental *to*

show patient that you support and accept his response to trauma.

Evaluations for expected outcomes
• Patient resumes usual activities of daily living to extent possible.
• Patient expresses feelings associated with traumatic event.
• Patient expresses feeling of safety.
• Patient interacts with supportive people to alleviate distress.
• Patient demonstrates use of at least one fear-reducing behavior (specify).
• Patient interacts with family members in beneficial manner.

Documentation
• Patient's perception of traumatic event
• Observations of patient's behavior
• Observations of patient's social interaction with others
• Interventions
• Patient's responses to nursing interventions
• Referrals to other support persons or groups
• Evaluations for expected outcomes

■ Posttrauma syndrome, risk for

Definition
Potential for feelings of fear, helplessness, or horror related to an overwhelming, unexpected event outside the usual range of one's experience, such as experiencing a serious life-threatening injury or witnessing the injury or death of a loved one

Assessment
• Age and sex
• History of traumatic event, including circumstances, losses incurred (financial, property, physical integrity, close relationships), effect of trauma on social interactions, and grief reaction
• Health history, including previous traumatic events, patient's characteristic perception of such events and coping responses, and alcohol or substance abuse
• Mental status, including cognitive and emotional function, problems with concentration, memory, orientation, mood, and behavior
• Changes in appetite, self-image, sleep pattern, or sexual drive
• Available sources of support, including friends, family, caregivers, and community resources

Risk factors
• Demoralization and isolation following a traumatic event
• Emotional constriction or numbness (resulting from need to avoid feelings, thoughts, and situations reminding one of a trauma)
• Feelings of guilt, shame, or anger following a traumatic event
• Recent exposure to something that symbolizes a traumatic event, such as gunfire, certain smells, and an anniversary
• Sudden unexpected event outside the usual range of the patient's experience, in which the patient believes he or a loved one may not survive

Associated medical diagnoses (selected)
Generalized anxiety disorder, major depression, panic disorder, posttraumatic stress disorder, substance abuse

Expected outcomes
• Patient won't develop chronic posttrauma response, substance abuse, or other mental health disorders.
• Patient will express understanding of posttrauma response.

• Patient's response to trauma won't be characterized by avoidance, numbness, or intrusiveness.
• Patient will express feelings of safety.
• Patient will employ effective coping skills and will reach out to appropriate sources of support to reduce fear.

Interventions and rationales

• Follow medical regimen *to treat any medical problems associated with the traumatic event.*
• Assess baseline mental status and monitor changes in cognitive and psychosocial function *to detect the need for intervention as soon as possible.*
• Listen actively to patient's statements about the traumatic event *to encourage a trusting relationship and open discussion.*
• Communicate to patient that you accept his fears and feelings related to traumatic event *to reassure patient that his feelings are appropriate and valid.*
• Reassure patient that he's in a safe environment. *Patient may be reluctant to express lingering fears and require reassurance.*
• Avoid nursing care or environmental stimuli that may worsen or initiate symptoms (such as loud noise, bright lights, and painful procedures) *to avoid triggering flashbacks to the traumatic event.* Also, warn patient to avoid disruptive stimuli.
• Caution patient before you touch him and avoid approaching him from behind *to avoid actions that may be misinterpreted and trigger reexperience of the traumatic event.*
• Explore with patient strategies to reduce the traumatic response, such as having a support person call the patient on a regular basis and using stress-reducing techniques when experiencing increased fear and anxiety,

to strengthen coping skills and foster a sense of control.
• Teach patient that a posttrauma response may occur immediately or days, weeks, or years after a trauma *to alert him to the risk of posttrauma response.*
• Help patient to increase his awareness of people, places, and events that trigger or reduce a posttrauma response *to encourage him to take an active role in treatment.*
• Provide opportunities for patient to discuss the trauma periodically, based on the patient's needs and his willingness to talk *to prevent the development of posttrauma response.*
• Encourage family members and friends to express their perceptions and feelings about the traumatic event and reactions they see in the patient *to aid assessment.*
• Provide teaching to family members, friends, and caregivers about the signs and symptoms of posttrauma response and interventions they can use *to promote involvement with rather than withdrawal from the patient.*
• Explore uses of appropriate community resources and make referrals according to the patient's and family members' needs *to ensure continuity of care and decrease patient's isolation.*

Evaluation of expected outcomes

• Patient doesn't develop chronic posttrauma response, substance abuse, or other mental health disorders.
• Patient expresses understanding of posttrauma response.
• Patient's response to trauma isn't characterized by avoidance, numbness, or intrusiveness.
• Patient expresses feelings of safety.

• Patient employs effective coping skills and reaches out to appropriate sources of support to reduce fear.

Documentation
• Patient's perception of the traumatic event
• Observation of the patient's behavior, coping skills, and use of support systems
• Patient's response to nursing care activities
• Patient's communication patterns with friends, family, and others and their responses
• Teaching provided to the patient and family
• Referrals for ongoing support
• Evaluations for expected outcomes

■ Powerlessness

related to chronic illness

Definition
Perceived loss of control over what happens to oneself and one's environment

Assessment
• Nature of medical diagnosis
• Mobility
• Behavioral responses (verbal and nonverbal), including calmness or agitation, anger, anxiety, depression, independence or dependence, interest or apathy, and satisfaction or dissatisfaction
• Coping strategies, including passage through grieving process
• Past experiences with illness
• Knowledge, including current understanding of physical condition and physical, mental, and emotional readiness to learn

• Environment, including equipment and supplies, health care professionals and personnel, lighting, location of patient's personal belongings, noise, privacy, and space
• Number and types of stressors
• Social factors
• Spiritual beliefs and value system

Defining characteristics
• Apathy
• Depression over physical deterioration
• Failure to monitor progress
• Failure to seek information about care
• Irritability because of dependence on others
• Passivity
• Resentment, anger, and guilt
• Reluctance to express true feelings because of fear of alienating caregivers
• Reluctance to participate in decisions about health
• Uncertainty about fluctuating energy levels
• Expressed dissatisfaction over inability to perform previous tasks
• Expressed self-doubt
• Expressed lack of control over self-care, current situation, and outcome

Associated medical diagnoses (selected)
Acquired immunodeficiency syndrome, blindness, chronic renal failure, diabetes mellitus, genital herpes, lung cancer, panic disorder, Parkinson's disease, pemphigus, psoriasis, spinal cord injury

Expected outcomes
• Patient will acknowledge fears, feelings, and concerns about current situation.
• Patient will make decisions regarding course of treatment.

• Patient will decrease level of anxiety by changing response to stressors.
• Patient will participate in self-care activities (specify).
• Patient will express feeling of regained control.
• Patient will accept and adapt to lifestyle changes.

Interventions and rationales

• Encourage patient to express feelings and concerns. Set aside time for discussions with patient about daily events. *This helps patient bring vaguely understood emotions into focus.*
• Accept patient's feelings of powerlessness as normal. *This indicates respect for patient and enhances patient's feelings of self-worth.*
• Try to be present during situations where feelings of powerlessness are likely to be greatest *to help patient cope.*
• Identify and develop patient's coping mechanisms, strengths, and resources for support. *By making use of coping skills, patient can reduce anxiety and fears and successfully undergo grieving necessary to come to terms with chronic illness.*
• Discuss situations that provoke feelings of anger, anxiety, and powerlessness *to identify areas patient can control and to prevent anger from being inappropriately directed at self or others.*
• Encourage participation in self-care. Provide positive reinforcement for patient's activities. Encourage patient to take active role as member of health care team. *This enhances patient's sense of control and reduces passive and dependent behavior.*
• Provide as many opportunities as possible for patient to make decisions about self-care (for instance, positioning, choosing an injection site, and visiting) *to communicate respect for patient and enhance feelings of independence.*
• Help patient learn as much as possible about health condition, treatment, and prognosis *to help patient feel in control.*
• Modify environment when possible to meet patient's self-care needs *to promote patient's sense of control over environment.*
• Decrease unpredictable events by discussing rules, policies, procedures, and schedules with patient. *Fear of unknown interferes with patient's ability to cope.*
• Encourage family members to support patient without taking control *to increase patient's feelings of self-worth.*
• Reinforce patient's rights as stated in Patient's Bill of Rights *to protect patient's right to make decisions about health care treatment.*
• Identify and arrange to accommodate patient's spiritual needs. *Spirituality enables patient to gain courage and resist despair.*
• Respect and show your acceptance of patient's cultural beliefs about health. *The belief that each patient has the personal authority and responsibility to try to reach optimal well-being is a Western value not shared by all cultures.*

Evaluations for expected outcomes

• Patient verbalizes positive and negative feelings about current situation.
• Patient demonstrates increased control by participating in decisions related to health care.
• Patient describes strategies for decreasing anxiety.
• Patient actively participates in planning and executing aspects of care.

• Patient communicates renewed sense of power and control of current situation.
• Patient demonstrates ability to adapt to and accept lifestyle changes.

Documentation
• Observations and interactions related to disease process and health care environment
• Patient's responses to opportunities to participate in own care
• Patient's feelings about chronic illness and situations that can't be changed
• Teaching and counseling to enhance patient's decision-making ability
• Interventions to help patient gain sense of control
• Patient's response to nursing interventions
• Evaluations for expected outcomes

■ Powerlessness

related to health care environment

Definition
Perceived loss of control over what happens to oneself and one's environment

Assessment
• Nature of the medical diagnosis
• Mobility
• Behavioral responses (verbal and nonverbal), including calmness or agitation, anger, independence or dependence, interest or apathy, and satisfaction or dissatisfaction
• Usual coping strategies
• Past experiences with hospitalization
• Knowledge, including current understanding of physical condition and physical, mental, and emotional readiness to learn
• Environment, including equipment and supplies, health care professionals and personnel, lighting, location of patient's personal belongings, noise, privacy, and space

Defining characteristics
• Apathy
• Depression over physical deterioration
• Failure to defend self-care practices
• Failure to monitor progress
• Failure to seek information about care
• Irritability because of dependence on others
• Passivity
• Resentment, anger, and guilt
• Reluctance to express true feelings because of fear of alienating caregivers
• Reluctance to participate in decisions about health
• Uncertainty about fluctuating energy levels
• Expressed dissatisfaction over inability to perform previous tasks
• Expressed self-doubt
• Expressed lack of control over self-care, current situation, and outcome

Associated medical diagnoses (selected)
This diagnosis is best identified by considering problems that restrict or confine patients rather than by medical diagnosis. Examples include blindness, confinement to an intensive care or cardiac care unit, isolation, language barrier, multiple I.V. lines, multisystem trauma, paralysis, restrictions caused by dependence on ventilators, and traction.

Expected outcomes

• Patient will identify feelings of powerlessness associated with the environment.
• Patient will describe modifications or adjustments to the environment that allow feelings of control.
• Patient will participate in self-care activities (specify).
• Patient will state feelings of regained control.

Interventions and rationales

• Visit with patient 15 minutes each shift *to allow patient to express concerns and feelings.*
• Acknowledge importance of patient's space:
– Verbally delineate patient's space.
– Orient patient to space.
– If patient is immobilized, ask for instructions regarding placement of personal belongings.
– If possible, allow patient to walk around the space and arrange personal belongings.
These measures enhance patient's potential for regaining sense of power.
• Place call light, television controls, bedside table, telephone, urinal, and other items within easy reach. Improvise wherever possible to give patient control over use of these objects. Attend to patient's ability or inability to use hands and arms. *These measures help reduce patient's frustration over inability to reach items in immediate area.*
• Reduce irritating noises, if possible, and explain reasons for alarms and other disturbances. *Excessive sensory stimuli can cause disorientation, hallucinations, and delusional thinking.*
• Explain all treatments and procedures and encourage patient to participate in planning care. Provide choices for when and how activities will occur (such as bathing, eating, and

getting out of bed). *This increases patient's feeling of powerfulness and reduces passivity and dependence on caregiver.*
• Provide as many situations as possible where patient can take control (such as positioning, choosing an injection site, and visiting) *to help reduce potential for maladaptive coping behaviors.*
• Encourage participation in self-care. Provide positive reinforcement for patient's activities *to encourage increasing participation in self-care in the future.*
• Help patient learn as much about current health problem as possible. *The greater his understanding, the more patient will feel in control.*

Evaluations for expected outcomes

• Patient expresses feelings of lack of control.
• Patient's environment is adjusted to enhance his feelings of control.
• Patient performs self-care measures to extent possible.
• Patient expresses feelings of regained control.

Documentation

• Patient's expressions of anger, frustration, and sense of lack of control over environment
• Patient's interest in surroundings, participation in self-care, verbalization of understanding, and demonstration of skill in relation to medical diagnosis
• Interventions to promote patent's control over environment
• Patient's response to nursing interventions
• Evaluations for expected outcomes

■ Powerlessness

related to illness-related regimen

Definition

Perceived loss of control over what happens to oneself and one's environment

Assessment

- Nature of medical diagnosis
- Mobility
- Behavioral responses (verbal and nonverbal), including calmness or agitation, anger, independence or dependence, interest or apathy, and satisfaction or dissatisfaction
- Past experiences with hospitalization
- Environment, including equipment and supplies, health care professionals and personnel, lighting, location of patient's personal belongings, noise, privacy, and space
- Knowledge, including current understanding of physical condition and physical, mental, and emotional readiness to learn

Defining characteristics

- Apathy
- Depression over physical deterioration
- Failure to monitor progress
- Failure to seek information about care
- Irritability because of dependence on others
- Passivity
- Resentment, anger, and guilt
- Reluctance to express true feelings because of fear of alienating caregivers
- Reluctance to participate in decisions about health
- Uncertainty about fluctuating energy levels

- Expressed dissatisfaction over inability to perform previous tasks
- Expressed self-doubt
- Expressed lack of control over self-care, current situation, and outcome

Associated medical diagnoses (selected)

Alcohol addiction, burns, heart failure, hypertension, maternal psychological stress, melanoma, osteoporosis, paralysis

Expected outcomes

- Patient will acknowledge feelings of powerlessness over regimen.
- Patient will participate in planning care.
- Patient will participate in self-care activities (specify).
- Patient will enumerate factors in illness-related regimen that he can control.
- Patient will demonstrate ability to plan for controllable factors.
- Patient will communicate sense of having regained control.

Interventions and rationales

- Encourage patient to express feelings about present situation. *This helps patient bring vaguely expressed emotions into clear awareness and acceptance.*
- Accept patient's feelings of powerlessness as normal. *This indicates respect for patient and enhances patient's feelings of self-worth.*
- Allow patient to make decisions about care (such as positioning and times for ambulation). *This helps patient maintain sense of control and reduces potential for maladaptive coping behaviors.*
- Encourage participation in self-care. Provide positive reinforcement for patient's activities. *This enhances patient's sense of control and reduces passive and dependent behavior.*

• Begin teaching patient how to regain and maintain optimal health. *In this teaching relationship, nurse presents information to patient on need-to-know basis.*
• Help identify specific areas where patient can maintain control *to reduce patient's feelings of helplessness.*
• Have patient demonstrate ways to consciously maintain some degree of control. *Repetitive demonstrations of skills and behaviors enhance learning.*
• Help patient learn as much as possible about present health problem. *The greater his understanding, the more patient will feel in control.*
• Respect and show your acceptance of patient's cultural beliefs about health. *The belief that each patient has the personal authority and responsibility to try to reach optimal well-being is a Western value not shared by all cultures.*

Evaluations for expected outcomes
• Patient expresses feelings of lack of control over health care regimen.
• Patient specifies preferences for care.
• Patient performs specified daily self-care measures.
• Patient identifies specific factors in illness-related regimen that he can control and plans appropriate action.
• Patient demonstrates ability to plan for controllable factors.
• Patient expresses feelings of regained control.

Documentation
• Patient's expressions of powerlessness
• Patient's behaviors that show evidence of feeling of powerlessness
• Interventions performed to help patient regain sense of control

• Patient's degree of participation in planning care
• Evaluations for expected outcomes

■ Relocation stress syndrome

related to inadequate preparation for admission, transfer, or discharge

Definition
Physiologic or psychosocial disturbances caused by change in health care environment

Assessment
• Reason for transfer or relocation
• Past experiences with relocation
• Nature of relocation
• Physical and mental status of patient, including health condition, cognitive functioning, and functional abilities
• Financial resources
• Support systems, including family, friends, and health care workers
• Resources available to help prepare for relocation
• Conditions in original environment versus conditions in new environment
• Coping and problem-solving abilities, including educational level, past experiences with relocation, and participation in recreational activities or hobbies

Defining characteristics
• Anxiety
• Apprehension
• Change in eating habits
• Change in environment
• Dependency
• Depression
• Expressed concern or anxiety about transfer

- Expressed unwillingness to relocate
- GI disturbances
- Increased confusion
- Increased expression of needs
- Insecurity
- Lack of trust
- Loneliness
- Restlessness
- Sad affect
- Sleep disturbance
- Unfavorable comparison of original and new staff or environment
- Vigilance
- Weight change
- Withdrawal

Associated medical diagnoses (selected)
Any change in physical, functional, or cognitive status that also requires a change in patient's environment, such as admission to hospital, transfer from one unit or institution to another, and discharge.

Expected outcomes
- Patient will request information about new environment.
- Patient will communicate understanding of relocation.
- Patient and family members will take steps to prepare for relocation.
- Patient will use available resources.
- Patient will express satisfaction with adjustment to new environment.

Interventions and rationales
- Assign primary nurse to patient *to provide consistent, caring, and accepting environment that enhances patient's adjustment and well-being.*
- Help patient and family members prepare for relocation. Conduct group discussions, provide pictures of new setting, and communicate any additional information that will ease transition *to help patient cope with new environment.*

- If possible, allow patient and family members to visit new location and provide introductions to new staff. *The more familiar the environment, the less stress patient will experience during relocation.*
- Assess patient's needs for additional health care services before relocation *to ensure that patient receives appropriate care in new environment.*
- Communicate all aspects of patient's discharge plan to appropriate staff members at new location *to ensure continuity of care.*
- Educate family members about relocation stress syndrome and its potential effects *to encourage family members to provide needed emotional support throughout transition period.*
- Encourage patient to express emotions associated with relocation *to provide opportunity to correct misconceptions, answer questions, and reduce anxiety.*
- Reassure patient that family members and friends know his new location and will continue to visit *to reduce feelings of abandonment and anxiety.*

Evaluations for expected outcomes
- Patient requests information about new environment.
- Patient expresses understanding of relocation process.
- Patient and family members complete preparations for relocation.
- Patient makes use of available resources to smooth transition to new environment.
- Patient expresses feelings associated with adjustment to new environment.

Documentation
- Evidence of patient's emotional distress over relocation
- Patient's needs in preparing for relocation

• Available resources and support systems
• Intervention to prepare patient and family members for relocation and patient's and family members' responses
• Discharge plan instructions communicated to new staff
• Evaluations for expected outcomes

■ Role performance alteration

related to ineffective coping

Definition
Disruption in the ability to perform usual social, vocational, or family roles

Assessment
• Health history, including medical diagnosis, course and severity of illness, and reason for hospitalization
• Patient's perception of illness and its effect on social, cultural, and vocational roles
• Psychosocial status, including current stressors, support systems, hobbies, interests, work history, educational background, and changes in role function
• Family status, including roles of family members, effect of illness on patient's family, and family's understanding of patient's illness

Defining characteristics
• Ambivalence, denial, or confusion about role or responsibility
• Anxiety, depression, dissatisfaction, pessimism, or uncertainty
• Change in perception of role (by self and others)
• Change in capacity to resume role
• Change in usual responsibilities

• Conflict among vocational, family, cultural, and social roles
• Discrimination
• Domestic violence or harassment
• Inadequate adaptation to change or transition
• Inadequate self-management, motivation, confidence, competence, or coping skills for fulfilling role
• Inappropriate developmental expectations
• Lack of external support for enacting role
• Lack of opportunities for enacting role
• Lack of knowledge about roles and responsibilities
• Powerlessness
• Role overload or strain

Associated medical diagnoses (selected)
This diagnosis may be associated with any illness that results in long-term disability or incapacitation. Examples include affective disorders, Alzheimer's disease, angina pectoris, blindness, bursitis, coronary artery disease, deafness, diabetes mellitus, fractures, heart failure, myocardial infarction, paralysis, schizophrenia, and tendinitis.

Expected outcomes
• Patient will express feelings about diminished ability to perform usual roles.
• Patient and family members will recognize and state feelings about limitations imposed by illness.
• Patient will make decisions about course of treatment and management of illness.
• Patient will continue to function in usual roles as much as possible.
• Patient will express feeling of making productive contribution to self-care, to others, or to environment.

Interventions and rationales

• If possible, assign same nurse to patient each shift *to establish rapport and foster development of therapeutic relationship.*

• Spend ample time with patient each shift *to foster sense of safety and decrease loneliness.*

• Provide opportunities for patient to express thoughts and feelings *to help patient identify how altered role performance has affected his life.*

• Convey belief in patient's ability to develop necessary coping skills. *By projecting positive attitude, you can help patient gain confidence.*

• Be aware of patient's emotional vulnerability, and allow open expression of all emotions. *An accepting attitude will help patient deal with effects of chronic illness and loss of functioning.*

• Provide opportunities for patient to make decisions, and encourage patient to maintain personal responsibilities. *Showing respect for patient's decision-making ability enhances feelings of independence.*

• Encourage patient to participate in self-care activities, keeping in mind physical and emotional limitations. *Involvement in self-care promotes optimal functioning.*

• Assess patient's knowledge of illness, and educate patient about condition, treatment, and prognosis. *Education helps patient cope with effects of illness more effectively.*

• Encourage patient to recognize personal strengths and to use them. *This will help maintain optimal functioning and foster healthier self-image.*

• Encourage patient to continue to fulfill life roles within constraints posed by illness. *This will help patient maintain sense of purpose and preserve connections with other people.*

• Encourage patient to participate in care as active member of health care team. *This will help establish mutually accepted goals between patient and caregivers. Patient who participates in care is more likely to take active role in other aspects of life.*

• Help family members identify feelings about patient's decreased role functioning. Encourage participation in support group. *Relatives of patient may need social support, information, and an outlet for ventilating feelings.*

• Offer patient and family members realistic assessment of patient's illness, and communicate hope for immediate future. *Education helps promote patient safety and security and helps family members plan for future health care requirements.*

• Educate patient and family members about managing illness, controlling environmental factors that affect patient's health, and redefining roles to promote optimal functioning. *Through education, family members may become resources in patient's care.*

Evaluations for expected outcomes

• Patient shares feelings about illness and altered role performance in constructive manner.

• Patient and family members understand role changes that are occurring because of chronic illness and express their feelings about these limitations.

• Patient demonstrates increased functioning by making decisions about health care and participating in planning and implementing aspects of personal care.

• Patient demonstrates ability to perceive options and uses options to function in usual roles as much as possible.

• Patient expresses feeling of having made productive contribution to self-care, to others, or to the environment.

Documentation
• Observations of patient's physical, emotional, and mental status
• Patient's thoughts and feelings about illness and diminished role capacity
• Nursing interventions performed to help patient understand change in role functioning
• Patient's response to nursing interventions
• All health teaching, counseling, and precautions taken to maintain or enhance patient's level of functioning
• Referrals to sources of support for patient and family members
• Evaluations for expected outcomes

■ Self-care deficit: Bathing and hygiene

related to musculoskeletal impairment

Definition
Inability to carry out activities associated with bathing and hygiene

Assessment
• History of injury or disease associated with musculoskeletal impairment
• Self-care abilities, including knowledge and use of adaptive equipment, preparation of equipment and supplies, and technical or mechanical skills
• Musculoskeletal status, including coordination; functional ability; gait; mechanical restriction (such as cast, splint, and traction); muscle tone, size, and strength; range of motion; and tremors

• Psychosocial status, including coping mechanisms, family members, lifestyle, patient's perceptions of health problem and self, and personality

Defining characteristics
• Inability to dry body
• Inability to get into and out of bathroom
• Inability to obtain bath supplies
• Inability to obtain or get to water source
• Inability to regulate water temperature or flow
• Inability to wash body or body parts

Associated medical diagnoses (selected)
Acute renal failure, adult respiratory distress syndrome, amyotrophic lateral sclerosis, asthma, atelectasis, cerebrovascular accident, chronic obstructive pulmonary disease, chronic renal failure, craniotomy, empyema, fractures, glomerulonephritis, gout, Guillain-Barré syndrome, head injury, meningitis, multiple sclerosis, multisystem trauma, muscular dystrophy, myasthenia gravis (crisis), osteoarthritis, Parkinson's disease, pneumonia, pulmonary edema, spinal cord injury or tumor

Expected outcomes
• Patient will have his self-care needs met.
• Patient will have few if any complications.
• Patient will communicate feelings about limitations.
• Patient and family members will demonstrate correct use of assistive devices.
• Patient and family members will carry out bathing and hygiene program daily.

Interventions and rationales

• Observe patient's functional level every shift; document and report any changes. *Careful observation helps you adjust nursing actions to meet patient's needs.*

• Perform prescribed treatment for underlying musculoskeletal impairment. Monitor progress, reporting favorable and adverse responses to treatment. *Applying therapy consistently aids patient's independence.*

• Encourage patient to voice feelings and concerns about self-care deficits *to help patient achieve highest functional level possible.*

• Monitor completion of bathing and hygiene daily. Praise accomplishments. *Reinforcement and rewards may encourage renewed effort.*

• Provide assistive devices, such as long-handled toothbrush, for bathing and hygiene; instruct on use. *Appropriate assistive devices encourage independence.*

• Assist with or perform bathing and hygiene daily. Assist only when patient has difficulty *to promote feeling of independence.*

• Instruct patient and family members in bathing and hygiene techniques (you can give family members written instructions). Have patient and family members demonstrate bathing and hygiene under supervision. *Return demonstration identifies problem areas and increases patients' and family members' self-confidence.*

• As needed, refer patient to psychiatric liaison nurse, support group, or home health care agency. *These extra resources will reinforce activities planned to meet patient's needs.*

Evaluations for expected outcomes

• Patient meets self-care needs with help of staff.

• Patient participates in activities that minimize risk of such complications as infection and skin integrity alteration.

• Patient expresses feelings about self-care deficit. If unable to meet own needs, patient seeks assistance from family member or staff within 24 hours.

• Patient or family members demonstrate appropriate use of assistive devices.

• Patient follows daily self-care plans. Family members assist as needed.

Documentation

• Patient's expression of feelings and concerns about self-care limitations and their impact on body image and lifestyle

• Patient's willingness to participate in bathing and hygiene routine

• Observations of patient's impaired ability to perform self-care

• Patient's response to treatment for underlying condition

• Interventions to provide supportive care

• Patient's response to nursing interventions

• Instructions to patient and family members and their understanding of instructions and demonstrated skill in carrying out self-care functions

• Evaluations for expected outcomes

■ Self-care deficit: Bathing and hygiene

related to perceptual or cognitive impairment

Definition

Inability to carry out activities associated with bathing and hygiene

Assessment
• History of neurologic, sensory, or psychological impairment
• Age
• Self-care abilities, including knowledge and use of adaptive equipment, preparation of equipment and supplies, and technical and mechanical skills
• Neurologic status, including cognition, communication ability, insight or judgment, level of consciousness, memory, motor ability, orientation, and sensory ability
• Psychosocial status, including coping mechanisms, family members, lifestyle, patient's perceptions of self, and personality

Defining characteristics
• Inability to dry body
• Inability to get into and out of bathroom
• Inability to obtain bath supplies
• Inability to obtain or get to water source
• Inability to regulate water temperature or flow
• Inability to wash body or body parts

Associated medical diagnoses (selected)
Alcohol addiction, Alzheimer's disease, bipolar disease (manic or depressive phase), Down syndrome, Huntington's disease, schizophrenia

Expected outcomes
• Patient will have his self-care needs met.
• Patient will have few if any complications.
• Patient and family members will carry out self-care program daily.
• Patient and family members will communicate feelings and concerns.
• Patient and family members will identify resources to help cope with problems after discharge.

Interventions and rationales
• Observe, document, and report patient's functional and perceptual or cognitive ability daily. *Careful observation helps you adjust nursing actions to meet patient's needs.*
• Perform prescribed treatment for underlying condition. Monitor progress and report favorable and adverse responses. *Applying therapy consistently aids patient's independence.*
• Allow patient to express frustration, anger, or feelings of inadequacy. Provide emotional support *to help patient achieve highest functional level.*
• Provide privacy *to enhance patient's self-esteem.*
• Monitor completion of bathing and hygiene daily. Remind patient of what he needs to accomplish. Offer praise. *Reinforcement and rewards may encourage daily activities.*
• Allow ample time for patient to perform bathing and hygiene. *Rushing creates unnecessary stress and promotes failure.*
• Direct patient in bathing and hygiene measures, giving simple instructions one at a time, *to aid comprehension.*
• Assist with bathing and hygiene daily only when patient has difficulty *to encourage independence and self-reliance.*
• Give written instructions to family members in bathing and hygiene techniques and supervise return demonstration. *Return demonstration identifies problem areas and increases family members' self-confidence.*
• Discuss normal aspects of bathing. Reassure patient with such statements as "You're in the tub" and "The water is only 3 inches deep" *to guard against panic reaction caused by fear of being drowned.*

• Refer patient to psychiatric liaison nurse, support group, or home health care agency, as needed. *These extra resources will reinforce activities planned to meet patient's needs.*

Evaluations for expected outcomes
• Patient meets self-care needs with help of staff.
• Patient doesn't experience infection, skin integrity alteration, or other complications of altered self-care.
• Patient and family members become more active in carrying out self-care program; need for staff assistance decreases.
• Patient and family members express feelings about patient's self-care deficit. If unable to meet own needs, patient seeks help from family members or staff within 24 hours.
• Patient and family members identify and contact support resources as needed.

Documentation
• Patient's and family members' expression of feelings and concern about self-care deficits
• Observations of patient's impaired ability to perform bathing and hygiene
• Patient's response to treatment for underlying condition
• Interventions to provide supportive care
• Instructions to patient (if capable) and family members, their understanding of instructions, and their demonstrated skill in carrying out self-care functions
• Patient's response to nursing interventions
• Evaluations for expected outcomes

■ Self-care deficit: Dressing and grooming

related to musculoskeletal impairment

Definition
Inability to perform activities associated with dressing and grooming

Assessment
• History of injury or disease associated with musculoskeletal impairment
• Self-care abilities, including knowledge and use of adaptive equipment, preparation of equipment and supplies, and technical or mechanical skills
• Musculoskeletal status, including coordination; functional ability; gait; mechanical restriction (such as cast, splint, and traction); muscle tone, size, and strength; range of motion; and tremors
• Psychosocial status, including coping mechanisms, family members, lifestyle, patient's perceptions of health problem and self, and personality

Defining characteristics
• Impaired ability to clothe part or all of body
• Impaired ability to fasten clothing (such as inability to use zippers)
• Impaired ability to obtain or replace items of clothing
• Impaired ability to put on or take off specific articles of clothing (such as socks and shoes)
• Inability to choose clothing
• Inability to maintain appearance at satisfactory level
• Inability to pick up clothing
• Inability to use assistive devices

Associated medical diagnoses (selected)
Acute renal failure, adult respiratory
distress syndrome, amyotrophic lateral sclerosis, asthma, atelectasis, cerebrovascular accident, chronic obstructive pulmonary disease, chronic renal
failure, empyema, fractures, glomerulonephritis, gout, Guillain-Barré syndrome, head injury, meningitis, multiple sclerosis, multisystem trauma,
muscular dystrophy, myasthenia
gravis (crisis), osteoarthritis, Parkinson's disease, pneumonia, pulmonary
edema, spinal cord injury or tumor

Expected outcomes
• Patient will have his self-care needs
met.
• Patient will have few if any complications.
• Patient will communicate feelings
about limitations.
• Patient and family members will
demonstrate correct use of assistive
devices.
• Patient and family members will
carry out dressing and grooming program daily.

Interventions and rationales
• Observe patient's functional level
every shift; document and report any
changes. *Careful observation helps
you adjust nursing actions to meet
patient's needs.*
• Perform prescribed treatment for
underlying musculoskeletal impairment. Monitor progress, reporting favorable and adverse responses to
treatment. *Applying therapy consistently aids patient's independence.*
• Encourage patient to voice feelings
and concerns about self-care deficits
to help patient achieve highest functional level.
• Provide enough time for patient to
perform dressing and grooming.

*Rushing creates unnecessary stress
and promotes failure.*
• Monitor patient's abilities to dress
and groom daily. *This identifies problem areas before they become sources
of frustration.*
• Encourage family members to provide clothing patient can easily manage. Patient may benefit from clothing slightly larger than regular size
and Velcro straps. *Such clothing
makes independent dressing easier.*
• Provide necessary assistive devices,
such as long-handled shoehorn and
zipper pull, as needed. Instruct on
use. *Appropriate assistive devices encourage independence.*
• Assist with or perform dressing and
grooming: fasten clothes, comb hair,
and clean nails. Provide help only
when patient has difficulty *to promote
feeling of independence.*
• Instruct patient and family members
in dressing and grooming techniques
(you can give family members written
instructions). Have patient and family
members demonstrate dressing and
grooming techniques under supervision. *Return demonstration reveals
problem areas and increases self-confidence.*
• As needed, refer patient to psychiatric liaison nurse, support group, or
home health care agency. *Extra resources reinforce activities planned to
meet patient's needs.*

Evaluations for expected outcomes
• Patient meets self-care needs with
help of staff.
• Patient participates in activities designed to minimize risk of complications, such as complying with treatment.
• Patient expresses feelings about
self-care limitations.

• Patient and family members demonstrate appropriate use of assistive devices.
• Patient follows daily self-care plans. Family members assist as needed.

Documentation
• Patient's expression of feelings and concerns about self-care limitations and their impact on body image and lifestyle
• Patient's willingness to participate in dressing and grooming
• Observations of patient's impaired ability to perform dressing and grooming
• Interventions to provide supportive care
• Patient's response to nursing interventions
• Instructions given to patient and family members, their understanding of instructions, and their demonstrated skill in carrying out self-care functions
• Evaluations for expected outcomes

■ Self-care deficit: Dressing and grooming

related to perceptual or cognitive impairment

Definition
Inability to carry out activities associated with dressing and grooming

Assessment
• History of neurologic, sensory, or psychological impairment
• Age
• Self-care abilities, including knowledge and use of adaptive equipment, preparation of equipment and supplies, and technical and mechanical skills

• Neurologic status, including cognition, communication ability, insight or judgment, level of consciousness, memory, motor ability, orientation, and sensory ability
• Psychosocial status, including coping mechanisms, family members, lifestyle, patient's perceptions of self, and personality

Defining characteristics
• Impaired ability to clothe part or all of body
• Impaired ability to fasten clothing (such as inability to use zippers)
• Impaired ability to obtain or replace items of clothing
• Impaired ability to put on or take off specific articles of clothing (such as socks and shoes)
• Inability to choose clothing
• Inability to maintain appearance at satisfactory level
• Inability to pick up clothing
• Inability to use assistive devices

Associated medical diagnoses (selected)
Alcohol addiction, Alzheimer's disease, bipolar disease (manic or depressive phase), Down syndrome, Huntington's disease, schizophrenia

Expected outcomes
• Patient will have his self-care needs met.
• Patient will have few if any complications.
• Patient and family members will carry out self-care program daily.
• Patient and family members will communicate feelings and concerns.
• Patient and family members will identify resources to help cope with problems and discharge.

Interventions and rationales
• Observe, document, and report patient's functional and perceptual or

cognitive ability daily. *Careful observation helps you adjust nursing actions to meet patient's needs.*
• Perform prescribed treatment for underlying condition. Monitor progress, and report favorable and adverse responses. *Applying therapy consistently aids patient's independence.*
• Allow patient to express frustration, anger, or feelings of inadequacy. Provide emotional support *to help patient achieve highest functional level.*
• Provide privacy *to enhance patient's self-esteem.*
• Monitor dressing and grooming daily. *This identifies problem areas before they become sources of frustration.*
• Provide assistive devices as needed. *Appropriate assistive devices can encourage independence.*
• Don't rush patient. *Rushing creates unnecessary anxiety and promotes failure.*
• Remind patient of what he needs to accomplish while performing actual task. Praise accomplishments *to foster self-confidence.*
• Assist with dressing and grooming daily: fasten clothes, clean nails, and comb hair. Select clothes and hand garments to patient one at a time in appropriate order. Provide help only when patient has difficulty *to promote feeling of independence.*
• Direct patient in grooming measures, giving simple instructions one at a time, *to aid comprehension.*
• Encourage patient to complete dressing and grooming measures. Provide positive feedback during task performance. *Reinforcement and rewards may encourage effort.*
• Encourage family member to provide clothing patient can easily manage: Patient may benefit from clothing slightly larger than regular size

and Velcro straps. *Such clothing makes independent dressing easier.*
• Give written instructions to family member in dressing and grooming technique, and supervise return demonstration *to identify problem areas and increase family member's self-confidence*
• As needed, refer patient to psychiatric liaison nurse, support group, or home health care agency. *These extra resources will reinforce activities planned to meet patient's needs.*

Evaluations for expected outcomes
• Patient meets self-care needs with help of staff.
• Patient doesn't experience infection, skin integrity alteration, or other complications of altered self-care.
• Patient and family members become more active in carrying out self-care program; need for staff assistance decreases.
• Patient and family members discuss feelings about patient's self-care deficit. If unable to meet own needs, patient seeks help from family member or staff within 24 hours.
• Patient and family members identify and contact available support resources as needed.

Documentation
• Patient's and family members' expression of feelings and concern about self-care deficits
• Observations of patient's impaired ability to perform dressing and grooming activities
• Patient's response to underlying treatment
• Interventions to provide supportive care
• Instructions to patient (if capable) and family members, their understanding of instructions, and their

demonstrated skill in carrying out self-care functions
• Patient's response to nursing interventions
• Evaluations for expected outcomes

■ Self-care deficit: Feeding
related to musculoskeletal impairment

Definition
Inability to carry out the self-care activity of feeding

Assessment
• History of injury or disease associated with musculoskeletal impairment
• Self-care abilities, including knowledge and use of adaptive equipment, preparation of equipment and supplies, and technical and mechanical skills
• Musculoskeletal status, including coordination; functional ability; gait; mechanical restriction (such as cast, splint, and traction); muscle tone, size, and strength; range of motion; and tremors
• Psychosocial status, including coping mechanisms, family members, lifestyle, motivation, patient's perception of health problem and self, and personality

Defining characteristics
Inability to perform one or more of the following:
• prepare food
• open containers
• use assistive devices
• handle utensils
• handle cup or glass
• get food onto utensil
• bring food from receptacle to mouth
• chew food

• swallow food
• ingest food safely and in socially acceptable manner
• ingest sufficient food
• complete meals

Associated medical diagnoses (selected)
Acute renal failure, adult respiratory distress syndrome, amyotrophic lateral sclerosis, atelectasis, cerebrovascular accident, chronic obstructive pulmonary disease, chronic renal failure, craniotomy, empyema, fractures, glomerulonephritis, Guillain-Barré syndrome, head injury, meningitis, multiple sclerosis, multisystem trauma, muscular dystrophy, myasthenia gravis (crisis), osteoarthritis, Parkinson's disease, pneumonia, pulmonary edema, rheumatoid arthritis, spinal cord injury or tumor

Expected outcomes
• Patient will express feelings about feeding limitations.
• Patient will maintain weight at ___ lb.
• Patient will have no evidence of aspiration.
• Patient will consume ___ % of diet.
• Patient and family members will demonstrate correct use of assistive devices.
• Patient and family members will carry out feeding program daily.

Interventions and rationales
• Observe patient's functional level every shift; document and report any changes. *Careful observation helps you adjust nursing actions to meet patient's needs.*
• Perform prescribed treatment for underlying musculoskeletal impairment. Monitor progress and report responses. *Applying therapy consistently aids patient's independence.*

• Weigh patient weekly and record weight. Report change of more than 1 lb/week *to ensure adequate nutrition and fluid balance.*
• Monitor and record breath sounds every 4 hours *to check for aspiration of food.* Report crackles, wheezes, or rhonchi.
• Encourage patient to express feelings and concerns about feeding deficits *to help patient achieve highest functional level.*
• Initiate ordered feeding program:
– Determine types of food best handled by patient *to encourage patient's feelings of independence.*
– Place patient in high Fowler's position to feed *to aid swallowing and digestion.* Support weakened extremities, and wash patient's face and hands before meals.
– Provide assistive devices; instruct patient on use *to allow more independence.*
– Supervise or assist at each meal — for example, cut food into small pieces. *This aids chewing, swallowing, and digestion and reduces risk of choking or aspiration.*
– Feed patient slowly. *Rushing causes stress, reducing digestive activity and causing intestinal spasms.*
– Keep suction equipment at bedside *to remove aspirated foods if necessary.*
– Instruct patient and family members in feeding techniques and equipment. *This aids understanding and encourages compliance.*
– Record percentage of food consumed *to ensure adequate nutrition.*
• Encourage patient to carry out aspects of feeding according to abilities. *This gives patient sense of achievement and control.*
• Refer patient to psychiatric liaison nurse, support group, or such community agencies as Visiting Nurse Association and Meals on Wheels. *Additional resources reinforce activities planned to meet patient's needs.*

Evaluations for expected outcomes
• Patient expresses frustration with feeding limitations.
• Patient obtains adequate fluid and nutritional intake and maintains weight at or above established limit.
• Patient doesn't experience aspiration.
• Patient consumes established percentage of diet.
• Patient adapts to use of assistive devices. Family members can explain use of assistive devices.
• Patient follows self-care feeding program daily. Family members provide assistance as needed.

Documentation
• Patient's expression of feelings and concerns about inability to feed self
• Observations of patient's impaired ability to perform self-care
• Patient's response to treatment
• Patient's weight
• Patient's intake
• Interventions to provide supportive care
• Instructions given to patient and family members, their understanding of instructions, and their demonstrated skill in carrying out self-care functions
• Patient's response to interventions
• Evaluations for expected outcomes

■ Self-care deficit: Feeding
related to perceptual or cognitive impairment

Definition
Inability to feed self

Assessment
• History of neurologic, sensory, or psychological impairment
• Age
• Self-care abilities, including knowledge and use of adaptive equipment, preparation of equipment and supplies, and technical and mechanical skills
• Neurologic status, including cognition, communication ability, insight or judgment, level of consciousness, memory, motor ability, orientation, and sensory ability
• Psychosocial status, including coping mechanisms, family members, lifestyle, patient's perceptions of self, and personality

Defining characteristics
Inability to perform one or more of the following:
• prepare food
• open containers
• use assistive devices
• handle utensils
• handle cup or glass
• get food onto utensil
• bring food from receptacle to mouth
• chew food
• swallow food
• ingest food safely and in socially acceptable manner
• ingest sufficient food
• complete meals

Associated medical diagnoses (selected)
Alcohol addiction, Alzheimer's disease, bipolar disease (manic or depressive phase), Huntington's disease, schizophrenia

Expected outcomes
• Patient will have his self-care needs met.
• Patient will have few if any complications.
• Patient and family members will carry out feeding program daily.
• Patient will maintain weight.
• Patient and family members will communicate feelings and concerns.
• Patient and family members will identify resources to help cope with problems and discharge.

Interventions and rationales
• Observe, document, and report patient's functional and perceptual or cognitive ability daily. *Careful observation helps you adjust nursing actions to meet patient's needs.*
• Weigh patient weekly and record results. Report loss of 2 lb or more *to ensure adequate nutrition and fluid balance.*
• Perform prescribed treatment for underlying condition. Monitor progress and report favorable and adverse responses. *Applying therapy consistently aids patient's independence.*
• Allow patient to express frustration, anger, or feelings of inadequacy. Provide emotional support *to help patient come to terms with self-care deficit and achieve highest functional level.*
• Determine types of food best handled by patient — for example, finger foods or soft or liquid diet. *Easily handled foods encourage patient's feelings of independence.*
• Provide assistive devices at each meal as needed. *These allow patient to do as much as possible for self.*
• Place patient in high Fowler's position *to reduce swallowing difficulty and aid digestion.*
• Supervise or assist at each meal; for example, cut food into small pieces. *Cutting food into small bites aids chewing, swallowing, and digestion and reduces risk of choking or aspiration.*

• Feed patient slowly. Don't rush. *Rushing causes stress, reducing digestive activity and causing intestinal spasms.*
• Encourage patient to do as much for self as possible, giving simple instructions one at a time, *to aid comprehension.*
• Keep suction equipment at bedside *to remove aspirated foods if necessary.*
• Instruct patient and family members in feeding techniques and use of equipment. Have patient and family members give return demonstration of feeding and equipment use under supervision. *This aids understanding and encourages compliance.*
• As needed, refer patient to psychiatric liaison nurse, support group, or home health care agency. *These extra resources will reinforce activities planned to meet patient's needs.*

Evaluations for expected outcomes
• Patient meets self-care needs with help of staff.
• Patient doesn't experience infection, skin integrity alteration, weight loss, or other complications of altered self-care.
• Patient and family members become more active in carrying out self-care program; need for staff assistance decreases.
• Patient maintains weight at designated level.
• Patient and family members express feelings about patient's self-care deficit. If unable to meet own needs, patient seeks help from family member or staff within 24 hours.
• Patient and family members identify and contact available support resources as needed.

Documentation
• Patient's and family members' expression of feelings and concerns about difficulty with feeding
• Observations of patient's impaired ability to feed self
• Weight
• Patient's response to treatment
• Interventions to provide supportive care
• Instructions to patient (if capable) and family members, their understanding of instructions, and their demonstrated skill in carrying out instructions
• Patient's response to nursing interventions
• Evaluations for expected outcomes

■ Self-care deficit: Toileting

related to musculoskeletal impairment

Definition
Inability to carry out toileting routine

Assessment
• History of injury or disease associated with musculoskeletal impairment
• Self-care abilities, including knowledge and use of adaptive equipment, preparation of equipment and supplies, and technical or mechanical skills
• Musculoskeletal status, including coordination; functional ability; gait; mechanical restriction (such as cast, splint, and traction); muscle tone, size, and strength; range of motion; and tremors
• Psychosocial status, including coping mechanisms, family members, lifestyle, patient's perceptions of health problem and self, and personality

Defining characteristics
• Inability to carry out proper toilet hygiene
• Inability to flush toilet or empty commode
• Inability to get to toilet or commode
• Inability to manipulate clothing for toileting
• Inability to sit on or rise from toilet or commode

Associated medical diagnoses (selected)
Acute renal failure, adult respiratory distress syndrome, amyotrophic lateral sclerosis, atelectasis, cerebrovascular accident, chronic obstructive pulmonary disease, chronic renal failure, craniotomy, empyema, fractures, glomerulonephritis, Guillain-Barré syndrome, head injury, meningitis, multiple sclerosis, multisystem trauma, muscular dystrophy, myasthenia gravis (crisis), Parkinson's disease, pneumonia, pulmonary edema, rheumatoid arthritis, spinal cord injury or tumor

Expected outcomes
• Patient will have his self-care needs met.
• Patient will have few if any complications.
• Patient will communicate feelings about limitations.
• Patient will maintain continence.
• Patient and family members will demonstrate correct use of assistive devices.
• Patient and family members will carry out toileting program daily.

Interventions and rationales
• Observe patient's functional level every shift; document and report any changes. *Careful observation helps you adjust nursing actions to meet patient's needs.*

• Perform prescribed treatment for underlying musculoskeletal impairment. Monitor progress, reporting favorable and adverse responses to treatment. *Applying therapy consistently aids patient's independence.*
• Encourage patient to voice feelings and concerns about self-care deficits *to help patient achieve highest functional level possible.*
• Monitor intake and output and skin condition; record episodes of incontinence. *Accurate intake and output records can identify potential imbalances.*
• Use assistive devices as needed, such as external catheter at night, bedpan or urinal every 2 hours during day, and adaptive equipment for bowel care. Instruct on use. As control improves, reduce use of assistive devices. *Assisting at appropriate level helps maintain patient's self-esteem.*
• Assist with toileting only if needed. Allow patient to perform independently as much as possible *to promote independence.*
• Perform urinary and bowel care if needed. Follow urinary or bowel elimination plans. *Monitoring success or failure of toileting plans helps identify and resolve problem areas.*
• Instruct patient and family members in toileting routine (you can give family members written instructions). Have patient and family members demonstrate toileting routine under supervision. *Return demonstration identifies problem areas and increases patient's self-confidence.*
• As needed, refer patient to psychiatric liaison nurse, support group, or home health care agency. *Extra resources reinforce activities planned to meet patient's needs.*

Evaluations for expected outcomes

• Patient meets self-care needs with help of staff.
• Patient doesn't experience constipation, infection, skin integrity alteration, weight loss, or other complications of altered self-care.
• Patient expresses feelings about self-care deficit. If unable to meet own needs, patient seeks assistance from family member or staff within 24 hours.
• Patient maintains continence.
• Patient and family members demonstrate appropriate use of assistive devices.
• Patient follows daily self-care plan. Family members assist as needed.

Documentation

• Patient's expression of feelings and concerns about self-care limitations and their impact on body image and lifestyle
• Patient's willingness to participate in self-care
• Observations of patient's impaired ability to perform toileting routine and patient's response to treatment
• Patient's intake and output
• Interventions to provide supportive care
• Instructions given to patient and family members, their understanding of instructions, and their demonstrated skill in carrying out self-care functions
• Patient's response to nursing interventions
• Evaluations for expected outcomes

■ Self-care deficit: Toileting

related to perceptual or cognitive impairment

Definition

Inability to carry out toileting routine

Assessment

• History of neurologic, sensory, or psychological impairment
• Age
• Self-care abilities, including knowledge and use of adaptive equipment, preparation of equipment and supplies, and technical or mechanical skills
• Neurologic status, including cognition, communication ability, insight or judgment, level of consciousness, memory, motor ability, orientation, and sensory ability
• Psychosocial status, including coping mechanisms, family members, lifestyle, patient's perceptions of self, and personality

Defining characteristics

• Inability to carry out proper toilet hygiene
• Inability to flush toilet or empty commode
• Inability to get to toilet or commode
• Inability to manipulate clothing for toileting
• Inability to sit on or rise from toilet or commode

Associated medical diagnoses (selected)

Alcohol addiction, Alzheimer's disease, Huntington's disease, schizophrenia

Expected outcomes

• Patient will have his self-care needs met.

• Patient will have few if any complications.
• Patient and family members will carry out toileting program daily.
• Patient will maintain continence.
• Patient and family members will communicate feelings and concerns.
• Patient and family members will identify resources to help cope with problems and discharge from facility.

Interventions and rationales

• Observe, document, and report patient's functional and perceptual or cognitive ability daily. *Careful observation helps you adjust nursing actions to meet patient's needs.*
• Perform prescribed treatment for underlying condition. Monitor progress and report favorable and adverse responses. *Applying therapy consistently aids patient's independence.*
• Allow patient to express frustration, anger, and feelings of inadequacy. Provide emotional support *to help patient achieve highest functional level.*
• Monitor intake and output; record episodes of incontinence. *Accurate intake and output records can identify potential imbalances.*
• Use assistive devices as needed, such as external catheter at night, bedpan or urinal every 2 hours during day, and adaptive equipment for bowel care. As control improves, reduce use of assistive devices. *Assisting at appropriate level helps maintain patient's self-esteem.*
• Assist with toileting, if needed, using visual and auditory cues to stimulate urination. *This allows patient to perform independently as much as possible.*
• Allow ample time for patient to perform toileting routine. *Rushing creates unnecessary stress and promotes failure.*

• Provide positive, constructive feedback when assisting with toileting. *Reinforcement and rewards may enhance self-esteem.*
• Assist with toileting, giving simple instructions one at a time, *to aid comprehension.*
• Complete urinary and bowel care if patient can't do so. Follow urinary and bowel elimination plans. *Monitoring success or failure of toileting plans helps identify and resolve problem areas.*
• Give written instructions in toileting routine to family members, and supervise return demonstration. *Return demonstration identifies problem areas and increases family members' self-confidence.*
• Refer patient to psychiatric liaison nurse, support group, or community agency, as needed. *These extra resources will reinforce activities planned to meet patient's needs.*

Evaluations for expected outcomes

• Patient meets self-care needs with help of staff.
• Patient doesn't experience constipation, infection, skin integrity alteration, weight loss, or other complications of altered self-care.
• Patient and family members become more active in carrying out self-care program; need for staff assistance decreases.
• Patient maintains continence.
• Patient and family members express feelings about patient's self-care deficit. If unable to meet own needs, patient seeks help from family member or staff within 24 hours.
• Patient and family members identify and contact available support resources as needed.

Documentation
• Patient's and family members' expressions of feelings and concerns about self-care deficits
• Observations of patient's impaired ability to perform toileting routine
• Patient's intake and output
• Patient's response to treatment for underlying condition
• Interventions to provide supportive care
• Instructions given to patient (if capable) and family members, their understanding of instructions, and their demonstrated skill in carrying out self-care functions
• Patient's response to nursing interventions
• Evaluations for expected outcomes

■ Self-esteem, chronic low

Definition
Long-standing negative self-evaluation or feelings about self or capabilities

Assessment
• Reason for hospitalization or outpatient treatment
• Age
• Sex
• Developmental stage
• Family system, including marital status, role in the family, and sibling position
• Perception of health problem
• Past experience with health care system
• Mental status, including abstract thinking, affect, communication, general appearance, judgment or insight, memory, mood, orientation, perception, and thinking process
• Belief system, including norms, religion, and values
• Social interaction pattern
• Social and occupational history
• Perception of self (past and present), including body image, coping mechanisms, problem-solving ability, and self-worth
• Past experience with crisis
• Past history of treatment for psychosocial disturbance, including hospitalization, medication, psychotherapy, and suicidal ideation, plans, and attempts
• Neurovegetative signs, including ability to experience pleasure, appetite, energy level, and sleep

Defining characteristics
• Expressions of self-negating thoughts
• Expressions of shame or guilt
• Extreme conformity or dependency on others' opinions
• Hesitation to try new things or situations
• Indecisiveness
• Need for excessive reassurance
• Nonassertive or passive tendencies
• Perception of self as unable to deal with events
• Poor eye contact
• Repeated experience of failure in career or other aspects of life
• Rejection of positive feedback and exaggeration of negative feedback

Associated medical diagnoses (selected)
Adrenal insufficiency, Alzheimer's disease, amyotrophic lateral sclerosis, antisocial personality disorder, anxiety disorder, Bell's palsy, bipolar disorder (manic or depressive phase), borderline personality disorder, brain abscess, cerebrovascular accident, chronic pain, depression, diabetes mellitus, end-stage renal disease, hemophilia, multiple sclerosis, myasthenia gravis, panic disorder, Parkinson's disease, seizure disorders, self-

destructive behaviors, spinal cord defect or tumor, suicidal behavior

Expected outcomes
• Patient will voice feelings related to self-esteem.
• Patient will report feeling safe in facility environment.
• Patient will make verbal contract not to harm self while in facility.
• Patient will gradually join in self-care and decision-making process.
• Patient will engage in social interaction with others.
• Patient will demonstrate verbal and behavioral decrease in negative self-evaluation.
• Patient will voice acceptance of positive and negative feedback without exaggeration.

Interventions and rationales
• Provide for specific amount of uninterrupted non-care-related time to engage patient in conversation. *This gives patient time for self-exploration.*
• Listen to patient with understanding, responding with nonjudgmental acceptance, genuine interest, and sincerity. *This expands patient's self-awareness and reduces element of threat.*
• Assess patient's mental status through interview and observation at least once weekly. *High anxiety from self-rejection may cause cognitive, sensory, and perceptual disturbances.*
• Assess suicide risk and lethal potential as indicated. *Extremely low levels of self-esteem may lead to suicide.*
• Institute suicidal precautions according to protocol. *Patient needs supervision until he demonstrates adequate self-control to ensure his own safety.*
• Provide patient with simple, structured daily routine. *Structured activity limits patient's anxious behaviors.*

• Encourage patient to care for self to extent possible. *Patient may neglect or reject aspects of self-care because of feelings of self-hate.*
• Involve patient in decisions about care on gradual basis *to reduce feelings of ambivalence, prevent procrastination, and promote confidence in decision making.*
• Arrange situations to encourage social interaction between patient and others. *Disturbed interpersonal relationships are direct expression of self-hate.*
• Provide patient with positive feedback for verbal reports and behaviors that indicate improved self-esteem. *This encourages future adaptive coping behaviors.*
• Help patient mobilize resources for assistance when discharged *to help patient replace maladaptive coping behaviors with more adaptive ones.*
• Refer patient to mental health professional as indicated. *Severity of symptoms accompanying chronic low self-esteem may require long-term psychotherapy.*

Evaluations for expected outcomes
• Patient expresses feelings about self.
• Patient doesn't feel threatened by facility environment.
• At least once daily, patient reiterates commitment not to harm self.
• Patient participates in at least one aspect of self-care daily.
• Patient converses with others on daily basis.
• Patient states at least two positive aspects about self.
• Patient accepts positive feedback and constructive criticism.

Documentation
• Patient's verbal expressions and behaviors that indicate low self-esteem

• Mental status examination (baseline and ongoing)
• Suicide assessment, interventions, and patient's response
• All nursing interventions implemented to promote self-esteem
• Patient's response to interventions
• Evaluations for expected outcomes

■ Self-esteem, situational low

Definition

Negative feelings about oneself that develop in response to a loss or change in an individual who previously had a positive self-evaluation

Assessment

• Age
• Sex
• Developmental stage
• Family system, including marital status, role in family, and sibling position
• Reason for health care visit
• Mental status, including affect, general appearance, and mood
• Cognitive ability
• Behavior
• Perception of self (past and present), including body image, coping mechanisms, and self-worth

Defining characteristics

• Difficulty making decisions
• Evaluation of self as unable to handle life events
• Expressions of self-negating thoughts
• Expressions of shame or guilt
• Expression of negative feelings about self (such as helplessness and uselessness)

• Negative self-appraisal in response to life events in a patient who previously exhibited positive self-evaluation

Associated medical diagnoses (selected)

This nursing diagnosis can be used with any patient experiencing an anticipated or actual loss (body part, normal body function, control over environment, threat to life). Diagnoses include end-stage cardiac disease, cerebrovascular accident, Down syndrome, impotence, infertility, spinal tumor, and any injury or illness resulting in prolonged hospitalization.

Expected outcomes

• Patient will voice feelings related to current situation and its effect on self-esteem.
• Patient will verbally appraise self before and during current health problem.
• Patient will participate in decisions related to care and therapies.
• Patient will report sense of control over life events.
• Patient will articulate return to previous positive feelings about self.

Interventions and rationales

• Encourage patient to express feelings about self (past and present). *Self-exploration encourages patient to consider future change.*
• Provide specific amount of uninterrupted non-care-related time to engage patient in conversation. *Such discussions help patient assume ultimate responsibility for coping responses.*
• Assess patient's mental status through interview and observation at least once daily. *If anxiety resulting from self-rejection becomes severe, patient may experience disorientation and psychotic symptoms.*

• Involve patient in decision-making process. *Making such decisions can help combat ambivalence and procrastination associated with low self-esteem.*
• Provide patient with positive feedback for verbal reports or behaviors that indicate return to positive self-appraisal. *This gives patient feelings of significance, approval, and competence, which can help him cope effectively with stressful situations.*

Evaluations for expected outcomes
• Patient expresses feelings about self in relation to recent stressful events.
• Patient describes how feelings about self have changed since current health problem began.
• Each day, patient makes decisions related to care.
• Patient reports feeling more self-confident in managing current situation.
• Patient states at least two positive feelings about self.

Documentation
• Patient's expressions of lowered self-esteem
• Mental status assessment (baseline and ongoing)
• Nursing interventions directed toward return to previous positive self-esteem
• Patient's response to interventions
• Evaluations for expected outcomes

■ Self-esteem disturbance

Definition
Negative self-evaluation or feelings about self or self-capabilities that may be directly or indirectly expressed

Assessment
• Age
• Developmental stage
• Sex
• Family system, including marital status and sibling position
• Reason for hospitalization or outpatient treatment
• Patient's perception of current health problem
• Patient's past experience with health problems
• Mental status, including affect, behavior, cognitive ability, general appearance, and mood
• Usual coping behaviors during stress
• Social interaction pattern

Defining characteristics
• Denial of problems that are evident to others
• Exhibitions of grandiosity
• Expressions of self-negating thoughts
• Expressions of shame or guilt
• Hesitation to try new things or situations
• Hypersensitivity to slights or criticism
• Perception of self as unable to deal with events
• Projection of blame or responsibility for problems onto others
• Rationalization of personal failures
• Rejection of positive feedback and exaggeration of negative feedback about self

Associated medical diagnoses (selected)
Self-esteem affects all patients. Possible diagnoses include abortion, amputation, colostomy, deafness, ileostomy, infertility, menopause, and rape.

Expected outcomes
• Patient will voice feelings related to self-esteem.

• Patient will participate in decisions related to care and therapies.
• Patient will engage in social interaction with others.
• Patient will voice acceptance of positive or negative feedback without exaggeration.
• Patient will initiate action to attain higher level of wellness, both physically and emotionally.
• Patient will articulate at least two positive qualities about self.

Interventions and rationales
• Encourage patient to express feelings about self. *Active listening is the most basic therapeutic skill.*
• Allow specific amount of uninterrupted, non-care-related time to engage patient in conversation. *This creates environment that encourages patient to express feelings at his own pace.*
• Assess patient's mental status through interview and observation at least once daily. *This helps detect abnormal feelings and behaviors.*
• Involve patient in decision-making process *to reduce patient's feelings of dependence on others.*
• Arrange situations to encourage social interaction between patient and others. *Improving social environment helps restore confidence and self-esteem.*
• Provide patient with positive feedback for verbal reports or behaviors indicating improved self-esteem. *This encourages future effective coping behaviors.*
• Refer patient to mental health professional if indicated. *Consultation can ease frustration, increase objectivity, and foster collaborative approach to patient's care.*

Evaluations for expected outcomes
• Patient expresses feelings about self.

• Patient makes at least two care-related decisions daily.
• Patient interacts with others at least once daily.
• Patient accepts responsibility for behavior and is open to constructive criticism.
• Patient performs self-care activities and undergoes therapy without prompting.
• Patient states at least two personal assets.

Documentation
• Patient's expressions of lowered self-esteem
• Mental status assessment (baseline and ongoing)
• Interventions directed toward improved self-esteem
• Patient's response to nursing interventions
• Evaluations for expected outcomes

■ Sensory or perceptual alteration
related to hallucinations

Definition
Perceptions of images or sensations that occur in the absence of external stimuli

Assessment
• Age
• Sex
• Reason for hospitalization or outpatient visit, including patient's perception of problem, recent stressors, changes in somatic functioning, circumstances surrounding onset of hallucinations, duration and diurnal nature of experiences, and delusional beliefs

• Mental status, including insight about current situation, judgment, abstract thinking, general information, mood, affect, recent and remote memory, thought processes, thought content, and orientation to time, place, and person
• Physical characteristics, including manner of dress, personal hygiene, posture, and gait
• Communication skills, including attitude toward interviewer, body language, and facial expressions
• Psychosocial assessment, including coping mechanisms, support systems, willingness to cooperate with treatment, ability to perform activities of daily living, and social interactions
• Health history, including medication history (response, effectiveness, and adverse reactions), substance abuse history (type and effect on mental status), sleep habits, and dietary and nutritional status
• Laboratory studies, including blood chemistry and toxicology screening
• Diagnostic tests, including computed tomography scan and electroencephalogram

Defining characteristics
• Acting out of hallucinatory experience (command hallucinations)
• Perception of images that occur in absence of external stimuli (visual hallucinations)
• Perception of odors of specific or unknown origin (olfactory hallucinations)
• Perception of taste sensations with no basis in reality (gustatory hallucinations)
• Perception of voices or sounds not heard by others and unrelated to objective reality (auditory hallucinations)
• Preoccupation and lack of awareness of surroundings

• Strange body sensations, including misperceptions about body parts (tactile hallucinations)
• Talking to self
• Watchfulness and listening in absence of external stimuli

Associated medical diagnoses (selected)
Affective disorders, dementia, intoxication, schizophrenia

Expected outcomes
• Patient will report decrease in number of hallucinatory experiences.
• Patient will report decrease in anxiety levels that lead to hallucinations.
• Patient will demonstrate increased ability to test reality at onset of hallucinations.
• Patient will meet interpersonal needs in realistic ways.

Interventions and rationales
• Provide safe and structured environment. Identify and reduce as many stressors as possible. Be honest and consistent in all interactions with patient. *These measures will help decrease patient's anxiety.*
• Encourage patient to identify and initiate anxiety-reducing measures *to give patient sense of control.*
• In organic hallucinations, use reality orientation and factual information to help patient cope. Tell patient that hallucination results from organic causes and can be reversed. *This will reduce anxiety.* In nonorganic hallucinations, don't attempt to reason with patient or challenge hallucination. Instead, provide comfort and support. *Attempts at reasoning only increase anxiety, which exacerbates hallucinations.*
• When speaking to patient, use directive statements such as "Look at me and listen; try not to pay attention to the voices right now." *Reacting ver-*

bally forces patient to focus on you rather than on internal stimuli.
• Provide regular physical activity that requires use of concentration and large muscles *to distract patient from internal stimuli.*
• Help patient to identify situations that evoke hallucinatory experiences *to enable patient to anticipate hallucinations and possibly prevent their onset.*
• Teach patient to intervene in hallucinatory experience. Encourage patient to speak out against hallucination, using such statements as "Go away; you aren't real." *Such responses foster sense of control and help distract patient, thereby reducing frequency and duration of hallucinations.*
• Teach patient to use consensual validation of perceptual experiences to test reality. *Having other people validate experiences will increase patient's orientation to reality.*
• As patient's anxiety level decreases, encourage participation in group-oriented activities and involvement in the community *to increase patient's level of functioning.*
• Refer patient to psychiatric liaison nurse, social service, or support group, as appropriate, *to provide additional support for patient and family members.*

Evaluations for expected outcomes
• Within 2 weeks, patient states that hallucinatory experiences have decreased in intensity and frequency.
• Patient reports reduced anxiety levels that lead to hallucination.
• Patient employs self-control measures to reduce hallucinations.
• Patient demonstrates improved social skills.

Documentation
• Patient's statements about type, frequency, and intensity of hallucinations
• Observations about environmental factors that precipitate hallucinatory experiences
• Patient's anxiety level
• Interventions to help patient cope
• Patient's response to nursing interventions
• Referrals
• Evaluations for expected outcomes

■ Sensory or perceptual alteration

related to sensory deprivation

Definition
Change in characteristics of incoming stimuli

Assessment
• Nature of medical diagnosis
• Mobility
• Neurologic status, including cognition (insight or judgment and recent and remote memory), level of consciousness, orientation, and sensory function
• Diagnostic tests, including electroencephalogram and computed tomography scan
• Communication status, including adaptive responses (such as gestures, lipreading, and signing), level of comprehension and expression, and speech pattern
• Environmental status, including equipment and supplies, lighting, location of patient's personal belongings, noise, privacy, and space
• Psychosocial status, including alcohol and drug use, behavior and personality, coping mechanisms, history of depression, and support systems

Defining characteristics
• Altered communication pattern
• Auditory distortions
• Change in behavior pattern
• Change in problem-solving abilities
• Change in usual response to stimuli
• Disorientation
• Hallucinations
• Irritability
• Poor concentration
• Reported or measured change in sensory acuity
• Restlessness
• Visual distortions

Associated medical diagnoses (selected)
This diagnosis is often seen in elderly patients who are hospitalized or institutionalized, and in patients who are on isolation precautions. It may also occur in Alzheimer's disease, bipolar disease (depressive phase), dementia, and depression.

Expected outcomes
• Patient will use adaptive equipment (such as glasses and hearing aid) as needed.
• Patient will remain oriented to person, place, and time.
• Patient will remain safe in environment.
• Patient will respond to environmental stimuli.
• Patient or family members will communicate understanding of sensory stimulation exercises.
• Patient or family members will take active role in preventing sensory deprivation and isolation.

Interventions and rationales
• Assist or encourage patient to use glasses, hearing aid, or other adaptive devices *to help reduce sensory deprivation.*
• Reorient patient to reality:
– Call patient by name.
– Tell patient your name.
– Give background information (time, place, and date) frequently throughout day.
– Orient to environment, including sights and sounds.
– Use large signs as visual cues.
– Post photo of patient on door if patient is ambulatory and disoriented.
– Provide visual contrast in environment.
These measures help reduce patient's sensory deprivation.
• Arrange environment to offset deficit:
– Place patient in room that allows him full view of his environment.
– Encourage family to bring in personal articles, such as books, cards, and photos.
– Keep articles in same place to promote sense of identity.
– Use such safety precautions as a night-light when needed.
These measures reduce sensory deprivation.
• Communicate patient's response level to family members and staff; record on plan of care and update as needed. *Patient's response to stimuli allows evaluation of his sensory deprivation level.*
• Talk to patient while providing care; encourage family members to discuss past and present events with patient. *Verbal stimuli can improve patient's reality orientation.*
• Arrange to be with patient at predetermined times during day *to avoid isolation.*
• Turn on television and radio for short periods of time based on patient's interests *to help orient patient to reality.*
• Hold patient's hand when talking. Discuss interests with patient and family members. Obtain needed items such as talking books. *Sensory stimuli*

help reduce patient's sensory deprivation.

• Assist patient and family members in planning short trips outside facility or health care environment. Educate about mobility, toileting, feeding, suctioning, and other requirements. *Trips help reduce patient's sensory deprivation.*

Evaluations for expected outcomes
• Patient uses adaptive equipment to alleviate sensory deprivation.
• Patient demonstrates ability to correctly identify people, places, and the time and to recall past events.
• Patient uses safety precautions to remain free of injury.
• Patient responds to environmental stimuli.
• Patient or family members communicate understanding of sensory stimulation exercises.
• Patient or family members identify and use techniques to prevent sensory deprivation.

Documentation
• Patient's or family members' expressions of concern about sensory deprivation
• Observations of patient's orientation, response to environmental stimuli, and safety
• Patient's or family members' response to nursing interventions
• Instructions and demonstration of skill in providing sensory stimuli
• Evaluations for expected outcomes

■ Sensory or perceptual alteration

related to sensory overload

Definition
Change in characteristics of incoming stimuli

Assessment
• History of major trauma or surgery, seizures, alcoholism, or psychiatric disorders
• Mobility status
• Neurologic status, including cognition (recent and remote memory and insight or judgment), level of consciousness, orientation, and sensory function
• Sleep-wake status
• Communication status, including adaptive responses (such as gestures, lipreading, and signing), level of comprehension and expression, and speech pattern
• Environmental status, including equipment and supplies, lighting, location of patient's personal belongings, noise, privacy, and space
• Psychosocial status, including alcohol and drug use, behavior and personality, coping mechanisms, history of depression, and support systems

Defining characteristics
• Altered communication pattern
• Auditory distortions
• Change in behavior pattern
• Change in problem-solving abilities
• Change in usual response to stimuli
• Disorientation
• Hallucinations
• Irritability
• Poor concentration
• Reported or measured change in sensory acuity
• Restlessness

• Visual distortions

Associated medical diagnoses (selected)
Acute respiratory failure, anxiety disorder, bipolar disorder (manic phase), craniotomy, hepatic coma, posttraumatic stress disorder

Expected outcomes
• Patient will remain oriented to person, place, and time.
• Patient will voice decreased anxiety and irritability.
• Patient will communicate in a lucid manner.
• Patient will recognize when sensory stimuli are excessive.
• Patient will reestablish usual sleep-wake cycle.
• Patient will state measures to reduce sensory overload.
• Patient will demonstrate positive coping behavior when sensory overload situation arises.

Interventions and rationales
• Reorient patient to reality: call patient by name, tell patient your name, give background information (time, place, and date) frequently, and orient to environment, including sights, sounds, and smells. *These measures will reduce susceptibility to sensory overload.*
• Provide nonthreatening environment, reduce excessive noise and lights, and keep environment uncluttered *to reduce sensory overload.*
• Accept patient's perception of stimuli. Don't challenge hallucinations or delusions; don't ridicule or tease. *Challenging patient's perceptions doesn't reduce sensory overload.*
• Help patient interpret environment (for example, "This is the hospital," "I am a nurse," "You're hearing the food cart go down the hall"). *This helps reduce anxiety.*

• Simulate "normal" environment: keep lights off (or dim) at night, let in light during day, provide clock and calendar, and place family photos at bedside. *This reduces sensory overload.*
• Explain procedures, tests, special equipment, and unusual sounds (such as alarms). Prepare patient for procedures in advance. *Increased knowledge reduces sensory overload.*
• Cluster procedures and treatments. Avoid disturbing patient unnecessarily. Always approach in calm, gentle manner to avoid startling patient. *Approaching patient in compassionate manner helps reduce sensory overload.*
• Help patient use coping strategies, such as talking to someone, when sensory overload occurs. *This provides sense of control.*
• Teach patient how to limit sensory overload — for example, turning off television and removing self from stimulating environment. *Knowledgeable patient is better able to reduce sensory overload.*
• Encourage regular sleep pattern and routines, possibly including milk or warm bath before bedtime. *Sufficient rest improves tolerance to stimuli.*
• Encourage family members to visit frequently; provide reassurance and explanations to aid understanding of patient's condition. *Orientation to reality through family visits helps to promote relaxation.*

Evaluations for expected outcomes
• Patient demonstrates ability to correctly identify people, places, and the time and to recall past events.
• Patient reports feeling less irritable and anxious.
• Patient communicates clearly.

• Patient recognizes when sensory stimuli are becoming excessive and requests time in quiet area.
• Patient states that he feels rested.
• Patient identifies measures to avoid sensory overload.
• Patient demonstrates positive coping behavior to handle sensory overload.

Documentation
• Patient's and family members' expressions of concern about sensory overload
• Observations of orientation, response to environment, anxiety level, and sleep pattern
• Patient's or family members' responses to nursing interventions
• Instructions and demonstration of skill in managing sensory overload
• Evaluations for expected outcomes

■ Sensory or perceptual alteration (auditory)

related to altered sensory reception, transmission, or integration

Definition
Change in characteristics of auditory stimuli

Assessment
• History of ear disorders, trauma, or surgery
• Age
• Auditory status, including ear position, size, and symmetry; skin color and texture; tympanic membrane (cerumen, color of canal, deformities, discharge, intactness or tension, and landmarks); and use of hearing aid
• Rinne test
• Weber's test

• Communication status, including adaptive responses (such as gestures, lipreading, and signing), level of comprehension and expression, and speech pattern
• Environmental factors such as factory noise
• Activities of daily living
• Behavioral assessment, including coping mechanisms and willingness to cooperate with treatment

Defining characteristics
• Altered communication pattern
• Auditory distortions
• Change in behavior pattern
• Change in problem-solving abilities
• Change in usual response to auditory stimuli
• Disorientation
• Hallucinations
• Irritability
• Poor concentration
• Reported or measured change in auditory acuity
• Restlessness

Associated medical diagnoses (selected)
Acoustic neuroma, brain tumors, chemotherapy, deafness, diabetes mellitus, disseminated intravascular coagulation, head injury, intoxication, Ménière's disease, meningitis

Expected outcomes
• Patient will discuss impact of hearing loss on lifestyle.
• Patient will remain oriented to person, place, and time.
• Patient will express feeling of comfort and security.
• Patient will show interest in external environment.
• Patient will compensate for auditory loss by using signing, gestures, lipreading, hearing aid, or other measures.

• Patient will plan to use community resources to assist with auditory deficit.

Interventions and rationales
• Allow patient to express feelings about hearing loss. Convey willingness to listen, but don't pressure patient to talk. *Giving patient chance to talk about hearing loss enhances acceptance of loss.*
• Determine how to communicate effectively with patient, using gestures, written words, signing, or lipreading. If patient has hearing aid, encourage its use. *Planned communication with patient improves care delivery.*
• Give patient clear, concise explanations of treatments and procedures. Avoid information overload. Face patient when speaking; enunciate words clearly, slowly, and in normal speaking voice; avoid putting hands to mouth when speaking. Wearing red lipstick helps to define mouth. *Patient will be better able to join in care with better understanding of treatment plan.*
• Provide sensory stimulation by using tactile and visual stimuli to help compensate for hearing loss. Encourage family members to bring familiar objects from home. *Sensory stimulation of patient's other senses helps compensate for hearing loss.*
• Provide reality orientation if patient is confused or disoriented *to permit more effective patient-staff interaction.*
• Make sure other staff members are aware of patient's hearing deficit. Record information on patient's plan of care and chart cover. *This ensures effective nursing care delivery by all staff members.*
• Respond to call light by going to patient's room as soon as possible. If feasible, assign same staff members

to care for patient. *These measures reduce patient's fears.*
• Teach patient alternative ways to cope with hearing loss; care of hearing aid, if prescribed; and safety and protective measures to avoid harm or injury (such as amplifier or signal devices on telephone and visual cues in environment). *Knowledgeable patient can better cope with hearing loss.*
• Refer to appropriate community resources, such as Self-help for Hard of Hearing People, to help patient adapt to loss. Involve family members in planning, and encourage their participation. *These measures help patient and family cope better with hearing loss.*

Evaluations for expected outcomes
• Patient discusses impact of hearing loss on lifestyle.
• Patient demonstrates ability to correctly identify people, places, and the time and to recall past events.
• Because of reduction in environmental risk factors, patient expresses comfort in surroundings.
• Patient expresses interest in interacting with others.
• Patient identifies and uses alternative methods of communication.
• Patient recognizes need for support during transition from facility to outside environment and states plans to use community resources to help him cope with auditory deficit.

Documentation
• Patient's statements of feelings about auditory loss
• Observations of patient's behavior or response to auditory loss and use of adaptive aids
• Instructions about safety and protective measures and patient's intent to use appropriate resources

• Patient's response to nursing interventions
• Evaluations for expected outcomes

■ Sensory or perceptual alteration (gustatory)

Definition
Change in sense of taste

Assessment
• Taste sensation, including change from baseline and ability to differentiate sweet, salty, sour, and bitter tastes
• Health history, including trauma, infection, vitamin or mineral deficiency, neurologic or oral disorders, and chemotherapy or radiation therapy
• Medication history, including use of certain antidepressants (such as clomipramine), antineoplastics, penicillamine, captopril, lithium, interferon alfa-2a, levamisole, or zidovudine
• Evidence of loss of appetite
• Weight change from baseline
• Mouth dryness
• Smoking history
• Sense of smell

Defining characteristics
• Altered taste sense:
– complete loss of taste (ageusia)
– distorted sense of taste (dysgeusia)
– partial loss of taste (hypogeusia)
• Loss of appetite
• Reported or measured change in sensory acuity
• Weight loss

Associated medical diagnoses (selected)
Bell's palsy, fractures, head injury, head or neck cancer, Sjögren's syndrome

Expected outcomes
• Patient will report changes in sense of taste.
• Patient will identify ways to enhance enjoyment of food.
• Patient will consume ___ % of diet.
• Patient will maintain weight.

Interventions and rationales
• Assess changes in sense of taste *to establish baseline.*
– Gently raise patient's tongue slightly with gauze sponge. Use moistened applicator to place a few crystals of salt or sugar on one side of tongue. Wipe tongue clean and ask patient to identify taste sensation *to test sweet and salt taste sensation.*
– Apply tiny amount of quinine to base of tongue *to test bitter taste sensation.*
– Place small piece of sour pickle on patient's tongue *to test sour taste sensation.*
• Pinch off one nostril and ask patient to close his eyes and sniff through open nostril to identify nonirritating odors, such as coffee, lime, and wintergreen, *to evaluate sense of smell; much of what constitutes taste is actually smell.* Repeat test on opposite nostril.
• Monitor and record patient's weight each week *to detect signs of weight loss.*
• Modify patient's diet *so he can distinguish and enjoy as many tastes as possible.* Identify ways to emphasize smell and enhance flavor of food, such as using herbs and spices, *to compensate for loss of taste.*
• Serve food in attractive surroundings. Prepare meals in attractive manner, using variety of different-colored foods, *to appeal to patient's visual sense.*

Evaluations for expected outcomes
• Patient reports changes in sense of taste.
• Patient identifies ways to make meals more appealing.
• Patient consumes __ % of diet.
• Patient maintains weight.

Documentation
• Evidence of changes in patient's sense of taste
• Patient's weight
• Techniques used to modify patient's diet
• Evaluations for expected outcomes

■ Sensory or perceptual alteration (kinesthetic)

Definition
Diminished ability to perceive position or location of body parts, especially changes in angles of joints

Assessment
• Health history, including presence of neurologic or musculoskeletal conditions
• Musculoskeletal status, including motor coordination and muscular weakness
• Use of safety devices
• Presence of other sensory impairments
• Neurologic status, including cognition (insight, judgment, and memory), level of consciousness, and orientation
• Coping behaviors
• Emotional response to illness
• Self-concept, including self-esteem and body image

Defining characteristics
• Diminished motor coordination

• Inability to identify position or location of body parts
• Inability to perceive changes in angles of joints
• Muscular weakness, flaccidity, rigidity, or atrophy
• Paralysis

Associated medical diagnoses (selected)
Joint replacement, multiple sclerosis, muscular dystrophy, spinal cord injury, spinal tumor

Expected outcomes
• Patient will express feelings associated with changes in kinesthetic perception.
• Patient will implement safety precautions.
• Patient will not experience skin breakdown, especially in areas around vulnerable joints.
• Patient will participate in self-care activities to maximum ability.
• Patient will participate in appropriate exercise program.
• Patient will not experience injury.

Interventions and rationales
• Encourage patient to express feelings related to diminished kinesthetic perception *to promote acceptance of perceptual impairment.*
• Assess changes in motor coordination, paralysis, or muscular weakness and report observations to health care team *to ensure appropriate care.*
• Implement appropriate safety measures, such as installing padded bed rails, maintaining bed in low position, and using wheelchair lapboard, *to avoid patient injury.*
• Remind patient to regularly check placement of his hands and feet *to avoid injury.*
• Teach staff members to remind patient of need to check positioning of hands and feet *to ensure safety and*

avoid injury. Emphasize importance of communicating supportive and accepting attitude *to enhance patient's emotional well-being.*
• Inspect skin daily, especially areas around vulnerable joints, *to detect signs of skin breakdown.*
• Encourage use of letter board, electric wheelchair, and feeding and dressing devices *to promote independence.*
• Provide patient with exercise program that includes active and passive range-of-motion routines *to maintain range of motion and prevent musculoskeletal degeneration.*

Evaluations for expected outcomes
• Patient describes feelings brought on by changes in kinesthetic perception.
• Patient implements safety precautions.
• Patient doesn't exhibit signs of skin breakdown.
• Patient participates in self-care activities to maximum ability.
• Patient participates in selected exercise program.
• Patient doesn't experience injury.

Documentation
• Observations of diminished kinesthetic perception
• Evidence of patient's understanding of instructions about safety and protective measures and intent to use appropriate safety devices
• Patient's response to nursing interventions
• Evaluations for expected outcomes

■ Sensory or perceptual alteration (olfactory)

Definition
Change in sense of smell

Assessment
• Alterations in olfactory sense and related symptoms, including nosebleeds, foul taste in mouth, sneezing, postnasal drip, dry or sore mouth or throat, loss of sense of taste or appetite, excessive tearing, and facial or eye pain
• Nutritional status, including weight, usual dietary intake, and nausea
• Medication history, including use of phenothiazines, estrogen, metronidazole, or antineoplastics and prolonged use of nasal decongestants or topical anesthetics
• History of intranasal drug abuse, such as cocaine and amphetamines
• Respiratory status, including nasal drainage, sputum characteristics, and history of colds, hay fever, or polyps
• Health status, including presence of any condition that causes irritation and swelling of nasal mucosa and obstruction of olfactory area (such as nasal disease and allergies) and any condition that may cause lesion in olfactory nerve pathway (such as head trauma)
• Smoking history
• Inhalation of irritants such as chlorine fumes
• Physical examination, including inspection and palpation of nasal structures, contour and color of nasal mucosa, size and color of turbinates, presence of polyps, source and character of nasal discharge, and olfactory nerve (cranial nerve I) function
• Home environment, including presence of gas or propane heating sys-

tems, smoke detectors, and chemical substances

Defining characteristics
• Altered sense of smell: diminished (hyposmia) or absent (anosmia)
• Diminished sense of taste and loss of appetite
• Weight changes

Associated medical diagnoses (selected)
Diabetes mellitus, fractures, head injury, nasal polyps, poisoning

Expected outcomes
• If appropriate, patient will state that decreased olfactory perception is temporary.
• If appropriate, patient will report improvements in olfactory perception.
• Patient will maintain weight.
• Patient will describe how to identify noxious odors and maintain safe home environment.

Interventions and rationales
• Assess patient's ability to smell and document findings *to establish baseline.*
• Prepare foods the patient likes and serve them in attractive manner *to stimulate patient's appetite.* Use variety of different-colored foods with each meal *to appeal to patient's visual sense.*
• Weigh patient weekly *to detect weight loss and monitor for possible malnutrition.*
• If altered olfactory perception results from nasal congestion, follow these steps:
– Reassure patient that condition is temporary and sense of smell should return *to diminish anxiety.*
– Tell patient with nasal packing that sense of smell will return after packing is removed and swelling decreases *to provide reassurance.*

– Administer prescribed medications, such as antihistamines and nose drops or sprays, *to relieve nasal congestion.*
– Monitor laboratory values and vital signs *to detect signs of infection.*
– Record nasal drainage characteristics, including amount, color, consistency, and odor, *to assess for changes in olfactory condition.*
– Ensure adequate hydration, and provide for humidification in patient's room *to prevent drying of mucous membranes.*
• If altered olfactory perception doesn't result from simple nasal congestion, prepare patient for diagnostic tests, such as sinus transillumination, skull X-ray, and computed tomography scan, as ordered, *to guide further treatment.*
• Provide home care instructions as necessary. Teach patient to:
– contact utility company *to implement measures for protecting against possible gas leaks.*
– place smoke detectors throughout home *to signal danger of fire.*
– discard food according to dates on packages rather than relying on sense of smell *to avoid eating spoiled food.*

Evaluations for expected outcomes
• Patient expresses understanding that change in olfactory perception is temporary.
• Patient reports improvement in olfactory perception.
• Patient's weight stabilizes.
• Patient demonstrates ability to identify noxious odors and maintain safe home environment.

Documentation
• Evidence of changes in patient's olfactory perception
• Nursing interventions performed and patient's response
• Patient's dietary preferences

- Patient's weight
- Instructions for home care and patient's or caregiver's response
- Evaluations for expected outcomes

■ Sensory or perceptual alteration (tactile)

Definition
Change in sense of touch

Assessment
- Vital signs
- Evidence of impaired tactile perception, including complaints of tingling, pain, or numbness; response to sharp and dull stimuli; and signs of bruises, cuts, scrapes, and other injury
- Neurologic status, including level of consciousness, cranial nerve function, muscle strength, deep tendon reflexes, and light touch, pain, temperature, vibration, and position sensation
- Skin color and temperature
- History of chemotherapy treatment
- History of alcohol abuse
- Medication history, including use of clomipramine, ceftizoxime, amiodarone, dichlorphenamide, guanadrel, anistreplase, interferon alfa-2b, or zidovudine

Defining characteristics
- Altered sense of touch:
– abnormal sensation, such as numbness, prickling, and tingling (paresthesia)
– decreased sensitivity to stimulation (hypoesthesia)
– diminished sensitivity to pain (hypalgesia)
– impaired sense of touch (dysesthesia)

Associated medical diagnoses (selected)
Arterial occlusion, brain tumor, cerebrovascular accident, diabetes mellitus, head injury, juvenile rheumatoid arthritis, multiple sclerosis, Parkinson's disease, poisoning, Raynaud's disease, seizure disorders, spinal cord injury, transient ischemic attacks

Expected outcomes
- Patient will express feelings about changes in tactile perception.
- Patient will not experience falls or injury.
- Patient will not experience skin breakdown.
- Patient will describe safety measures to avoid injury.
- Family member or caregiver will describe program to provide patient with increased tactile stimulation.

Interventions and rationales
- Allow patient to express feelings associated with altered tactile perception. Be willing to listen, but don't pressure patient to talk. *Providing chance to talk will help patient cope with sensory deficits.*
- Teach patient to regularly check placement of his hands and feet *to avoid injury.*
- Inspect skin daily, especially on patient's feet, *to detect signs of skin breakdown.*
- Use padded side rails or lapboard on wheelchair if appropriate. Make any other environmental modifications as needed *to promote safe tactile experiences and prevent accidental injury.*
- Teach patient safety measures, such as testing bath water with thermometer, *to prevent injury.*
- Teach family members or caregiver to touch patient in areas with preserved sensation, using variety of textures, *to promote sensory input.* For example, suggest family members

provide satin pillowcase, wrap soft scarf around patient's neck, or give gentle massage with scented lotion.

Evaluations for expected outcomes
• Patient expresses feelings associated with changes in tactile perception.
• Patient doesn't experience falls or injury.
• Patient's skin remains intact.
• Patient lists ways to protect against risk of injury caused by diminished tactile sensation.
• Family member or caregiver describes program to provide patient with increased tactile sensation.

Documentation
• Evidence of diminished tactile sensation
• Patient's expression of feelings about diminished tactile perception
• Instructions about safety and protective measures
• Patient's response to nursing interventions
• Evaluations for expected outcomes

■ Sensory or perceptual alteration (visual)

related to altered sensory reception, transmission, or integration

Definition
Change in characteristics of visual stimuli

Assessment
• History of eye disorders, trauma, or surgery
• Age
• Visual status, including corneal reflex, extraocular movement, inspection of lid and eyeball, ophthal-
moscopy, palpation of lid and eyeball, pupil size and accommodation, tonometry, use of glasses or contact lenses, visual acuity (near and distant), and visual fields
• Environmental and occupational factors
• Activities of daily living
• Behavioral assessment, including coping mechanisms, support system, and willingness to cooperate with treatment

Defining characteristics
• Altered communication pattern
• Change in behavior pattern
• Change in problem-solving abilities
• Change in usual response to stimuli
• Disorientation
• Hallucinations
• Irritability
• Poor concentration
• Reported or measured change in visual acuity
• Restlessness
• Visual distortions

Associated medical diagnoses (selected)
Blindness, brain tumors, cataracts, detached retina, diabetes mellitus, disseminated intravascular coagulation, food poisoning, glaucoma, head injury, intoxication, macular degeneration, meningitis, polycythemia vera, pregnancy-induced hypertension

Expected outcomes
• Patient will discuss impact of vision loss on lifestyle.
• Patient will express a feeling of safety, comfort, and security.
• Patient will maintain orientation to person, place, and time.
• Patient will show interest in external environment.
• Patient will regain visual functioning and will come to terms with any vision loss.

• Patient will compensate for vision loss by use of adaptive devices.
• Patient will plan to use appropriate resources.

Interventions and rationales
• Allow patient to express feelings about vision loss such as its impact on lifestyle. Convey willingness to listen, but don't pressure patient to talk. *Allowing patient to voice fears aids acceptance of vision loss.*
• Provide safe environment by removing excess furniture or equipment from patient's room. Orient patient to room. Show patient how to use call light. Don't move furniture or leave objects in hallway. *Orienting patient to surroundings reduces risk of injury.*
• If patient is blind on admission, allow patient to direct arrangement of room; walk with patient to bathroom and other key areas until he becomes familiar with environment. If patient has seeing-eye dog, make arrangements for dog's needs. *Maintaining patient's optimal level of independence fosters sense of control.*
• Modify environment to maximize any vision patient may have. For example, with hemianopia, place patient in room to maximize visual field, approach patient from best visual angle, remind patient to scan environment to pick up visual cues, and place objects within visual field. *Modifying environment helps patient meet self-care needs.*
• If patient has diplopia, patch one eye *to ameliorate double vision.*
• Always introduce yourself or announce your presence on entering patient's room; let patient know when you're leaving. *Familiarizing patient with caregiver aids reality orientation and conveys respect.*
• Provide sensory stimulation by using tactile, auditory, and gustatory stimuli to help compensate for vision loss. Obtain large-print books, talking books, audiotapes, or radio, as preferred by patient. *Nonvisual sensory stimulation helps patient adjust to vision loss.*
• Provide reality orientation if patient is confused or disoriented *to allow for more effective patient-staff interaction.*
• Give patient clear, concise explanations of treatments and procedures. Avoid information overload. When speaking to patient, enunciate words clearly, slowly, and in normal speaking voice. *A knowledgeable patient will be better able to participate in treatment plan.*
• Encourage family and friends to visit patient and bring familiar objects to leave in patient's room. *Presence of familiar objects aids reality orientation.*
• Make sure that health care personnel are aware of vision loss. Record information on patient's plan of care and chart cover or post in patient's room. *Nursing care is improved if staff is aware of patient's vision loss.*
• Respond to call light as soon as possible. Provide for continuity by assigning same staff members to care for patient if possible. *These measures help reduce patient's fears.*
• If patient has had eye surgery, provide appropriate care as indicated. Be aware of and take steps to limit activities that increase intraocular pressure, such as bending, stooping, getting on and off bedpan, coughing, and vomiting. *Avoiding postoperative activities that increase intraocular pressure helps reduce complications.*
• Administer and monitor effectiveness of medications. Report any adverse effects. *Medications help reduce pain and may control disease process.*

• Educate patient in alternative ways of coping with vision loss; care of such adaptive devices as eyeglasses, magnifying glass, contact lenses, and artificial eye; and administration of eyedrops, including name, dosage, and therapeutic and adverse effects. *A knowledgeable patient will be better able to cope with vision loss.*
• Refer to appropriate community resources to help patient and family adapt to vision loss — for example, American Foundation for the Blind or other community agencies or support groups. *Postdischarge support will help patient and family cope better with patient's vision loss.*

Evaluations for expected outcomes
• Patient discusses effects of vision loss on lifestyle.
• Because of reduction in environmental risk factors, patient reports comfort in surroundings.
• Patient demonstrates ability to correctly identify people, places, and the time and to recall past events.
• Patient expresses interest in interacting with others.
• Patient regains visual functioning to the extent possible and begins to come to terms with any permanent vision loss.
• Patient uses adaptive devices to compensate for vision loss.
• Patient recognizes need for support during transition from facility to outside environment and plans to use appropriate resources as needed.

Documentation
• Patient's feelings about visual deficits
• Observations of patient's behavior and response to visual deficit and use of adaptive equipment or devices

• Instructions about safety and protective measures, coping strategies, and postoperative management
• Patient's and family members' intent to use appropriate resources
• Patient's response to nursing interventions
• Evaluations for expected outcomes

■ Sexual dysfunction
related to altered body structure or function

Definition
Presence of physiologic or emotional factors that alter one's usual pattern of sexual function

Assessment
• History of problem that caused change in structure or function
• Patient's perception of change's effect
• Marital status and attitude of spouse or significant other
• Living arrangement
• Usual sexual patterns
• Sexual problems before current health problem
• Patient's attitude toward modifying sexual patterns
• Patient's present knowledge about appropriate options available

Defining characteristics
• Actual or perceived limitation imposed by disease or therapy
• Change in achieving perceived sex role
• Change in relationship with spouse or significant other
• Change of interest in self and others
• Conflicts involving values
• Inability or change in ability to achieve sexual satisfaction

• Need for confirmation of sexual desirability
• Verbal expression of problem

Associated medical diagnoses (selected)

Acute renal failure, adrenal insufficiency, benign prostatic hypertrophy, chemotherapy, chronic renal failure, diabetes mellitus, endometriosis, interstitial cystitis, menopause, myocardial infarction, pelvic inflammatory disease, radiation therapy, rheumatoid arthritis, spinal cord injury or tumor, testicular cancer, urinary diversion

Expected outcomes

• Patient will acknowledge problem or potential problem in sexual function.
• Patient will voice feelings about changes in sexual identity.
• Patient will explain reason for sexual dysfunction.
• Patient will express willingness to obtain counseling.
• Patient will reestablish sexual activity at pre-illness level.

Interventions and rationales

• Provide nonthreatening atmosphere and encourage patient to ask questions about personal sexuality. *This encourages patient to ask questions specifically related to current situation.*
• Allow patient to express feelings openly in nonjudgmental atmosphere. *This enhances communication and understanding between patient and caregiver.*
• Provide answers to specific questions. *This helps patient focus on specific issues, clarifies misconceptions, and builds trust in caregiver.*
• Provide time for privacy. *This demonstrates respect for patient, allows time for introspection, and gives patient control over time spent interacting with others.*
• Suggest that patient discuss concerns with partner. *This fosters sharing of concerns and strengthens relationships.*
• Provide support for partner. *Supportive interventions such as active listening communicate concern, interest, and acceptance.*
• Educate patient and partner about limitations imposed by patient's current physical condition. *Education about limitations imposed on sexual activity by illness helps patient avoid complications or injury.*
• Suggest referral to sex counselor or other appropriate professional for future guidance *to provide patient with resource for postdischarge support.*

Evaluations for expected outcomes

• Patient acknowledges existence of problem or potential problem in sexual function.
• Patient expresses anxiety, anger, depression, or frustration over changes in sexual function.
• Patient explains relationship between illness or treatment and sexual dysfunction.
• Patient expresses willingness to obtain counseling.
• Patient resumes usual level of sexual activity.

Documentation

• Patient's perception of problem
• Subtle comments made by patient about inability to cope with change in structure or function
• Observations of patient's behavior
• Interventions performed to assist patient and spouse or significant other; response to interventions
• Evaluations for expected outcomes

■ Sexual dysfunction

related to impotence

Definition

Presence of physiologic or emotional factors that alter a man's usual pattern of sexual function

Assessment

• Age
• Type of impotence:
– organic (anatomic or central nervous system defect)
– functional (physiologic alterations in nervous and cardiovascular systems)
– psychogenic (inhibition by emotions of neural transmission from brain to sexual organs)
– primary (failure to ever achieve satisfactory erection for coitus)
– secondary (at least one successful coitus)
• History of organic impotence or physiologic disorders that interfere with erection
• Anatomic anomalies of penis
• Psychological variables, including patient's perception of sexual performance, relationships, desire for erection, guilt, shame, relationship with parents (presence of overbearing mother), and family or social pressures
• Physiologic status, including medication history (response, effectiveness, and adverse reactions) and history of substance abuse (type and effect on mental status)
• Sociocultural factors, including educational level, socioeconomic status, ethnic group, and religious beliefs and practices
• Sexual history, including sexual drive, sexual preference, frequency of impotence, premature ejaculation, spontaneous morning erections, positive coital experiences, types of erotic stimulation used, past professional counseling or sex therapy, homosexual experiences, affairs (other partners or prostitutes), and feelings of anger, hostility, or disgust toward partner

Defining characteristics

• Actual or perceived limitation imposed by disease or therapy
• Change in achieving perceived sex role
• Change in relationship with spouse or significant other
• Change of interest in self and others
• Conflicts involving values
• Inability or change in ability to achieve sexual satisfaction
• Need for confirmation of sexual desirability
• Verbal expression of problem

Associated medical diagnoses (selected)

Alcohol or drug addiction, impotence, prostate cancer

Expected outcomes

• Patient will acknowledge problem in sexual function.
• Patient will voluntarily discuss his problem.
• Patient and partner will discuss their feelings and perceptions about changes in sexual performance.
• Patient will learn methods to enhance sexual pleasure for himself and his partner and incorporate them into his sexual activities.
• Patient will continue to communicate with partner about sexual issues and needs.
• Patient will agree to obtain sexual evaluation and therapy if needed.
• Patient will develop and maintain positive attitude toward his sexuality and sexual performance.

Interventions and rationales
• Establish therapeutic relationship with patient *to provide safe, comfortable atmosphere for discussing sexual concerns.*
• Encourage patient to discuss feelings and perceptions about his sexual dysfunction *to help him validate perceptions and reduce emotional distress through catharsis.*
• Encourage partner to discuss feelings and perceptions *to help couple clarify issues about their relationship and improve communication.*
• Educate patient and partner about alternative methods of lovemaking and expressing affection. *Alternative expressions of love and intimacy can raise patient's self-esteem until impotence is evaluated and treated.*
• Encourage use of sexual fantasies and erotica to promote sexual stimulation and erection. *This helps patient and partner achieve sexual satisfaction and decreases "spectatoring" (watching oneself during sexual activity with partner), which can inhibit performance.*
• Encourage patient to seek professional evaluation and therapy *to obtain proper diagnosis and treatment.*

Evaluations for expected outcomes
• Patient states that he has problem in sexual function.
• Patient states that he feels comfortable discussing his sexual concerns.
• Patient and partner communicate with each other about their sexual relationship.
• Patient states specific ways in which he will enhance sexual pleasure with his partner.
• Patient continues to talk with partner about sexual issues and needs
• Patient participates in sexual evaluation and sex therapy if needed.

• Patient makes positive comments about self.

Documentation
• Patient's perception of sexual problem
• Overt and covert remarks made by patient that indicate his difficulty dealing with impotence
• Observations of patient's behavior in response to his inability to perform
• Interventions performed to assist patient and his partner
• Responses to nursing interventions
• Evaluations for expected outcomes

■ Sexuality pattern alteration

related to illness or medical treatment

Definition
State in which an individual expresses concern about personal sexuality

Assessment
• History of current illness
• Current treatment regimen (medications and therapies)
• Marital status and family members
• Patient's perception of sexual identity and role
• Usual sexual activity pattern
• Patient's perception of changes in sexual activity resulting from illness or treatment
• Significance of sexual relationship to patient and partner
• Emotional reactions (affect and mood)
• Behavioral reactions (specify)

Defining characteristics
• Reported difficulties, limitations, or changes in sexual activity

Associated medical diagnoses (selected)
Acquired immunodeficiency syndrome, Alzheimer's disease, amyotrophic lateral sclerosis, angina pectoris, benign prostatic hypertrophy, Bell's palsy, brain abscess, cardiac arrhythmias, cerebrovascular accident, chlamydia, colostomy, coronary artery disease, diabetes mellitus, end-stage renal disease, genital herpes, gonorrhea, hypertension, ileostomy, multiple sclerosis, myocardial infarction, orthopedic injuries, osteoporosis, Parkinson's disease, prolonged hospitalization, spinal cord injury, syphilis, urinary diversion

Expected outcomes
• Patient will voice feelings about potential or actual changes in sexual activity.
• Patient will express concern about self-concept, self-esteem, and body image.
• Patient will state at least one effect of illness or treatment on sexual behavior.
• Patient and partner will resume effective communication patterns.
• Patient and partner will use available counseling referrals or support groups.

Interventions and rationales
• Allow for specific amount of uninterrupted time to talk with patient. *This demonstrates your comfort with sexuality issues and reassures patient that his concerns are acceptable for discussion.*
• Provide nonthreatening, nonjudgmental atmosphere for patient to verbalize feelings about perceived changes in sexual identity and behaviors. *This demonstrates unconditional positive regard for patient and his concerns about sexuality patterns.*

• Provide patient and partner with information about illness and treatment. Answer any questions and clarify any misconceptions they may have. *This helps them focus on specific concerns, encourages questions, and avoids misunderstandings.*
• Provide time for privacy. *This demonstrates respect for patient, allows time for introspection, and gives patient control over time spent interacting with others.*
• Encourage social interaction and communication between patient and partner. *This fosters sharing of concerns and strengthens relationships.*
• Offer referral to counselors or support persons, such as mental health professional, sex counselor, and illness-related support groups (such as "I Can Cope," Reach for Recovery, and Ostomy Association) *to provide patient with resources for postdischarge support.*

Evaluations for expected outcomes
• Patient expresses concerns and fears related to altered sexuality pattern.
• Patient expresses feelings about change in self-image resulting from illness or medical treatment.
• Patient identifies specific physical symptom that has negative effect on sexual behavior.
• Patient and partner communicate effectively.
• Patient and partner participate in therapy with appropriate counselor.

Documentation
• Patient's perception of changes in sexual patterns
• Patient's ability to interact with other people
• Interventions to support and educate patient and partner
• Response to nursing interventions
• Evaluations for expected outcomes

■ Sexuality pattern alteration

related to separation from spouse or partner

Definition
State in which an individual expresses concern about personal sexuality

Assessment
• Reason for hospitalization
• Current and anticipated length of stay
• Marital status and family members
• Living arrangement
• Patient's perception of sexual identity and role
• Usual sexual activity pattern
• Patient's perception of limitation on sexual activity resulting from hospitalization
• Significance of sexual relationship to patient and partner
• Emotional reactions (affect and mood)
• Behavioral reactions (specify)

Defining characteristics
• Reported difficulties, limitations, or changes in sexual activity

Associated medical diagnoses (selected)
This nursing diagnosis can occur in any hospitalized patient separated from partner for prolonged period. Examples include patients with infectious diseases, neurologic illnesses, orthopedic injuries, postoperative complications, and terminal illnesses.

Expected outcomes
• Patient will voice feelings about changes in usual sexual activity.
• Patient will alter inappropriate behaviors if indicated.
• Patient and partner will discuss possible realistic alternatives for intimacy within hospital setting.
• Patient and partner will use available counseling referrals.

Interventions and rationales
• Allow specific amount of uninterrupted, non-care-related time to talk with patient. *This demonstrates your comfort with sexuality issues and reassures patient that his concerns are acceptable for discussion.*
• Display an accepting, nonjudgmental manner *to encourage patient to discuss concerns about sexuality.* Approach partner in same manner and include in discussions with patient, if agreeable to both. *A nonjudgmental approach demonstrates unconditional positive regard for both patient and partner.*
• Include patient in plan for setting limits on inappropriate behavior, if indicated by behavioral assessment.
– Explain aspects of patient's behavior that are inappropriate.
– Share proposed plan of care with patient, including expectations, goals, and approaches for reducing bothersome behavior.
– Request patient's cooperation, but be willing to compromise if he offers acceptable alternatives.
Working together to set limits allows patient to take part in planning to reduce undesirable behaviors.
• Discuss with patient and partner realistic, acceptable alternatives for intimacy needs. *This encourages open communication between them as sexual partners.*
• Explain to patient and partner limitations related to illness and facility environment *to establish standard for realistic and acceptable behavior.*
• Provide time for privacy. *This allows patient and partner to discuss*

feelings about sexuality and to engage in alternatives for intimacy while patient is hospitalized.
• Offer referral for counseling, such as mental health professional and sex counselor, if indicated. *Referrals provide opportunities for additional ongoing therapy during hospitalization and after discharge.*

Evaluations for expected outcomes
• Patient describes usual sexual activity pattern and expresses feelings resulting from changes in pattern.
• Patient demonstrates ability to decrease or eliminate inappropriate behavior. For example, patient avoids making comments with sexual or abusive overtones, maintains appropriate grooming and attire, and finds outlet for angry feelings to lessen potential for acting out.
• Patient and partner request privacy and seek permission to use acceptable alternatives for intimacy, such as holding and kissing.
• Patient and partner seek counseling.

Documentation
• Patient's verbal and nonverbal behaviors
• Patient's and partner's perception of current situation
• Specific nursing interventions to reduce emotional and behavioral reactions, such as active listening, limit setting, and counseling referrals
• Patient's and partner's response to nursing interventions
• Evaluations for expected outcomes

■ Skin integrity impairment

related to external (environmental) factors

Definition
Interruption in skin integrity

Assessment
• History of skin problems, trauma, surgery, or immobility
• Age
• Integumentary status, including color, elasticity, hygiene, lesions, moisture, quantity and distribution of hair, sensation, temperature and blood pressure, texture, and turgor
• Musculoskeletal status, including anesthetic area, joint mobility, muscle strength and mass, paralysis, and range of motion
• Nutritional status, including appetite, dietary intake, hydration, current weight, and change from normal weight
• Hemoglobin and hematocrit
• Serum albumin
• Psychosocial status, including coping skills, family members, mental status, self-concept, and body image
• Occupational hazards
• Patient's current understanding of physical condition and physical, mental, and emotional readiness to learn

Defining characteristics
• Destruction of skin layers
• Disruption of skin surface
• Invasion of body structures

Associated medical diagnoses (selected)
Accidental radiation exposure, acoustic neuroma, adult respiratory distress syndrome, amyotrophic lateral sclerosis, anemias, appendicitis, bone marrow transplantation, brain

abscess, breast cancer, breast engorgement, burns, cerebral aneurysm, cervical cancer, colostomy, craniotomy, Crohn's disease, dermatomyositis and polymyositis, fractures, hepatic coma, Hodgkin's disease, ileostomy, lesions, Lyme disease, neuromuscular trauma, open wounds, osteomyelitis, paralysis, postmaturity, pressure ulcers, pseudomembranous colitis, Reiter's syndrome, tracheostomy, urinary diversion, urinary incontinence, viral hepatitis

Expected outcomes

• Patient will exhibit no evidence of skin breakdown.
• Patient will show normal skin turgor.
• Patient will regain skin integrity — for example, pressure ulcer will decrease in size (specify).
• Patient's surgical wound will heal.
• Patient will communicate understanding of skin protection measures.
• Patient will demonstrate skill in care of wound, burn, or incision.
• Patient will demonstrate skin inspection technique.
• Patient will perform skin care routine.
• Patient will communicate feelings about change in body image.

Interventions and rationales

• Inspect skin every shift, describe and document skin condition, and report changes. *This provides evidence of effectiveness of skin care regimen.*
• Perform prescribed treatment regimen for skin condition involved; monitor progress. Report responses to treatment regimen *to maintain or modify current therapy.*
• Provide supportive measures as indicated.

– Assist with general hygiene and comfort measures *to promote comfort and sense of well-being.*
– Administer pain medication and monitor its effectiveness. *Patient needs pain relief to maintain health.*
– Maintain proper environmental conditions *to promote patient's sense of well-being.*
– Use foam mattress, bed cradle, or other devices *to avoid skin breakdown.*
– Warn against tampering with wound or dressings *to avoid potential for infection.*
– Maintain infection control standards *to reduce risk of spreading disease.*
• Position patient for comfort and minimal pressure on bony prominences. Change position at least every 2 hours. Monitor frequency of turning and skin condition. *These measures reduce pressure, promote circulation, and avoid skin breakdown.*
• Explain therapy to patient and family members *to encourage compliance.*
• Allow patient to express feelings about skin problem. *This helps allay anxiety and develops coping skills.*
• Instruct patient and family members in skin care regimen *to encourage compliance.*
• Supervise patient and family members in skin care management. Provide feedback *to improve skill in managing skin care.*
• Make referral to psychiatric liaison nurse, social service, or other support groups, as indicated. *These provide additional support for patient and family.*

Evaluations for expected outcomes

• Patient's skin remains intact.
• Patient's skin turgor remains normal.

• Patient's pressure ulcer heals, as evidenced by presence of granulation tissue and decreased size and depth of ulcer.
• Patient's surgical wound heals, as evidenced by clean suture line and absence of scar discoloration and skin breakdown.
• Patient understands necessity of avoiding prolonged pressure, obtaining adequate nutrition, and using protective devices.
• Patient demonstrates skill in care of wound, burn, or incision.
• Patient demonstrates skin inspection techniques.
• Patient performs skin care routine.
• Patient expresses feelings about changes in body image.

Documentation
• Patient's concerns about change in skin integrity, willingness to accept treatment, and participation in treatment regimen
• Observations of wound, pressure ulcer, and incision healing and response to treatment regimen
• Interventions to provide supportive care and prescribed treatment
• Patient's response to nursing interventions
• Patient's and family members' understanding and skill in performing skin care measures
• Evaluations for expected outcomes

■ Skin integrity impairment

related to internal (somatic) factors

Definition
Interruption in skin integrity

Assessment
• History of skin problems, trauma, chronic debilitating disease, or immobility
• Age
• Integumentary status, including color, elasticity, hygiene, lesions, moisture, quantity and distribution of hair, sensation, temperature and blood pressure, texture, and turgor
• Musculoskeletal status, including anesthetic area, joint mobility, muscle strength and mass, paralysis, and range of motion
• Nutritional status, including appetite, dietary intake, hydration, current weight, and change from normal weight
• Hemoglobin and hematocrit
• Serum albumin
• Psychosocial status, including coping patterns, family members, mental status, occupation, self-concept, and body image
• Knowledge, including patient's current understanding of physical condition and physical, mental, and emotional readiness to learn

Defining characteristics
• Destruction of skin layers
• Disruption of skin surfaces
• Invasion of body structures

Associated medical diagnoses (selected)
Acute renal failure, arterial occlusion, cellulitis, Cushing's syndrome, diabetes mellitus, hyperosmolar hyperglycemic nonketotic syndrome, nutritional deficiencies, pemphigus, peripheral vascular disease, polycythemia vera, prostatectomy, psoriasis, rubella, thrombophlebitis

Expected outcomes
• Patient will exhibit no evidence of skin breakdown.

• Patient will exhibit improved or healed lesions or wounds.
• Patient will report increased comfort.
• Patient will have few if any complications.
• Patient will correlate precipitating factors with appropriate skin care regimen.
• Patient will explain skin care regimen.
• Patient and family members will demonstrate skin care regimen.
• Patient will voice feelings about changed body image.

Interventions and rationales

• Inspect skin every shift, describe and document skin condition, and report changes. *This provides evidence of effectiveness of skin care regimen.*
• Perform prescribed treatment regimen for skin condition involved; monitor progress. Report favorable and adverse responses to treatment regimen *to maintain or modify current therapies as needed.*
• Provide supportive measures as indicated.
– Assist with general hygiene and comfort measures *to promote comfort and general sense of well-being.*
– Administer pain medications and monitor effectiveness. *Patient needs pain relief to maintain health.*
– Maintain proper environmental conditions, including room temperature and ventilation. *Providing comfortable environment promotes sense of well-being.*
– Apply bed cradle *to protect lesions from bed covers.*
– Remind patient not to scratch *to avoid skin injury.*
– Administer and monitor effectiveness of antipruritic medications. *Antipruritics reduce itching sensation.*

– Explain dietary restrictions — for example, explain that certain foods may cause skin allergy, leading to pruritus and skin breakdown. *Avoiding foods that cause skin allergy helps prevent skin breakdown.*
• Encourage patient to express feelings about skin condition *to enhance coping.*
• Explain therapy to patient and family *to encourage compliance.*
• Discuss precipitating factors, if known, and long-term effects of skin integrity interruption. *Knowledge of precipitating factors helps patient reduce their occurrence and severity.*
• Instruct patient and family in skin care regimen *to ensure compliance.*
• Supervise patient and family in skin care regimen. Provide feedback. *Practice helps improve skill in managing patient's skin care regimen.*
• Encourage adherence to other aspects of health care management *to control or minimize effects on skin.*
• Refer patient to psychiatric liaison nurse, social service, or support group, as appropriate. *These resources provide additional support for patient and family.*

Evaluations for expected outcomes

• Patient's skin remains intact.
• Patient's wounds or lesions heal.
• Patient reports feeling of comfort.
• Patient doesn't experience further skin breakdown or other complications.
• Patient lists factors precipitating skin breakdown.
• Patient explains skin care regimen.
• Patient and family members demonstrate skin integrity regimen.
• Patient expresses feelings about body image changes.

Documentation

- Patient's concerns about skin disorder and its impact on body image and lifestyle
- Patient's willingness to participate in care
- Observations of skin condition, healing, and response to treatment regimen
- Interventions to provide supportive care
- Instructions about treatment regimen
- Patient's or family members' understanding of and skill in carrying out instructions
- Patient's response to nursing interventions
- Evaluations for expected outcomes

■ Skin integrity impairment, risk for

Definition

Presence of risk factors for interruption or destruction of skin surface

Assessment

- History of skin problems, trauma, chronic debilitating disease, or immobility
- Age
- Integumentary status, including color, elasticity, hygiene, lesions, moisture, sensation, quantity and distribution of hair, temperature and blood pressure, texture, and turgor
- Musculoskeletal status, including anesthetic area, muscle strength and mass, joint mobility, paralysis, and range of motion
- Nutritional status, including appetite, dietary intake, hydration, current weight, and change from normal weight
- Hemoglobin and hematocrit

- Serum albumin
- Psychosocial status, including activities of daily living, mental status, occupation (sun exposure), and recreational activities

Risk factors

- External factors, including pressure, friction and shearing, restraints, physical immobilization, humidity and moisture, chemical substances, radiation, excretions and secretions, hypothermia or hyperthermia, and extreme youth or age
- Internal factors, including effects of medications, skeletal prominences, and altered nutritional status (obesity or emaciation), sensation, pigmentation, metabolic state, circulation, or skin turgor

Associated medical diagnoses (selected)

This diagnosis may occur in any patient who's on prolonged bed rest or is immobilized. Specific conditions include chemotherapy, chronic renal failure, diabetes mellitus, esophageal varices, hydrocephalus, paralysis, peripheral vascular disease, Raynaud's disease, spinal cord injury or tumor, thrombophlebitis, and viral hepatitis.

Expected outcomes

- Patient will experience no skin breakdown.
- Patient will maintain muscle strength and joint range of motion.
- Patient will sustain adequate food and fluid intake.
- Patient's mucous membranes will remain intact.
- Patient will maintain adequate skin circulation.
- Patient will communicate understanding of preventive skin care measures.

• Patient and family members will demonstrate preventive skin care measures.
• Patient and family members will correlate risk factors and preventive measures.

Interventions and rationales
• Inspect skin every shift; document skin condition and report any status changes. *Early detection of changes prevents or minimizes skin breakdown.*
• Change patient's position at least every 2 hours; follow turning schedule posted at bedside. Monitor frequency of turning. *These measures reduce pressure on tissues, promote circulation, and avoid skin breakdown.*
• Encourage ambulation or perform or assist with active range-of-motion exercises at least every 4 hours while patient is awake. *Exercises prevent muscle atrophy and contracture; ambulation promotes circulation and relieves pressure.*
• Use preventive skin care devices as needed, such as foam mattress, alternating pressure mattress, sheepskin, pillows, and padding, *to avoid discomfort and skin breakdown.*
• Keep patient's skin clean and dry; lubricate as needed. Don't use irritating soap, and rinse skin well. *These measures alleviate skin dryness, promote comfort, and reduce risk of irritation and skin breakdown.*
• Protect bony prominences with foam padding. *Prominences have little subcutaneous fat and are prone to breakdown; using foam padding may help promote skin integrity.*
• Lift patient's body when moving him, using a lifting sheet if needed. Avoid shearing force. *Shearing force results when tissues slide against each other; a lifting sheet reduces sliding.*

• Keep linen dry, clean, and free of wrinkles or crumbs. Change wet bed linens and incontinence pads immediately. *Dry, smooth linens help prevent excoriation and skin breakdown.*
• Monitor nutritional intake; maintain adequate hydration. *Anemia (less than 10 mg hemoglobin) and low serum albumin concentrations (less than 2 mg) are associated with development of pressure ulcers. Hydration helps maintain skin integrity.*
• Educate patient and family in preventive skin care. Teach them how to maintain good personal hygiene; use nonirritating (nonalkaline) soap; pat rather than rub skin dry; inspect skin regularly; avoid prolonged exposure to water, sun, cold, and wind; avoid rubber rings; recognize beginning of skin breakdown (redness, blisters, and discoloration); and report signs and symptoms. *These measures encourage compliance with patient's skin care regimen.*
• Indicate risk factor potential on patient's chart and plan of care, and reevaluate weekly, using an accepted form such as Braden Scale. *Risk factor score helps evaluate treatment progress.*
• Explain importance of practicing preventive skin care measures *to encourage compliance with skin care regimen.*
• Supervise patient and family in preventive skin care measures. Give constructive feedback. *Practice helps improve skill in managing skin care regimen.*

Evaluations for expected outcomes
• Patient's skin will remain intact.
• Patient will not show evidence of contracture or muscle atrophy.
• Patient's weight will remain within established limits.

• Patient's mucous membranes will remain intact.
• Patient will not show evidence of poor circulation.
• Patient will list preventive skin care measures.
• Patient and family members will demonstrate skin care measures.
• Patient and family members will understand need to avoid prolonged pressure, obtain adequate nutrition, prevent incontinence, and consistently perform skin care measures.

Documentation
• Patient's and family members' expression of concern about potential skin breakdown
• Observations of risk factors and skin condition
• Use of preventive skin care devices and their effectiveness
• Instructions about preventive skin care; patient's and family members' understanding of instructions
• Patient's and family members' demonstrated skill in carrying out preventive skin care measures
• Results of Braden Scale
• Patient's response to nursing interventions
• Evaluations for expected outcomes

■ Sleep deprivation

Definition
Prolonged periods of time without sustained natural, periodic suspension of relative unconsciousness

Assessment
• Number of hours of sleep patient usually needs to feel rested
• Premorbid sleep patterns and current sleep patterns
• Daytime activity and work patterns
• Recent changes in health status or lifestyle
• Sleep environment, including recent changes to environment
• Activities that promote sleep
• Quality of sleep, as described by patient
• Dietary and drug history, including ingestion of caffeine or other stimulants, nicotine, alcohol, and sedative-hypnotics

Defining characteristics
• Irritability, lethargy, listlessness, restlessness, anxiety, malaise, apathy
• Decreased ability to function
• Daytime drowsiness
• Hand tremors
• Heightened sensitivity to pain
• Inability to concentrate
• Perceptual disorders (for example, disturbed body sensation, delusions, feeling afloat)
• Agitated or combative
• Hallucination
• Acute confusion
• Transient paranoia
• Mild, fleeting nystagmus

Associated medical diagnoses (selected)
This diagnosis may affect the elderly, patients with chronic illness, individuals with altered neuromuscular function, hospitalized patients, patients sharing a room, and patients requiring frequent monitoring of vital signs, frequent position changes, frequent catheterization, mechanical ventilation, medication administration, and other treatments during the night. Associated medical diagnoses include head injury, pulmonary disease, rheumatoid arthritis, spinal cord injury, and stroke.

Expected outcomes
• Patient will identify factors that prevent or disrupt sleep.

• Patient will sleep ___ (specify) hours without interruption.
• Patient will express feeling of being well rested.
• Patient will show no physical signs of sleep deprivation.
• Patient will not exhibit complications associated with sleep deprivation, such as sleep apnea and nocturnal hypoxic episodes.
• Patient will alter diet and habits to promote sleep — for example, by reducing caffeine intake and limiting alcohol intake.
• Patient will not exhibit such sleep-related behavioral symptoms as irritability, lethargy, listlessness, restlessness, anxiety, worry, or depression.
• Patient will perform relaxation exercises at bedtime.
• Health care providers will schedule nighttime treatments to allow for maximum restful sleep.

Interventions and rationales
• Encourage patient to identify factors in the environment that make sleeping difficult. *A strange or new environment may affect rapid eye movement (REM) and non-rapid eye movement (NREM) sleep.*
• Ask the patient what changes would help promote sleep *to encourage the patient to play an active role in care.*
• Advise the patient to avoid daytime naps if they interfere with nocturnal sleep *to promote restful nocturnal sleep.*
• Tell the patient to avoid spending long periods of time in bed without sleep. *Activity produces healthy fatigue, which promotes restful sleep.*
• Make immediate changes to accommodate the patient — for example, reduce noise; change catheterization, medication, or treatment schedule; change lighting; and close door.

These measures promote rest and sleep.
• Develop a plan to allow the patient to have ___ hours of uninterrupted sleep, if possible. *This provides consistent nursing care and provides patient with maximum hours of uninterrupted sleep.*
• Perform interventions to promote sleep, such as giving the patient a bath or back rub, ensuring that the patient is positioned properly, or providing pillows, food, or drink. *Personal hygiene routine precedes sleep for many individuals. Milk and some high-protein snacks, such as cheese or nuts, contain L-tryptophan, a sleep promoter.*
• Assess the patient each morning to determine quality of sleep the night before *to help detect sleep-related behavioral symptoms.*
• Teach the patient relaxation techniques, such as guided imagery, meditation, and progressive muscle relaxation. Practice them with the patient at bedtime. *Purposeful relaxation efforts commonly promote sleep.*
• Instruct patient to limit alcohol and caffeine intake and avoid foods that interfere with sleep (such as spicy foods). Foods and beverages with caffeine should be avoided for 4 to 5 hours before bedtime. *Dietary changes may help to promote restful sleep.*
• Avoid quick, unanticipated movements when turning and positioning patients with neuromuscular dysfunction *to prevent spasticity, which may interrupt sleep.*
• In stroke patients with muscle tone problems, plan to position the patient on the affected side during the last turn of the night. *This promotes restful sleep and helps normalize the patient's muscle tone for morning activities.*

• Refer the patient experiencing sleep deprivation to a sleep disorder center especially if activities of daily living are affected or sleep apnea occurs. *A specialist may be required to assist in treatment.*

• Assess daytime schedule to ensure adequate time for rest. *Excessive fatigue can result in insomnia.*

• Help patient with chronic illness or disability find resources for addressing psychosocial issues. *Fears and concerns about future prevent restful sleep.*

Evaluations for expected outcomes

• Patient identifies factors that prevent or disrupt sleep.

• Patient sleeps ___ (specify) hours without interruption.

• Patient expresses feeling of being well rested.

• Patient shows no physical signs of sleep deprivation.

• Patient doesn't exhibit complications associated with sleep deprivation, such as sleep apnea and nocturnal hypoxic episodes.

• Patient alters diet and habits to promote sleep — for example, by reducing caffeine intake and limiting alcohol intake.

• Patient doesn't exhibit such sleep-related behavioral symptoms as irritability, lethargy, listlessness, restlessness, anxiety, worry, or depression.

• Patient performs relaxation exercises at bedtime.

• Health care providers schedule nighttime treatments to allow for maximum restful sleep.

Documentation

• Patient's reports of sleep disturbances

• Patient's expressions of feelings related to sleep deprivation

• Observations of behaviors that indicate sleep deprivation

• Nursing interventions to alleviate sleep deprivation

• Patient's response to nursing interventions

• Evaluations for expected outcomes

■ Sleep pattern disturbance

related to external factors

Definition

Inability to meet individual need for sleep or rest arising from external factors

Assessment

• Daytime activity and work patterns

• Normal bedtime

• Usual number of hours of sleep required

• Problems associated with sleep, including early morning awakening, falling asleep, nightmares, sleepwalking, and staying asleep

• Quality of sleep

• Sleeping environment

• Activities associated with sleep

• Personal beliefs about sleep

• Chemical ingestion, including alcohol, caffeine, hypnotics, and nicotine

Defining characteristics

• Decreased ability to function

• Difficulty either awakening or staying asleep

• Dissatisfaction with sleep

• Earlier- or later-than-desired awakenings

• Increased Stage 1 sleep, decreased Stage 3 or 4 sleep, or decreased rapid eye movement (REM) sleep

• Less than age-normal total sleep time

• Self-induced impairment of normal sleep pattern
• Sleep onset greater than 30 minutes
• Verbal complaints of difficulty falling asleep or not feeling well rested
• Three or more nighttime awakenings

Associated medical diagnoses (selected)

This diagnosis may affect elderly, hospitalized patients, patients sharing a room with someone confused and noisy, and patients whose treatment involves any of the following: frequent monitoring of vital signs, intensive care, mechanical ventilation, medications during the night, treatments given during the night. Examples of medical diagnoses include acute respiratory failure, craniotomy, and panic disorder.

Expected outcomes

• Patient will identify factors that prevent or promote sleep.
• Patient will sleep ___ hours without interruption.
• Patient will express feeling of being well rested.
• Patient will show no physical signs of sleep deprivation.
• Patient will alter diet and habits to promote sleep — for example, reducing caffeine and alcohol intake.
• Patient will exhibit no sleep-related behavioral symptoms, such as restlessness, irritability, lethargy, and disorientation.
• Patient will perform relaxation exercises at bedtime.

Interventions and rationales

• Ask patient what environmental factors make sleep difficult. *Sleeping in strange or new environment tends to influence both REM and non-REM sleep.*

• Ask patient what changes would promote sleep. *This allows patient to take active role in treatment.*
• Make whatever immediate changes are possible to accommodate patient; for example, reduce noise, change lighting, and close door. *These measures promote rest and sleep.*
• Plan medication administration schedules *to allow for maximum rest.* If patient requires diuretics in evening, give far enough in advance *to allow peak effect before bedtime.*
• Make a detailed plan to provide patient with a set number of hours of uninterrupted sleep if possible. *This allows consistent nursing care and gives patient uninterrupted sleep time.*
• Provide patient with normal sleep aids, such as pillow, bath, back rub, food, and drink. *Milk and some high-protein snacks, such as cheese and nuts, contain L-tryptophan, a sleep promoter. Personal hygiene routine precedes sleep in many patients.*
• Ask patient to describe in specific terms each morning quality of sleep during previous night. *This helps detect presence of sleep-related behavioral symptoms.*
• Teach patient such relaxation techniques as guided imagery, meditation, and progressive muscle relaxation. Practice them with patient at bedtime. *Purposeful relaxation efforts often help promote sleep.*
• Instruct patient to eliminate caffeine from diet, limit alcohol intake, and avoid foods that interfere with sleep (for example, spicy foods). *Foods and beverages containing caffeine consumed less than 4 hours before bedtime may interfere with sleep.*

Evaluations for expected outcomes

• Patient describes factors that prevent or promote sleep.

• Patient sleeps specified number of hours without interruption.
• Patient expresses feeling of being well rested.
• Patient doesn't exhibit physical signs of sleep deprivation.
• Patient reports changing diet habits and making lifestyle changes to promote sleep.
• Patient doesn't exhibit sleep-related behavioral symptoms.
• Patient performs relaxation exercises at bedtime.

Documentation
• Patient's complaints about sleep disturbances
• Patient's verbalization of feelings about sleep
• Observations of behavior that indicates sleep deprivation
• Interventions to alleviate sleep disturbance
• Patient's response to nursing interventions
• Evaluations for expected outcomes

■ Sleep pattern disturbance

related to internal factors

Definition
Inability to meet individual need for sleep or rest arising from internal factors

Assessment
• Age
• Daytime activity and work patterns
• Time patient usually retires
• Number of hours of sleep patient usually needs to feel rested
• Problems associated with sleep, including early morning awakening,

difficulty falling asleep, nightmares, sleepwalking, and staying asleep
• Quality of sleep
• Sleeping environment
• Activities associated with sleep, including bath, drink, food, and medication
• Personal beliefs about sleep

Defining characteristics
• Decreased ability to function
• Difficulty either awakening or staying asleep
• Dissatisfaction with sleep
• Earlier- or later-than-desired awakenings
• Early morning insomnia
• Increased Stage 1 sleep, decreased Stage 3 or 4 sleep, or decreased rapid eye movement (REM) sleep
• Less than age-normal total sleep time
• Self-induced impairment of normal sleep pattern
• Sleep onset greater than 30 minutes
• Verbal complaints of difficulty falling asleep or not feeling well rested
• Three or more nighttime awakenings

Associated medical diagnoses (selected)
Acute renal failure, adrenal insufficiency, anorexia nervosa, bipolar disorder (manic or depressive phase), bulimia nervosa, chronic fatigue syndrome, chronic obstructive pulmonary disease, cystitis, depression, drug or alcohol addiction, hyperthyroidism, myocardial infarction, obsessive-compulsive disorder, rheumatoid arthritis, schizophrenia

Expected outcomes
• Patient will identify factors that prevent or disrupt sleep.
• Patient will sleep ____ hours a night.
• Patient will express feeling of being well rested.

• Patient will show no physical signs of sleep deprivation.
• Patient will exhibit no sleep-related behavioral symptoms, such as restlessness, irritability, lethargy, and disorientation.
• Patient will perform relaxation exercises at bedtime.

Interventions and rationales
• Allow patient to discuss any concerns that may be preventing sleep. *Active listening helps you determine causes of difficulty with sleep.*
• Plan nursing care routines to allow ____ hours of uninterrupted sleep. *This allows consistent nursing care and gives patient uninterrupted sleep time.*
• Provide patient with usual sleep aids, such as pillows, bath before sleep, food or drink, and reading materials. *Milk and some high-protein snacks (such as cheese and nuts) contain L-tryptophan, a sleep promoter. Personal hygiene routine precedes sleep in many patients.*
• Create quiet environment conducive to sleep; for example, close curtains, adjust lighting, and close door. *These measures promote rest and sleep.*
• Administer medications that promote normal sleep patterns as ordered. Monitor and record adverse effects and effectiveness. *Hypnotic agents induce sleep; tranquilizers reduce anxiety.*
• Promote involvement in diversional activities or exercise program during day. Discuss relationship of exercise and activity to improved sleep. Discourage excessive napping. *Activity and exercise promote sleep by increasing fatigue and relaxation.*
• Ask patient to describe in specific terms each morning quality of sleep during previous night. *This helps de-*

tect sleep-related behavioral symptoms.
• Educate patient in such relaxation techniques as imagery, progressive muscle relaxation, and meditation. *Purposeful relaxation efforts often help promote sleep.*

Evaluations for expected outcomes
• Patient identifies factors that prevent or disrupt sleep.
• Patient sleeps specified number of hours nightly.
• Patient expresses feeling of being well rested.
• Patient doesn't exhibit signs of sleep deprivation.
• Patient doesn't exhibit sleep-related behavioral symptoms.
• Patient performs relaxation exercises at bedtime.

Documentation
• Patient's complaints about sleep disturbances
• Patient's report of improvement in sleep patterns
• Observations of physical and behavioral sleep-related disturbances
• Interventions to alleviate sleep disturbances
• Patient's response to nursing interventions
• Evaluations for expected outcomes

■ Social interaction impairment
related to altered thought processes

Definition
Insufficient quantity or ineffective quality of social exchange

Assessment
• Reason for hospitalization (physiologic or psychiatric)
• Usual pattern of social interaction (nonverbal behaviors and verbal communication)
• Neurologic functioning, including level of consciousness, orientation, and sensory and motor ability
• Mental status, including abstract ability, affect, concentration ability, insight and judgment, memory, mood, and thought content
• History of substance abuse
• Education and intelligence level
• Sociocultural background, including beliefs, norms, religion, and values
• Support systems, including clergy, family members, and friends

Defining characteristics
• Discomfort in social situations
• Family report of change in style of interaction
• Inability to receive or communicate satisfying sense of belonging, caring, interest, or shared history
• Use of unsuccessful or dysfunctional social interaction skills

Associated medical diagnoses (selected)
Alzheimer's disease, cerebrovascular accident, head injury, schizophrenia

Expected outcomes
• Patient will remain free of injury.
• Patient and family members will report concern about difficulties in social interaction.
• Patient will maintain orientation to person, place, and time.
• Patient's perceptions will be reality based.
• Patient and family members will participate in care and prescribed therapies.
• Patient will express needs and will communicate whether needs are met.

• Patient will regain appropriate neurologic function to extent possible.
• Patient will demonstrate effective social interaction skills in one-on-one and group settings.
• Patient and family members will identify and mobilize resources for rehabilitation and discharge planning as necessary.

Interventions and rationales
• Follow medical regimen to treat underlying condition. *Nurse is responsible for following medical regimen and working with doctor to plan appropriate care.*
• Take precautions to ensure safe and protected environment (provide side rails, help with out-of-bed activities, keep room free of clutter, and use physical restraints as necessary). *This reduces potential for patient injury.*
• Assess neurologic function and mental status every shift *to monitor changes in patient's status;* reorient patient as often as necessary:
– Call patient by name and say your name each time you interact with patient.
– Tell patient correct day, date, time, and place at least once a shift.
– Teach family members how to reorient patient, and help them do so.
– Ask family members to bring patient familiar objects from home, such as clock, radio, and photographs.
– Post structured schedule of daily activities in patient's room within visual range.
– Explain schedule to family members and other caregivers to provide consistency and continuity.
Reorienting patient and involving family members enhances patient's reality-testing ability and overall mental status. Scheduling daily routine narrows patient's frame of

reference, thereby decreasing potential for increased confusion.
• If delusions and hallucinations occur, don't focus on them; provide patient with reality-based information and reassure patient of safety. *This increases patient's ability to grasp reality and reduces fears associated with these disturbances.*
• Provide specific, non-care-related time with patient each shift to encourage social interaction. Begin with one-on-one interaction and increase to group interaction as patient's skills indicate. *Gradually increasing social interaction reduces patient's feeling of being overwhelmed and eliminates sensory input that may renew cognitive or perceptual disturbance.*
• Give positive reinforcement for appropriate and effective interaction behaviors (verbal and nonverbal). *This helps patient recognize progress and enhances feelings of self-worth.*
• Assist patient and family members in progressive participation in care and therapies. *This reduces feelings of helplessness and enhances patient's feeling of control and independence.*
• Initiate or participate in multidisciplinary patient-centered conferences to evaluate progress and plan discharge. In addition to patient and family members, conferences may include physical, occupational, and speech therapists; social worker; attending doctor; and other consultants, as necessary. *These conferences involve patient and family in cooperative effort to develop strategies for altering plan of care as necessary.*

Evaluations for expected outcomes
• Patient doesn't exhibit physical evidence of injury.
• Patient and family members express concern about patient's inability to interact normally.

• Neurologic assessment reveals that patient is oriented to person, place, and time.
• Patient's verbal responses and behavior don't indicate delusions or hallucinations.
• Patient and family members perform care-related procedures to extent possible.
• Patient uses words, gestures, or writing to communicate needs and whether needs are met.
• Patient maintains appropriate cognitive and perceptual functioning to extent possible.
• Patient communicates effectively in one-on-one and group settings.
• Patient and family members identify and contact available support resources as needed.

Documentation
• Patient's verbal and nonverbal behaviors
• Neurologic and mental status assessment
• Observations of patient's social interaction skills
• Interventions to facilitate appropriate and effective social interaction
• Patient's responses to nursing interventions
• Evaluations for expected outcomes

■ Social interaction impairment
related to sociocultural dissonance

Definition
Insufficient quantity or ineffective quality of social exchange

Assessment
• Reason for hospitalization (physiologic or psychiatric)

• Sociocultural background (beliefs, norms, rituals, and values)
• Usual pattern of social interaction, including dominant language, group participation, level of comprehension, nonverbal communication skills (such as drawing and gestures), and speech pattern
• Patient's position in family
• Support systems, including clergy, family members, and friends
• Education and intelligence level

Defining characteristics
• Discomfort in social situations
• Family report of change in style of interaction
• Inability to receive or communicate satisfying sense of belonging, caring, interest, or shared history
• Use of unsuccessful or dysfunctional social interaction skills

Associated medical diagnoses (selected)
This diagnosis can occur in any hospitalized patient separated from usual sociocultural environment. For example, in some European and Asian cultures, nonverbal means of communication (eye contact, touch) are considered an invasion of privacy; many Native Americans consider social interaction outside the family to be disloyal.

Expected outcomes
• Patient will provide information concerning cultural background.
• Patient will identify needs and will communicate (verbally or through behavior) whether needs are met.
• Patient will express understanding of care-related instruction.
• Patient and family members will participate in planning care.
• Patient will identify effective coping techniques to deal with sociocultural differences.

• Patient will express feelings of comfort and trust in interaction with caregivers.
• Patient will use resources outside normal sociocultural group as necessary.

Interventions and rationales
• Assign primary nurse to patient if possible. *Primary nursing provides consistency, enhances trust, and decreases potential for fragmented care.*
• Provide specific time (for example, 10 minutes each shift) to talk with patient and family members about sociocultural background. *In many cultural groups, trust develops slowly and may be hampered by lengthy interviews.*
• Explain care-related activities clearly, answering questions as accurately as possible. *This enhances patient's understanding of care-related procedures and facility routine.*
• Use an interpreter when necessary *to ensure effective communication for non-English-speaking patients.*
• Involve patient and family members in planning care, and encourage patient's participation in self-care on continuing basis. *This increases their sense of control and reduces feelings of helplessness and isolation.*
• Help patient identify and use effective social-interaction behaviors, such as increased eye contact, calling people by name, and asking questions. *Teaching patient effective interpersonal communication helps him function more effectively in social environment.*
• Demonstrate respect for patient's privacy, personal belongings, cultural norms, and religious beliefs and practices *to provide sensitive care to patients from varied cultural backgrounds.*

• Offer referral to other support systems (such as social services, financial counseling, home health care, mental health care, and professional care) if indicated. *This ensures comprehensive approach to patient's care.*

Evaluations for expected outcomes
• Patient provides information about culture, including values, attitudes, roles, and beliefs.
• Patient reports needs and gratification of these needs, either verbally or through behavior.
• Patient demonstrates care-related procedures.
• Patient and family members help develop plan of care.
• Patient specifies positive ways to cope with cultural differences.
• Patient communicates sense of security and demonstrates decrease in anxiety-related behaviors.
• Patient uses appropriate resources outside normal sociocultural group as needed.

Documentation
• Patient's and family members' perceptions of current situation
• Interventions to promote effective social interaction
• Patient's verbal and nonverbal responses to nursing interventions
• Evaluations for expected outcomes

■ Social isolation
related to altered state of wellness

Definition
Aloneness that patient perceives negatively; may be self-imposed or be perceived as being imposed by others; alternatively, may result from environmental factors

Assessment
• Reason for hospitalization (physiologic or psychiatric)
• Support systems available, including clergy, family members, and friends
• Functional ability
• Diversional interests
• Attitudes of family or friends toward patient
• Financial resources
• Occupation
• Education level
• Coping and problem-solving ability
• Self-esteem

Defining characteristics
• Culturally unacceptable behavior
• Description of lifestyle as solitary or circumscribed by membership in subculture
• Evidence of physical or mental handicap or altered state of wellness
• Expressed feelings of being different from others
• Expressed feelings of rejection or aloneness
• Expressed frustration over inability to meet expectations of others
• Inappropriate or immature interests or activities
• Insecurity in public
• Lack of family, friends, and social groups
• Lack of purpose in life
• Preoccupation with own thoughts
• Projection of hostility in voice and behavior
• Repetitive, meaningless actions
• Sad, dull affect
• Uncommunicative and withdrawn behavior, with poor eye contact

Associated medical diagnoses (selected)
Acquired immunodeficiency syndrome, Alzheimer's disease, amyotrophic lateral sclerosis, anorexia nervosa, Bell's palsy, bipolar disease (depressive phase), bulimia nervosa,

cerebrovascular accident, depression, diabetes mellitus, genital herpes, osteoporosis, Parkinson's disease, psoriasis, seizure disorders, spinal cord injuries, tuberculosis, urinary incontinence, viral hepatitis

Expected outcomes
• Patient will express feelings associated with social isolation.
• Patient will identify causes of social isolation and participate in developing plan for increasing social activity.
• Patient will interact with family members or friends.
• Patient will interact with caregivers.
• Patient will perform self-care activities independently.
• Patient will participate daily in meaningful diversional activity (specify).
• Patient will indicate social relationships have improved and negative feelings have diminished.
• Patient will achieve expected state of wellness.

Interventions and rationales
• Assign primary nurse to patient, if possible, *to provide continuity, enhance trust, and decrease potential for fragmented care.*
• Initiate trusting nurse-patient relationship *to help gain patient's confidence.*
• Provide honest and immediate feedback about patient's behavior *to help patient become aware of effects of behavior and to modify, verify, or correct patient's perceptions.*
• Help patient identify causes of social isolation *to identify patient's needs and guide planning of care.* Involve patient and family or friends in setting goals and planning care *to individualize plan of care and decrease patient's feelings of helplessness and isolation.*

• Encourage patient to perform such self-care activities as bathing, grooming, dressing, eating, and ambulating *to reduce feelings of helplessness and foster independent action.*
• Spend at least 15 minutes each shift with patient. Sit with patient and listen. *Listening communicates concern, interest, and acceptance and allows time for patient to collect thoughts and express feelings.*
• Arrange with patient for specific periods of appropriate planned diversional activity *to provide pleasure, increase feelings of self-worth, and decrease negative self-absorption.*
• Allow ample private time for patient to spend with family or friends *to demonstrate respect for patient and for patient's relationships with others.*
• Identify appropriate social agencies and support groups for patient and provide referrals *to ensure ongoing opportunities for patient to increase social interaction.*
• Educate patient and family about health care needs and treatment *to promote optimal health and well-being, thereby allowing for greater social activity.*

Evaluations for expected outcomes
• Patient expresses sadness, frustration, anxiety, and other feelings associated with social isolation.
• Patient identifies causes of social isolation and helps develop plan for increasing social activity.
• Patient interacts with family members or friends.
• Patient interacts with caregivers.
• Patient initiates self-care activities, such as bathing, dressing, eating, and grooming, to extent possible.
• Patient identifies at least three activities that provide enjoyment and participates in one activity daily.

• Patient reports decreased feelings of isolation and increased social interaction.
• Patient reports regaining physical and psychological health. Assessment data and perceptions of doctors and other caregivers confirm patient's reports.

Documentation
• Observations of patient's social interaction skills
• Causes of social isolation identified by patient
• Resources identified to help patient increase social interaction
• Interventions to encourage social interaction and patient's response
• Evaluations for expected outcomes

■ Spiritual distress

related to separation from religious and cultural ties

Definition
Separation or alienation from religious traditions or values

Assessment
• Religious ties and practices
• Religious commitment
• Visits (church members, family members, or clergy)

Defining characteristics
• Anger toward God
• Change in behavior and mood (anger, crying, withdrawal, anxiety)
• Desire for spiritual assistance
• Displaced anger toward religious representatives
• Expressed concern about meaning of life and death, belief systems, and relationship with deity

• Expressed inner conflicts about beliefs
• Inability to participate in usual religious practices
• Questioning of meaning of own existence
• Questioning of meaning of suffering
• Questioning of moral and ethical implications of therapeutic regimen

Associated medical diagnoses (selected)
This diagnosis may be seen in any hospitalized patient, depending on the individual and circumstances.

Expected outcomes
• Patient will communicate conflict about beliefs.
• Patient will identify source of spiritual conflict.
• Patient will specify whatever spiritual assistance he needs.
• Patient will discuss beliefs about religious practices.
• Patient will identify coping techniques to deal with spiritual discomfort.
• Patient will express feelings of spiritual comfort.

Interventions and rationales
• Listen for cues about patient's feelings ("Why did God do this to me?" or "God is punishing me"). *Active listening demonstrates involvement with patient and allows you to hear important messages indicating spiritual distress.*
• Approach patient in nonjudgmental way *to focus on patient's feelings without evaluating them as right or wrong, good or bad.*
• Acknowledge patient's spiritual concerns, and encourage expression of thoughts and feelings *to help build therapeutic relationship.*
• Help patient concretely define problem causing inner conflict. *This is first*

step in developing strategies for resolving conflicts.

• Arrange for visits by clergy, as appropriate, *thereby using spiritual care resources to help patient.*

• Encourage patient to continue religious practices during hospitalization; do whatever you must to facilitate this. For example:

– If patient is accustomed to reading Scripture and doesn't have Bible, try to get one.

– If Jewish male wears yarmulke, allow him to continue wearing it if possible.

– In cases in which patient's religious traditions prohibit or require certain foods, make every effort to communicate these needs to dietary department and see that they're honored.

These measures demonstrate support and convey caring and acceptance to patient.

• Communicate and collaborate with patient's clergy person or with hospital chaplain, when this is appropriate. *This ensures consistent care and provides more complete database.*

• Arrange for patient to have at bedside objects that provide spiritual comfort (such as Bible, prayer shawl, pictures, statues, and rosary beads). *Items of spiritual significance may influence patient's ability to reduce conflict.*

• Provide privacy during patient's visits with clergy person or chaplain *to demonstrate respect for patient's relationship with clergy.*

Evaluations for expected outcomes

• Patient expresses feelings of uncertainty or ambivalence related to spiritual beliefs.

• Patient states specific causes of spiritual distress.

• Patient requests spiritual assistance if needed.

• Patient discusses usual religious practices, including rituals, prayers, values, and beliefs.

• Patient reports decreased spiritual discomfort.

• Patient expresses desire to resume usual religious practices.

Documentation

• Patient's expressions of concern about spiritual matters, whether direct or indirect

• Observations about patient's spiritual distress or well-being

• Interventions carried out to promote spiritual comfort

• Observations about patient's responses to interventions

• Evaluations for expected outcomes

■ Spiritual distress

related to situational crisis

Definition

Separation or alienation from religious tradition or values

Assessment

• Reason for hospitalization

• Religion or church affiliation

• Patient's usual and current perception of faith and religious practices

• Available spiritual support persons (such as minister, priest, and rabbi)

Defining characteristics

• Anger toward God

• Change in behavior and mood (anger, crying, withdrawal, anxiety)

• Desire for spiritual assistance

• Displaced anger toward religious representatives

• Display of gallows humor

• Expressed concern about meaning of life and death, belief systems, and relationship with deity
• Expressed inner conflicts about beliefs
• Questioning of meaning of own existence
• Questioning of meaning of suffering
• Questioning of moral and ethical implications of therapeutic regimen

Associated medical diagnoses (selected)
This nursing diagnosis can apply to any individual with strong religious beliefs and practices. It's particularly evident in those experiencing the threat of death. Examples of medical diagnoses include acute respiratory failure, end-stage renal disease, melanoma, metastatic disease, and myocardial infarction.

Expected outcomes
• Patient will express feelings about usual and current religious beliefs.
• Patient will identify areas of ambivalence and conflict resulting from current situation.
• Patient will state an understanding of grief process and its stages.
• Patient will use effective coping strategies to ease spiritual discomfort.
• Patient will seek appropriate support persons (family members, priest, minister, or rabbi) for assistance.

Interventions and rationales
• Approach patient in an accepting, nonjudgmental manner *to demonstrate unconditional positive regard for patient.*
• Acknowledge patient's spiritual concerns and encourage expression of feelings *to help build therapeutic relationship.*
• Encourage patient to provide information about religious beliefs and practices. *Acquiring this initial database is first step in nursing process.*
• Instruct patient on stages of grieving and on emotions and behaviors common to each stage. *This promotes understanding and encourages feelings of normalcy.*
• Provide for continuation of patient's religious practices (allow for specific religious materials or clothing; respect dietary restrictions if possible). *These measures demonstrate support and convey caring and acceptance to patient.*
• Facilitate visits from clergy and provide privacy during visits *to demonstrate respect for patient's relationship with clergy.*
• Encourage patient to discuss concerns with clergy, *thereby using expert spiritual care resources to help patient.*

Evaluations for expected outcomes
• Patient discusses feelings about spiritual or religious beliefs.
• Patient specifies areas of spiritual conflict, such as anger toward God, questioning of usual beliefs about life after death, and guilt associated with loss of faith.
• Patient communicates understanding of grief process and its stages.
• Patient continues religious practices that ease spiritual distress.
• Patient makes use of available resources for spiritual assistance.

Documentation
• Patient's verbal and nonverbal communication of spiritual discomfort
• Stage of anticipatory grief as indicated by behavior
• Interventions to promote spiritual comfort
• Patient's response to nursing interventions
• Evaluations for expected outcomes

■ Spiritual distress, risk for

Definition
Potential for separation from religious and cultural ties

Assessment
• Health history, including debilitating disease (for example, rheumatoid arthritis); terminal illness; recurrent cancer; conditions that alter body image (for example, burns and scars); relapse or exacerbation of neurologic disease (for example, multiple sclerosis); alcoholism, depression, and drug abuse; and major traumatic injury
• Impact of current illness, injury, or disability on lifestyle
• Spiritual status, religious affiliation, beliefs, and practices; relationship with spiritual authority (minister, priest, or rabbi); and beliefs about life, death, and suffering
• Psychological status, including perception of self, body image, problem-solving ability, and coping mechanisms; sources of support (family, partner, friends, caregivers); perception of medical diagnosis or health problem (progression, severity, prognosis, and treatment options); reaction to illness, injury, or disability; self-image, mood, behavior, motivation, and energy level; stressors (finances, job, marital or partner discord, losses through death or separation); expressions of grief; and changes in sleep pattern
• Family status, including socioeconomic status; quality of relationships; communication patterns; methods of conflict resolution; ability of family members to meet patient's physical, emotional, and social needs; and family goals

Risk factors
• Altered ability to carry out religious practices because of illness or hospitalization
• Disturbance in belief system
• Lack of support with regard to religious beliefs and practices
• Loss of appetite, disturbed sleep pattern, and changes in exercise and eating patterns
• Recent experience with a life-threatening event (such as major traumatic injury or burn) with resulting disability
• Statements indicating doubt and spiritual emptiness
• Strong religious beliefs or practices

Associated medical diagnoses (selected)
Advanced metastatic disease, end-stage renal disease, exacerbation or relapse of multiple sclerosis, myocardial infarction, recurrent cancer, terminal illness, uncontrolled seizure disorder

Expected outcomes
• Patient will discuss current religious beliefs.
• Patient will discuss effects of illness, injury, or disability on beliefs and spiritual practices.
• Patient will use healthy coping techniques to maintain his spiritual well-being.
• Patient will express feelings of spiritual well-being.
• Patient will be supported in efforts to pursue spirituality in coping with illness, injury, or disability.
• Patient will reach out to family members, partner, priest, minister, rabbi, or others for assistance.

Interventions and rationales
• Assess importance of spirituality in patient's life and in coping with illness. Note participation in religious

rituals and practices and patient's desire to discuss spiritual beliefs. Assess impact of illness, injury, or disability on patient's spiritual outlook. *Accurate assessment of meaning of spirituality for patient is necessary before intervening.*
• Assess patient's desire for help in coping with spiritual concerns *to determine extent to which patient is motivated to address spiritual concerns and open to help from others.*
• Express your willingness to discuss spirituality if patient desires *to reduce isolation and to bring spiritual issues into open.*
• Encourage patient to talk about religious beliefs and practices. Listen actively to patient's discussion of spiritual concerns *to foster open discussion.*
• Encourage patient to express feelings related to his recent life-threatening experience *to help him clarify and cope with his feelings.*
• Communicate to patient that you accept his expression of spiritual concerns, even if his feelings are angry and negative *to reassure him that his feelings are valid.*
• Show willingness to pray with patient, if he wishes, *to provide spiritual support.*
• Maintain nonjudgmental manner. Keep conversation focused on patient's spiritual values *to maintain therapeutic value of your interaction with patient.*
• Provide for continuation of patient's religious practices (for example, help patient obtain ritual items and respect dietary restrictions, if possible) *to demonstrate support and convey caring and acceptance to patient.*
• Arrange for visits by clergy, as appropriate, *to provide patient with expert spiritual support.* Provide privacy during visits.

• Collaborate with patient's clergyman or facility's chaplain to develop a plan to integrate spiritual interventions into patient's care *to ensure continuity of care.*

Evaluations for expected outcomes
• Patient discusses current religious beliefs.
• Patient discusses effects of illness, injury, or disability on beliefs and spiritual practices.
• Patient uses healthy coping techniques to maintain spiritual well-being.
• Patient expresses feelings of spiritual well-being.
• Patient is supported in efforts to pursue spirituality in coping with illness, injury, or disability.
• Patient reaches out to family members, partner, priest, minister, rabbi, or others for assistance.

Documentation
• Patient's statements regarding religious beliefs and practices
• Patient's statements indicating effect of current crisis on spiritual outlook
• Patient's statements indicating which rituals and practices help maintain spiritual well-being
• Patient's statements indicating effectiveness of interventions to promote spiritual well-being
• Visits with selected spiritual authority
• Additional referrals to clergy or chaplain
• Evaluations for expected outcomes

■ Suffocation, risk for

related to external factors

Definition

Accentuated risk of accidental suffocation (inadequate air available for inhalation)

Assessment

• Health history, including accidents, allergies, exposure to pollutants, falls, hyperthermia, hypothermia, poisoning, seizures, sensory or perceptual changes (auditory, gustatory, kinesthetic, olfactory, tactile, or visual), and trauma
• Circumstances of current situation that might lead to injury
• Neurologic status, including level of consciousness, mental status, and orientation
• Laboratory studies, including clotting factors, hemoglobin and hematocrit, platelet count, and white blood cell count

Risk factors

• Access to unattended bathtub or pool (children)
• Consumption of large mouthfuls of food
• Discarded refrigerators or freezers with doors still in place
• Fuel-burning heater used in area without ventilation
• Habit of smoking in bed
• Household gas leaks
• Low-strung clotheslines
• Pacifier hung around neck (infant)
• Plastic bags or small objects within reach of children
• Propped bottle or pillow in infant's crib
• Vehicle left running in closed garage

Associated medical diagnoses (selected)

Acute respiratory failure, asphyxia, chronic obstructive pulmonary disease, drug overdose, inhalation injuries, near-drowning episode

Expected outcomes

• Patient's airway will remain patent at all times.
• Patient's vital signs will remain within normal parameters.
• Patient and family members will demonstrate knowledge of safety measures to prevent suffocation.

Interventions and rationales

• Monitor and record respiratory status. *Changes in parameters (such as respiratory rate, cough, sputum production, and skin color) may indicate airway obstruction.*
• Monitor and record neurologic status. *Headache, depression, apathy, memory loss, poor muscle coordination, fatigue, stupor, and loss of consciousness may indicate hypoxia.*
• Monitor vital signs and report changes. *Tachycardia and slight rise in blood pressure may indicate hypoxia. Reduced heart rate and loss of consciousness indicate advanced hypoxia.*
• Position patient on side or position head and neck to prevent relaxed neck muscles from obstructing airway. *This allows maximal chest expansion and prevents aspiration and airway obstruction.*
• Check all ventilator connections every 30 minutes if patient on mechanical ventilation *to ensure patient receives proper amount of oxygen at appropriate volume and rate.*
• Check ventilator alarms every 30 minutes and after suctioning *to ensure proper alarm function.*
• Suction airway as needed *to prevent secretion accumulation.* Do this only

as needed *to prevent tracheal irritation.*
• Provide patient and family members with information about safety practices *to enable patient and family members to take active role in care and ensure performance of safety measures.*

Evaluations for expected outcomes
• Patient's airway remains free of obstruction.
• Patient's vital signs remain within normal parameters.
• Patient and family members demonstrate safety measures to prevent suffocation.

Documentation
• Patient's statements that indicate potential for injury
• Physical findings
• Observations or knowledge of unsafe practices
• Interventions performed to prevent injury
• Patient's response to nursing interventions
• Evaluations for expected outcomes

■ Suffocation, risk for

related to internal factors

Definition
Accentuated risk of accidental suffocation (inadequate air available for inhalation)

Assessment
• Health history, including accidents, allergies, exposure to pollutants, falls, hyperthermia, hypothermia, poisoning, seizures, sensory or perceptual changes (auditory, gustatory, kines-

thetic, olfactory, tactile, or visual), and trauma
• Circumstances of current situation that might lead to injury
• Neurologic status, including level of consciousness, mental status, and orientation
• Laboratory studies, including clotting factors, hemoglobin and hematocrit, platelet count, and white blood cell count

Risk factors
• Cognitive or emotional difficulties
• Injury or disease process
• Lack of safety education
• Lack of safety precautions
• Reduced motor abilities
• Reduced olfactory sensation

Associated medical diagnoses (selected)
Multisystem trauma, placement under general anesthesia, sedation

Expected outcomes
• Patient will avoid accidental suffocation.
• Patient's vital signs will remain within normal parameters.
• Patient and family members will demonstrate knowledge of safety measures to prevent suffocation.

Interventions and rationales
• Observe, record, and report falls, seizures, and unsafe practices *to ensure implementation of appropriate interventions.*
• Monitor and record respiratory status. *Changes in parameters (such as respiratory rate, cough, sputum production, and skin color) may indicate airway obstruction.*
• Monitor and record neurologic status. *Headache, depression, apathy, memory loss, poor muscle coordination, fatigue, stupor, and loss of consciousness may indicate hypoxia.*

• Monitor vital signs and report changes. *Tachycardia and slight rise in blood pressure may indicate hypoxia. Reduced heart rate and loss of consciousness indicate advanced hypoxia.*

• Position patient on side or position head and neck to prevent relaxed neck muscles from obstructing airway. *This allows maximal chest expansion and prevents aspiration and airway obstruction.*

• Obtain suction equipment, assemble, and keep at bedside *to assure equipment readiness in case of need.*

• Suction as needed *to keep upper and lower airways clear and to stimulate cough reflex to enhance sputum removal.* Do this only as needed *to prevent tracheal irritation.*

• Provide patient and family members with information about safety practices *to enable patient and family members to take active role in care and ensure performance of safety measures.*

Evaluations for expected outcomes

• Patient doesn't experience accidental suffocation.

• Patient's vital signs remain within normal parameters.

• Patient or caregiver demonstrates safety measures that prevent suffocation.

Documentation

• Patient's statements about situation that indicate potential for injury

• Physical findings

• Record of falls, seizures, and unsafe practices

• Interventions that reduce risk of injury

• Patient's response to nursing interventions

• Evaluations for expected outcomes

■ Surgical recovery, delayed

Definition

Following surgery, a delay in recovery due to postoperative complications or patient's preoperative condition

Assessment

• Age

• Sex

• Reason for surgery

• Type and length of surgical procedure

• Current health status, including weight, vital signs, temperature, nutritional status, integumentary status, neurologic status, cardiovascular status, musculoskeletal status, and pain status

• Laboratory studies, including complete blood count, electrolyte studies, urinalysis, blood cultures, blood coagulation studies, immunologic and serologic tests, liver function tests, cardiac enzyme studies, and arterial blood gas levels

• Health history, including past surgical procedures, food or drug allergies, substance abuse, mental illness, and chronic metabolic or systemic disease (diabetes mellitus; cardiovascular, hepatic, renal, or immunologic disease; coagulation disorders; and splenic or bone marrow disorders)

• Mobility status

• Complications during surgical procedure, such as hemorrhage, drop in blood pressure, and cardiac arrhythmias

• Current medical treatments, including radiation therapy, chemotherapy, antibiotic or antifungal therapy, steroid treatment, anticoagulant or thrombolytic therapy, and immunosuppressive therapy

• Social support, including family status and presence of caregiver and health care provider

Defining characteristics
• Delay in resumption of activities such as eating
• Delay in return to normal bowel and bladder habits
• Delay in return to usual mobility level
• Less than optimal nutritional status
• One or more postoperative complications, including shock, hemorrhage, deep vein thrombosis, pulmonary embolism, respiratory complications, urine retention, intestinal obstruction, postoperative psychosis or depression, severe pain, or infection

Associated medical diagnoses (selected)
Amputation, bowel resection, craniotomy, gastrectomy, hip replacement, open heart surgery, organ transplantation

Expected outcomes
• Vital signs and laboratory values will return to patient's normal limits.
• Wound healing will begin; incision site will appear free from signs and symptoms of infection.
• Patient will exhibit improved nutritional status.
• Postoperative complications will be resolved.
• Patient will resume normal mobility status.
• Patient will seek and obtain emotional support from family and friends.
• Patient will resume normal eating, bowel, and bladder habits.
• Patient and family members will use community resources that are available to assist after discharge.

Interventions and rationales
• Assess for factors that may be related to delay in recovery, such as respiratory complications and infection. Document and report assessment findings *to facilitate development of an individualized plan of care.*
• Monitor wound healing. Assess surgical site for signs of infection, such as erythema, edema, pain, drainage, odor, incision approximation, and intact sutures. *Infection may delay surgical recovery.*
• Monitor nutritional status by evaluating intake, output, and integumentary status. Consult dietitian regarding changes to diet *to promote optimal nutritional status. Optimal nutritional status promotes wound healing and provides energy for recovery.*
• Assess all body systems *to detect signs and symptoms of postoperative complications that can delay surgical recovery.*
• Follow proper pulmonary regimen *to facilitate resolution of respiratory complications, if present. Respiratory complications can lead to decreased oxygen levels, which can slow wound healing and delay mobility.*
• Following postoperative bleeding, monitor hemoglobin and hematocrit levels. *Bleeding can lead to low hemoglobin and hematocrit levels, reducing the ability of red blood cells to carry oxygen, which can hinder wound healing and diminish patient's energy level.*
• If patient is suffering from psychosis, continue to reorient him during the postoperative recovery period. Report any psychological reaction, such as development of depression-like symptoms. *Psychosis or depression may delay recovery.*
• Administer pain medication as prescribed. *A patient in pain will not move or cough and deep breathe as*

needed for timely recovery from surgery.

• As appropriate, make sure someone is available to walk with patient or that such devices as walkers or canes are available. Don't allow patient to ambulate alone until steady. *Assistance (from staff or with devices) enhances safety and encourages patient to improve mobility without fear of falling. Mobility will facilitate improved strength, help prevent such complications as deep vein thrombosis and, ultimately, enhance recovery.*

• Make sure patient wears support stockings or a sequential compression device, such as Venodyne, *to facilitate venous return and prevent deep vein thrombosis.*

• Monitor bowel and bladder activity. Report urine retention and absent or decreased bowel sounds. *Abnormal bowel and bladder patterns slow surgical recovery. Continual assessment ensures prompt treatment and enhances recovery.*

• Make sure patient and family members have access to community resources to assist with recovery when patient returns home *to ensure ongoing recovery.*

• Educate patient and family members regarding appropriate care after discharge *to help them carry out medication and treatment regimens.*

Evaluations for expected outcomes

• Vital signs and laboratory values return to patient's normal limits.

• Wound healing begins; incision site appears free from signs and symptoms of infection.

• Patient exhibits improved nutritional status.

• Postoperative complications are resolved.

• Patient resumes normal mobility status.

• Patient seeks and obtains emotional support from family and friends.

• Patient resumes normal eating, bowel, and bladder habits.

• Patient and family members use community resources that are available to assist after discharge.

Documentation

• Assessment findings
• Type and length of operation
• Type of anesthesia
• Intraoperative complications
• Postoperative complications (as they occur)
• Results of ongoing multisystem assessment
• Treatment regimen (for normal recovery and complications)
• Patient's and family members' progress in following treatment regimen
• Teaching provided to patient and family members
• Discharge plans
• Evaluations for expected outcomes

■ Swallowing impairment

related to neuromuscular impairment

Definition

Inability to move food, fluid, or saliva from mouth through esophagus

Assessment

• History of neuromuscular, cerebral, or respiratory disease
• Age
• Sex
• Nutritional status, including appetite, dietary intake, hydration, current weight, and change from normal weight

• Neurologic status, including barium swallow; chest X-ray; cognition; esophageal video fluoroscopy; gag reflex; level of consciousness; memory; motor ability; orientation; symmetry of face, mouth, and neck; sensory function; and tongue movement

Defining characteristics
• Evidence of aspiration, nasal reflux, heartburn, or epigastric pain
• Observed evidence of difficulty in swallowing, including choking, coughing, vomiting, decreased gag reflex, and stasis of food in oral cavity

Associated medical diagnoses (selected)
Bell's palsy, cerebrovascular accident, head injury, laryngectomy, maxillofacial trauma

Expected outcomes
• Patient will show no evidence of aspiration pneumonia.
• Patient will achieve adequate nutritional intake.
• Patient will maintain weight.
• Patient will maintain oral hygiene.
• Patient and caregiver will demonstrate correct feeding techniques to maximize swallowing.
• Patient and caregiver will list strategies to prevent aspiration.

Interventions and rationales
• Elevate head of bed 90 degrees during mealtimes and for 30 minutes after completion of meal *to decrease risk of aspiration.*
• Position patient on side when recumbent *to decrease risk of aspiration.*
• Keep suction apparatus at bedside; observe and report instances of cyanosis, dyspnea, or choking. *Symptoms indicate presence of material in lungs.*

• Monitor intake and output and weight daily until stabilized. Establish intake goal — for example, "Patient consumes ___ ml of fluid and ___% of solid food." Record and report any deviation from this. *Evaluating calorie and protein intake daily allows any necessary modifications to begin quickly.*
• Consult with dietitian to modify patient's diet, and conduct calorie count as needed *to establish nutritional requirements.*
• Consult with dysphagia rehabilitation team, if available, *to obtain expert advice.*
• Provide mouth care three times daily *to promote comfort and enhance appetite.*
• Keep oral mucous membrane moist by frequent rinses; use bulb syringe or suction, if necessary, *to promote comfort.*
• Lubricate patient's lips *to prevent cracking and blisters.*
• Encourage patient to wear properly fitted dentures *to enhance chewing ability.*
• Serve food in attractive surroundings; encourage patient to smell and look at food. Remove soiled equipment, control smells, and provide quiet atmosphere for eating. *A pleasant atmosphere stimulates appetite; food aroma stimulates salivation.*
• Teach patient and family about positioning, dietary requirements, and specific feeding techniques, including facial exercises (such as whistling), using a short straw to provide sensory stimulation to lips, tipping head forward to decrease aspiration, applying pressure above lip to stimulate mouth closure and swallowing reflex, and checking oral cavity frequently for food particles (remove if present). *These measures allow patient to take an active role in maintaining health.*

Evaluations for expected outcomes
• Patient shows no evidence of aspiration pneumonia. Breath sounds remain bilaterally clear; fever, chills, purulent sputum, and rapid shallow respirations are absent.
• Patient's fluid and dietary intake remains within established daily limits.
• Patient's weight remains stable.
• Patient demonstrates appropriate oral hygiene practices.
• Patient and caregiver demonstrate feeding techniques to maximize swallowing and minimize risk of complications.
• Patient and caregiver list strategies to prevent aspiration.

Documentation
• Patient's expressions of feelings about current situation
• Observations of weight, swallowing ability, intake and output, and oral hygiene
• Patient's response to nursing interventions
• Instructions about diet monitoring and feeding techniques
• Evaluations for expected outcomes

■ Thermoregulation, ineffective

related to trauma or illness

Definition
Fluctuations in body temperature caused by thermoregulatory disturbances

Assessment
• History of current illness
• Medication history
• Neurologic status, including level of consciousness, mental status, motor status, and sensory status
• Cardiovascular status, including blood pressure, capillary refill time, electrocardiogram, heart rate and rhythm, pulses (apical and peripheral), and temperature
• Respiratory status, including arterial blood gas measurements, breath sounds, and rate, depth, and character of respirations
• Integumentary status, including color, temperature, and turgor
• Fluid and electrolyte status, including blood urea nitrogen, intake and output, serum electrolytes, and urine specific gravity
• Laboratory studies, including clotting factors, hemoglobin and hematocrit, platelet count, and white blood cell count

Defining characteristics
• Cyanotic nail beds
• Increased capillary refill time
• Fluctuations in body temperature above or below normal range
• Flushed skin
• Hypertension
• Increased respiratory or heart rate
• Mild shivering
• Moderate pallor
• Piloerection
• Seizures or convulsions
• Warm or cool skin

Associated medical diagnoses (selected)
Cerebrovascular accident, drug overdose, encephalitis, head injury, heart failure, hemorrhage, hyperthermia, hypothermia, inhalation injuries, near-drowning episode, Reye's syndrome, sepsis

Expected outcomes
• Patient will maintain body temperature at normothermic levels.
• Patient will not shiver.
• Patient will express feelings of comfort.

• Patient will have warm, dry skin.
• Patient will maintain heart rate and blood pressure within normal range.
• Patient will exhibit no signs of compromised neurologic status.
• Patient and family members will voice an understanding of health problem.

Interventions and rationales

• Monitor body temperature every 4 hours, more often if indicated. Record temperature and route (keep in mind that baseline depends on route). *Monitoring determines effectiveness of therapy or if intervention is required and allows accurate comparison of data.*
• Monitor and record neurologic status every 8 hours. Report any changes to doctor. *Changes in level of consciousness can result from tissue hypoxia related to altered tissue perfusion. Hyperthermia increases cerebral edema and thus intracranial pressure (ICP); hypothermia depresses metabolic rate.*
• Monitor and record heart rate and rhythm, blood pressure, and respiratory rate every 4 hours. *Hyperthermia may create hypoxia by increasing oxygen demand, which results from increased tissue metabolism (metabolism increases 7% with each increase of 1° F [0.56° C]). This, in turn, results in faster breathing and rising pulse rate.*
• Administer analgesics, antipyretics, and medications that prevent shivering, as indicated. Monitor and record effectiveness. *Antipyretics help reduce fever. Shivering tends to retard lowering of body temperature.*
• If patient develops excessive fever, take the following steps:
– Remove blankets; place loincloth over patient.
– Apply ice bags to axilla and groin.

– Initiate tepid water sponge bath.
– Use cooling blanket if temperature rises above ____. Cool patient to ____.
These measures help to reduce excessive fever.
• Maintain hydration:
– Monitor intake and output.
– Administer parenteral fluids as ordered.
– Determine patient's fluid preference. Keep oral fluids at bedside and encourage patient to drink. *These measures help maintain fluid balance. Keeping preferred fluids at bedside allows patient to actively participate in prescribed treatment.*
• Maintain environmental temperature at comfortable setting:
– Ensure that all metal and plastic surfaces that come into contact with patient's body are covered.
– Use warm blankets.
– Ensure that linen and clothing are clean and dry.
Temperature of external environment affects ease of body temperature regulation.
• Instruct patient and family members about the following:
– signs and symptoms of altered body temperature
– precautionary measures to avoid hypothermia or hyperthermia
– adherence to other aspects of health care management to help normalize temperature (such as dietary habits and measures to prevent increased ICP)
– rationale for treatment.
These measures allow patient to take active role in health maintenance.

Evaluations for expected outcomes

• Patient's temperature remains within normal parameters.
• Patient doesn't shiver.

• Patient indicates feeling of comfort, either verbally or through behavior.
• Patient's skin remains warm and dry.
• Patient's heart rate and blood pressure remain within normal parameters.
• Patient doesn't exhibit signs of neurologic complications associated with extremes in temperature.
• Patient and family state understanding of health problem.

Documentation
• Patient's needs and perceptions of current problem
• Physical findings
• Intake and output
• Patient's response to nursing interventions
• Evaluations for expected outcomes

■ Thought process alteration

related to loss of memory

Definition
Inability to process thoughts accurately and correctly

Assessment
• History of neurologic disorder, head injury, or psychiatric disorder
• Neurologic status, including cognition, insight and judgment, memory, motor ability, orientation, and sensory ability
• Self-care status, including ability to perform activities of daily living and safety practices
• Psychosocial status, including coping mechanisms, family members, occupation, personality, and stressors (finances, job, or marital discord)

Defining characteristics
• Cognitive dissonance
• Distractibility
• Egocentricity
• Hypervigilance or hypovigilance
• Inaccurate interpretation of environment
• Inappropriate, fantasy-based thinking
• Memory impairment

Associated medical diagnoses (selected)
Alzheimer's disease, Cushing's syndrome, dissociative disorder

Expected outcomes
• Patient will maintain orientation to person, place, and time.
• Patient will sustain no harm or injury.
• Patient will maintain current health status.
• Patient and family members will voice feelings and concerns.
• Family members will communicate understanding of care required by patient.
• Family members will demonstrate appropriate coping skills.
• Family members will identify available health resources.

Interventions and rationales
• Observe patient's thought processes every shift. Document and report any changes. *Changes may indicate progressive improvement or decline in underlying condition.*
• Perform prescribed treatment for underlying condition; monitor progress. Report any favorable or adverse responses to treatment *to assess effectiveness of treatment.*
• Orient patient to reality as needed:
– Call patient by name.
– Tell patient your name.
– Provide background information (place, time, and date) frequently

throughout day. Reinforce verbal reports with visual aids such as reality orientation board.
– Orient patient to environment, including sights, sounds, and smells.
– Use television or radio purposefully to augment orientation.
Reality orientation techniques foster patient's awareness of self and environment.
• Keep items in same places. *Consistent, stable environment reduces confusion, decreases frustration, and aids successful completion of activities of daily living.*
• Ask family members to provide patient with photos (labeled with name and relationship on back), favorite belongings, and cards. *Belongings promote sense of continuity and memory and create sense of security and comfort.*
• Protect patient from sensory overload; allow frequent rest periods. *Sensory overload may increase confusion; frequent rest periods help avoid fatigue.*
• Provide structured environment for patient. List daily routine and post in patient's room *to provide continuity of care.*
• Communicate patient's skill level to all personnel *to preserve level of independent functioning.*
• Spend time daily with patient to encourage memories and discussion of past events. Encourage patient's participation in reminiscence groups. *Remote memory may be intact. Discussion of past events promotes sense of continuity, aids memory, and promotes feelings of security. Joining in reminiscence groups provides diversional activity and may increase socialization skills.*
• Correct patient privately for inappropriate behavior; walk patient to room or initiate another behavior.

This avoids feelings of embarrassment and frustration. Redirection and engagement in previously successful activities increase patient's sense of accomplishment and reinforce desirable behavior.
• Provide close supervision *to prevent patient from wandering off or incurring harm.* Instruct family members on how to maintain safe home environment for patient. *Patient may be unable to consider own safety needs or risks.* Place patient's photo or name on door to room *to aid memory and help patient find room.*
• Encourage patient to voice feelings and concerns about loss of memory. *This helps reduce anxiety and ventilate frustrations and promotes acceptance of need for supervision and treatment regimen.*
• Help family members develop necessary coping skills to deal with patient. *Family members need these skills to deal with patient's neurologic or psychiatric impairment and potential for deterioration in patient's condition.*
• Demonstrate reorientation techniques to family members, and provide time for supervised return demonstrations. *Informed family members are better prepared to cope with patient with altered thought processes.*
• Help family members identify community support group (such as stroke club and Alzheimer's group) *to assist in coping with effects of illness.*

Evaluations for expected outcomes
• Neurologic assessment indicates that patient is oriented to person, place, and time.
• Patient doesn't show evidence of harm or injury.
• Patient maintains current health status.

• Patient and family members express concerns about loss of memory and effect on patient's lifestyle.
• Family members report understanding of care required by patient.
• Family members demonstrate appropriate interventions, reorientation techniques, and coping skills.
• Family members identify and contact at least one support group to assist in coping with effects of illness.

Documentation
• Patient's and family members' expressions of concern and feelings about patient's altered thought processes
• Observations of patient's altered thought processes and response to treatment for underlying condition
• Patient's response to nursing interventions
• Instructions to family members and their understanding of instructions and demonstrated ability to care for patient
• Referrals made for patient and family members
• Evaluations for expected outcomes

■ Thought process alteration
related to physiologic causes

Definition
Inability to process thoughts accurately and correctly

Assessment
• Reason for hospitalization
• Mental status, including abstract thinking (ask patient to interpret a proverb); general information (ask patient to name five states); insight concerning the present situation; judg-

ment (ask patient to solve a simple problem); memory for recent and remote past; and orientation to person, place, and time
• Neurologic status, including level of consciousness, motor ability, and sensory ability
• Sleep habits
• Ability to perform activities of daily living
• Safety hazards
• Medication history
• Dietary and nutritional status
• History of alcohol consumption

Defining characteristics
• Cognitive dissonance
• Distractibility
• Egocentricity
• Hypervigilance or hypovigilance
• Inaccurate interpretation of environment
• Inappropriate, fantasy-based thinking
• Memory impairment

Associated medical diagnoses   (selected)
Acute renal failure, acute respiratory failure, brain tumor, cirrhosis, diabetic ketoacidosis, drug overdose, encephalitis, esophageal varices, head injury, hemodialysis, hepatic coma, hyperosmolar hyperglycemic nonketotic syndrome, hypothyroidism, metabolic acidosis, metabolic alkalosis, nutritional deficiencies

Expected outcomes
• Patient will remain safe and protected from injury.
• Patient will maintain awareness of need for assistance.
• Patient will maintain orientation to person, place, and time.
• Patient will perform activities of daily living with assistance.
• Patient's laboratory values will stay within normal range.

• Patient will receive treatment for physiologic causes of altered thought processes, resulting in restoration of thought processes.
• Family members will identify partial or complete confusion.
• Family members will make arrangements for home care.

Interventions and rationales
• Monitor and record vital signs every 4 hours, neurologic status every shift, and laboratory values as ordered (including blood glucose and alcohol, arterial blood gases, and electrolytes). *Vital signs allow assessment of patient for indications of infection or complication. Neurologic assessment and laboratory studies may reveal progressive improvement or decline of underlying condition.*
• Carry out medical regimen to treat underlying causes of mental status deterioration. *Medical regimen aims to alleviate causes of mental status deterioration.*
• Address patient by name and tell him your name. *Reality orientation techniques foster patient's awareness of self and environment.*
• Give short, simple explanations to patient each time you do something *to avoid confusion and aid successful task completion.*
• Schedule nursing care to provide quiet times. *Rest periods help prevent sensory overload.*
• Mention time, place, and date frequently throughout day. Have clock and calendar where patient can easily see them; refer to these aids when orienting patient. *Reality orientation techniques foster patient's awareness of self and environment.*
• Keep patient's things in same places as much as possible. *A consistent, stable environment reduces confusion and frustration and aids successful*
completion of activities of daily living.
• Use appropriate safety measures to protect patient from injury. Avoid physical restraints if possible. *Patient may be unable to consider own safety needs or risks. Restraints may agitate patient.*
• Ask family members to bring photos (label with name and relationship on back), favorite articles, and cards. *Familiar items help create more secure environment for patient.*
• Plan patient's routine, and follow it as consistently as possible. *A consistent daily plan aids task completion and reduces confusion and frustration.*
• Speak slowly and clearly. Allow ample time for patient to respond. *This reduces confusion and frustration and aids task completion.*
• Encourage patient to perform activities of daily living. Be patient and specific in providing instructions. Allow time for patient to perform each task. *This enhances patient's self-esteem and helps prevent complications of inactivity.* Limit new skills or tasks to small, critical units *to aid learning.* If needed, provide extensive supervision and repetition *to allow patient to master new tasks.*
• Encourage family members to share stories and discuss familiar things with patient. *Remote memory often remains intact. Sharing stories and familiar things promotes sense of continuity, aids memory, and creates a sense of security and comfort.*
• Support family members in attempts to interact with patient. *Family members need positive reinforcement for visiting and attempting to interact with patient.*
• Allow time before and after visits for family members to express feelings. *Expression of feelings in sup-*

portive environment helps family members cope with patient's illness.
• Refer family members to appropriate resources to plan for patient care after discharge. *This helps provide comprehensive approach to postdischarge care.*

Evaluations for expected outcomes
• Patient remains free from injury.
• Patient maintains awareness of need for assistance.
• Neurologic assessment reveals that patient is oriented to person, place, and time.
• Patient performs activities of daily living with assistance.
• Patient's laboratory values remain within set limits.
• Patient receives treatment for physiologic causes of altered thought processes.
• Family members identify partial or complete confusion as indicator of patient's changing physiologic state.
• Family members contact appropriate resources to arrange for home care.

Documentation
• Patient's verbal responses
• Observations of patient's behavior indicating altered thought processes
• Interventions that focus on helping patient maintain reality orientation
• Responses of patient to nursing interventions
• Evaluations for expected outcomes

■ Thought process alteration

related to psychological causes

Definition
Inability to process thoughts accurately and correctly because of a fixed, false belief that can't be corrected by logic

Assessment
• Age
• Reason for hospitalization, including patient's perception of problem, recent stressors, and changes in somatic functioning
• Mental status, including insight about current situation, judgment (ask patient to solve a simple problem), abstract thinking (ask patient to interpret a proverb), general information (ask patient to name five states), mood, affect, recent and remote memory, thought processes, thought content, and orientation to person, place, and time
• Physical appearance, including manner of dress, personal hygiene, posture, and gait
• Communication status, including attitude toward interviewer, body language, and facial expressions
• Sleep habits
• Self-care status, including ability to perform activities of daily living and safety practices
• Physiologic status, including medication history (response, effectiveness, and adverse reactions) and history of substance abuse (type and effect on mental status)
• Dietary and nutritional status
• Laboratory studies, including toxicology screening and blood chemistry
• Diagnostic tests, including computed tomography scan and electroencephalogram

Defining characteristics
• Cognitive dissonance
• Distractibility
• Egocentricity
• Hypervigilance or hypovigilance
• Inaccurate interpretation of environment

• Inappropriate, fantasy-based thinking
• Memory impairment

Associated medical diagnoses (selected)

Affective disorders, anxiety disorder, bipolar disease (manic or depressive phase), delusional disorder, dementia, hyperthyroidism, hypochondriasis, intoxication, posttraumatic stress disorder, schizophrenia

Expected outcomes

• Patient will identify internal and external factors that trigger delusional episodes.
• Patient will identify and perform activities that decrease delusions.
• Patient will practice distraction techniques to reduce anxiety before the onset of delusion.
• Patient will interact with others without becoming delusional.
• Patient will consider alternative interpretation of situation without becoming unduly hostile or anxious.
• Patient will recognize how delusional system meets his interpersonal needs.
• Patient will recognize symptoms and comply with therapeutic regimen.

Interventions and rationales

• Project nonjudgmental and trusting attitude toward patient through active listening. *Patient must trust you to talk openly about delusions and feelings.*
• Orient patient to reality as needed:
– Call patient by name.
– Tell patient your name.
– Provide background information (place, time, and date) frequently throughout day, verbally and visually, using reality orientation board.
– Orient patient to environment, including sights, sounds, and smells.

Reality orientation techniques foster patient's awareness of self and environment.
• Explain to patient with organic delusions that distorted thinking is caused by temporary biochemical changes *to help decrease patient's anxiety level.*
• Don't argue, reason with, or challenge patient with nonorganic delusions; instead, provide comfort and support. *Attempts to correct delusional beliefs will increase anxiety.*
• Explore events that trigger delusions. Discuss anxiety associated with triggering events. *Exploring these topics will help you understand dynamics of patient's delusional system.*
• Without arguing or agreeing, acknowledge plausible elements of delusion. Make such statements as "I don't doubt that your family brought you to the hospital. However, I have no reason to believe that they're cooperating with the CIA to kill you." *Delusions usually have some basis in reality. By conveying acceptance of delusions but not belief in them, you can better help patient.*
• Once dynamics of delusions are understood, discourage repetitive talk about delusions and refocus conversation on patient's underlying feelings. *As patient begins to learn to cope with underlying feelings, delusions will become less necessary.*
• Help patient find other means to meet emotional needs that he attempts to fulfill through delusions. *Delusions usually decrease when needs are met in other ways.*
• Educate patient and family members about signs and symptoms of illness and effects of medication. *Collaboration with family members promotes continuity of care.*
• Refer family members to appropriate resources to plan for patient care after discharge. *This helps provide*

comprehensive approach to postdis-charge care.

Evaluations for expected outcomes
• Patient describes at least two situations that increase delusions.
• Patient describes two self-initiated activities to decrease delusions.
• Patient gives two concrete examples of anxiety-reducing techniques.
• Patient interacts with primary nurse 30 minutes per day without delusional content.
• Patient discusses two reality-based interpretations of events that are validated by others.
• Patient communicates insight about his delusional system.
• Patient and family members discuss delusional symptoms and adverse effects of medication.

Documentation
• Patient's statements indicating type, number, and intensity of delusions
• Observations about environmental factors that precipitate delusional behavior
• Interventions that focus on helping patient maintain reality orientation
• Patient's response to nursing interventions
• Referrals
• Evaluations for expected outcomes

■ Tissue integrity impairment

related to peripheral vascular changes

Definition
Damage to mucous membranes or to corneal, integumentary, or subcutaneous tissue

Assessment
• History of peripheral vascular disease or surgery
• Age
• Sex
• Integumentary status, including color, skin care practices, temperature, tenderness, texture, turgor, and edema
• Cardiovascular status, including blood pressure, cardiac output, occupation, patient and family history of cardiovascular disease, peripheral pulses, and smoking history
• Nutritional status, including dietary patterns, laboratory tests, serum lipids level, serum protein level, and change from normal weight
• Neurologic status, including motor function and sensory pattern

Defining characteristics
• Damaged or destroyed tissue

Associated medical diagnoses (selected)
Buerger's disease (thromboangiitis obliterans), chronic or acute arterial insufficiency, peripheral vascular disease, pregnancy, pressure ulcer, Raynaud's disease, venous insufficiency or venous stasis

Expected outcomes
• Patient will attain relief from immediate signs and symptoms (pain, ulcers, color changes, and edema).
• Patient will maintain collateral circulation.
• Patient will voice intent to stop smoking.
• Patient will voice intent to follow specific management routines after discharge.

Interventions and rationales
• Provide scrupulous foot care. Administer and monitor treatments according to institutional protocols. *Foot care prevents fungal infections*

and ingrown toenails, stimulates circulation, and allows detection of signs and symptoms you should report to doctor immediately.
• Instruct patient to avoid pressure on popliteal space. For example, say "Don't cross your legs or wear constrictive clothing." *This avoids reducing arterial blood supply and increasing venous congestion.*
• Encourage adherence to exercise regimen as tolerated. *Exercise improves arterial circulation and venous return by promoting muscle contraction and relaxation.*
• Educate patient about risk factors and prevention of injury. Refer patient to smoking cessation program. *Teaching about factors influencing peripheral vascular disease and prevention of tissue damage helps prevent complications.*
• Maintain adequate hydration. Monitor intake and output and record daily weights. *Adequate hydration reduces blood viscosity and decreases risk of clot formation.*
• If patient has venous insufficiency, apply antiembolism stockings or intermittent pneumatic compression stockings, removing them for 1 hour every 8 hours or according to institutional protocol. Elevate patient's feet when sitting and elevate foot of bed 6″ to 8″ when lying down. *These measures promote venous return and decrease venous congestion in lower extremities.*
• If patient has arterial insufficiency, elevate head of bed 6″ to 8″ when lying down. *This increases arterial blood supply to extremities.*

Evaluations for expected outcomes
• Patient attains relief from immediate symptoms:

– Patient's feet don't show signs of infection, ingrown toenails, or impaired circulation.
– Patient maintains normal skin turgor.
– Patient's mucous membranes remain moist.
– Patient maintains balanced intake and output.
– Patient's weight remains stable.
– Patient's vital signs remain within normal parameters.
• Patient uses interventions (antiembolism stockings or intermittent pneumatic compression stockings, elevation of feet, and elevation of head of bed) to promote arterial and venous circulation.
• Patient states rationale for quitting smoking and begins program to stop smoking.
• Patient describes plan to incorporate prescribed treatment program into postdischarge routine, including avoiding risk factors and activities that contribute to vascular compression (such as popliteal compression, leg crossing, and wearing constrictive clothing), following exercise program, and practicing foot care.

Documentation
• Patient's expressions of feelings about current situation
• Observations of skin color, turgor, temperature, and ulcer size
• Patient's response to nursing interventions
• Evaluations for expected outcomes

■ Tissue integrity impairment

related to physical, chemical, or electrical hazards during surgery

Definition
Damage to mucous membranes or to corneal, integumentary, or subcutaneous tissue

Assessment
• Reason for, type of, and anticipated length of surgery
• Health status, including age, sex, weight, vital signs, and nutritional, integumentary, cardiovascular, neurologic, respiratory, and psychosocial status
• Mobility status, including range of motion
• Patient's description of pain, numbness, and tingling
• Laboratory studies, including hematocrit and hemoglobin, complete blood count, blood coagulation studies, immunologic and serologic tests, electrolytes, urinalysis, liver function tests, and serum protein levels
• Wound classification (clean, clean-contaminated, contaminated, or dirty)
• Allergies to medications, irrigation solutions, or cleaning solutions
• Health history, including altered immunologic status, malnutrition, and chronic metabolic or systemic disease (diabetes mellitus; cancer; cardiovascular, renal, or hepatic diseases; coagulation disorders; blood dyscrasias; or hematopoietic diseases)
• Current medical treatments, including chemotherapy and radiation, steroid, immunosuppressive, anticoagulant, thrombolytic, and antibiotic therapy

• Presence of infection, draining wounds, bruises, shear ulcers, or pressure ulcers

Defining characteristics
• Damaged or destroyed tissue

Associated medical diagnoses (selected)
This diagnosis may occur in conjunction with any surgical procedure.

Expected outcomes
• Patient will express feelings of comfort.
• Patient will remain free from alteration in tissue integrity related to physical hazards.
• Patient will remain free from alteration in tissue integrity related to chemical hazards.
• Patient will remain free from alteration in tissue integrity related to electrical hazards.

Interventions and rationales
• Document and report results of preoperative nursing assessment. Identify factors that predispose patient to impaired tissue integrity. *Complete nursing assessment allows development of individualized plan of care.*
• Classify surgical wound according to degree of contamination of wound and surrounding tissue. *Classifying surgical wound facilitates assessment of risk of wound infection and subsequent tissue injury.*
• Use padding, special mattresses, and support devices during surgery. *These measures reduce undue pressure and decrease risk of impaired tissue integrity.*
• Maintain environmental temperature at comfortable setting. Offer blankets if needed. *Comfortable environment reduces shivering, muscle tension, and reactive pain. These metabolic*

stressors can affect rate of cellular repair.
• Monitor patient for signs of hypothermia (shivering, cool skin, pallor, piloerection, and increased heart rate) *to determine need to implement warming measures.*
• Warm prepping and irrigation solutions *to prevent reduction in patient's temperature.*
• For infants (1 year old or younger), use warming unit and head covering. *Infants have immature thermoregulatory mechanisms and don't retain adequate body heat.*
• When using pneumatic tourniquets, pad skin, place cuff so skin is free of wrinkles, set to proper pressure, and monitor inflation time. *Improper tourniquet use can impair circulatory status of affected limb.*
• Check patient history for sensitivity or allergy to prepping solution. Clean and prepare skin incision site with nonirritating solutions. *Nonallergenic, physiologic prepping and cleaning solutions reduce risk of tissue reaction and injury.*
• To avoid pooling of solutions, use towels or pads during prep. When using sprays, shield patient's face and eyes. *Pooled solutions can produce skin maceration. Sprays may damage cornea and mucous membranes.*
• Ensure adequate aeration of items sterilized by ethylene oxide gas. *Residual gas is toxic to tissue.*
• Rinse chemosterilized items adequately. *Residual chemosterilization solutions are toxic to tissue.*
• Remove powder from gloves. *Glove powder may cause granulomas and other reactions.*
• Perform sponge, sharp, and instrument counts according to protocol, account for other items (such as bulldogs, umbilical tapes, and vessel loops), and document results. *Re-tained objects may produce foreign body reaction or injury to tissue.*
• Follow manufacturer's instructions for applying medications and chemical agents, such as glutaraldehyde and methylmethacrylate. *Agents may be toxic when applied directly to tissue.*
• Use physiologic solutions or prescribed medications for irrigation or topical application. *Nonphysiologic solutions may cause interstitial edema and cellular injury or death.*
• Check label, route, dose, and expiration date of each medication with scrub nurse *to reduce risk of error.*
• When administering medications, record drug, dosage, and route. Document verbal orders and have doctor cosign. *Documentation helps to reduce medication errors.*
• Inspect all electrical, mechanical, and air-powered equipment before use. Operate equipment according to manufacturers' instruction *to reduce chances of patient injury.*
• Apply electrosurgical dispersive pad to clean, dry skin near operative site. Avoid bony prominences, hairy surfaces, scar tissue, and areas of poor circulation. *Proper placement reduces risk of burn injury.*
• When using hypothermia or hyperthermia blanket, avoid creases, place sheet between skin and blanket, and set and maintain correct temperature. Pad extremities during hypothermia therapy. *Proper use protects against tissue injury.*

Evaluations for expected outcomes
• Patient has minimal or no shivering, muscle tension, or reactive pain.
• Patient doesn't develop rash, edema, bruises, discoloration, redness, skin breakdown, or other signs of altered tissue integrity related to physical hazards.

• Patient doesn't develop allergic or toxic reaction to sterilizing agents, glove powder, irrigating solutions, medications, or chemical agents and has little or no reaction to cleaning procedure.
• Patient doesn't develop reddened or discolored areas at site of electrosurgical grounding pad or adjacent tissue or any other signs of postoperative alteration in tissue integrity related to electrical hazards.

Documentation
• Results of preoperative nursing assessment
• Surgical procedure
• Type of anesthesia
• Preoperative and postoperative diagnosis
• Wound classification
• Preexisting conditions that increase risk of tissue injury
• Nursing interventions performed to protect tissue integrity
• Medications administered
• Patient's status on discharge to postanesthesia care unit
• Skin condition on discharge to postanesthesia care unit
• Presence of lines, tubes, catheters, and drains
• Type of wound closure and dressing
• Evaluations for expected outcomes

■ Tissue integrity impairment

related to radiation

Definition
Damage to mucous membranes or to corneal, integumentary, or subcutaneous tissue

Assessment
• History of radiation therapy or exposure
• Age
• Sex
• Integumentary status, including color, distribution of hair, mucous membranes, skin care practices, temperature, tenderness, texture, turgor, scars, lesions, and wounds
• Nutritional status, including dietary patterns and change from normal weight

Defining characteristics
• Damaged or destroyed tissue

Associated medical diagnoses (selected)
Accidental radiation exposure, bladder cancer, bone sarcomas, brain tumors, endometrial cancer, head or neck cancer, Hodgkin's disease, leukemia, lung cancer, lymphomas, ovarian cancer, prostate cancer, radiation therapy

Expected outcomes
• Patient will show no irritation or skin breakdown in irradiated areas.
• Patient's ulcerated areas will heal.
• Patient will maintain adequate fluid and nutritional intake.
• Patient and family members will communicate understanding of skin care regimen, medication use, and need for adequate fluid and nutritional intake.

Interventions and rationales
• Keep skin clean, dry, and exposed to air as much as possible *to promote healing of excoriated areas and prevent infection.*
• Avoid constrictive clothing *to reduce risk of friction and decreased blood flow.* Avoid exposure to sun *to reduce risk of sunburn and possible skin cancer.*

• Avoid nonprescription ointments, creams, and warm packs *because they may increase skin irritation and possible radiation (if they contain heavy metals).*
• Avoid extremes of hot and cold on affected skin areas *to prevent further irritation and skin breakdown.*
• Avoid vigorous scrubbing of irradiated areas *to minimize skin breakdown.*
• Use nonadhesive dressings *to avoid pulling on affected skin.*
• Provide oral hygiene as indicated *to promote comfort and reduce risk of infection.* Use soft toothbrush *to reduce risk of bleeding.*
• Use cornstarch over unbroken areas *to decrease itching and friction.*
• Provide regular change of position, bed cradle, or pressure-relieving devices, when indicated. *These measures reduce friction and risk of skin breakdown on affected body parts.*
• Inspect skin every shift. Report areas of breakdown and signs of infection *to ensure early treatment.*
• Follow institutional protocol for treating infected lesions. Administer creams, antibiotic ointments, and irrigation solutions, as ordered, and monitor effectiveness. *Protocols are established to meet specific patient needs.*
• Administer analgesics as ordered, and monitor effectiveness. *Analgesics reduce pain resulting from skin problems.*
• Consult dietitian to assist with diet, emphasizing diet high in protein, calories, vitamins, and minerals to promote tissue repair and prevent catabolism. *Positive nitrogen balance promotes wound healing.*
• Administer antiemetics as ordered *to promote patient comfort and adequate nutrition.* Monitor effectiveness.

• Educate family and patient in skin care regimen, medication administration, and nutritional needs *to promote compliance and maintain tissue integrity.*

Evaluations for expected outcomes
• Irradiated areas don't show signs of cracking, oozing, sloughing, or infection.
• Patient's ulcerated areas heal.
• Patient maintains adequate fluid and nutritional intake.
• Patient and family members demonstrate proper skin care and medication administration techniques and communicate understanding of importance of maintaining nutritional intake.

Documentation
• Patient's expression of feelings
• Physical findings
• Interventions performed to prevent irritation or breakdown and to promote healing
• Patient's response to nursing interventions
• Patient's and family members' response to education
• Evaluations for expected outcomes

■ Tissue perfusion alteration

related to hypovolemia

Definition
Decrease in cellular nutrition and respiration because of decreased capillary blood flow

Assessment
• History of trauma, surgery, or condition resulting in fluid volume depletion

• Cardiovascular status, including blood pressure, capillary refill time, central venous pressure (CVP), electrocardiogram, heart rate and rhythm, heart sounds, hemoglobin (Hb) and hematocrit (HCT), jugular filling, peripheral pulses, and tilt test
• Respiratory status, including breath sounds and respiratory rate and rhythm
• Renal status, including intake and output, urine specific gravity, and weight
• Neurologic status, including level of consciousness (LOC), mental status, and orientation
• Integumentary status, including color, moisture, and temperature

Defining characteristics
• Alterations of cardiopulmonary, cerebral, gastrointestinal, peripheral, or renal tissue perfusion

Associated medical diagnoses (selected)
Hemothorax, hyperosmolar hyperglycemic nonketotic syndrome, osteomyelitis, spontaneous or therapeutic abortion

Expected outcomes
• Patient will maintain hemodynamic stability: pulse greater than _____ and less than _____; systolic blood pressure greater than _____; CVP greater than _____; and mean arterial pressure greater than _____.
• Patient will maintain fluid balance, with intake equal to output.
• Patient will maintain urine specific gravity within normal parameters.
• Patient will maintain respiratory rate within ±5 of baseline.
• Patient will maintain skin integrity.
• Patient will remain oriented to person, place, and time.
• Patient will not have crackles or rhonchi.

• Patient will exhibit improved circulation.
• Patient's Hb, HCT, white blood cell (WBC) count, and coagulation studies will remain within normal parameters.
• Patient will communicate understanding of medical regimen, diet, medications, and activity restrictions.

Interventions and rationales
• Monitor heart rate and rhythm, CVP, and blood pressure every hour until stable, then every 2 hours; record and report any changes above or below established limits. Monitor skin color and temperature every 2 hours. *Decreased heart rate, CVP, and blood pressure can indicate hypovolemia, which leads to increased tissue perfusion. Blanched or mottled, cool skin indicates decreased tissue perfusion.*
• Monitor respiratory rate and depth every hour until stable, then every 2 to 4 hours. Record and report changes outside established limits. *Increased respiratory rate is a compensatory mechanism of tissue hypoxia that can result from decreased tissue perfusion.*
• Measure and record urine output every hour until output exceeds 30 ml/hour, then every 2 to 4 hours. *If patient has no history of renal disease, urine output is a good indicator of tissue perfusion. Decreased or absent urine output usually indicates poor renal perfusion.*
• Perform appropriate measures to treat underlying cause of hypovolemia. *Patient must receive treatment for underlying cause to avoid continued or worsening hypovolemia.*
• Administer fluid or blood as ordered. Monitor for such adverse reactions as fluid overload and transfusion reactions. *Vigorous fluid or blood resuscitation can cause fluid overload,*

cardiac decompensation, or both. Transfusion reactions can occur during blood administration and may further compromise patient's condition.
• Initiate measures to help improve perfusion:
– Keep patient warm, but don't overheat. *Warmth aids vasodilation, which improves tissue perfusion.*
– Relieve anxiety and pain. *Anxiety and pain can cause sympathetic reaction that results in vasoconstriction and decreased tissue perfusion.*
– Elevate lower extremities *to increase arterial blood supply and improve tissue perfusion.*
• Perform pulmonary toilet as ordered; follow facility policies. *Properly performed pulmonary toilet helps prevent pulmonary edema, respiratory complications, and possible respiratory failure.*
• Test urine specific gravity every shift; record and report abnormalities. *Concentrated urine with increased specific gravity indicates hypovolemia.*
• Weigh patient daily before breakfast and record weight. *Weighing patient daily helps predict total fluid status; weighing at regular times gives better indication of weight changes.*
• Change patient's position regularly, follow turning schedule, inspect skin every shift, and record and report any potential areas of breakdown. *These measures avoid decreased tissue perfusion and risk of skin breakdown.*
• Watch for signs of confusion and disorientation. Reorient patient to reality frequently: call him by name; tell him your name; and orient him to surroundings (sounds, smells, and sights). *Change in LOC may result from decreased tissue perfusion. Reorientation helps patient recall person, place, and time and may also reduce fear and anxiety.*
• Monitor Hb, HCT, WBC count, and coagulation studies. Frequency depends on severity of patient's problem. *Monitoring helps establish blood replacement requirements, fluid status, blood viscosity level, and anticoagulation therapy parameters and allows detection of infection.*
• Educate patient in medical regimen (diet, medications, and activity restrictions). *This allows patient to take active role in health maintenance.*

Evaluations for expected outcomes
• Patient's hemodynamic measurements remain within established limits.
• Patient's daily fluid intake equals output.
• Patient's urine specific gravity remains within normal parameters.
• Patient maintains respiratory rate within established limits.
• Patient maintains normal skin color and doesn't exhibit redness or skin breakdown.
• Patient can identify self and state time of day, date, and location.
• Patient has clear lung fields on auscultation.
• Patient exhibits improved circulation as evidenced by strong, palpable peripheral pulses; normal skin color and temperature; and normal blood pressure and other hemodynamic measurements.
• Patient's Hb, HCT, WBC count, and coagulation studies remain within normal parameters.
• Patient communicates understanding of medical regimen, diet, medications, and activity restrictions.

Documentation
• Patient's expression of concern about hemodynamic status

• Observations of vital signs, intake and output, status of skin, and level of orientation
• Patient's response to nursing interventions
• Instructions about diet, monitoring, and medical regimen
• Evaluations for expected outcomes

■ Tissue perfusion alteration (cardiopulmonary)

related to decreased cellular exchange

Definition

Decrease in cellular nutrition and respiration because of decreased capillary blood flow

Assessment

• Health history, including presence of diabetes mellitus, high cholesterol, hypertension, obesity, smoking, stressful lifestyle, and family history of heart disease
• Neurologic status, including level of consciousness, mental status, and orientation
• Cardiovascular status, including blood pressure; heart rate and rhythm; heart sounds; peripheral pulses; skin color, temperature, and turgor; hepatojugular reflux; jugular vein distention; and history of congenital heart disease or valvular disorder
• Diagnostic tests, including chest X-ray, regular and exercise electrocardiogram (ECG), echocardiogram, nuclear isotope studies, and cardiac angiography
• Respiratory status, including arterial blood gas (ABG) levels, auscultation of breath sounds, and respiratory rate and depth

• Renal status, including intake and output, serum electrolyte levels, urine specific gravity, and weight
• Integumentary system, including cyanosis, pallor, and peripheral edema

Defining characteristics

• Abnormal ABG levels
• Arrhythmias
• Bronchospasms
• Capillary refill time greater than 3 seconds
• Chest pain
• Chest retraction
• Dyspnea
• Nasal flaring
• Respiratory rate outside of acceptable parameters
• Sense of impending doom
• Use of accessory muscles

Associated medical diagnoses (selected)

Abruptio placentae, acute respiratory failure, adult respiratory distress syndrome, anaphylactic shock, anemia, aortic aneurysm, aortic stenosis or insufficiency, cardiac arrhythmias, cardiogenic shock, cerebral aneurysm, chemotherapy, chronic obstructive pulmonary disease, coronary artery disease, cyanotic maternal cardiac disease, ectopic pregnancy, esophageal varices, head injury, heart failure, hemothorax, joint replacement, leukemia, liver transplantation, lung abscess, mitral stenosis or insufficiency, mitral valve prolapse, multisystem trauma, myocardial infarction, pericarditis, pneumonia, pneumothorax, postpartum hemorrhage, pseudomembranous colitis, pulmonary edema, pulmonary embolus, shock, uterine rupture

Expected outcomes

• Patient will attain hemodynamic stability, with pulse not less than _____

beats/minute and not greater than ____ beats/minute and blood pressure not less than ____ mm Hg and not greater than ____ mm Hg.
• Patient won't exhibit arrhythmias.
• Patient's skin will remain warm and dry.
• Patient's heart rate will remain within prescribed limits while he carries out activities of daily living.
• Patient will maintain adequate cardiac output.
• Patient will modify lifestyle to minimize risk of decreased tissue perfusion.

Interventions and rationales
• Monitor and document vital signs (heart rate, blood pressure, and pulmonary artery pressure) every 1 hour until stable, then every 2 hours. Report any findings outside prescribed limits. *Decreased heart rate and blood pressure may indicate increased arteriovenous exchange, which leads to decreased tissue perfusion.*
• Administer fluids as needed *to maintain preload.*
• Monitor skin color and temperature every 2 hours. Assess for signs of skin breakdown. *Cool, blanched, mottled skin and cyanosis may indicate decreased tissue perfusion.*
• Monitor respiratory rate and breath sounds. Document findings. *Increased respiratory rate may indicate that patient is compensating for tissue hypoxia.*
• Monitor ECG for changes in heart rate and rhythm. *Altered heart rate and rhythm may affect tissue perfusion and possibly indicate a life-threatening crisis.*
• Maintain oxygen therapy, as ordered, *to maximize oxygen exchange in alveoli and at cellular level.*

• Encourage patient to change position and participate in activity, as condition permits, *to enhance vital capacity and avoid lung congestion and skin breakdown.*
• Encourage frequent rest periods *to conserve energy and maximize tissue perfusion.*
• Monitor creatine kinase, lactate dehydrogenase, and ABG levels. *Abnormal findings may indicate tissue damage or decreased oxygen exchange in lungs.*
• Inform patient about:
– risk factors for heart and lung disease
– proper use of nitroglycerin
– proper use of medications and possible adverse reactions
– benefits of a low-fat, low-cholesterol diet
– need to avoid straining with bowel movements
– benefits of quitting smoking.
Effective teaching encourages patient to take active role in health maintenance.

Evaluations for expected outcomes
• Patient attains hemodynamic stability within specified parameters.
• Patient shows no signs of arrhythmias.
• Patient's skin remains warm, dry, and intact.
• Patient's heart rate remains within prescribed parameters while he carries out activities of daily living.
• Patient maintains adequate cardiac output.
• Patient describes plans to modify lifestyle to minimize cause of decreased tissue perfusion.

Documentation
• Observations of physical findings
• Observation of patient's response to activity

• Verbal statements and behavior indicating patient's perception of health problems and health needs
• Nursing interventions performed and patient's response
• Patient's demonstration of skills associated with maintaining diet, adhering to medication regimen, maintaining activity level, and managing stress
• Evaluations for expected outcomes

■ Tissue perfusion alteration (cerebral)

related to decreased cellular exchange

Definition

Decrease in cellular nutrition and respiration because of decreased capillary blood flow

Assessment

• Vital signs
• History of the event, including presenting problem, history of development, chief complaint, associated vascular problems, and associated psychosocial problems (which may contribute to behavioral changes)
• Neurologic status, including level of consciousness; Glasgow Coma Scale score (eye, motor, and verbal response); orientation; pupil size; response to light and accommodation; motor activity; strength, positioning, and appearance of all four extremities; presence of reflexes (corneal, gag, swallowing, and Babinski's); nuchal rigidity; weakness; numbness; headaches; dizziness; dysphagia; slurred speech; seizure activity; posturing; and Cushing's triad (increased systolic pressure, decreased diastolic pressure, and decreased heart rate)

• Respiratory status, including shallow or irregular breathing pattern

Defining characteristics

• Altered mental status
• Behavioral changes
• Change in motor response
• Difficulty swallowing
• Pupillary changes
• Speech abnormalities
• Weakness or paralysis in extremity

Associated medical diagnoses (selected)

Acoustic neuroma, brain abscess, cerebral aneurysm, cerebrovascular accident, craniotomy, esophageal varices, head injury, lupus erythematosus, multiple myeloma, multisystem trauma, postpartum hemorrhage, pregnancy-induced hypertension, shock, transient ischemic attack, uterine rupture

Expected outcomes

• Patient will maintain or improve current level of consciousness.
• Patient's intracranial pressure (ICP) will remain between ____ mm Hg and ____ mm Hg.
• Patient's blood pressure will remain high enough to maintain cerebral perfusion pressure but low enough to prevent increased bleeding or cerebral swelling.
• Patient will not develop hypercarbia.
• Patient will remain free from pain.
• Patient will stay in quiet environment.
• Patient will maintain balanced intake and output.
• Patient will perform activities of daily living with maximum level of mobility and independence.
• Risk factors for altered cerebral perfusion and complications will be reduced as much as possible.

Interventions and rationales

• Conduct neurologic assessment every 1 to 2 hours initially, then every 4 hours once patient becomes stable *to screen for changes in level of consciousness and neurologic status.*

• Take vital signs every 1 to 2 hours initially, then every 4 hours once patient becomes stable *to detect early signs of decreased cerebral perfusion pressure or ICP.*

• Take patient's temperature at least every 4 hours. *Hyperthermia causes increased ICP; hypothermia causes decreased cerebral perfusion pressure.*

• Elevate head of patient's bed 30 degrees *to promote venous drainage, thereby reducing cerebral edema.*

• Keep head in neutral alignment *to keep carotid flow unobstructed, thereby promoting perfusion.*

• If patient score of less than 10 on Glasgow Coma Scale, hyperventilate patient on ventilator in accordance with facility policy *to increase oxygenation and prevent cerebral swelling and hypercarbia.*

• Monitor for Cushing's triad, *which indicates impending herniation.*

• Keep environment and patient quiet. Sedate patient if necessary. Space nursing actions. *These measures reduce increased ICP.*

• If patient has potentially compromised airway, use antiemetics or nasogastric suction *to prevent nausea and vomiting, which may lead to increased ICP and aspiration.*

• Institute physical and occupational rehabilitation *to increase patient's ability for independent functioning.*

• Prepare patient's discharge plan *to make sure patient continues to receive necessary rehabilitative care after discharge.*

• Maintain adequate nutrition *to promote tissue healing, oxygenation, and metabolism.*

• Maintain routine bowel and bladder function and administer diuretics such as mannitol, as ordered, *to prevent increased ICP.*

• Monitor hematocrit and hemoglobin and report abnormalities *to prevent ischemia.*

• Take measures to ward off infection *to prevent increased metabolic and oxygen demands that can interfere with brain's metabolic needs.*

• Measure accurate intake and output *to prevent volume overload or deficit.*

• Instruct patient and family members in ways to minimize risk factors for altered tissue perfusion *to increase probability that healthy adaptation will continue.*

• Administer histamine$_2$-receptor antagonists, as ordered, *to prevent development of stress ulcers.*

Evaluations for expected outcomes

• Patient regains sense of orientation.
• Patient's ICP remains within prescribed limits.
• Patient's blood pressure remains high enough to maintain cerebral perfusion pressure but low enough to prevent increased bleeding or cerebral swelling.
• Patient doesn't develop hypercarbia.
• Patient will remain free from pain.
• Patient's environment remains quiet.
• Patient maintains balanced intake and output.
• Patient performs activities of daily living with maximum level of mobility and independence.
• Risk factors are reduced as much as possible.

Documentation

• Observations of vital signs and neurologic findings

- Intake and output
- Patient's response to treatment of underlying condition
- Medications administered and patient's response
- Nursing interventions performed and patient's response
- Family members' response to education and nursing interventions
- Patient's response to physical and occupational therapy
- Evaluation of plan of care
- Evaluations for expected outcomes

■ Tissue perfusion alteration (gastrointestinal)

related to decreased cellular exchange

Definition

Decrease in cellular nutrition and respiration caused by decreased capillary blood flow

Assessment

- Vital signs
- GI status, including abdominal distention; nausea and vomiting; usual bowel habits; change in bowel habits; stool characteristics (color and consistency); presence or absence of occult blood; history of GI problems, disease, or surgery; pain; inspection of abdomen; palpation for tenderness; auscultation of bowel sounds; and abdominal girth
- Nutritional status, including dietary intake, change from normal diet, current weight, and change from normal weight
- Laboratory studies, including complete blood count, serum electrolytes, and liver profile
- Medications (especially those with vasoconstrictive properties)

Defining characteristics

- Abdominal distention
- Abdominal pain or tenderness
- Hypoactive or absent bowel sounds
- Nausea

Associated medical diagnoses (selected)

Colitis, colostomy, duodenal ulcer, gastric cancer, gastric ulcer, ileostomy, intestinal obstruction, liver transplantation, multisystem trauma, pseudomembranous colitis

Expected outcomes

- Patient's intake and output will remain within normal limits.
- Patient's normal bowel function will return.
- Patient will have no more nausea and vomiting.
- Patient and family members will express understanding of need to modify dietary habits.
- Patient will discuss with doctor possible need to alter medication regimen.
- Patient will express understanding of benefits of regular exercise in maintaining routine bowel habits.
- Patient's abdominal pain will subside.
- Patient's laboratory values will return to normal.
- Patient's vital signs will remain stable.
- Patient will express understanding of need to check stools for occult blood.

Interventions and rationales

- Monitor intake and output every 4 hours *to prevent hypovolemia, which may cause poor perfusion and subsequent ischemia.*
- Monitor patient's vital signs, including temperature, every 4 hours *to detect possible hypovolemia and screen for infection.*

• Monitor for increased abdominal tenderness *to detect early signs of increased ischemia.*
• Monitor bowel sounds and report changes. *Changes in bowel sounds may signal impending obstruction or return to normal bowel function.*
• Monitor complete blood count, serum electrolytes, and liver functions daily, as ordered, *to detect ischemia caused by low hematocrit and hemoglobin, monitor for improvement in organ function, and screen for infection.*
• Administer prescribed pain medications sparingly. *Many narcotics decrease gastric motility.* Use pain distraction techniques if possible *to provide relief with nonpharmacologic methods.*
• Implement nasogastric suctioning *to eliminate nausea and vomiting, thereby reducing risk of inflammation.*
• Establish bowel regimen *to prevent constipation.*
• When appropriate, provide alternative methods of nutrition, such as total parenteral nutrition, *to allow bowel rest and recovery and to prevent ischemic episodes after meals.*
• Start enteral feedings slowly and increase them gradually *to allow recovering bowel to adapt to increased tissue demands.*
• Teach patient and family members about dietary habits that may have contributed to poor perfusion *to prevent future episodes of altered GI tissue perfusion.*
• Encourage patient to eat small, frequent meals, to increase fluid intake, and to eat more high-fiber foods (such as cruciferous vegetables and whole grains) *to prevent constipation and potential obstruction.*
• Teach patient importance of routine exercise. *Routine exercise stimulates peristalsis.*

• Instruct patient to limit alcohol and fat intake *to preserve adequate liver function.*
• Teach patient to check all stools for occult blood *to monitor for blood loss, which may indicate anemia.*
• Encourage patient to discuss with doctor need to avoid medications that have vasoconstrictive properties or that decrease peristalsis. *Such medications may contribute to decreased perfusion.*
• Teach patient to rest after meals *to allow adequate blood circulation, thereby assuring oxygen supply for increased metabolic demands.*

Evaluations for expected outcomes
• Patient's intake and output stay within normal limits.
• Patient's normal bowel function returns.
• Patient's nausea and vomiting cease.
• Patient and family members recognize need to modify dietary habits
• Patient expresses understanding of need to alter medication regimen.
• Patient recognizes benefits of regular exercise in maintaining routine bowel habits.
• Patient's abdominal pain subsides.
• Patient's laboratory values return to normal.
• Patient's vital signs remain stable.
• Patient recognizes need to check stools for occult blood.

Documentation
• Observations of physical findings
• Results of laboratory studies
• Intake and output
• Nursing interventions to treat altered tissue perfusion
• Patient's and family members' response to teaching
• Effectiveness of nursing interventions

• Stool characteristics, including color, consistency, and presence of occult blood
• Evaluations for expected outcomes

■ Tissue perfusion alteration (peripheral)

related to reduced arterial blood flow

Definition

Decrease in cellular nutrition and respiration because of decreased capillary blood flow

Assessment

• History of vascular problems and disease (self or family)
• Age
• Sex
• Integumentary status, including color, condition of nails, distribution of hair, lesions, temperature, texture, and edema
• Cardiovascular status, including blood pressure, capillary refill time, clotting profile, Doppler studies, exercise test, heart rate and rhythm, pulses (brachial, femoral, pedal, peripheral, popliteal space, posterior tibial, and radial), serum cholesterol and triglyceride levels, and venogram or arteriogram
• Neurovascular status, including activity tolerance, mobility, and sensation
• Nutritional status, including dietary patterns and weight
• Psychosocial status, including alcohol intake, family support, history of smoking, occupation, and stressors

Defining characteristics

• Altered condition of hair and nails
• Altered sensation

• Edema
• Positive Homans' sign
• Weak or absent pulses
• Skin discoloration, temperature changes, and moisture

Associated medical diagnoses (selected)

Aortic aneurysm, arterial occlusion, carpal tunnel syndrome, diabetes mellitus, heart failure, myocardial infarction, Raynaud's disease, thrombophlebitis

Expected outcomes

• Patient will express feeling of comfort or absence of pain at rest.
• Patient will not develop arrhythmias.
• Patient's peripheral pulses will remain present and strong.
• Patient's skin color and temperature will remain unchanged.
• Patient's feet will remain clean and free of pressure areas.
• Patient will perform Buerger-Allen exercises.
• Patient will lose ___ lb/week.
• Patient will have a prothrombin time of 35 to 60 seconds.
• Patient will practice relaxation techniques at least once every 8 hours.
• Patient's ulcerated areas will heal.
• Patient will demonstrate ability to perform skills needed to follow prescribed care regimen.
• Patient will identify risk factors that exacerbate problem.
• Patient will maintain tissue perfusion and cellular oxygenation.
• Patient will reduce metabolic needs.

Interventions and rationales

• Elevate head of bed 30 degrees or place head of bed on 6″ to 8″ blocks *to promote circulation to lower extremities.*

• Change patient's position every 2 hours *to reduce risk of skin breakdown.*

• Administer analgesics and monitor effectiveness *to help reduce ischemic pain. Recording effectiveness guides further analgesic administration.*

• Monitor vital signs and heart rhythm every 4 hours. Report development of rapid, irregular pulse. *Rapid, irregular pulse can cause decreased cardiac output, which results in decreased tissue perfusion.*

• Check peripheral pulses every 4 hours. Document presence or absence and intensity of each. Use an ultrasonic blood flow detector if one is available. *Palpable, strong peripheral pulses indicate good arterial flow. Documentation reveals changes from one assessment to the next.*

• Assess skin color, temperature, and texture at least every 4 hours. Note, record, and report development of mottling or black-and-blue areas. *Decreased tissue perfusion causes mottling; skin also becomes cooler and skin texture changes.*

• Don't apply direct heat to extremities. You may apply heat to abdomen; this causes reflex dilation of arteries of lower extremities. *Directly heating extremities causes increased tissue metabolism; if arteries don't dilate normally, tissue perfusion decreases and ischemia may occur.*

• Use light cotton blankets to cover legs. *These provide insulation from cold but don't exert pressure on extremities.*

• Use bed cradle when patient has ulcerations or gangrene. *This helps prevent heavy sheets and blankets from resting on affected extremities.*

• Provide meticulous foot care daily: soak patient's feet in warm water; trim nails carefully; rub feet with lanolin-based lotion; dry feet thoroughly; apply heel protectors; and instruct patient to wear white cotton socks. *These measures prevent cracking of dry skin and other complications.*

• Teach patient to perform Buerger-Allen exercises twice a day: Raise affected extremity above heart level and hold for 2 minutes; then lower extremity to dependent position and hold for 3 minutes. Repeat. *These exercises aid collateral circulation to legs.*

• Encourage ambulation to level of tolerance *to encourage circulation to extremities.*

• Provide diet low in saturated fat *to reduce risk of atherosclerosis, which further decreases circulation and tissue perfusion.*

• Reduce patient's caloric intake to promote weight reduction. *Extra weight can stress heart and decrease circulation.*

• Help patient set goals for weight reduction. *This gives patient sense of control and provides motivation.*

• Consult dietitian *to help patient modify eating patterns and habits.*

• Administer anticoagulants, as ordered, to prevent thrombi. *Thrombi and emboli can further reduce arterial circulation and decrease tissue perfusion.*

• Monitor clotting data *to guide administration of anticoagulants.*

• Administer vasodilators, alpha-blocking agents, and other medications, as ordered. Monitor effectiveness and document patient response. *These agents aid vessel dilation, which promotes increased circulation. They work only if vessels are capable of dilating.*

• Teach patient relaxation techniques *to help improve vasodilation and help prevent vasoconstriction caused by anxiety.*

• For patients with leg ulcers, follow prescribed regimen. *Collaborative practice enhances overall patient care.*
• Educate patient about:
– foot care
– importance of exercise
– need for low-cholesterol, low-calorie diet
– need to avoid tight clothes, crossing legs, and keeping legs dependent
– need to avoid vasoconstrictors (such as cold, stress, and smoking)
– precautionary measures to prevent injury.
These measures enable patient and family members to join actively in care and allow patient to make more informed decisions about his health status.

Evaluations for expected outcomes
• Patient indicates feeling of comfort, either verbally or through behavior.
• Patient doesn't display arrhythmias during monitoring or examination.
• Patient's radial, brachial, pedal, and popliteal pulses are present and palpable.
• Patient's skin remains warm and dry, with normal color.
• Patient's feet remain clean and don't exhibit signs of redness or breakdown.
• Patient performs Buerger-Allen exercises.
• Patient's weight decreases by established amount weekly.
• Patient's prothrombin time remains between 35 and 60 seconds.
• Patient practices relaxation techniques at least once every 8 hours.
• Patient's ulcerated areas heal and don't require dressings.
• Patient demonstrates skills needed to follow self-care regimen.
• Patient states risk factors that may exacerbate problem.

• Patient maintains tissue perfusion and cellular oxygenation.
• Patient reduces metabolic needs.

Documentation
• Patient's expressions of symptoms, such as pain, numbness, and muscle weakness
• Observations of physical findings
• Nursing interventions performed for patient
• Patient's response to nursing interventions
• Patient's response to education
• Evaluations for expected outcomes

■ Tissue perfusion alteration (peripheral)

related to reduced venous blood flow

Definition
Decrease in cellular nutrition and respiration because of decreased capillary blood flow

Assessment
• History of vascular problems or disease (self or family)
• Age
• Sex
• Medication history
• Integumentary status, including color, condition of nails, distribution of hair, lesions, temperature, and texture
• Cardiovascular status, including capillary refill time, clotting profile, Doppler studies, exercise test, heart rate and rhythm, pulses (brachial, femoral, pedal, peripheral, popliteal, posterior tibial, and radial), serum cholesterol and triglyceride levels, and venogram or arteriogram

• Neurovascular status, including activity tolerance, mobility, and sensation
• Nutritional status, including dietary patterns and weight
• Psychosocial status, including alcohol intake, family support, history of smoking, occupation, and stressors

Defining characteristics
• Altered condition of hair and nails
• Altered sensation
• Edema
• Positive Homans' sign
• Weak or absent pulses
• Skin discoloration, temperature changes, and moisture

Associated medical diagnoses (selected)
Pregnancy, pulmonary embolus, sickle cell anemia. Also any condition requiring prolonged bed rest, multiple venipunctures, or long-term I.V. therapy

Expected outcomes
• Patient will not develop embolization of thrombi.
• Patient will have less inflammation and improved venous blood flow.
• Patient's clotting studies will remain within therapeutic range.
• Patient will explain reasons for measures used to prevent pooling of blood in lower extremities.
• Patient will move bowels without straining.
• Patient will demonstrate ability to perform skills needed for prescribed care regimen.
• Patient will identify risk factors that exacerbate problem.

Interventions and rationales
• Monitor and record temperature, pulse, respiration, and blood pressure at least every 4 hours. *Accurate monitoring of vital signs allows detection of increased respiratory rate, pulse rate, and blood pressure, which may indicate pulmonary embolus.*
• Auscultate and record breath sounds every 4 hours. *Decreased, absent, or adventitious breath sounds may result from pulmonary embolus.*
• Observe for development of pulmonary emboli. Report immediately any increase in temperature, pulse, or respiratory rate; decrease in blood pressure; anxious, apprehensive behavior; complaints of dyspnea, cough, or hemoptysis; or development of crackles or red, frothy sputum. *Embolization of thrombi from deep veins (legs and pelvis) frequently causes pulmonary embolus.*
• Monitor clotting profile as ordered. *This guides anticoagulant therapy and indicates potential for clot formation.*
• Administer anticoagulant therapy, monitor effectiveness, and observe for bleeding (epistaxis, bleeding gums, and petechiae). *This reduces further thrombosis by preventing clot propagation.*
• Measure and compare size of calves every 4 hours. *Venous pooling and stasis can cause fluid to move into interstitial space to cause edema.*
• Apply antiembolism stockings or intermittent pneumatic compression stockings, as ordered. Remove stockings for 1 hour every 8 hours or according to policy. *Stockings may decrease venous stasis, but they can also cause edema from constriction. Monitor their use closely.*
• Apply moist heat to affected extremity as ordered (may be contraindicated in chronic venous insufficiency). *Moist heat may aid vasodilation, reduce vasospasm, and enhance venous return.*
• Elevate affected extremity. Don't use knee gatch or pillows under

knees, and explain reasons for not using them to patient. *Elevation aids venous return; knee gatch or pillows under knees hinder venous return because they elevate knees above feet.*

• Instruct patient not to cross legs or lie in fetal position. Explain importance of remembering not to cross legs. *Crossing legs constricts popliteal vessels, thus reducing venous return and promoting venous stasis.*

• Increase patient's activity as ordered. *This helps prevent venous pooling and stasis and promotes venous return.*

• Urge patient to elevate legs when sitting in chair, supporting entire length of legs. *Elevating legs aids venous return. Supporting entire leg ensures blood flow.*

• Encourage patient to walk. Discourage prolonged standing in one place. *Walking promotes venous blood flow by causing muscles to compress veins. Standing promotes venous stasis.*

• Use stool softeners *to avoid constipation and straining during bowel movement. Valsalva's maneuver, used in straining during bowel movement, decreases venous blood return.*

• Educate patient about anticoagulant therapy; importance of having blood work done as ordered; need to report bleeding gums and blood in urine and secretions; and dietary precautions while on anticoagulant therapy, such as minimizing intake of green, leafy vegetables if on oral agent. *Leafy vegetables contain vitamin K, which inhibits anticoagulants such as coumadin.*

• Educate patient about use of antiembolism stockings or intermittent pneumatic compression stockings; avoidance of crossing legs, wearing constrictive clothing, or standing in one place; and importance of protecting extremities from injury. *Education allows patient and family members to take active role in health maintenance.*

Evaluations for expected outcomes

• Patient doesn't exhibit indications of embolization, such as increased respiratory rate, pulse rate, and blood pressure; decreased, absent, or adventitious breath sounds; and signs and symptoms of pulmonary embolus.

• Patient's inflammation decreases and venous blood flow improves.

• Patient's prothrombin time and partial thromboplastin time remain within established limits.

• Patient explains reasons for measures used to prevent pooling of blood in lower extremities.

• Patient moves bowels without straining.

• Patient demonstrates ability to perform skills needed for prescribed care regimen.

• Patient lists risk factors that exacerbate reduced venous blood flow or demonstrates understanding of risk factors through behavior.

Documentation

• Patient's expression of feelings about hospitalization and current situation

• Observations of physical findings

• Clotting profile

• Administration of anticoagulant therapy, including adverse effects

• Nursing interventions performed to promote circulation to lower extremities

• Patient's response to nursing interventions

• Patient's response to education

• Evaluations for expected outcomes

■ Tissue perfusion alteration (renal)

related to decreased cellular exchange

Definition
Decrease in cellular nutrition and respiration caused by decreased capillary blood flow

Assessment
• Health history, including surgery, any condition resulting in fluid volume depletion, and use of nephrotoxic drugs
• Renal status, including color of urine, intake and output, presence of anuria or oliguria, urine specific gravity, and weight
• Cardiovascular status, including blood pressure, central venous pressure, hemodynamic readings, jugular filling, and presence of dependent edema, fluid retention, or palpitations
• Respiratory status, including auscultation of breath sounds, respiratory rate and rhythm, and shortness of breath
• Neurologic status, including level of consciousness (LOC), mental status, orientation, decreased tolerance to activity, fatigue, and weakness
• Integumentary status, including color, moisture, and presence of edema and secondary skin ulcerations from edema.
• Nutritional status, including thirst and signs of anorexia
• Laboratory studies, including blood urea nitrogen (BUN), creatinine, creatinine clearance, hemoglobin, serum electrolytes, and urine osmolality

Defining characteristics
• Blood pressure readings outside acceptable parameters

• Bruits
• Claudication
• Diminished arterial pulses
• Elevated BUN and creatinine levels
• Hematuria
• Oliguria or anuria
• Pallor in elevated legs that doesn't return to normal after lowering legs
• Slow healing of lesions

Associated medical diagnoses (selected)
Acute renal failure, anaphylactic shock, aortic aneurysm, burns, cardiogenic shock, cerebral aneurysm, chemotherapy, chronic renal failure, diabetes mellitus, esophageal varices, glomerulonephritis, head injury, hemorrhage, joint replacement, leukemia, liver transplantation, lupus erythematosus, multisystem trauma, myocardial infarction, poisoning, polycystic kidney disease, pseudomembranous colitis, shock, sickle cell anemia, urinary calculi, uterine rupture

Expected outcomes
• Patient will maintain fluid balance.
• Patient will maintain urine specific gravity within normal limits (specify).
• Patient's weight won't fluctuate.
• Patient will report increased comfort.
• Patient will maintain hemodynamic stability.
• Patient will identify risk factors that exacerbate decreased tissue perfusion and will modify lifestyle appropriately.
• Patient will communicate understanding of medical regimen, medications, diet, and activity restrictions.

Interventions and rationales
• Monitor and document intake and output every hour until output exceeds 30 ml/hour, then every 2 to 4 hours. *If patient has no history of re-*

nal disease, urine output is good indicator of tissue perfusion. Decreased or absent urine output usually indicates poor renal perfusion.

• Document urine color and characteristics. Report any changes. *Concentrated urine may indicate poor kidney function or dehydration.*

• Weigh patient daily before breakfast and record weight. *Weighing patient daily helps predict total fluid status; weight gain may indicate fluid overload. Weighing at regular times gives better indication of weight changes.*

• Assess for dependent edema. *Dependent edema may indicate lack of kidney function.*

• Observe voiding patterns *to note deviations from normal.*

• Monitor urine specific gravity, serum electrolytes, BUN, and creatinine levels. *Rising levels may indicate decreased kidney function.*

• Monitor hemodynamic status and vital signs. Notify doctor of any changes. *Increase from baseline may indicate fluid overload caused by lack of kidney function.*

• Explain reasons for therapy and its intended effects to patient and family *to encourage patient to take active role in health maintenance.*

• Allow for frequent rest periods *to enable patient to conserve energy.*

• Refer patient to dietitian for special diet for renal impairment *to help patient avoid foods that place increased demands on kidneys.*

• Instruct patient to check with doctor before taking over-the-counter medications. *Some may be nephrotoxic.*

• Provide patient and family members with psychological support if renal failure becomes chronic *to encourage healthy adaptation.*

Evaluations for expected outcomes

• Patient maintains fluid balance.

• Patient maintains urine specific gravity within normal limits (specify).

• Patient's weight doesn't fluctuate.

• Patient reports achieving increased comfort level.

• Patient maintains hemodynamic stability.

• Patient recognizes risk factors that exacerbate problem and changes lifestyle appropriately.

• Patient communicates understanding of medical regimen, medications, diet, and activity restrictions.

Documentation

• Patient's expressions of concern over signs and symptoms of decreased tissue perfusion

• Vital signs, intake and output, LOC, and other clinical findings

• Nursing interventions performed to maintain fluid balance and hemodynamic stability

• Patient's response to nursing interventions

• Patient's response to education

• Evaluations for expected outcomes

■ Transfer ability, impaired

related to neuromuscular dysfunction

Definition

Limitation of independent movement between two nearby surfaces

Assessment

• Age

• Sex

• Vital signs

• Drug history

• History of neuromuscular disorder or dysfunction

• Musculoskeletal status, including coordination, muscle size and strength, muscle tone, range of motion (ROM), functional mobility as follows:

0 = completely independent

1 = requires use of equipment or device

2 = requires help, supervision, or teaching from another person

3 = requires help from another person and equipment or device

4 = dependent; doesn't participate in activity

• Neurologic status, including level of consciousness, motor ability, and sensory ability

• Endurance — for example, how long the patient can remain sitting in wheelchair before becoming fatigued

• Knowledge of wheelchair transfer techniques

Defining characteristics
• Altered postural reflexes
• Fatigue
• Flaccidity
• Impaired ability to transfer from bed, chair, or floor to wheelchair
• Inability to coordinate movement
• Lack of knowledge of wheelchair transfer techniques
• Paraplegia
• Paresis
• Quadriplegia
• Spasticity
• Weakness

Associated medical diagnoses (selected)
Brain abscess, cerebral aneurysm, cerebrovascular accident, Guillain-Barré syndrome, head injury, multiple sclerosis, muscular dystrophy, myasthenia gravis, paralysis, paresis, Parkinson's disease, spinal cord injury or tumor

Expected outcomes
• Patient will not exhibit complications associated with impaired wheel-

chair transfer mobility, such as depression, altered health maintenance, and falls.

• Patient will maintain or improve muscle strength and joint ROM.

• Patient will achieve highest level of mobility possible (independence with regard to wheelchair transfer, ability to transfer to wheelchair with assistance, verbalization of needs regarding wheelchair transfer).

• Patient will maintain safety during wheelchair transfer.

• Patient will adapt to alteration in ability to perform wheelchair transfer.

• Patient will demonstrate understanding of wheelchair transfer techniques.

• Patient will participate in social and occupational activities to the greatest extent possible.

Interventions and rationales
• Perform ROM exercises to joints of affected limbs, unless contraindicated, at least once per shift. Progress from passive to active ROM, as tolerated, *to prevent joint contractures and muscle atrophy.*

• Identify patient's level of independence using functional mobility scale. Report findings to staff *to provide continuity and preserve documented level of independence.*

• Monitor and record daily evidence of complications related to altered mobility or decreased ability to perform wheelchair transfer (contractures, venous stasis, skin breakdown, thrombus formation, depression, altered health maintenance, or self-care deficit). *Patients with neuromuscular dysfunction are at risk for complications.*

• Teach patient wheelchair transfer techniques, such as performing a standing or sitting transfer, *to maintain muscle tone, prevent complications of immobility, and promote inde-*

pendence. Adapt teaching to limits imposed by his condition *to prevent injury.*
• Refer to physical therapist for development of wheelchair mobility program to *assist with rehabilitation of musculoskeletal deficits.*
• Encourage patient to attend physical therapy. Request written copy of wheelchair transfer instructions to use as a reference *to maintain continuity of care and foster safety.*
• Assess patient's skin upon his return to bed and request a wheelchair cushion, if necessary, *to maintain skin integrity.*
• As part of your teaching plan, demonstrate transfer techniques to family members and note the date. Have them perform return demonstration *to ensure use of proper technique and to promote continuity of care.*
• Identify resources (stroke program, sports association for disabled, National Multiple Sclerosis Society) *to promote patient's reintegration into community.*

Evaluations for expected outcomes
• Patient doesn't exhibit complications associated with impaired wheelchair transfer mobility, such as depression, altered health maintenance, and falls.
• Patient maintains or improves muscle strength and joint ROM.
• Patient achieves highest level of mobility possible (independence with regard to wheelchair transfer, ability to transfer to wheelchair with assistance, verbalization of needs regarding wheelchair transfer).
• Patient maintains safety during wheelchair transfer.
• Patient adapts to alteration in ability to perform wheelchair transfer.
• Patient demonstrates understanding of wheelchair transfer techniques.

• Patient participates in social and occupational activities to the greatest extent possible.

Documentation
• Patient's mobility status
• Presence of complications
• Evidence of alterations in patient's ability to perform wheelchair transfer
• Patient's statements regarding difficulties in wheelchair transfer
• Instruction of transfer techniques
• Patient's and family members' return demonstration of skills
• Patient's response to nursing interventions
• Evaluations for expected outcomes

Trauma, risk for

related to external factors (environmental, physical, chemical agents)

Definition
Accentuated risk of accidental tissue injury, such as burns and fractures

Assessment
• Health history, including accidents, allergies, exposure to pollutants, falls, hyperthermia, hypothermia, poisoning, sensory or perceptual changes (auditory, gustatory, kinesthetic, olfactory, tactile, and visual), seizures, and trauma
• Circumstances of current situation that might lead to injury from surgery or from chemical, physical, or human agents
• Neurologic status, including level of consciousness, mental status, and orientation
• Laboratory studies, including clotting factors, hemoglobin and hemat-

ocrit, and platelet and white blood cell counts

Risk factors
• Unsafe home environment
• Lack of safety precautions

Associated medical diagnoses (selected)
Alzheimer's disease, cerebrovascular accident, craniotomy, drug overdose, fractures, head injury, hemophilia, osteoporosis, Parkinson's disease

Expected outcomes
• Patient will avoid injury.
• Patient will state understanding of safety precautions.
• Patient will use assistive devices correctly (walker or cane, for example).

Interventions and rationales
• Observe, record, and report falls, seizures, and unsafe practices. *Accurate assessment promotes appropriate interventions; documentation ensures continuity of care.*
• Monitor and record respiratory status. *Trauma increases respiratory rate; other respiratory effects depend on nature of trauma.*
• Monitor and record neurologic status *to detect changes and to report deteriorated status.*
• If patient has seizure, remain with him, loosen restrictive clothing, and protect him from environmental hazards. Don't restrain him or pry mouth open. Keep oral airway at bedside and maintain patent airway. Turn patient to side after seizure stops and suction if secretions occlude airway. Record seizure characteristics, including onset, duration, and body movements. Reorient patient to surroundings and allow rest period. *Remaining with patient provides safety and information for accurate documentation of event.*

Loosening clothing and proper positioning may prevent further harm.
• Keep side rails up at all times *to protect patient and provide sense of security.*
• Keep bed in low position except when providing direct care. *This minimizes effects of possible fall.*
• Emphasize importance of asking for help before getting up. *Illness or injury may have weakened patient.*
• Help debilitated, weak, or unsteady patient to get out of bed. Ensure that floor is dry and that furniture and litter don't block patient's way. *This helps prevent falls.*
• When using soft restraints, don't secure them too tightly *to avoid skin burns.*
• Use leather restraints following facility policy; pad them well before applying. Release each extremity on rotation basis every hour; check for skin burns. *Such restraints should be used only when other kinds are ineffective.*
• Instruct patient and family members in safety practices such as correct use of walker, crutches, or cane. *These enable patient and family members to take active role in health care and maintain safe environment.*

Evaluations for expected outcomes
• Patient remains free of injury.
• Patient identifies specific safety precautions.
• Patient demonstrates proper use of assistive device (specify).

Documentation
• Patient's statements that indicate potential for injury
• Physical findings
• Observations or knowledge of unsafe practices
• Interventions performed to prevent injury

• Patient's response to nursing interventions
• Evaluations for expected outcomes

■ Trauma, risk for

related to internal factors

Definition
Accentuated risk of accidental tissue injury, such as burns and fractures

Assessment
• Health history, including accidents, allergies, exposure to pollutants, falls, hyperthermia, hypothermia, poisoning, sensory or perceptual changes (auditory, gustatory, kinesthetic, olfactory, tactile, and visual), seizures, and trauma
• Circumstances of current situation that might lead to injury
• Neurologic status, including level of consciousness, mental status, and orientation
• Laboratory studies, including albumin and globulin levels, clotting factors, hemoglobin and hematocrit, and platelet and white blood cell counts

Risk factors
• Cognitive or emotional difficulties
• History of previous trauma
• Lack of money to purchase safety equipment or effect repairs
• Lack of safety education and safety precautions
• Poor balance
• Poor coordination
• Poor vision
• Reduced tactile sensation
• Reduced temperature
• Weakness

Associated medical diagnoses (selected)
Cerebrovascular accident, hypoparathyroidism, Ménière's disease, multisystem trauma, seizure disorder, spinal cord injury

Expected outcomes
• Patient will avoid injury.
• Patient will voice need for understanding safety precautions.
• Patient will use safety devices correctly (walker or cane, for example).

Interventions and rationales
• Observe, record, and report falls, seizures, and unsafe practices. *Accurate assessment promotes appropriate interventions; documentation ensures continuity of care.*
• Monitor and record respiratory status. *Trauma increases respiratory rate; other respiratory effects depend on nature of trauma.*
• Monitor and record neurologic status *to assess changes and to report deteriorated status.*
• For seizures:
– Keep side rails up *to protect patient and provide sense of security.*
– Pad side rails *to protect patient.*
– Protect patient from further injury during seizure *to ensure well-being.*
– Position patient on side *to prevent aspiration.*
– Record such seizure characteristics as onset, duration, and body movements *to help pinpoint involved area of brain and guide treatment.*
– If patient is confused and walking about after seizure ends, walk with him and guide him back to his bed; don't try to restrain him *to prevent injury.*
• To prevent falls:
– Keep bed rails up *to enhance safety.*
– Maintain bed in low position except when providing direct care *to reduce risk of injury.*

– Emphasize importance of asking for help before getting up. *Illness or injury may have weakened patient.*
– Provide help in ambulating and going to bathroom *to ensure safety.*
– Anticipate times when falls occur (during night, after administering diuretic, while patient is sitting in chair) and monitor patient closely *to prevent injuries.*
• Instruct patient and family members in use of such assistive devices as cane, walker, crutches, and wheelchair *to ensure their proper use and to provide patient with feeling of security.*
• Provide patient and family members with information about necessary safety precautions *to enable patient and family members to take active role in health care and maintain safe environment.*

Evaluations for expected outcomes
• Patient remains free from injury during specific time frame.
• Patient identifies need for specific safety precautions.
• Patient demonstrates proper use of assistive device (specify).

Documentation
• Patient's statements about situation that indicate potential for injury
• Physical findings
• Record of falls, seizures, and unsafe practices
• Interventions that reduce risk of injury
• Patient's response to nursing interventions
• Evaluations for expected outcomes

■ Urinary elimination alteration

related to obstruction

Definition
Alteration or impairment of urinary function

Assessment
• History of urinary tract disease, trauma, surgery, or previous urethral infection
• Age
• Sex
• Vital signs
• Genitourinary status, including characteristics of urine, excretory urography, pain or discomfort, palpation of bladder, urinalysis, and voiding patterns
• Fluid and electrolyte status, including blood urea nitrogen, creatinine, intake and output, mucous membranes (inspection), serum electrolytes, skin turgor, and urine specific gravity
• Nutritional status, including appetite, constipation, dietary intake, elimination habits, current weight and change from normal, and rectal examination
• Sexuality status, including capability, concerns, habits, and sexual partners
• Psychosocial status, including coping skills, patient's perception of health problem, self-concept (body image), family members, and stressors (such as finances and job)

Defining characteristics
• Dysuria
• Frequency
• Hesitancy
• Incontinence
• Nocturia

• Retention
• Urgency

Associated medical diagnoses (selected)
Benign prostatic hypertrophy, bladder cancer, cystitis, interstitial cystitis, metastatic disease, ovarian cancer, prostate cancer, prostatectomy, renal calculi, urinary calculi, urinary tract infection

Expected outcomes
• Patient will maintain fluid balance; intake will equal output.
• Patient will voice increased comfort.
• Patient will voice understanding of treatment.
• Patient will have few if any complications.
• Patient will discuss impact of urologic disorder on self and family members.
• Patient will demonstrate skill in managing urinary elimination problem.
• Patient will maintain urinary continence.

Interventions and rationales
• Observe voiding pattern. Document urine color and characteristics, intake and output, and patient's daily weight. Report any changes. *Accurate intake and output measurements are essential for correct fluid replacement therapy. Urine characteristics help verify diagnosis.*
• Administer appropriate care for urologic condition and monitor progress (for example, strain urine). Report favorable and adverse responses to treatment regimen. *Appropriate care helps patient recover from underlying disorder. Reporting responses to treatment allows modification of treatment as needed.*
• Observe bowel habits:
– Check for constipation.

– Check for fecal impaction; if present, disimpact and institute bowel regimen. *This promotes comfort and prevents loss of rectal muscle tone from prolonged distention.*
• If patient requires surgery, give appropriate preoperative and postoperative instructions and care. *Accurate information allows patient to understand procedure and builds trust in caregivers.*
• Explain reasons for therapy and intended effects to patient and family members *to increase patient's understanding and build trust in caregivers.* If patient needs urinary diversion, prepare him for change in body appearance (instruct patient and family members how to care for ostomy site postoperatively). *Preparation and appropriate information helps patient and family members cope with changes.*
• Provide supportive measures as indicated.
– Administer pain medication and monitor patient *to reduce pain and assess effects of medication.*
– Force fluids, as ordered, *to moisten mucous membranes and dilute chemical materials within body.*
– Refer to dietitian for instructions on diet. *Dietary changes may decrease urinary infections.*
– Assist with general hygiene and comfort measures as needed. *Cleanliness prevents bacterial growth and promotes comfort.*
– Maintain patency of catheters, drainage bags, and other urinary elimination equipment *to avoid reflux and risk of infection and ensure effectiveness of therapy.*
– Provide meatal care according to facility procedure *to promote cleanliness and comfort and reduce risk of infection.*

• Encourage patient to ventilate feelings and concerns related to urologic problem. *Active listening conveys respect for patient; ventilation helps pinpoint patient's fears.*
• Refer patient and family members to psychiatric liaison nurse, sex counselor, or support group, when appropriate. *These resources help patient gain knowledge of self and situation, reduce anxiety, and promote personal growth. Community resources often provide support and care not available in other health agencies.*
• Explain urologic condition to patient and family members, including instructions on preventive measures if appropriate. Prepare for discharge according to individual needs. *Accurate health knowledge increases patient's ability to maintain health. Involving family members assures patient that he will be cared for.*

Evaluations for expected outcomes
• Patient's fluid intake equals output.
• Patient expresses feelings of comfort.
• Patient voices understanding of treatment, including urinary diversion therapy if appropriate.
• Patient doesn't show evidence of skin breakdown, infection, or other complications.
• Patient discusses disease, signs and symptoms, complications, treatments, and adjustments to lifestyle caused by altered urinary pattern.
• Patient demonstrates proficiency in steps necessary to manage urinary elimination problems.
• Patient maintains urinary continence.

Documentation
• Observations of urologic condition and response to treatment regimen

• Interventions to provide supportive care and patient's response
• Instructions given to patient and family members on urologic problem, response to instructions, and demonstrated ability to manage patient's urinary elimination needs
• Patient's expression of concern about urologic problem and its impact on body image and lifestyle; patient's motivation to participate in self-care
• Evaluations for expected outcomes

■ Urinary elimination alteration

related to sensory or neuromuscular impairment

Definition
Alteration or impairment of urinary function

Assessment
• History of urinary tract disease, trauma, surgery, or infection
• History of sensory or neuromuscular impairment
• Vital signs
• Genitourinary status, including characteristics of urine, cystometry, pain or discomfort, palpation of bladder, postcatheterization, presence and amount of residual urine, use of urinary assistive devices, urinalysis, and voiding pattern
• Fluid and electrolyte status, including blood urea nitrogen, creatinine, and serum electrolyte levels; inspection of mucous membranes; intake and output; skin turgor; and urine specific gravity
• Neuromuscular status, including degree of neuromuscular function, motor ability to start and stop urinary

stream, and sensory ability to perceive bladder fullness
• Sexuality status, including capability, concerns, habits, and sexual partners
• Psychosocial status, including coping skills, family members, patient's perception of health problem, self-concept, and stressors (such as finances and job)

Defining characteristics
• Dysuria
• Frequency
• Hesitancy
• Incontinence
• Nocturia
• Retention
• Urgency

Associated medical diagnoses (selected)
Brain tumors, cerebrovascular accident, diabetes mellitus, disseminated intravascular coagulation, hydronephrosis, multiple sclerosis, prolapsed intervertebral disk, Reiter's syndrome, salmonella, spinal cord defect, spinal cord injury, spinal tumor

Expected outcomes
• Patient will maintain fluid balance; intake will equal output.
• Patient will voice increased comfort.
• Patient will have few if any complications.
• Patient and family members will demonstrate skill in managing urinary elimination problem.
• Patient will express feelings about condition.
• Patient will discuss impact of urologic disorder on self and family members.
• Patient and family members will identify resources to assist with care following discharge.

Interventions and rationales
• Monitor patient's neuromuscular status and voiding pattern; document and report intake and output. *Accurate intake and output measurements are essential for correct fluid replacement therapy. Data form basis for complete evaluation to diagnose cause.*
• Provide appropriate care for urologic condition and monitor progress. Report responses to treatment. *Appropriate care helps patient recover from underlying disorder. Reporting responses to treatment allows modification of treatment as needed.*
• Assist with ordered bladder elimination procedure as indicated.
– For bladder training, place patient on commode or toilet every 2 hours while awake and once during the night. Maintain regular fluid intake while patient is awake. Provide privacy. Teach patient how to perform Kegel exercises to strengthen sphincter control. *These measures aid adaptation to routine physiologic function. Women with good muscle tone may improve levator muscle action significantly if they perform Kegel exercises regularly.*
– For intermittent catheterization, catheterize patient using clean or sterile technique every ___ hours. Record amount voided spontaneously and amount obtained with catheterization (for example: 7 a.m., spontaneous void of 200 ml; catheter void of 150 ml). Record bladder balance every (day or week). *These measures promote normal voiding, prevent infection, and help maintain integrity of ureterovesical function. Catheterization schedule is based on flow sheet data and can provide baseline chart.*
– Bladder balance = Amount of residual urine/Amount of voided urine

– For external catheterization (in male patient), monitor patency. Apply condom catheter according to established policy. *Applying foam strip in spiral fashion increases adhesive surface and reduces risk of impairing circulation.* Avoid constriction. Observe skin condition of penis, and clean with soap and water at least twice daily. *These measures prevent infection and ensure therapeutic effectiveness.*

– For indwelling urinary catheter, monitor patency. Keep tubing free of kinks and keep drainage bag below level of bladder *to avoid urine reflux.* Clean urinary meatus according to established policy, and maintain closed drainage system *to prevent skin irritation and bacteriuria.* Secure catheter to leg (female) or abdomen (male); avoid tension on sphincter. *Anchoring catheter avoids straining trigone muscle of bladder and prevents friction leading to inflammation.*

– For suprapubic catheter, monitor patency. Change dressing and clean catheter site according to policy. Keep tubing free of kinks; keep drainage bag below bladder level. Maintain closed drainage system. *Suprapubic drainage allows increased patient mobility and reduces risk of bladder infection.*

• Provide supportive measures:
– Administer pain medication and monitor patient *to reduce pain and assess effects of medication.*
– Encourage fluid intake up to 3,000 ml every 24 hours (unless contraindicated) *to moisten mucous membranes and dilute chemical materials within body.*
– Provide privacy during toileting procedure. *This avoids inhibiting elimination.*
– Respond to patient's call light quickly, assign patient to bed next to bathroom, and have patient wear easily removed clothing (such as gown rather than pajamas). *These measures reduce delay and impediments to voiding routine.*

• Alert patient and family members to signs and symptoms of full bladder: restlessness, abdominal discomfort, sweating, and chills. *Adequate education increases patient's and family members' ability to maintain health level and to prevent patient from harming self.*

• Instruct patient and family members on catheterization techniques to be used at home; provide time for return demonstrations until they can perform procedure well. *Knowledge of procedures and rationales reduces anxiety and promotes comfort. Demonstrations may progress through several sessions until patient can perform independently.*

• Instruct patient and family members on signs and symptoms of autonomic dysreflexia (headache, cold sweat, nausea, and elevated blood pressure) and and how to manage it (by checking for kinked indwelling catheter, catheterizing, and elevating head of bed). Instruct patient and family members to call doctor or facility immediately if symptoms don't subside with initial treatment. *Autonomic dysreflexia, a medical emergency, is pathologic reflex condition characterized by exaggerated autonomic responses to stimuli.*

• Encourage patient to ventilate feelings and concerns related to urologic problem. *Active listening conveys respect for patient; ventilation helps pinpoint patient's fears.*

• Refer patient and family members to psychiatric liaison nurse, sex counselor, visiting nurses' society, or support group, when appropriate. *These resources help patient gain knowledge of self and situation, reduce anx-*

iety, and help promote personal growth. Community resources often provide care and support not available in other health agencies.

Evaluations for expected outcomes
• Patient's fluid intake equals output.
• Patient expresses feeling of comfort.
• Patient doesn't develop infection, swelling of penis, skin breakdown, or other complications, and urinalysis remains normal.
• Patient and family members demonstrate skill in managing urinary elimination problem, including catheterization techniques to be used at home.
• Patient expresses feelings about condition.
• Patient expresses understanding of urologic disorder and its effect on family and lifestyle after discharge.
• Patient and family members identify and contact visiting nurse, support group, or other resources as needed.

Documentation
• Observations of urologic condition and response to treatment regimen
• Interventions to provide supportive care and patient's response
• Instructions given to patient and family members, their understanding of instructions, and demonstrated ability to manage patient's urinary elimination
• Patient's expression of concern about urologic problem and impact on body image and lifestyle; patient's motivation to participate in self-care
• Evaluations for expected outcomes

■ Urinary retention
related to obstruction, sensory or neuromuscular impairment

Definition
Incomplete emptying of bladder

Assessment
• History of sensory or neuromuscular impairment, prostate enlargement, surgery, urethral trauma or tumor, or urinary tract disease
• Age
• Sex
• Vital signs
• Genitourinary status, including pain or discomfort, palpation of bladder, residual urine volume after voiding, urethral obstruction (prostate hypertrophy or masses, fecal impaction, masses, and swelling), urinalysis, urine characteristics, and voiding patterns
• Fluid and electrolyte status, including inspection of mucous membranes, intake and output, skin turgor, urine specific gravity, serum electrolytes, blood urea nitrogen, and creatinine
• Medication history
• Neuromuscular status, including anal sphincter tone, motor ability to start and stop stream, neuromuscular function, and sensory ability to perceive bladder fullness and voiding
• Sexuality status, including capability and concerns or partner's concerns
• Psychosocial status, including coping skills, patient's or family members' perception of problem, self-concept, and stressors (such as finances and job)

Defining characteristics
• Bladder distention
• Dysuria
• High residual urine

• Overflow incontinence (continuous dribbling)
• Sensation of bladder fullness
• Small, frequent voiding or no urine output

Associated medical diagnoses (selected)

Benign prostatic hypertrophy, impotence, intestinal obstruction, spinal cord injury

Expected outcomes

• Patient will maintain fluid balance, with intake equal to output.
• Patient will voice increased comfort.
• Patient will voice understanding of treatment.
• Patient will have few if any complications.
• Patient's urinalysis will remain normal.
• Patient will avoid bladder distention.
• Patient and family members will demonstrate skill in managing urine retention.
• Patient will discuss impact of urologic disorder on self and family members.
• Patient and family members will identify resources to assist with care following discharge.

Interventions and rationales

• Monitor intake and output. Report if intake exceeds output. *Accurate intake and output measurements are essential for correct fluid replacement therapy.*
• Monitor voiding pattern. *Data on time, place, amount, and patient's awareness of micturition are needed to establish pattern of incontinence.*
• Assist with ordered bladder elimination procedure as follows:
– voiding techniques. Perform Credé's or Valsalva's maneuver every 2 to 3 hours *to increase bladder pres-*

sure to pass urine. Repeat until empty.
– intermittent catheterization. Catheterize using clean or sterile technique every 2 hours. Record amount voided spontaneously and amount obtained with catheterization. *These measures promote normal voiding, prevent infection, and help maintain integrity of ureterovesical function.*
– use of indwelling urinary catheter. Monitor patency and avoid kinks in tubing. Keep drainage bag below bladder level *to avoid urine reflux.* Perform catheter care according to established policy and maintain closed drainage system *to prevent skin irritation and bacteriuria.* Secure catheter to leg (female) or abdomen (male), avoiding tension on sphincter. *Anchoring catheter prevents straining of trigone muscle of bladder and prevents friction leading to inflammation.*
– use of suprapubic catheter. Change dressings according to facility policy. Monitor patency and avoid kinks in tubing. Keep drainage bag below bladder level. Maintain closed drainage system. *Suprapubic drainage allows for increased mobility and reduces risk of bladder infection.*
• Administer pain medication as ordered and monitor patient *to reduce pain and assess effects of medication.*
• For fecal impaction, disimpact and institute bowel regimen. *This promotes comfort and prevents loss of rectal muscle tone from prolonged distention.*
• Encourage high fluid intake (2,500 ml/day), unless contraindicated, *to moisten mucous membranes and dilute chemical materials within body.* Limit fluid intake after 7 p.m. *to prevent nocturia.*

• Monitor therapeutic and adverse effects of prescribed medications *for early recognition and treatment of drug reactions.*
• If patient requires surgery, give appropriate preoperative and postoperative instructions and care *to increase patient's understanding.* If he will undergo urinary diversions, prepare him for change in body image. *Preparation and appropriate information helps patient and family members cope with changes.*
• Instruct patient and family members on voiding techniques to be used at home. Provide for return demonstrations until they can perform procedure well. *Knowledge of procedures and rationales reduces anxiety and promotes comfort. Demonstrations may progress through several sessions until patient can perform independently.*
• Encourage patient and family members to share feelings and concerns related to urologic problems. *Ventilation helps pinpoint patient's fears and establishes environment of trust in which patient and family members can begin to deal with the situation.*
• Refer patient and family members to psychiatric liaison nurse, enterostomal therapist, sex counselor, support group, or visiting nurse's association, when appropriate. *These resources help patient gain knowledge of self and situation, reduce anxiety, and help promote personal growth. Community resources often provide services not available at other health agencies.*

Evaluations for expected outcomes
• Patient's intake equals output.
• Patient expresses absence of pain.
• Patient voices understanding of treatment, including ordered bladder

elimination procedure and surgery, if appropriate.
• Patient doesn't experience skin breakdown or other complications.
• Patient's urinalysis remains normal.
• Patient avoids bladder distention.
• Patient and family members demonstrate skill in managing urine retention, including voiding techniques to be used at home.
• Patient expresses at least one fear, one concern, and one positive feeling about urologic problem. If appropriate, patient expresses feelings and fears about surgery.
• Patient or family contacts visiting nurse, support group, or other resources, as needed.

Documentation
• Observations of urologic condition and response to treatment regimen
• Interventions to provide supportive care and patient's response
• Instructions given to patient and family members on urologic problem and their returned response and demonstrated ability to manage patient's urinary elimination
• Patient's concerns about urologic problem and its impact on body image and lifestyle; motivation to participate in self-care
• Evaluations for expected outcomes

■ Ventilation, spontaneous: Inability to sustain

Definition
Inability to breathe adequately

Assessment
• Health history, including previous respiratory problems
• Respiratory status, including rate, rhythm, and depth of respirations;

chest excursion and symmetry; presence of cyanosis; and use of accessory muscles
• Effectiveness of cough in clearing secretions
• Suctioning demands, including frequency and tolerance
• Sputum characteristics, including appearance, consistency, color, and odor
• Neuromuscular strength and endurance
• Mental and emotional status, including cognitive state and ability to follow directions
• Laboratory values, including arterial blood gas (ABG) levels (baseline and ongoing), complete blood count, serum electrolyte levels, coagulation studies, serum and sputum cultures, and sensitivity tests
• Vital signs
• Functional status, including ability to perform activities of daily living
• Related or concurrent events that may contribute to respiratory distress, such as bleeding, hypervolemia, hypovolemia, and sepsis

Defining characteristics
• Apprehension
• Decreased cooperation
• Decreased arterial oxygen saturation
• Decreased partial pressure of arterial oxygen (Pao_2)
• Decreased tidal volume
• Dyspnea
• Increased metabolic rate
• Increased partial pressure of arterial carbon dioxide
• Increased restlessness
• Increased use of accessory muscles
• Tachycardia

Associated medical diagnoses (selected)
Adult respiratory distress syndrome, amyotrophic lateral sclerosis, burns, chest trauma, chronic bronchitis, chronic obstructive pulmonary disease, emphysema, Guillain-Barré syndrome, hemothorax, multiple sclerosis, Parkinson's disease, pneumonia, pneumothorax, sepsis, shock

Expected outcomes
• Patient's respiratory rate will remain within ±5 breaths/minute of baseline.
• Patient's ABG levels will be normal.
• Patient will indicate feeling comfortable and will not report pain, dyspnea, or fatigue.
• Patient will carry out activities of daily living with minimal supplemental oxygen.
• Patient's breathing pattern will return to baseline.
• Patient's Pao_2 will remain within normal limits as his activity level increases.
• Patient will breathe spontaneously after ventilator support is withdrawn.

Interventions and rationales
• Monitor patient's vital signs every 15 minutes to 1 hour *to detect tachypnea and tachycardia, early indicators of respiratory distress.*
• Monitor patient for nasal flaring, change in depth and pattern of breathing, use of accessory muscles, and cyanosis *to detect signs of severe respiratory distress.*
• Monitor ABG levels and report deviations promptly *to determine need for changes to therapeutic regimen.*
• Monitor hemoglobin (Hb) and hematocrit (HCT) level. *Low Hb and HCT level indicate decreased oxygen-carrying capacity of the blood.*
• Begin oxygen support using smallest concentration needed to make patient comfortable. Monitor closely *to avoid oxygen toxicity.*
• Place patient in Fowler's position *to increase comfort and to promote adequate chest expansion and diaphrag-*

matic excursion, thereby decreasing work of breathing.

• Help patient progress gradually from bed rest to increased activity to improve patient's sense of well-being. Monitor vital signs and ABG levels closely. If respiratory status is compromised, return patient to bed rest to decrease basal metabolic rate and lower oxygen demands.

• Explain all procedures to patient. Describe specific sensations he may experience during each procedure to decrease anxiety.

• Anticipate possible complications. Keep in mind that if patient decompensates while on 100% fraction of inspired oxygen nonrebreather mask, he may require endotracheal intubation. Anticipating complications facilitates prompt intervention.

• If patient requires intubation, monitor him for spontaneous breathing and gradually wean him from ventilator. Progressive weaning helps patient to adjust physiologically and emotionally to increased work of breathing.

• Avoid respiratory depressants, such as narcotics, sedatives, and paralytics, to facilitate patient's recovery.

Evaluations for expected outcomes

• Patient's respiratory rate is within ±5 breaths/minute of baseline.

• Patient's ABG levels are normal.

• Patient doesn't report pain, dyspnea, or fatigue.

• Patient carries out activities of daily living with minimal supplemental oxygen.

• Patient's breathing pattern returns to baseline.

• Patient's Pao_2 remains within normal limits when his activity level increases.

• Patient breathes spontaneously after ventilator support is withdrawn.

Documentation

• Patient's reports of malaise, dyspnea, restlessness, chest pain, dizziness, or lightheadedness

• Patient's response to nursing interventions

• Patient's response to initiation of oxygen therapy and progressive changes in therapy

• Laboratory data, including ABG levels

• Respiratory status (baseline and ongoing)

• Subtle personality changes

• Changes in lung sounds revealed by auscultation

• Evaluations for expected outcomes

■ Ventilatory weaning response, dysfunctional

related to diminished ventilator support

Definition

Difficulty adjusting to lowered levels of mechanical ventilator support

Assessment

• Health history, including previous respiratory problems

• Nutritional status, including caloric intake and type of and tolerance for feeding

• Neurologic status, including mental status and level of consciousness (LOC)

• Emotional status, including signs of anxiety or stress

• Laboratory values, including arterial blood gas (ABG) levels (baseline and ongoing), serum electrolyte and blood glucose levels, complete blood count, blood and sputum culture, and sensitivity tests

• Weaning parameters and current ventilator settings
• Respiratory status, including respiratory rate, pattern, character, and depth; chest expansion and symmetry; sputum characteristics (color, amount, odor, and consistency); cough effectiveness; presence of cyanosis in mucous membranes and nail beds; and auscultation of lung sounds
• Need for suctioning, including frequency and patient's response
• Musculoskeletal status, including muscle mass, strength, and endurance level
• Cognitive state, including patient's ability to follow directions and readiness to learn
• Recent administration of potential respiratory-depressant medications, such as narcotics, sedatives, and neuromuscular blockers
• Vital signs
• Pulse oximetry readings

Defining characteristics
• Mild dysfunctional weaning response:
– breathing discomfort
– expressed increased need for oxygen
– fatigue
– increased concentration on breathing
– queries about possible machine malfunction
– restlessness
– slight increase in respiratory response above baseline
• Moderate dysfunctional weaning response:
– apprehension
– changes in skin color (paleness and mild cyanosis)
– decreased air entry on auscultation
– diaphoresis

– hypervigilance to activities related to ventilator functioning
– inability to cooperate
– inability to respond to coaching
– increase in blood pressure (no more than 20 mm Hg above baseline)
– increase in heart rate (no more than 20 beats/minute above baseline)
– increase in respiratory rate (no more than 5 breaths/minute above baseline)
– slight respiratory accessory muscle use
– wide-eyed look
• Severe dysfunctional weaning response:
– adventitious breath sounds
– agitation
– audible airway secretions
– breathing uncoordinated with ventilator
– cyanosis
– decreased LOC
– deteriorating ABG levels
– full use of respiratory accessory muscle
– increased blood pressure (more than 20 mm Hg above baseline)
– increased heart rate (more than 20 beats/minute above baseline)
– paradoxical abdominal breathing
– profuse diaphoresis
– shallow, gasping breaths
– significant increase in respiratory rate

Associated medical diagnoses (selected)
Adult respiratory distress syndrome, amyotrophic lateral sclerosis, burns, chest trauma, chronic obstructive pulmonary disease, multisystem trauma, myasthenia gravis, Parkinson's disease, pleural effusion, pulmonary edema, sepsis

Expected outcomes
• Patient will maintain respiratory rate within ±5 breaths/minute of baseline during weaning period.

• Patient's ABG levels will remain within acceptable limits (specify).
• Patient's mental status and emotional state will remain stable during gradual withdrawal of ventilatory support.
• Patient will express comfort with progressive ventilator changes.
• Patient won't experience dyspnea, fatigue, or pain during progressive ventilator changes.
• Patient will remain within adequate weaning parameters:
– Tidal volume: 4 to 5 cc/kg.
– Negative inspiratory force: greater than or equal to –20 cm H_2O.
– Vital capacity: 10 to 15 cc/kg.
– Minute ventilation: 6 to 10 liters.
• Patient's cough effectively clears secretions.

Interventions and rationales

• Monitor patient's vital signs every hour when changing ventilator settings. *Fever, tachycardia, tachypnea, and elevated blood pressure may indicate hypoxemia.*
• Auscultate for lung sounds every 2 hours and report deviations. *Adventitious sounds may precede respiratory failure.*
• Place patient in comfortable position (preferably Fowler's) *to facilitate adequate chest expansion and drainage.*
• Describe all weaning procedures to patient. Explain to patient that he may experience changes in breathing rate and pattern, increased difficulty breathing, and fatigue *to decrease anxiety.*
• If patient is receiving intermittent mandatory ventilation (IMV), begin to decrease IMV by increments of 2 breaths/minute. This process may take place over days or weeks. *Lowering IMV encourages patient to take*

his own breaths, thereby exercising respiratory muscles.
• Monitor ABG levels with every ventilator change *to assess for adequate oxygenation and acid-base balance.*
• Include periods of rest between ventilator changes, especially at night, *to reduce tissue oxygen demand.*
• If patient tolerates IMV of 2 to 4 breaths/minute, try pressure support ventilation (PSV). *PSV prolongs positive airway pressure during inspiration, allowing patient to regulate his own respiratory rate and tidal volume.*
• Once patient is breathing adequately without IMV, place him on continuous positive airway pressure (CPAP) of 5 cm H_2O *to prevent alveolar collapse.*
• When patient tolerates CPAP, place him on T-piece (T-bar) of 30% to 50% fraction of inspired oxygen. *This allows patient to breathe on his own, continue to receive oxygen, and remain intubated in event of respiratory compromise.*
• Once patient tolerates longer weaning periods, incorporate activities of daily living into daily routine *to increase muscular strength and endurance.*
• When patient has satisfactory respiratory status, weaning parameters, and ABG levels, assist with removal of ventilator tubes and keep oxygen mask on hand *to prevent respiratory compromise.*
• Assess patient for stridor, respiratory distress, and dysphonia and report these findings to doctor *to monitor need for renewed ventilatory assistance.*
• Perform chest physiotherapy and suctioning as needed *to maintain patent airway.*
• Monitor respiratory effects of medications closely and evaluate response

to bronchodilators *to detect respiratory status compromise.* Avoid respiratory depressants.

Evaluations for expected outcomes
• Patient's respiratory rate is within ±5 breaths/minute of baseline during weaning period.
• Patient's ABG levels are within specified acceptable limits.
• Patient maintains stable mental and emotional status during withdrawal of ventilatory support.
• Patient expresses comfort with progressive ventilator changes.
• Patient doesn't experience dyspnea, fatigue, or pain during progressive ventilator changes.
• Patient remains within adequate weaning parameters.
• Patient's cough effectively clears secretions.

Documentation
• Patient's reports of malaise, anxiety, restlessness, breathlessness, and unusual pain
• Patient's response to ventilator changes
• Subtle changes in patient's mental or emotional status
• Laboratory data, including ABG levels
• Patient's response to nursing interventions, including positioning, chest physiotherapy, and suctioning
• Patient responses to medications, including narcotics, bronchodilators, and neuromuscular blockers
• Respiratory rate, pattern, and depth, including changes from baseline
• Evaluations for expected outcomes

■ Verbal communication impairment

related to decreased circulation to brain

Definition
Decreased ability to speak, understand, or use words appropriately

Assessment
• Neurologic status, including level of consciousness, orientation, cognition, memory (recent and remote), insight, and judgment
• Speech characteristics, including pattern (garbled, incomprehensible, difficulty forming words), language and vocabulary, level of comprehension and expression, and ability to use other forms of communication (such as eye blinks, gestures, pictures, and nods)
• Motor ability
• Circulatory status, including a history of cardiac and circulatory problems, pulse, blood pressure, arteriogram, electroencephalogram, and computed tomography scan
• Respiratory status, including dyspnea and use of accessory muscles

Defining characteristics
• Disorientation
• Difficulty expressing thought verbally (aphasia, dysphasia, apraxia, dyslexia)
• Difficulty comprehending and maintaining usual communication pattern
• Difficulty forming words or sentences (aphonia, dyslalia, dysarthria)
• Difficulty using or inability to use facial expressions or body language
• Dyspnea
• Impaired articulation
• Inability or lack of desire to speak

• Inability to speak dominant language
• Inappropriate verbalizations
• Lack of eye contact or poor selective attention
• Stuttering or slurring
• Visual deficit (partial or total)

Associated medical diagnoses (selected)
Acute respiratory failure, arterial occlusion, cerebrovascular accident, food poisoning, head injury

Expected outcomes
• Staff members will meet patient's needs.
• Patient and family members will express satisfaction with level of communication ability.
• Patient will maintain orientation.
• Patient will maintain effective level of communication.
• Patient will answer direct questions correctly.

Interventions and rationales
• Observe patient closely for cues to needs and desires, such as gestures, pointing to objects, looking at items, and pantomime *to enhance understanding.* Don't continually respond to gestures if potential exists to improve speech *to avoid discouraging improvement.*
• Monitor and record changes in speech pattern or level of orientation. *Changes may indicate improvement or deterioration of condition.*
• Speak slowly and distinctly in normal tone when addressing patient, and stand where patient can see and hear you. *These actions promote comprehension.*
• Reorient patient to reality:
– Call patient by name.
– Tell patient your name.
– Give patient background information (place, date, and time).

– Use television or radio to augment orientation.
– Use large calendars and reality orientation boards.
These measures develop orientation skills through repetition and recognition of familiar objects.
• Use short, simple phrases and yes-or-no questions when patient is very frustrated *to reduce frustration.*
• Encourage attempts at communication and provide positive reinforcement *to aid comprehension.*
• Allow ample time for response. Don't answer questions yourself if patient has ability to respond. *This improves patient's self-concept and reduces frustration.*
• Repeat or rephrase questions if necessary *to improve communication.* Don't pretend to understand if you don't, *to avoid misunderstanding.*
• Remove distractions from environment during attempts at communication. *Reduced distractions improve comprehension.* Use communication boards (including alphabet and some common words and pictures) if appropriate *to aid comprehension.*
• Review diagnostic test results *to determine improvement or deterioration of disease process.* Adjust plan of care accordingly.

Evaluations for expected outcomes
• Staff members consistently meet patient's needs.
• Patient and family members communicate at satisfactory level.
• Patient demonstrates orientation by consistently communicating thoughts to staff and family.
• Patient communicates effectively____ times every 8 hours (specify).
• Patient correctly answers ____ direct questions (specify).

Documentation
• Patient's current level of communication, orientation, and satisfaction with communication efforts
• Observations of speech deficits, expressiveness and receptiveness, and ability to communicate
• Interventions carried out to promote effective communication
• Patient's observable response to nursing interventions
• Evaluations for expected outcomes

■ Verbal communication impairment

related to physical barriers

Definition
Decreased ability to speak, understand, or use words appropriately

Assessment
• History of respiratory, neurologic, or musculoskeletal disorder or surgery
• Respiratory status, including dyspnea, use of accessory muscles, and respiratory pattern
• Neurologic status, including mental status (level of consciousness, orientation, cognition, memory, insight, and judgment) and speech (pattern, signing, and such communication aids as artificial larynx, computer-assisted speech device, pen and pencil, slate, picture board, and alphabet board)
• Musculoskeletal status, including range of motion and manual dexterity

Defining characteristics
• Disorientation
• Difficulty expressing thought verbally (aphasia, dysphasia, apraxia, dyslexia)
• Difficulty comprehending and maintaining usual communication pattern
• Difficulty forming words or sentences (aphonia, dyslalia, dysarthria)
• Difficulty using or inability to use facial expressions or body language
• Dyspnea
• Impaired articulation
• Inability or lack of desire to speak
• Inability to speak dominant language
• Inappropriate verbalizations
• Lack of eye contact or poor selective attention
• Stuttering or slurring
• Visual deficit (partial or total)

Associated medical diagnoses (selected)
Acute respiratory failure, adult respiratory distress syndrome, amyotrophic lateral sclerosis, asthma, atelectasis, Bell's palsy, chronic obstructive pulmonary disease, cleft lip or palate, cor pulmonale, head or neck cancer, lung cancer, myasthenia gravis, pneumonia, pulmonary edema, pulmonary embolus, tracheostomy

Expected outcomes
• Patient will communicate needs and desires without undue frustration.
• Patient will use alternate means of communication.
• Patient will demonstrate correct use of adaptive equipment.
• Patient will express plans to use appropriate resources to maximize communication skills.

Interventions and rationales
• Maintain consistent daily schedule of activities as much as possible. Observe patient closely for cues to needs and desires, such as gestures, pointing to or looking at objects, and pantomime, *to enhance understanding.*
• Obtain communication aids for patient's use, such as an alphabet board,

slate, pen, paper, and picture board, *to provide alternative communication methods.*
• Use short, simple phrases and yes-or-no questions *to reduce frustration and anxiety.*
• Encourage communication attempts; allow time to select or write words or pictures *to reduce pressure and improve interaction with others.*
• Allow ample time for response; don't answer questions for patient *to reduce frustration.*
• Consult with speech therapist to suggest such communication aids as artificial larynx. Assist with use. *Appropriate early referral encourages use of communication aids.*
• Demonstrate communication techniques, such as gestures, sign language, and eye blinking, to patient and family members *to develop alternative communication skills.*
• Assist patient in energy-conserving techniques *to allow maximum breath for speech or use of communication aids.*
• Use tracheostomy plug *to facilitate speech,* if tolerated by patient.
• Provide patient with emergency call system (bell or call light), and respond to all calls immediately and in person. Place sign over intercom to alert all staff members of need to respond quickly. *Prompt responses reduce patient's fear and anxiety.*
• Encourage attendance at a laryngectomy club or other appropriate support groups *to provide additional support.*

Evaluations for expected outcomes
• Patient consistently communicates needs without frustration.
• Patient successfully uses alternate means of communication (specify).

• Patient uses adaptive equipment ____ times daily to improve communication (specify).
• Patient identifies and contacts appropriate support resources, such as speech therapist and laryngectomy club.

Documentation
• Patient's feelings about inability to communicate
• Observations of patient's attempts to communicate, response to and ability to use alternate communication means, and level of frustration or fatigue
• Patient's response to nursing interventions
• Patient's preferences in daily care activities, such as when to shave or bathe and what kind of razor to use
• Evaluations for expected outcomes

■ Walking, impaired

related to neuromuscular dysfunction

Definition
Alteration in ability to move feet properly with one foot clearing ground before other touches

Assessment
• Age
• Sex
• Vital signs
• History of cerebrovascular accident, spinal cord injury, head injury, multiple sclerosis, Guillain-Barré syndrome, or Parkinson's disease
• Medication history
• Musculoskeletal status, including coordination, gait, muscle size and strength, muscle tone, range of mo-

tion (ROM), and functional mobility as follows:

0 = completely independent

1 = requires use of equipment or device

2 = requires help, supervision, or teaching from another person

3 = requires help from another person and equipment or device

4 = dependent; doesn't participate in activity

• Neurologic status, including level of consciousness, motor ability, and sensory ability

• Endurance level — for example, how far the patient can walk before tiring

Defining characteristics

• Altered postural reflexes

• Ataxia

• Fatigue

• Flaccidity

• Inability to ambulate

• Paraplegia

• Paresis

• Quadriplegia

• Spasticity

• Weakness

Associated medical diagnoses (selected)

Brain abscess, cerebral aneurysm, cerebrovascular accident, Guillain-Barré syndrome, head injury, multiple sclerosis, muscular dystrophy, myasthenia gravis, paralysis, paresis, Parkinson's disease, spinal cord injury or tumor

Expected outcomes

• Patient will not exhibit complications associated with impaired walking, such as alteration in skin integrity, contractures, venous stasis, or thrombus formation.

• Patient will maintain or improve muscle strength and joint ROM

• Patient will achieve highest level of ambulation possible (independence using wheelchair, ambulation with device, ambulation without device).

• Patient will maintain safety during ambulation.

• Patient will demonstrate ability to use equipment or devices safely.

• Patient will adapt to alteration in walking.

• Patient will participate in social and occupational activities.

• Patient will demonstrate understanding of specific interventions related to coping with alteration in walking.

• Patient will utilize community resources to promote and maintain highest level of mobility.

Interventions and rationales

• Perform ROM exercises for joints of affected limbs, unless contraindicated, at least once per shift. Progress from passive to active ROM, as tolerated, *to prevent joint contractures and muscle atrophy.*

• Make sure that patient maintains anatomically correct and functional body positioning. Encourage repositioning every 2 hours when patient is in bed. Establish turning schedule for dependent patients. *Proper positioning relieves pressure, thereby preventing skin breakdown and fluid accumulation in dependent extremities.*

• Identify patient's level of independence using the functional mobility scale. Communicate findings to staff *to provide continuity and preserve documented level of independence.*

• Implement preambulation program (for example, turning in bed, sitting on side of bed, sitting up in chair) *to increase independence and patient's self-esteem.*

• Monitor and record daily evidence of complications related to altered walking, such as contractures, venous stasis, skin breakdown, or thrombus formation. *Patient with history of neuromuscular dysfunction is at risk for complications.*

• Perform medical regimen to manage or prevent complications (for example, administration of prophylactic heparin for venous thrombosis) *to promote patient's health and well-being.*

• Provide progressive ambulation up to limits imposed by patient's condition *to maintain muscle tone and prevent complications associated with immobility.*

• Refer patient to physical therapist for development of program to promote walking *to assist with rehabilitation of musculoskeletal deficits.*

• Encourage attendance at physical therapy sessions and reinforce prescribed activities by using the same equipment, devices, and techniques used in therapy sessions. Request a written copy of patient's ambulation program to use as reference. *This maintains continuity and helps ensure patient's safety.*

• Instruct patient and family members in ambulation techniques and measures to prevent complications *to help prepare patient and family for discharge.*

• Demonstrate ambulation regimen and note date. Have patient and family members perform return demonstration *to ensure continuity of care and use of proper technique.*

• Assist in identifying resources to promote and maintain highest level of mobility, such as community stroke program, sports associations for the disabled, or the National Multiple Sclerosis Society *to promote patient's reintegration into the community.*

Evaluations for expected outcomes

• Patient doesn't exhibit complications associated with impaired walking, such as alteration in skin integrity, contractures, venous stasis, or thrombus formation.

• Patient maintains or improves muscle strength and joint range of motion.

• Patient achieves highest level of ambulation possible (independence using wheelchair, ambulation with device, ambulation without device).

• Patient maintains safety during ambulation.

• Patient demonstrates ability to use equipment or devices safely.

• Patient adapts to alteration in walking.

• Patient participates in social and occupational activities.

• Patient demonstrates understanding of specific interventions related to coping with alteration in walking.

• Patient utilizes community resources to promote and maintain highest level of mobility.

Documentation

• Patient's ambulation status, presence of complications, and response to ambulation program

• Patient's statements regarding loss of ambulation ability, current ambulation ability, and goals set for improved ambulation ability

• Patient teaching

• Return demonstration of skills for carrying out ambulation program

• Patient's response to nursing interventions

• Evaluations for expected outcomes

ADOLESCENT HEALTH

INTRODUCTION

This section focuses on providing nursing care for adolescent patients. The tremendous physiologic and cognitive changes that occur between ages 10 and 18 are commonly accompanied by overpowering emotional turmoil.

The adolescent patient commonly struggles with issues of independence and identity. When taking his history, demonstrate respect for his struggle. Be alert to language; adolescents particularly resent being "talked down to." Let the patient decide the level of parental involvement. Although some adolescents prize their independence, others still need parental support during physical examination and history taking. If possible, perform at least part of the nursing assessment in private to allow for open discussion of highly personal issues such as sexuality.

Many adolescents feel invulnerable. This characteristic places them at high risk for such health problems as drug and alcohol abuse, sexually transmitted diseases, and trauma. When talking with the patient, explore feelings of personal invulnerability and discuss potential consequences.

When planning interventions, think of ways to foster independence and promote self-esteem while helping the adolescent obtain needed support from parents, health care providers, and others. Refer to plans of care included in the sections on Adult Health and Child Health as well. Use every opportunity to teach the patient about health promotion. Increased knowledge allows the adolescent to assume responsibility for himself.

Adolescence can be a trying time for families as well. In addition to asking direct questions about family relationships, be alert to nonverbal and verbal indications of conflict. Also be aware that parents may be struggling with their child's newly found independence and may need your help as well.

■ Body image disturbance

related to an eating disorder

Definition
Inaccurate self-perception that leads to weight loss in an attempt to conform to an idealized body image

Assessment
• Age
• Sex
• Health history, including previous eating disorders; dieting; physical, emotional, or sexual abuse; and episodes of emesis
• Exercise pattern, including type and duration
• Cardiovascular status, including skin color and temperature, heart rate and rhythm, blood pressure, and complete blood count
• Nutritional status, including daily food intake, food likes and dislikes, meal preparation, and knowledge of dietary requirements; height and weight and weight fluctuations over past year; and serum albumin, lymphocyte, and electrolyte levels
• Psychological status, including expressions of need for control or perceived loss of self-control, behavioral changes, expressions of helplessness, recent emotional crisis, stress, and body image
• Perception of ideal feminine form
• Family status, including role performance, perception of role within family, and attitudes and perceptions related to food, body image, success, and control
• Use of diuretics and laxatives

Defining characteristics
• Change in body structure, body weight, or function
• Denial of eating disorder

• Depression
• Excessive and ritualized exercise
• Excessive need for control of self and environment
• Fear of weight gain
• Hiding body in oversized clothing
• Obsession with food
• Ritualized eating patterns
• Verbalization of feelings or perceptions that reflect an altered view of one's physical appearance

Associated medical diagnoses (selected)
Anorexia nervosa, bulimia nervosa, cardiac arrhythmias, depression, diarrhea

Expected outcomes
• Adolescent will comply with prescribed treatment.
• Adolescent will express feelings associated with food, exercise, weight loss, and medical condition.
• Adolescent will describe her perception of personal daily caloric needs.
• Adolescent will express understanding that current eating and exercise patterns are self-destructive.
• Adolescent will consume appropriate number of calories each day.
• Adolescent will ask for help in controlling destructive behavior.
• Adolescent will participate in decisions about care and treatment.
• Adolescent will participate in support group for people with eating disorders.
• Adolescent will express insight into reasons behind current eating patterns and other self-destructive behaviors.
• Adolescent will learn and implement new coping behaviors.
• Adolescent will express positive feelings about self.
• Adolescent will express satisfaction with parental involvement in care.

Interventions and rationales

• Implement adolescent's prescribed therapy *to help restore health and body function.*

• Monitor and record adolescent's vital signs, weight, and electrolytes *to detect abnormal values and prevent complications.*

• Obtain referral for dietary consultation *to identify caloric intake, necessary diet modifications, and goals for weight gain and stabilization.*

• Obtain referral for psychiatric evaluation *to identify problems related to altered body image, poor self-esteem, and inappropriate coping.*

• Convey a positive, caring attitude to adolescent and take steps to ensure continuity of care throughout treatment *to ensure safety and foster trusting therapeutic relationship.*

• Encourage adolescent to participate in self-care and, as appropriate, to make decisions about therapy *to foster sense of control and involvement in restoring health.*

• Tell adolescent that you accept her as a person and provide reassurance that she can overcome her problems *to validate self-perception and enhance confidence.*

• Maintain communication throughout adolescent's course of treatment *to assess coping mechanisms and level of self-esteem.*

• Encourage adolescent to express feelings about self, eating, exercise, hospitalization, and medical condition *to correct misconceptions, help her clarify her thoughts, and reinforce realistic self-appraisal.*

• Reinforce appropriate behaviors *to encourage adolescent to comply with therapy and to participate in care.*

• Use behavior modification strategies consistently *to enable adolescent to predict consequences of behavior.*

• Avoid using coercive techniques to make adolescent participate in care or adhere to rules. *Use of coercion may encourage adolescent to view manipulative behavior as acceptable.*

• Monitor food consumption and record intake *to ensure that adolescent consumes prescribed calories.*

• Monitor adolescent in bathroom *to detect episodes of purging.*

• Without conveying attitude of distrust, watch for signs of noncompliance with medical regimen. Emphasize that prescribed caloric intake is necessary to maintain health and won't lead to obesity. *This promotes early detection of self-destructive behavior and may improve adolescent's sense of control.*

• Inform adolescent of her progress throughout hospitalization *to increase her awareness of achievements and motivate her to keep trying.*

• Help adolescent to identify positive aspects of her appearance *to improve self-esteem by correcting distorted perceptions about body image.*

• Help direct adolescent's need for control away from body image and eating behaviors by encouraging her participation in appropriate diversional activities *to channel her energies into new areas in which she can take pride.*

• Encourage adolescent's participation in group discussions with peers who also have eating disorders *to foster insight and group support.*

• Help adolescent identify appropriate coping strategies. Discuss previously effective strategies *to help her substitute them for maladaptive ones.*

• Encourage parents to demonstrate emotional support for adolescent throughout course of treatment *to strengthen family support system.*

• Encourage parents to participate in support group with other parents of children with eating disorders *to provide forum for expressing feelings and obtaining support from individuals who can understand their concerns.*

• Teach parents how to detect signs that their child may be relapsing into self-destructive behaviors *to help them identify need for early assistance and enhance their confidence in their ability to protect their child from harm.*

Evaluations for expected outcomes

• Adolescent complies with prescribed treatment regimen.
• Adolescent expresses feelings associated with food, exercise, weight loss, and medical condition.
• Adolescent describes her perception of personal daily caloric needs.
• Adolescent expresses understanding of the idea that her eating and exercise patterns are self-destructive.
• Adolescent consumes appropriate number of calories each day.
• Adolescent asks for help in controlling destructive behavior.
• Adolescent participates in decisions related to care and treatment.
• Adolescent participates in support group for people with eating disorders.
• Adolescent expresses insight into reasons behind her eating patterns and other self-destructive behaviors.
• Adolescent learns and implements new coping behaviors.
• Adolescent expresses positive feelings about self.
• Adolescent expresses satisfaction with parental involvement in care.

Documentation

• Vital signs
• Weight (recorded daily or weekly according to facility's protocol)

• Amount of food consumed at each meal
• Adolescent's description of herself
• Observations of rituals related to food and exercise
• Adolescent's participation in and response to support group
• Observations of self-destructive behaviors, such as forced emesis or use of laxatives or diuretics
• Observations of manipulative behaviors
• Coping mechanisms
• Exercise patterns
• Behavior modification techniques used by caregivers
• Adolescent's response to treatment protocol
• Adolescent's response to nursing interventions
• Evidence of changes in adolescent's self-perception
• Evaluations for expected outcomes

■ Caregiver role strain, risk for

related to developmental state

Definition
Adolescent's inability to meet developmental needs because of responsibilities to act as caregiver

Assessment
• Adolescent caregiver's physical and mental status, including age, sex, and developmental stage; level of cognitive functioning; emotional functioning; and self-care abilities
• Care recipient's physical and mental status, including age, sex, illness, self-care limitations, mobility limitations, level of cognitive functioning, and relationship to adolescent (parent, sibling, or other)

• Family status, including role performance and perception of role within family
• Available resources, including finances, emotional support system, community services, and health-related services, such as geriatric day care and home health aides
• Home environment, including structural barriers, layout of home, need for medical equipment or devices, and availability of transportation
• Cultural, ethnic, and religious background
• Perceived and actual obligations of adolescent
• Effect of caregiver responsibilities on adolescent
• Adolescent's coping skills, problem-solving abilities, and ability to participate in hobbies and preferred activities

Risk factors
• Codependency (between caregiver and recipient)
• Competing role commitments (caregiver)
• Developmental delay or disability (caregiver or recipient)
• Discharge of family member with significant home care needs (care recipient)
• Drug or alcohol addiction (caregiver or recipient)
• Inadequate housing, transportation, community services, or equipment for providing care
• Isolation (caregiver)
• Lack of developmental readiness for caregiver role
• Lack of experience (caregiver)
• Lack of respite or recreation (caregiver)
• Numerous, complex caregiving tasks
• Premature birth or congenital defect (recipient)

• Probability of long duration of caregiving
• Presence of abuse or violence (recipient)

Associated medical diagnoses (selected)
This diagnosis may occur in any chronic illness or disability. Examples include acquired immunodeficiency syndrome, Alzheimer's disease, amyotrophic lateral sclerosis, cerebral palsy, cerebrovascular accident, chronic obstructive pulmonary disease, dementia, end-stage renal or cardiac disease, heart failure, Huntington's disease, macular degeneration, multiple sclerosis, muscular dystrophy, paralysis, Parkinson's disease, and schizophrenia.

Expected outcomes
• Adolescent will identify current stressors.
• Adolescent will identify and implement adaptive coping strategies.
• Adolescent will identify personal developmental needs and tasks.
• Adolescent will contact sources of support to help provide care.
• Adolescent will allot time each day for respite, recreation, and personal development activities.
• Adolescent will report less stress related to caregiver duties.

Interventions and rationales
• Assess developmental stage and needs of adolescent caregiver *to provide basis for developing interventions that reduce caregiver role strain. During adolescence, individuals begin establishing their identity by trying various roles without assuming complete responsibility for them. The imposed role of caregiver impedes this developmental task.*
• Help adolescent identify current stressors. Discuss how her responsi-

bility to act as caregiver places limits on her lifestyle *to evaluate the degree of caregiver role strain.*

• Encourage adolescent to discuss coping skills used previously *to reinforce her confidence in her ability to manage current situation and explore new ways to apply coping strategies.*

• Help adolescent identify informal sources of support, such as family members, support groups, or church groups that can help with caregiver tasks, *to provide opportunities for respite from caregiver activities.*

• Teach adolescent about formal sources of support, such as home health care agencies, social workers, doctors, clinics, and day-care centers, *to allow adolescent to fulfill other obligations, such as attending school.*

• Encourage regular participation in enjoyable activities, such as sports, hobbies, reading, or social gatherings. *Incorporating enjoyable activities into daily schedule helps discipline adolescent to take needed breaks from caregiver responsibilities.*

• Provide adolescent with information about available support groups, and encourage participation. *Support groups provide outlet for expressing feelings and foster sense of support and belonging.*

• Assess adolescent's view of her actual and perceived responsibilities as caregiver and correct any misconceptions. *Emotional ties to care recipient, confusion about roles within family, or codependence may cloud adolescent caregiver's perceptions. Your input helps her develop more objective view of situation.*

Evaluations for expected outcomes

• Adolescent describes her emotional response to stressors in her life.
• Adolescent identifies and uses adaptive coping strategies.

• Adolescent identifies personal developmental needs and tasks.
• Adolescent uses available support systems.
• Adolescent schedules respite periods for personal developmental needs and recreation.
• Adolescent reports reduced stress from caregiver responsibilities.

Documentation

• Care recipient's physical and mental status and adolescent caregiver's responsibility for providing care
• Current stressors identified by adolescent
• Risk factors (developmental, situational, psychological, and pathophysiologic) for caregiver role strain
• Adolescent's statements indicating intention to take actions to minimize stress, such as joining support group, seeking help from support services, and scheduling respite
• Observations of adolescent's response to stress
• Coping strategies identified by adolescent and nurse
• Referrals provided
• Evaluations for expected outcomes

■ Decisional conflict

related to sexual activity

Definition

Uncertainty about whether to engage in sexual activity

Assessment

• Age
• Sex
• Developmental stage, including physical maturity, cognition, beliefs, values, and ethics

• Family system, including nuclear family, extended family, birth order, family roles, and evidence of conflict
• History of sexual experiences, including experimentation, trauma, and other experiences
• Psychological status, including level of function, coping mechanisms, support systems, self-image, self-esteem, and attitude toward physical appearance
• Sociocultural status, including level of education, ethnicity, and religious affiliation
• Sexual orientation

Defining characteristics
• Delayed decision making
• Expressed feelings of distress and questioning of values and beliefs while attempting to decide
• Expressed uncertainty
• Focus on self
• Lack of experience or interference with decision making
• Physical indications of distress (such as increased heart rate, muscle tension, and restlessness)
• Vacillation between choices
• Verbalization of undesired consequences of alternative decisions

Associated medical diagnoses (selected)
Depression, eating disorders, obsessive-compulsive disorder, personality disorders, psychiatric disorders

Expected outcomes
• Adolescent will express feelings about sexuality and sexual activity.
• Adolescent will discuss conflicts between personal values and social pressures to be sexually active.
• Adolescent will identify desirable and undesirable consequences of sexual activity.

• Adolescent will describe family conflicts and will explore their potential effect on sexual conduct.
• Adolescent will accept help from parents, other family members, friends, and health professionals.
• Adolescent will report confidence in choosing sexual behavior consistent with personal values.

Interventions and rationales
• Visit adolescent frequently and encourage frequent visits by family members *to promote trusting therapeutic relationship and ease anxiety and fears.*
• Encourage expressions of feelings about social and sexual patterns *to improve recognition of feelings and foster open discussion.*
• Assess adolescent's knowledge of sex and sexuality. Discuss sexual behavior and its potential consequences. Provide information about safer sex practices, birth control, and abstinence. *Correct information about sexual practices reduces adolescent's confusion about whether or not to be sexually active.*
• Listen attentively and remain nonjudgmental as adolescent describes personal fears, values, and desires. *Nonjudgmental, active listening demonstrates your unconditional positive regard for adolescent.*
• Provide guidance as adolescent explores options for sexual activity *to promote confidence in decision-making capabilities.*
• Discuss peer pressure. Ask if adolescent feels strong social pressure to be sexually active. Ask about other ways peers exert influence, and explore ways of coping with peer pressure. *Adolescents must learn to deal with peer pressure.*
• Discuss family conflicts. Ask adolescent if troubled family relation-

ships are pushing adolescent to become sexually active. *Adolescents may seek in sexual relationships love they don't receive from family members.*
• Respect adolescent's right to make choices based on personal values, desires, religious beliefs, cultural norms, and sexual preference *to foster autonomy and self-confidence.*
• Help adolescent identify support network (friends, family, community services, and church or synagogue groups) and encourage their use in decision making *to help adolescent make decisions and resolve conflicts in emotionally supportive environment.*

Evaluations for expected outcomes
• Adolescent expresses feelings related to sexuality and sexual activity.
• Adolescent describes conflicts between personal values and social pressure to become sexually active.
• Adolescent expresses increased understanding of options regarding sexual activity and their potential consequences.
• Adolescent discusses possible influences, including peer pressure and conflicts with family, on decision to be sexually active.
• Adolescent identifies support network and uses it to aid decision making.
• Adolescent reports feeling more comfortable with ability to make decisions regarding sexuality and sexual activity.

Documentation
• Adolescent's statements indicating conflict over decision about whether to be sexually active
• Adolescent's cognitive, emotional, and behavioral functioning

• Adolescent's knowledge of birth control and safer sex practices
• Nursing interventions to help adolescent make choices regarding sexuality and sexual conflict
• Adolescent's responses to interventions
• Evaluations for expected outcomes

■ Decisional conflict
related to substance use

Definition
Uncertainty about whether to use recreational drugs

Assessment
• Age
• Physical maturity
• Sociocultural factors, including level of education, financial status, and ethnic group
• Family history, including family roles, coping patterns, family's ability to meet adolescent's physical and emotional needs, and history of substance abuse in family members
• Level of functioning (cognitive, emotional, and behavioral)
• Coping mechanisms
• Available support systems
• Evidence of drug use, including drug toxicology screening, urinalysis, personality changes, and social withdrawal

Defining characteristics
• Delayed decision making
• Expressed feelings of distress and questioning of values and beliefs while attempting to decide
• Expressed uncertainty
• Focus on self
• Lack of experience or interference with decision making

• Physical indications of distress (such as increased heart rate, muscle tension, and restlessness)
• Vacillation between choices
• Verbalization of undesired consequences of alternative decisions

Associated medical diagnoses (selected)

This diagnosis commonly accompanies any diagnosis related to substance abuse or psychiatric illness and may coincide with many other diagnoses.

Expected outcomes

• Adolescent will discuss conflict over drug use.
• Adolescent will describe conflict between personal values and options and external value systems (parental, societal, peer, and legal).
• Adolescent will identify perceived desirable and undesirable consequences of drug use.
• Adolescent will accept assistance from parents, other family members, friends, and health care providers.
• Adolescent will report increased comfort with making choices about drug use that are consistent with personal values.

Interventions and rationales

• Visit adolescent frequently. Schedule specific amount of time each day for visits *to promote trust and provide time when adolescent can discuss feelings confidentially.*
• Make adolescent aware that you're willing to discuss all topics, including substance use. Assure that all information will be kept confidential *to encourage honest discussion of concerns.*
• Encourage adolescent to explore feelings related to drug use, school, family, friends, and other vital topics. Remain nonjudgmental and be will-

ing to listen to his values, beliefs, and concerns *to demonstrate that you regard him as a worthwhile person with valid values and beliefs.*
• Ask adolescent to describe family and home life *to assess for family conflict that may be creating emotional distress.* Provide referrals for family counseling, if needed.
• Ask adolescent if peers pressure him to use drugs. Explore ways of coping with peer pressure. *Adolescents must learn to deal with peer pressure.*
• Discuss adolescent's self-esteem and explore ways of building self-esteem *to strengthen adolescent's ability to deal with peer pressure.*
• Help adolescent explore alternative recreational activities, such as sports, art, music, community service, or participation in church or synagogue groups, *to help develop alternatives to substance use.*
• Teach adolescent about health and legal consequences of substance abuse. *Accurate information will help him make informed, rational decisions.*
• Encourage adolescent to identify and use support network (family, friends, clinics, school nurse, or other health care providers). *Support network can help adolescent make decisions and resolve conflicts in emotionally supportive environment.*
• Refer adolescent for long-term counseling, if necessary. *Long-standing emotional conflicts may require in-depth intervention.*

Evaluations for expected outcomes

• Adolescent discusses conflict over whether to use drugs.
• Adolescent discusses peer pressure, family conflict, or other factors that may be influencing him to use drugs.
• Adolescent identifies health and legal consequences of drug use.

• Adolescent identifies available sources of emotional support and requests help if needed.
• Adolescent reports increased self-esteem and ability to deal with peer pressure.

Documentation
• Evidence of drug use
• Adolescent's stated feelings about drug use
• Adolescent's level of cognitive, emotional, and behavioral functioning
• Interventions performed to help adolescent make choices about drug use
• Adolescent's responses to interventions
• Evaluations for expected outcomes

■ Health maintenance alteration

related to management of type 1 diabetes mellitus

Definition
Lack of knowledge or motivation regarding health practices, in this case adolescent's failure to properly manage type 1 diabetes mellitus

Assessment
• Age
• Sex
• Developmental stage, including cognitive ability and physical maturity
• Level of knowledge about type 1 diabetes mellitus, routine health practices, preventive needs and safety measures, and treatment and follow-up
• Level of motivation to perform self-care
• Current health status, including height, weight, recent illnesses, and adolescent's perception of personal health status
• Social status, including lifestyle, activity level, sports, interests, and socioeconomic status
• Family health history, including history of diabetes mellitus

Defining characteristics
• History of lack of health-seeking behaviors
• Impaired personal support systems
• Inability to take responsibility for meeting basic health needs
• Interest in improving health behaviors
• Lack of adaptive behaviors to internal or external changes
• Lack of knowledge regarding basic health practices
• Lack of necessary equipment or financial and other resources

Associated medical diagnoses (selected)
Type 1 diabetes mellitus

Expected outcomes
• Adolescent will describe feelings about self-management of type 1 diabetes mellitus.
• Adolescent will describe disease process.
• Adolescent will describe influence of peer pressure on his health care practices.
• Adolescent will describe proper techniques for managing signs and symptoms of hypoglycemia, hyperglycemia, and ketosis.
• Adolescent will demonstrate ability to perform self-care activities, such as properly administering insulin and choosing appropriate foods.
• Adolescent won't exhibit signs or symptoms of hypoglycemia, hyperglycemia, or ketosis.

Interventions and rationales

• Evaluate adolescent's understanding of type 1 diabetes mellitus and attitude about need to manage it. *This will help you determine which teaching interventions to use.*

• Correct any misconceptions about type 1 diabetes mellitus and therapeutic regimen. Use teaching materials appropriate for adolescent's age *to increase his knowledge of his condition and instill confidence in his ability to manage it.*

• Discuss peer pressure. Ask adolescent if he feels social pressure that causes him to ignore his diet or avoid self-administering insulin. Ask if he feels embarrassed about his disorder. Explore ways of coping with peer pressure. *Adolescents must learn to deal with peer pressure.*

• Observe as adolescent performs self-care activities *to assess his skills and overall progress.*

• Teach adolescent how to interpret glycosylated hemoglobin results and correlate these values with degree of metabolic control *to increase autonomy and decision-making skills.*

• Provide written materials that cover each teaching topic. *These materials help reinforce learning and can refresh adolescent's memory later.*

• Describe resources available to help adolescent manage his disorder. Consider arranging visit with hospital dietitian or diabetes counselor *to reinforce teaching.*

• Work with adolescent to develop exercise plan *to prevent hypoglycemia.* The plan should identify support person capable of assisting during hypoglycemic episode and should include:
– obtaining blood glucose level before and after exercise
– consuming extra food before exercise (if blood glucose falls between 80 and 180 mg/dl) in form of carbohydrates
– abstaining from strenuous exercise if blood glucose is elevated
– wearing medical identification bracelet
– carrying quick-acting sugar in case hypoglycemia occurs.
These measures ensure adolescent's safety while allowing participation in activities.

• Discuss how to manage diabetes during illness. For example, explain that infections may lead to hyperglycemia or ketosis and that early detection of infection can reduce severity of these episodes. Also, explain that fever, nausea, vomiting, and diarrhea require modifications in prescribed diet, such as substituting juice for raw fruits. Teach adolescent to check over-the-counter medications such as cold remedies for sugar content and to avoid products high in sugar. Explain importance of following prescribed regimen for increasing insulin dosage in relation to blood glucose test results. *These measures help provide a sense of control, ensure safety, and prevent complications.*

• Teach adolescent to recognize signs and symptoms he must report to his health care provider *to improve management skills and ensure safety.*

• Discuss possible complications, such as atherosclerosis, which most commonly affects eyes, kidneys, and lower extremities, and diabetic neuropathy, which may lead to loss of sensation, function, and paresthesia. *Understanding possible major complications may encourage adolescent to adhere to prescribed regimen.*

• Encourage adolescent to contact support group sponsored by Juvenile Diabetes Association *to provide peer support.*

Evaluations for expected outcomes
• Adolescent expresses feelings about self-management of diabetes.
• Adolescent accurately describes disease process of type 1 diabetes mellitus.
• Adolescent discusses influence of peer pressure on his health care practices.
• Adolescent demonstrates techniques for managing signs and symptoms of hypoglycemia, hyperglycemia, and ketosis.
• Adolescent demonstrates proficiency in self-care activities, including administering insulin and selecting foods.
• Adolescent doesn't exhibit signs or symptoms of hypoglycemia, hyperglycemia, or ketosis.

Documentation
• Adolescent's statements indicating his understanding of type 1 diabetes mellitus, health-promoting activities, management techniques during exercise and illness, and necessary self-care skills
• Adolescent's statements indicating disregard for consequences of failing to properly manage type 1 diabetes mellitus
• Adolescent's response to interventions and teaching
• Literature provided to adolescent about managing his disorder
• Observations of adolescent's demonstrations of self-care techniques
• Referrals to community resources or hospital services
• Evaluations for expected outcomes

■ Poisoning, risk for
related to substance abuse

Definition
Accentuated risk of accidental ingestion of drugs, alcohol, or other potentially hazardous substances in doses sufficient to cause poisoning

Assessment
• Age
• Sex
• Developmental stage, including cognitive ability and physical maturity
• Medication history (prescription and over-the-counter medications)
• Physical status, including evidence or history of renal or hepatic impairment, eating disorders, or substance abuse
• Family status, including living arrangement, family dynamics, history or current evidence of substance abuse, and financial status
• Social status, including peer group and related social pressures and level of activity
• Knowledge of risks associated with use of drugs, alcohol, or other potentially hazardous substances (such as fumes from glue, nitrous oxide propellants, or lighter fuel gases)
• Psychological status, including evidence of depression or depressive disorder, feelings of isolation, history of attempted suicide, and level of self-esteem
• Results of laboratory tests

Risk factors
• Cognitive or emotional difficulties
• Dangerous products stored within easy reach
• Drugs stored in unlocked cabinets or large supplies of drugs stored in home
• Insufficient finances

- Lack of proper precautions
- Lack of safety or drug education
- Use of illegal drugs contaminated with poisonous additives

Associated medical diagnoses (selected)
Depression, renal or hepatic impairment, substance abuse

Expected outcomes
- Adolescent will express understanding of harmful and potentially lethal effects of substance abuse.
- Adolescent will remain free from toxicity and other injuries during hospital stay.
- Adolescent will identify stressors and feelings that precipitate episodes of substance abuse.
- Adolescent will demonstrate two or more constructive techniques for coping with stressors.
- Adolescent will describe prescribed medication regimen, including dosage and administration schedule, and will demonstrate compliance.
- Adolescent will describe available community resources and will express intention to contact them.

Interventions and rationales
- Follow medical regimen to treat toxicity or other injury caused by substance abuse *to ensure adolescent's safety and promote recovery.*
- Teach adolescent about harmful and potentially lethal effects of abusing drugs, alcohol, or other dangerous substances *to enhance his knowledge, which may help him make better-informed decisions.* Provide appropriate written materials. *Written materials reinforce teaching and allow review after discharge.*
- Help adolescent identify stressors, such as depression, peer pressure, or family dysfunction, that may precipitate substance abuse *to provide basis*

for developing strategies to prevent future episodes.
- Describe available community resources to help prevent or treat substance abuse. *Support services and groups can provide adolescent with safe settings in which to explore problems and feelings and develop adaptive methods of coping.*
- If medication is prescribed for adolescent, explain reason for medication. Discuss administration techniques, schedule, dosage, cautions, and possible adverse effects *to promote compliance with medication regimen.*

Evaluations for expected outcomes
- Adolescent describes harmful and potentially lethal effects of substance abuse.
- Adolescent remains free from toxicity caused by use of drugs, alcohol, or other hazardous substances.
- Adolescent describes stressors and feelings that precipitate episodes of substance abuse.
- Adolescent demonstrates two or more constructive techniques for coping with such stressors as depression, peer pressure, and family dysfunction.
- Adolescent describes prescribed medication regimen and demonstrates compliance.
- Adolescent describes available community resources and expresses intention to contact appropriate support services.

Documentation
- Interventions to treat toxicity or other injury
- Factors that increase adolescent's risk of drug toxicity
- Knowledge deficits and learning objectives

• Teaching topics, materials, and methods
• Adolescent's response to nursing interventions
• Indications that adolescent is using adaptive techniques to cope with stress, anxiety, peer pressure, or dysfunctional family
• Referrals to community resources or professionals for ongoing counseling
• Evaluations for expected outcomes

■ Self-esteem disturbance

related to problematic relationship with parents

Definition
Presence of conflict with parents that disturbs adolescent's sense of self-esteem

Assessment
• Age
• Sex
• Level of education
• Family history, including marital status of parents, financial status, family rules, ability of family to modify rules, consequences when rules are broken, how family members communicate, quality of communication, methods of conflict resolution, family alliances, family stability, ability of family to meet adolescent's physical and emotional needs, and disparities between adolescent's needs and family's ability to meet them
• Goals and values, including extent to which family permits adolescent to pursue individual goals and values
• Family genogram
• Parental status, including level of education, knowledge of normal growth and development, ability to

agree on appropriate discipline, stability of parental relationship, and understanding of adolescent's self-esteem disturbance
• Adolescent's psychological status, including changes in appetite, energy level, motivation, personal hygiene, self-image, self-esteem, and sleep patterns; alcohol or drug abuse; reaction to puberty; quality of relationships with authority figures; and scholastic performance

Defining characteristics
• Denial of problems that are evident to others
• Exhibitions of grandiosity
• Expressions of self-negating thoughts
• Expressed feelings of shame or guilt
• Hesitation to try new things or situations
• Hypersensitivity to slights or criticism
• Perception of self as unable to deal with events
• Projection of blame or responsibility for problems onto others
• Rationalization of personal failures
• Rejection of positive feedback and exaggeration of negative feedback about self

Associated medical diagnoses (selected)
Communication disorders, conduct disorder, learning disabilities, mood disorders, oppositional defiant disorder, posttraumatic stress disorder

Expected outcomes
• Adolescent and parents will describe areas of conflict.
• Adolescent will begin to express feelings openly to family members.
• Parents will encourage and support adolescent's attempt at expression of feelings.

• Adolescent will describe positive qualities about self.
• Parents will describe positive qualities of adolescent and family unit.
• Adolescents and parents will state plans for continued outpatient family treatment.

Interventions and rationales
• Provide secure, structured environment for adolescent and parents *to foster open discussion of family conflicts.*
• Educate all family members about schedule, purpose, and goals of individual and family treatment. *Awareness of expectations and rationale for treatment will enhance cooperation.*
• Encourage adolescent to participate in group activities, group therapy, and individual counseling *to provide opportunities to develop enhanced self-esteem.*
• Encourage adolescent to express feelings directly, such as "I'm mad because of my curfew." *Such statements help him get in touch with his feelings and talk about them.*
• Tell parents that their child is learning to express his feelings directly. *Because family communication patterns are deeply ingrained, parents may need time to adjust to their child's assertiveness.*
• Help parents understand value of talking about feelings *to encourage them to express emotions appropriately and to discourage them from punishing their child for expressing his feelings toward them.*
• Provide adolescent with small notebook he can use to write down positive events as they occur *to encourage him to focus on his strengths and to enhance self-esteem.*
• Teach parents to reward and praise adolescent for expressing his feelings

appropriately *to encourage them to focus on child's strengths and to strengthen entire family system.*
• Use role-playing to teach adolescent different ways to respond to specific family conflicts. *This will help him develop problem-solving and negotiating skills.*
• Communicate with outpatient clinician *to plan continued treatment for family.*
• Emphasize to adolescent and parents need for continued support and family therapy after discharge *to enhance compliance.*

Evaluations for expected outcomes
• Adolescent and parents begin to talk about difficulties at home.
• Adolescent begins to express feelings directly to family members.
• Parents demonstrate support for adolescent's expression of feelings.
• Adolescent uses more positive statements about self.
• Parents make positive statements about adolescent and family as a whole.
• Parents and adolescent agree to participate in outpatient treatment.

Documentation
• Specific family conflicts as described by adolescent and parents
• Adolescent's and parents' behavior when interacting with each other
• Nursing interventions to facilitate family communication and expression of feelings
• Frequency of family visits and therapy appointments
• Adolescent's description of his own strengths
• Referrals for continued treatment after discharge
• Evaluations for expected outcomes

■ Social isolation

related to behavior that fails to conform to social norms

Definition

Negatively perceived loneliness imposed by oneself or others

Assessment

- Age
- Sex
- Developmental stage
- Level of education
- Reason for hospitalization (physiologic or psychiatric)
- Attitudes of family, friends, teachers, and other important individuals toward adolescent
- Available support systems
- Factors contributing to social isolation, including delayed physical development, immaturity, altered mental status, changes in behavior or cognition, illness, and history of trauma
- Self-esteem
- Coping and problem-solving ability
- Evidence of substance abuse
- Current and past stressors
- Sociocultural factors, including ethnic and religious background

Defining characteristics

- Culturally unacceptable behavior
- Description of lifestyle as solitary or circumscribed by membership in subculture
- Evidence of physical or mental handicap or altered state of wellness
- Expressed feelings of being different from others
- Expressed feelings of rejection or aloneness
- Expressed frustration over inability to meet expectations of others
- Inappropriate or immature interests or activities
- Insecurity in public
- Lack of family, friends, and social groups
- Lack of purpose in life
- Preoccupation with own thoughts
- Projection of hostility in voice and behavior
- Repetitive, meaningless actions
- Sad, dull affect
- Uncommunicative and withdrawn behavior, with poor eye contact

Associated medical diagnoses (selected)

This diagnosis may accompany any medical diagnosis requiring hospitalization, thereby separating adolescent from his usual environment. Other associated disorders include depression and rape.

Expected outcomes

- Adolescent will express feelings of social isolation.
- Adolescent will identify causes of social isolation.
- Adolescent will participate in planning social activities.
- Adolescent will identify personal behaviors that are considered socially unacceptable and will acknowledge the need for change.
- Adolescent will demonstrate more socially acceptable behaviors.
- Adolescent will exhibit effective interpersonal communication skills.
- Adolescent will report feeling less isolated as social interaction improves and will report improved sense of self-esteem.

Interventions and rationales

- Assign primary nurse to adolescent *to enhance continuity of care, establish trusting relationship, and provide opportunity to practice developing one-on-one relationship.*
- Arrange uninterrupted time to talk with adolescent during each visit.

Listen to his concerns and feelings. Provide honest feedback (positive and negative) about his behavior *to encourage appropriate behaviors and reinforce awareness of inappropriate ones. Feedback is essential to behavior modification.*

• Provide guidance as adolescent explores possible causes for his sense of social isolation. Help him identify inappropriate behaviors, and teach him ways to improve communication and interpersonal skills *to foster socially acceptable behavior. When adolescent becomes aware of connection between unacceptable behavior patterns and his feelings of isolation, he may be more willing to learn new skills and behaviors.*

• Make contract with adolescent that requires him to demonstrate one new behavior within specific period. Reward successful changes in behavior. *Contracts can enhance self-esteem by giving adolescent responsibility for making constructive changes and allowing enough time to practice new behavior and communication skills without fear of criticism if he falls short. Successful completion of contract provides positive reinforcement.*

• Demonstrate appropriate communication skills and behaviors in all interactions with adolescent *to provide example of appropriate behavior and reinforce teaching concepts.*

• Engage adolescent in role-playing activities that simulate social situations. Provide encouragement and positive reinforcement and avoid criticism *to provide opportunity to rehearse new skills in safe environment, which reduces anxiety and boosts self-confidence.*

• Encourage adolescent to participate in group activities and one-on-one interactions with staff members. *Gradual increases in social interaction*

help reduce adolescent's feelings of social isolation and instill confidence in newly developed communication and interpersonal skills.

• Talk to adolescent about community resources, such as social services or support groups, that can provide ongoing support. Provide names, addresses, and phone numbers whenever possible. *This provides adolescent with ongoing opportunities for social interaction in supportive environment.*

Evaluations for expected outcomes

• Adolescent expresses feelings of social isolation and desire for help.
• Adolescent identifies causes of social isolation.
• Adolescent takes part in planning social activities.
• Adolescent identifies socially unacceptable personal behaviors and acknowledges the need for change.
• Adolescent demonstrates more socially appropriate behaviors.
• Adolescent exhibits effective communication skills.
• Adolescent reports increased social interaction, decreased feelings of isolation, and improved self-esteem.

Documentation

• Observations of adolescent's behavior and communication skills
• Adolescent's description of causes for impaired social interaction
• Nursing interventions to promote behavior modification and improved socialization
• Adolescent's responses to interventions
• Resources and referrals provided to adolescent or family members
• Evaluations for expected outcomes

■ Trauma, risk for

related to feelings of personal invulnerability

Definition
Accentuated risk of accidental tissue injury such as burns or fractures

Assessment
• Age
• Sex
• Level of education
• Developmental factors, including tendency to test independence and take risks (especially in company of peers), feelings of indestructibility, high level of energy, need for peer approval, and access to potential safety hazards (such as complex machinery or tools, farm equipment, car, motorcycle, jet-ski, or snowmobile)
• Health history, including allergies, sports accidents, auditory or visual impairments, and seizure disorders
• Social history, including academic performance, sports, hobbies, social activities, and job
• Neurologic status, including level of consciousness and orientation

Risk factors
• Access to alcohol, drugs (prescription, over-the-counter, illicit), poisons, or other toxic substances
• Access to vehicles
• Adolescent developmental stage and level of maturity
• Frequent unsupervised activities with peers
• History of chronic or periodic substance abuse
• Lack of experience operating a car, motorcycle, or other vehicle or poor understanding of safety issues related to operating a vehicle (such as driving at excessive speed or after using alcohol or drugs)
• Participation in contact sports
• Use of complex power tools or machinery (at work, school, or home)

Associated medical diagnoses (selected)
Burns, fractures, head injury, psychiatric disorders, seizure disorders, spinal cord injury

Expected outcomes
• Adolescent will recover from injury while in hospital.
• Adolescent won't experience additional injury while in hospital.
• Adolescent will identify risks and behaviors he should avoid.
• Adolescent will state understanding of appropriate safety precautions (for example, obeying speed limits, following fire prevention precautions, never driving while intoxicated, wearing helmets or seat belts, and using protective clothing or equipment).
• Adolescent will state intention to adopt appropriate safety precautions.

Interventions and rationales
• Follow medical regimen to treat adolescent's injury *to promote recovery.*
• Document risk factors and unsafe practices discovered through observation or through discussions with adolescent *to plan effective interventions.*
• Select teaching topics that will help adolescent prevent future injuries and promote personal health — for example, automotive and motorcycle safety, proper use of protective equipment in sports, or alcohol and drug awareness. *Teaching adolescent increases his knowledge and reinforces notion that he is responsible for ensuring personal safety.*
• Demonstrate use of appropriate safety equipment such as protective

sports gear and have adolescent perform return demonstration *to reinforce learning.*
• Include adolescent's parents or guardian in teaching sessions. *If properly informed, family and friends can help adolescent improve safety practices.*

Evaluations for expected outcomes
• Adolescent recovers from existing injuries, if present.
• Adolescent remains free from further injury during hospital stay.
• Adolescent identifies risks and behaviors he should avoid.
• Adolescent demonstrates proper use of safety devices and equipment, as appropriate (for example, using protective sports gear, seat belt, and motorcycle helmet).
• Adolescent states intention to adopt safety precautions.

Documentation
• Adolescent's statements indicating lack of awareness of or disregard for safety practices
• Physical findings
• Observations of unsafe practices
• Medical treatment for existing injuries
• Nursing interventions to reduce adolescent's risk of future injury
• Adolescent's response to interventions
• Evaluations for expected outcomes

■ Violence, risk for: Self-directed

related to suicide attempt

Definition
Presence of risk factors for deliberate, self-directed violence

Assessment
• Age
• Sex
• Developmental stage
• Availability of weapons or toxic substances
• Mood and affect, including persistent depression; feelings of worthlessness, hopelessness, helplessness, isolation, inadequacy, and humiliation; deterioration in school work; and flat, distant, remote affect
• Behavioral changes, including loss of interest in personal appearance, overeating or eating too little, verbal or written cues or preoccupation with death, threats of suicide, acting out (such as sexual promiscuity, delinquency, or running away), low energy level, sleep disturbances, frequent naps, irritability, somatic and physical complaints, antisocial or self-destructive behavior, tendency to be accident-prone, and acts of self-mutilation
• Psychological status, including loss of interest in hobbies and preferred activities, refusal to attend school (cutting class and truancy), social withdrawal and isolation, academic problems, and feelings of rejection by peers and social group

Risk factors
• Access to lethal weapon
• Dysfunctional family
• Excessive stress and anxiety
• Expressed or implied statements indicating desire to commit suicide
• Feelings of worthlessness, hopelessness, loneliness, and helplessness
• History of suicide attempts
• Low self-esteem
• Poor impulse control
• Real or perceived threatened loss of important person or possession
• Recent stressful event, such as parents' divorce or death in family

• Recent suicide of close friend or relative
• Severe depression
• Substance abuse or withdrawal

Associated medical diagnoses (selected)
Any illness resulting in long-term or permanent disability or incapacity (terminal diseases, degenerative diseases, traumatic injury), depression, personality disorders, schizophrenia, substance abuse or withdrawal

Expected outcomes
• Adolescent won't harm self while in hospital.
• Adolescent will recover from suicidal episode.
• Adolescent will discuss feelings that precipitated suicide attempt.
• Adolescent will attend therapy sessions with mental health professional.
• Adolescent will describe available resources for crisis prevention and management.
• Adolescent will report improved feelings of self-worth.

Interventions and rationales
• Take all suicide threats seriously. *Early intervention reduces likelihood of suicide attempt.*
• Ask adolescent directly, "Have you thought about killing yourself?" If he says yes, ask, "What do you plan to do?" *Suicide risk increases if adolescent has definite plan.*
• Remove any objects that adolescent could use to injure self, such as razors, belts, glass objects, and pills, *to ensure his safety.*
• Arrange supervision (preferably one-on-one) for adolescent according to facility policy. *This ensures compliance with legal requirements to protect adolescent while demonstrating staff concern.*

• Make contract with adolescent that he won't harm himself for specific period. Continue negotiating until there is no evidence of suicidal ideation. *Contract puts subject of suicide in the open, places some responsibility for safety on adolescent, and demonstrates your regard for adolescent as worthwhile.*
• Supervise administration of all prescribed medications, and be aware of their actions and possible adverse effects. *Medications may be treatment alternative. By watching as they are administered, you prevent adolescent from hoarding doses (sometimes called "cheeking"), thus ensuring his safety.*
• Convey caring, nonjudgmental attitude when talking with adolescent. *This demonstrates your unconditional positive regard and helps establish trusting relationship.*
• Listen carefully to adolescent as he talks. Don't challenge his statements or reinforce denial of current situation. *This communicates caring, support, and understanding without reinforcing denial, which often masks underlying suicidal feelings.*
• Encourage adolescent to set goal of cooperating with psychiatric intervention. *Ambivalence about psychiatric care or refusal to attend sessions indicates that adolescent is still in denial.*
• Provide adolescent and family members with telephone numbers for crisis prevention centers, suicide hot lines, counselors, and other community support services. *Having many alternatives for support helps reduce adolescent's anxiety.*

Evaluations for expected outcomes
• Adolescent doesn't harm self during hospital stay.

• Adolescent recovers from suicide attempt.
• Adolescent discusses feelings and reasons for attempting suicide.
• Adolescent attends counseling sessions with mental health professional.
• Adolescent describes crisis prevention resources, such as hot-line telephone number, local crisis center, or name of therapist.
• Adolescent expresses improved sense of self-esteem.

Documentation
• Adolescent's description of his feelings before and after suicide attempt
• Observations of adolescent's behavior, mood, and affect
• Nursing interventions to reduce or prevent self-destructive behavior
• Adolescent's response to interventions
• Evaluations for expected outcomes

PART THREE

CHILD
HEALTH

INTRODUCTION

This section focuses on providing care for children, helping them to maintain optimal health and achieve their full developmental potential. Your first task is to establish rapport with the child and family under your care. When talking to the child, show understanding and use simple language. If he's frightened, turning portions of your examination into a game may help to calm him. Talk to the child about toys, hobbies, or other subjects of interest, and be generous with compliments.

Your plan of care should emphasize working with the entire family. Obtaining accurate assessment information, for example, usually requires the cooperation and trust of family members.

During each stage of growth and development, the child must master specific physical, cognitive, and developmental tasks. Assessment should include an evaluation of the child's growth and developmental level as well as an examination of body systems. Other assessment areas include family roles and relationships, parenting style, stressors, coping patterns, religion, cultural background, living conditions, and financial status. You'll also want to explore how the child and family members perceive the health problem.

After analyzing the assessment data, you'll formulate nursing diagnoses. Your diagnoses should state the child's actual health problems or health problems for which the child is at risk; they may take into account physiologic, psychosocial, or cognitive aspects of the child's well-being. Your nursing plan of care will stem from these diagnoses.

When developing interventions, include steps to encourage the child and family members to participate in care. Some families may need encouragement just to ask questions about the child's status; others may want to become involved in treatment-related decisions. To foster participation, be sensitive to the family's values, ideas, and beliefs. Provide referrals to appropriate social service agencies and other community resources. Keep in mind that your ultimate goal is to make the child and family as self-sufficient as possible in managing the health problem.

Periodically evaluate the child's and family's progress as you implement your plan of care. If you carefully monitor the effectiveness of interventions, you will readily see what revisions you need to make to the plan of care.

■ Aspiration, risk for

related to ineffective swallow reflex

Definition
State of being at risk for aspiration of secretions, food, or fluids into tracheo-bronchial passages

Assessment
• Respiratory status, including rate, depth, and pattern of respirations; auscultation of breath sounds; frequency and effectiveness of cough; ability to handle secretions; palpation for fremitus; percussion of lung fields; and sputum characteristics (color, consistency, amount, and odor)
• Neurologic status, including mental status and level of consciousness
• GI status, including presence or absence of gag and swallowing reflex, gastroesophageal reflux, and continuous or intermittent tube feedings
• Diagnostic studies, including arterial blood gas levels, chest X-rays, and cardiorespiratory monitoring

Risk factors
• Decreased GI motility
• Delayed gastric emptying
• Depressed cough and gag reflexes
• Feeding or GI tubes
• Impaired swallowing
• Incompetent lower esophageal sphincter
• Increased gastric residual
• Increased intragastric pressure
• Medication administration
• Reduced level of consciousness
• Situations hindering elevation of upper body
• Surgery or trauma to face, mouth, or neck
• Tracheostomy or endotracheal tube
• Wired jaws

Associated medical diagnoses (selected)
Cerebrovascular accident, chest trauma, cleft lip or palate, Down syndrome, head injury, neuromuscular disease, poisoning, tracheoesophageal fistula

Expected outcomes
• Auscultation will reveal clear breath sounds.
• Auscultation will reveal presence of bowel sounds.
• Child will maintain patent airway.
• Child will breathe easily, cough effectively, and show no signs of respiratory distress or infection.
• Family members will demonstrate measures to prevent aspiration.
• Child's respiratory rate will remain within normal limits for age.
• Family members will describe plan for home care (for example, removing objects that a child could choke on).

Interventions and rationales
• Assess child for gag and swallowing reflex. *Impaired reflexes may cause aspiration.*
• Assess respiratory status at least every 4 hours or according to established standards; begin cardiopulmonary monitoring *to detect signs of possible aspiration (increased respiratory rate, cough, sputum production, and diminished breath sounds).*
• Auscultate bowel sounds every 4 hours and report changes. *Delayed gastric emptying may cause regurgitation of stomach contents.*
• Elevate head of bed or place child in Fowler's position *to aid breathing.*
• Help child to turn, cough, and deep-breathe every 2 to 4 hours. Perform postural drainage, percussion, and vibration every 4 hours or as ordered. Suction as needed *to stimulate cough and clear upper and lower airways. These measures promote drainage of*

secretions and full expansion of lungs.
• Perform chest physiotherapy before feeding child *to decrease risk of emesis leading to aspiration.*
• Hold infant with head elevated during feeding and position in infant seat after feeding. *Such positioning uses gravity to prevent regurgitation of stomach contents and promotes lung expansion.*
• Recognize progression of airway compromise and report findings *to detect complications early.*
• Encourage fluids within prescribed restrictions. Provide humidification as ordered (such as oxygen tent or nebulizer). *Fluids and humidification liquefy secretions.*
• Place child in lateral or prone position. Change child's position at least every 2 hours *to reduce potential for aspiration by allowing secretions and blood to drain.*
• Instruct child and family members in home care plan. *Child and family members must demonstrate ability to ensure adequate home care before discharge.*

Evaluations for expected outcomes
• Auscultation reveals clear breath sounds.
• Auscultation reveals presence of bowel sounds.
• Child maintains airway patency.
• Child breathes easily, coughs effectively, and shows no signs of respiratory distress or infection.
• Family members demonstrate measures to prevent aspiration in child (for example, correct positioning of infant during and after feeding).
• Child's respiratory rate remains within normal limits for age.
• Family members describe plan for home care.

Documentation
• Child's ability to handle oral secretions and feedings
• Observation of respiratory status and response to treatment regimen
• Child's and family members' abilities to carry out home care plan
• Evaluations for expected outcomes

■ Body image disturbance
related to alterations in health or invasive medical procedures

Definition
Negative perception of one's body that interferes with healthful functioning

Assessment
• Physiologic changes
• Behavioral changes
• Child's and family members' perceptions of health problem
• Child's developmental stage
• Child's eating pattern, sleeping pattern, and usual play activities

Defining characteristics
• Behaviors of avoiding, monitoring, or acknowledging one's body
• Behavior of hiding or overexposing body part (intentional or unintentional)
• Change in social involvement
• Expressed negative feelings about body
• Expressions of actual or perceived change in appearance, structure, or function
• Extension of body boundary to incorporate environmental objects
• Loss of body part
• Refusal to look at or touch body part
• Preoccupation with change or loss
• Refusal to acknowledge change

• Trauma to nonfunctioning part

Associated medical diagnoses (selected)
Amputation, burns, colostomy, diabetes mellitus

Expected outcomes
• Child will acknowledge change in body appearance or function.
• Child will express positive feelings about self.
• Family members will acknowledge change in child's appearance or body functioning and will verbalize acceptance of child.

Interventions and rationales
• Hold, rock, or touch child frequently *to give child awareness of body integrity.*
• Provide opportunity for child to interact with peers who have experienced similar health problem *to decrease child's feelings of isolation and sense of being different from others.*
• Give child as much freedom as possible. If restraints are called for, use minimum restraint necessary to prevent injury. *Providing least restrictive environment enhances child's control over surroundings and provides opportunity to release feelings through physical activity.*
• Explain medical procedures in age-appropriate language. For child under age 7, use dolls and actual medical equipment to describe procedure. *Children in preoperational stage of development understand best by seeing and manipulating objects.* For older child, use body diagrams to illustrate what changes will and won't appear in body as result of medical treatment or disease progression. *Illustration is one technique to reinforce learning.*

• For young child, cover injection sites with adhesive bandages. *A child in preoperational stage of development may hold misconception that injections create holes that allow blood to drain out. Adhesive bandages may help reinforce child's sense of body integrity.*
• Encourage young child to participate in play activities *to allow child to act out feelings that he may not have verbal or cognitive skills to express.*
• Set aside time with older school-age child to discuss his feelings *to assess perceptions, clarify misconceptions, and provide opportunity to ventilate emotions.*
• Ensure privacy during procedures *to accommodate heightened sense of modesty that children develop beginning in early school-age years.*
• Encourage family members to express feelings and concerns about changes in child's body appearance or function. Provide accurate information and answer questions thoroughly. *Encouraging open discussion enables you to provide emotional support and may help ease family members' anxiety.*

Evaluations for expected outcomes
• Child expresses understanding of changes in body.
• Child expresses positive feelings about self.
• Family members acknowledge change, verbalize positive feelings about child, and display warmth and affection by holding, comforting, and hugging child as appropriate for child's age.

Documentation
• Child's statements about appearance
• Family members' statements about changes in child's body structure or function

• Account of child's behavior during medical procedures and in play activities
• Observations of family members' behavior toward child and participation in care
• Evaluations for expected outcomes

■ Body temperature alteration, risk for

related to dehydration

Definition

State of being at risk for failure to maintain body temperature within normal range

Assessment

• Age
• Vital signs, including pattern of temperature fluctuation
• Hydration status, including mucous membranes, skin turgor, and fontanels (in infants)
• Respiratory status, including respiratory rate and depth, dyspnea, and use of accessory muscles
• Neurologic health history, including seizures, cerebrospinal fluid infection, abscess, hemorrhage, and history of trauma or cranial surgery
• Nutritional status, including decreased intake and vomiting
• Medical history, including effects of drugs or toxins
• Evidence of disturbance in the temperature-regulating centers of brain

Risk factors

• Altered metabolic rate
• Clothing not appropriate for environmental temperature
• Dehydration
• Exposure to cold or hot environment
• Extremes of age or weight

• Illness or trauma that affects temperature regulation
• Inactivity or vigorous activity
• Use of medication that causes vasoconstriction or vasodilation
• Use of sedation

Associated medical diagnoses (selected)

Burns, colitis, cystic fibrosis, gastroenteritis, head injury, hemophilia, psoriasis, pyloric stenosis

Expected outcomes

• Child will maintain body temperature of 98.6° to 99.5° F (37° C to 37.5° C).
• Child will maintain weight within 5% of baseline.
• Child will maintain balanced intake and output within normal limits for age.
• Child's urine specific gravity will remain between 1.010 and 1.015.

Interventions and rationales

• Assess child's temperature every 4 hours. Use temperature-taking method appropriate for child's age and size (rectal or axillary for infant or toddler, axillary or oral for preschooler, and oral for school-age child). *Prolonged elevation of temperature above 104° F (40° C) may produce dehydration and harmful central nervous system effects.*
• Weigh child daily every morning and record results. *Decrease in weight may indicate dehydration.*
• Maintain adequate fluid intake by offering small amounts of flavored fluids at frequent intervals; record intake and output every shift. *Fever increases child's fluid requirements by increasing metabolic rate. High-calorie liquids, such as colas, fruit juices, and flavored water sweetened with corn syrup, help prevent dehydration.*

• Administer antipyretics as ordered and monitor effectiveness. *Antipyretics act on hypothalamus to regulate body temperature.*
• Check and record urine specific gravity with each voiding. *Urine specific gravity increases with dehydration.* Adequate urine output and urine specific gravity between 1.010 and 1.015 indicates sufficient hydration for children.
• Give tepid sponge bath for increased temperature *to increase vaporization from skin and decrease body temperature.*
• Teach parents to dress child in lightweight clothing when child has elevated body temperature *to allow perspiration to evaporate, thereby releasing body heat.*

Evaluations for expected outcomes
• Child maintains body temperature of 98.6° to 99.5° F (37° to 37.5° C).
• Child maintains baseline weight.
• Child maintains balanced intake and output within normal limits for age.
• Child maintains urine specific gravity of 1.010 to 1.015.

Documentation
• Observation of physical findings
• Nursing interventions, including administration of medications
• Child's body temperature (recorded every 4 hours)
• Child's weight, urine output, and urine specific gravity
• Child's response (behavioral, cognitive, and physiologic) to interventions, including administration of antipyretics
• Evaluations for expected outcomes

■ Breathing pattern, ineffective

related to inability to maintain adequate rate and depth of respirations

Definition
Change in rate, depth, or pattern of breathing that alters normal gas exchange

Assessment
• Age
• Allergies
• History of respiratory disorders
• Respiratory status, including rate and depth of respiration, symmetry of chest expansion, use of accessory muscles, nasal flaring, presence of cough, anterior-posterior chest diameter, palpation for fremitus, percussion of lung fields, auscultation of breath sounds, pulmonary function studies, arterial blood gas monitoring, and pulse oximetry readings
• Cardiovascular status, including history of congenital or acquired heart disease
• Neurologic status, including mental status and level of consciousness
• Emotional well-being
• Knowledge, including understanding of physical condition and physical, mental, and emotional readiness to learn

Defining characteristics
• Use of accessory muscles
• Altered chest excursion
• Altered respiratory rate or depth or both
• Dyspnea
• Nasal flaring
• Orthopnea
• Prolonged expiratory phase
• Pursed-lip breathing

• Shortness of breath

Associated medical diagnoses (selected)
Anemia, asthma, burns, congenital heart disease, cystic fibrosis, heart failure, metabolic alkalosis, prematurity, rheumatic fever

Expected outcomes
• Auscultation will reveal no abnormal breath sounds.
• Child's oxygen saturation (Sao$_2$) level will remain above 95%.
• Child's respiratory status will remain within normal limits for age.
• Child will demonstrate adequate breathing pattern, with easy, unlabored respirations.
• Child will demonstrate correct technique in pursed-lip breathing, abdominal breathing, and relaxation techniques.
• Child or family member will demonstrate correct technique to use in medication administration, oxygen administration, and airway suctioning.
• Child will participate in age-appropriate play activities without increased respiratory difficulty.
• Family members will develop effective plan of care for child's return home.

Interventions and rationales
• Assess respiratory rate and depth every 2 to 4 hours; monitor for nasal flaring, chest retractions, and cyanosis *to detect early signs of respiratory compromise.*
• Monitor arterial blood gas values and pulse oximetry readings *to evaluate oxygenation and respiratory status.*
• Auscultate breath sounds every 2 to 4 hours *to detect decreased or adventitious breath sounds;* report changes.

• Administer oxygen, as ordered, *to help reduce hypoxemia and relieve respiratory distress.*
• Force fluids *to liquefy secretions and prevent dehydration related to increased respiratory rate.*
• Provide nebulizer treatment, vaporizer, or mist tent, as ordered, *to liquefy secretions.*
• Provide postural drainage and chest percussion every 4 hours before meals *to facilitate removal of secretions.*
• Suction airway, as needed, *to remove secretions.*
• Place child in Fowler's position, raising head of bed. Place overbed table padded with pillow in front of child and have him extend his arms over table *to promote lung expansion.*
• Remain with child and offer reassurance during periods of respiratory difficulty *to relieve anxiety.*
• Administer bronchodilators and antibiotics as ordered. *Dilation of bronchi allows greater passageway for air. Antibiotics treat infection.* Monitor effectiveness and check for adverse reactions *to ensure safety and efficacy of therapy.*
• Prohibit parents and other visitors from smoking in child's room and explain why. *Smoking depletes room of its natural oxygen supply and poses serious fire hazard in room with oxygen equipment.*
• Schedule necessary care activities to provide frequent rest periods *to prevent fatigue and reduce oxygen demand.* Allow adequate playtime. *Children of all ages require play for normal growth and development.*
• Assist with activities of daily living, as necessary, *to help child conserve energy and avoid fatigue.*
• Identify child's developmental level and select appropriate teaching methods. For preschooler or early school-

age child, use stuffed animals, puppets, and drawings. *Preschoolers use sensory experiences to understand information.* For older school-age child, use demonstration and audiovisual materials, such as body outline. *Children in this age-group have ability to think logically but not abstractly.*

• Limit number of new skills taught each day according to child's age and ability. Teach preschooler one skill per day and school-age child, two skills per day. *Limiting daily teaching avoids overloading child with new information and enhances learning.*

• Teach child pursed-lip breathing, abdominal breathing, and relaxation techniques. *These measures allow child to participate in maintaining health status and improve ventilation.*

• Discuss with child and family members ways to conserve energy while carrying out daily routine *to prepare child for discharge from hospital.*

• Help family plan for care at home. Discuss medication administration, use of assistive equipment, and available community resources. Also discuss signs and symptoms of complications and when to report them. *Increasing family's knowledge improves likelihood of compliance with medical treatment, thereby decreasing risk of recurrence of breathing problem.*

Evaluations for expected outcomes

• Auscultation reveals normal breath sounds.

• Pulse oximetry readings reveal Sao_2 above 95%.

• Child's respiratory status remains within normal limits for age.

• Child demonstrates adequate breathing pattern and unlabored respirations.

• Child demonstrates correct technique in pursed-lip breathing, abdom-

inal breathing, and relaxation techniques.

• Family members demonstrate correct technique in medication administration, oxygen administration, and suctioning.

• Child participates in age-appropriate play activities without increased respiratory difficulty.

• Family members describe plan of care they will implement on child's return home.

Documentation

• Child's expressions of comfort in breathing

• Child's and family members' understanding of medical diagnosis and readiness to learn

• Child's and family members' responses to teaching

• Physical findings from pulmonary assessment

• Interventions performed

• Child's and family members' responses to nursing interventions

• Evaluations for expected outcomes

■ Coping, ineffective family: Disabling

related to long-term illness

Definition

Destructive behavior on the part of family members during a child's prolonged illness

Assessment

• Child's illness, including severity, duration, and impact on family

• Family process, including number and ages of children, usual patterns of interaction, roles of parents and children, communication patterns, relationship changes (such as separation,

divorce, or remarriage), and past response to crisis
• Family members' understanding of child's present health status
• Family resources (financial, social, and spiritual)
• Parental status, including perception of child's behavior, past responses to stress, child care provisions, history of inappropriate parenting, and history of destructive behavior or substance abuse
• Alteration in child's growth and development resulting from illness or dysfunctional parenting
• Transportation limitations, including geographic distances to health resources

Defining characteristics
• Agitation, depression, aggression, and hostility (child)
• Assumption of illness symptoms of child (family member)
• Decisions or actions that harm family's economic or social well-being (parent)
• Desertion of child (parent)
• Development of helplessness and dependence (child)
• Distorted perception of child's health problem, including extreme denial about its existence or severity (parent)
• Impaired individualization (child)
• Impaired restructuring of meaningful life for self (family member)
• Intolerance of child's physical ailments or psychological weaknesses (parent)
• Maintenance of usual routines (parent)
• Neglect of child's basic human needs and illness treatment (parent)
• Neglect of relationships with other family members (parent)
• Prolonged excessive concern for child (parent)

• Rejection of child (parent)

Associated medical diagnoses (selected)
Burns, cancer, chromosomal abnormalities, chronic endocrine disorders, chronic renal disorders, chronic respiratory disorders, congenital anomalies, degenerative disease, developmental disabilities, neuromuscular disorders, trauma

Expected outcomes
• Family members will identify factors that trigger stress and inappropriate behavior.
• Family members will make use of appropriate sources of support.
• Family members will interact appropriately with staff members and each other.
• Parents will meet developmental needs of their children.
• Family members will express feelings and individual needs.
• Children will meet developmental milestones appropriate for age.
• Family members will meet child's health care needs.

Interventions and rationales
• Assess family history *to identify family's strengths and limitations.*
• Determine if family members are prepared to accept help. *Changes in behavior won't take place until family members are ready.*
• Communicate only brief amounts of information to family members at any one time. *Family members under stress often can't grasp large amounts of information.*
• Help family identify which tasks to tackle now and which to put off until stress level decreases. *Performing easy, familiar activities decreases discomfort during times of stress.*
• Encourage family members to allow open expression of feelings and to

avoid passing judgment on one another. *Family members need to be able to communicate openly without putting each other on the defensive.*
• Identify instances of successful communication among family members *to single out and encourage positive behavior.*
• Use play activity to promote self-esteem in children. *Parents frequently forget developmental needs of children during crisis. If one child is seriously ill, parents may ignore siblings.*
• Help family members identify situations that trigger inappropriate behavior. *Family members must learn to recognize their tolerance threshold to react appropriately.*
• Help family members identify coping mechanisms used successfully in past *to enable them to develop appropriate responses without learning new behaviors.*
• Help family members identify options when confronted with difficult decisions. *Members of dysfunctional families commonly believe they lack choices.*
• Teach parents about health care and developmental needs of their child. *Family-centered care is essential for an ill child.*
• Provide referral to appropriate social service agencies *to help family members find additional resources.*

Evaluations for expected outcomes
• Family members state specific factors that lead to inappropriate behavior.
• Family members state their plans for contacting sources of support.
• Family members interact with appropriate verbal and nonverbal behavior.
• Parents meet developmental needs of their children.

• Family members express feelings and try to meet each others' emotional needs.
• Children show evidence of achieving age-appropriate developmental tasks.
• Family members meet health care needs of chronically ill child.

Documentation
• Observation of family members' interactions with each other and with outsiders
• Observations of family members' reactions to stress
• Examples of communication between family members
• Parents' understanding of normal childhood growth and development
• Interventions performed to help improve family members' coping skills
• Family members' level of participation in care of ill child
• Referrals to community resources
• Evaluations for expected outcomes

■ Dentition, altered

Definition
Deterioration in condition of teeth and gums as evidenced by presence of caries, extractions, plaque, malocclusion, or evulsion

Assessment
• Child's age (chronological and developmental) and sex
• Dental health history, including primary and secondary tooth development; frequency of visits to the dentist; frequency of brushing; condition of teeth (such as presence of caries, extractions, plaque, malocclusion, and evulsion), gums, lips, tongue, and mucous membranes; and signs of salivary dysfunction (such as fissuring

at corners of mouth, sore mucous membranes, dryness and cracking of lips, crusting of tongue and palate, and paresthesia of tongue or mucous membrane)
• Health history, including medication history, X-ray treatments, infection, allergies, trauma, lead poisoning, rubella, nephrotic illness, and malnutrition
• Nutritional status, including amount of sugar in diet
• Socioeconomic conditions, including access to dental health care
• Environmental conditions, including lack of fluoride in drinking water
• Family status, including willingness and ability of child's primary caregiver to supervise or perform dental health measures and to take child to dental appointments

Defining characteristics
• Caries
• Extractions
• Evidence of periodontal disease
• Evulsion
• Inability or unwillingness of parents or caregiver to provide child with dental care
• Lack of access to dental care
• Lack of knowledge of appropriate dental hygiene practices
• Malocclusion
• Plaque

Associated medical diagnoses (selected)
Acquired salivary dysfunction related to infection of salivary glands, psychiatric or emotional disturbances, tuberculosis, or vitamin B_{12} deficiency; enamel hypoplasia related to allergies, chronic pediatric lead poisoning, infection, malnutrition, nephrotic syndrome, or trauma; prolonged bottle-feeding; xerostomia (dry mouth, usually resulting from radiation treatment or medications)

Expected outcomes
• Child will brush teeth with minimal supervision.
• Child will demonstrate good brushing technique.
• Child won't show evidence of dental caries, periodontal disease, or malocclusion.
• Child will reduce quantity of cariogenic foods in his diet.
• Child's teeth will show evidence of good daily oral hygiene.

Interventions and rationales
• Teach child principles of good dental hygiene using teaching methods appropriate to age-group *to foster compliance.*
• Demonstrate good brushing technique. Stress importance of having teeth feel clean rather than need to follow a specific procedure. Help child establish a schedule for brushing. If necessary, provide direct assistance as well as demonstrations *to reinforce good dental hygiene habits.*
• Teach child and parents or caregiver, if necessary, about the relationship between diet and dental health. For example, show child pictures of foods that promote good dental health (such as milk) and pictures of foods that promote tooth decay (such as those containing refined sugar, honey, or molasses). If child is able to read food labels, teach him to identify and avoid products with excessive sucrose *to increase child's awareness of cariogenic foods and encourage better eating habits and more frequent brushing.*
• If assessment reveals evidence of dental caries, periodontal disease, malocclusion, or other conditions requiring dental care, contact child's parents *to ensure they are aware of altered dentition and the need for*

follow-up care. Provide a referral to a dentist *to ensure professional care.*
• Assess whether child's parents are able and willing to assist in meeting child's needs regarding dental health. Provide referrals to community resources that may help family members obtain dental care. *The high cost of dental care may cause some families to neglect dental care needs.*
• If child is prone to dental problems, emphasize need for more meticulous home dental care *to avoid further deterioration of child's teeth and gums.*
• Schedule appointment to determine whether child's parents or caregiver have followed up on your referral to dentist *to ensure continuity of care.*

Evaluations for expected outcomes
• Child assumes responsibility for brushing teeth with minimal supervision.
• Child demonstrates good brushing technique.
• Assessment of child's mouth reveals no evidence of dental caries, periodontal disease, or malocclusion.
• Child reduces quantity of cariogenic foods in his diet.
• Child's teeth show evidence of good daily oral hygiene.

Documentation
• Dental health history
• Evidence of dental problems
• Teaching sessions with child and parents or caregiver
• Evidence of improvement in child's dental hygiene
• Child's response to nursing interventions
• Evaluations for expected outcomes

■ Development, altered, risk for

Definition
Presence of risk factors that may cause child to deviate from developmental norms for age

Assessment
• Age and sex
• Physical development, including height and development of sensory capacities (touch, taste, smell, vision, hearing)
• Motor skills development, including gross and fine motor skills, head control, hand control, and locomotion
• Intellectual development, including perception, memory, learning, reasoning, thinking, and language skills
• Personality development, including activity level, response to a new stimulus (approach or withdrawal), adaptability, mood, attention span, distractibility, threshold of responsiveness (how much stimulation is needed to evoke a response), intensity of reaction to stimulation, and hunger, sleep, and elimination patterns
• Environmental factors, including toys, playmates, and supervision available for the promotion of age-appropriate activities
• Nutritional status, including dietary intake, appetite, ability to feed self (or availability of feeding assistance), and consumption of adequate calories and appropriate number and size of servings for child's age and sex (based on the U.S. Department of Agriculture's Food Guide Pyramid)
• Social status, including family structure, type and quality of parents' or guardian's interactions with child, peer relationships (if age appropriate), and socioeconomic status

• Cultural status, including nationality, ethnicity, religious affiliation, and beliefs and practices regarding health and child rearing
• Health history, including psychiatric or medical diagnoses, and use of over-the-counter or prescription medications

Risk factors
• Altered growth
• Altered mobility status
• Altered nutritional status
• Child abuse or neglect
• Environmental deprivation or lack of stimulation
• Interruption in loving and supportive interactions with caregivers
• Lack of age-appropriate recreational activities
• Prolonged illness

Associated medical diagnoses (selected)
Attention deficit hyperactivity disorder, autism, chromosomal abnormalities, congenital hypothyroidism, Down syndrome, failure to thrive, fragile X syndrome, head or spinal cord trauma, maternal alcohol or drug abuse, mental retardation, musculoskeletal disorders, myelomeningocele, phenylketonuria, physical or emotional abuse or neglect, prematurity, seizure disorders, and exposure to radiation, viruses, or chemicals such as lead

Expected outcomes
• Child will grow and gain weight in accordance with growth-chart norms for age and sex.
• Child will consume _____ calories and _____ ml of fluids representing ____ servings (specify for each food group).
• Parents or guardian will maintain loving and supportive relationship with child.

• Child will participate in activities in a supervised, unconfined environment that includes age-appropriate toys and fosters interaction with other children.
• Parents or guardian will identify risk factors that may interfere with child's development.
• Parents or guardian will express understanding of measures to reduce child's risk for altered development.
• Child will demonstrate progress in acquiring self-care skills (specify).
• Child won't experience alterations in development.

Interventions and rationales
• Weigh and measure child, and review growth chart curve *to establish current height and weight values for child and monitor growth history.*
• Collaborate with dietary department to establish a meal program to meet child's nutritional needs. Teach parents or guardian appropriate nutritional requirements based on child's age and sex. Discuss the various meal choices available to child *to ensure that daily nutritional requirements are met.*
• Educate parent or guardian about child's need for high-quality interactions with family members and others. Emphasize importance of communicating with child in a loving, supportive way *to encourage intellectual, language, and social development.*
• Help parents or guardian to identify age-appropriate activities and toys as well as potential playmates for child. Emphasize importance of providing an unconfined, supervised environment in which child can play *to promote motor skills, socialization, and intellectual development.*
• Educate parents or guardian about risk factors that may lead to altered development, such as lack of support-

ive interactions or age-appropriate activities, *so that they can identify and ameliorate environmental or stimulation deficiencies on their own.* Help parents or guardian identify preventive measures they may initiate at home *to ensure continuity of care.*
• Teach parents or guardian techniques for promoting their child's progress in acquiring self-care skills. Record child's progress on a chart or graph prominently displayed in child's room *to provide child and parents with positive reinforcement.*
• Provide parents or guardian with a written copy of child's teaching plan *to encourage consistent implementation of the plan at home.*

Evaluations for expected outcomes
• Child continues to grow and gain weight, in accordance with growth-chart norms for age and sex.
• Child consumes _____ calories and _____ ml of fluids representing _____ servings (specify for each food group).
• Parents or guardian maintain loving and supportive relationship with child.
• Child participates in activities and is provided with a supervised, unconfined environment that includes age-appropriate toys and fosters interaction with other children.
• Parents or guardian identify risk factors that may interfere with child's development.
• Parents or guardian express understanding of measures to reduce child's risk for altered development.
• Child demonstrates progress in acquiring self-care skills (specify).
• Child doesn't experience alterations in development.

Documentation
• Child's age, sex, height, and weight
• Growth history

• Presence of risk factors for altered development
• Input and output, daily dietary intake, and appetite
• Activities provided for child in the hospital, including type of activities, toys, and presence of supervision
• Teaching provided to parents or guardian regarding altered development
• Parents' or guardian's response to teaching, including statements indicating understanding of teaching, ability to identify risk factors for altered development, and understanding of need to make alterations in child's environment
• Follow-up care plan and referrals
• Evaluations for expected outcomes

■ Diarrhea

related to primary bowel pathology

Definition
Alteration of normal elimination pattern characterized by frequent, loose stools

Assessment
• History of bowel disorder or surgery
• GI status, including nausea and vomiting, usual bowel patterns, changes in bowel patterns, stool characteristics (color, amount, consistency, and presence of blood or mucus), pain, inspection of abdomen, auscultation of bowel sounds, and palpation for masses and tenderness
• Medication history, including use of antibiotics
• Nutritional status, including dietary intake, appetite, weight, and changes to usual diet
• Fluid and electrolyte status, including intake and output, urine specific

gravity, skin turgor, mucous membranes, and serum potassium and sodium levels
• Skin integrity

Defining characteristics
• Abdominal pain and cramping
• At least three loose, liquid stools per day
• Hyperactive bowel sounds
• Urgency

Associated medical diagnoses (selected)
Colitis, Crohn's disease, gastroenteritis, lactose intolerance, salmonella, shigellosis

Expected outcomes
• Child will exhibit normal elimination pattern for age.
• Child will maintain balanced intake and output within normal limits for age.
• Auscultation will reveal normal bowel sounds.
• Child's body temperature will remain normal.
• Child's urine specific gravity will be between 1.010 and 1.015.
• Child's skin will remain intact.
• Caregivers will demonstrate appropriate skin care techniques.

Interventions and rationales
• Assess frequency and characteristics of stool, and auscultate bowel sounds every 4 hours *to monitor effectiveness of treatment.*
• Monitor and record intake and output, urine specific gravity (with each voiding), skin turgor, condition of mucous membranes, presence of tears, and condition of fontanels (in infants) *to monitor hydration status and need for fluid replacement.*
• Record daily weight before first feeding each morning *to determine if child is suffering from dehydration.*

Weight loss of 5% or more in 1 day may indicate dehydration.
• As ordered, offer oral replacement solution such as Pedialyte or clear liquids in small amounts (5 to 15 ml) every 10 to 15 minutes, waiting 20 to 30 minutes after voiding of loose stool, *to decrease intestinal irritation and likelihood of further diarrhea.*
• Don't offer fruit juices or carbonated fluids. *High glucose content and osmolar load associated with these beverages may stimulate further episodes of diarrhea.*
• Offer child BRAT diet (banana, rice, apple, and toast) 4 hours after last loose stool *to help meet child's nutritional needs without exacerbating diarrhea.*
• Check skin in perianal area after each stool. Change diaper frequently and clean skin thoroughly *to prevent skin breakdown.*
• Apply protective ointment to diaper area *to provide barrier between child's skin and stool.*
• Monitor child's temperature every 2 to 4 hours *to detect fever, which may be associated with fluid loss and inflammation.* Measure temperature using axillary or oral routes *because use of rectal thermometer may stimulate further diarrhea.*
• Teach caregivers importance of frequent diaper changes and meticulous skin care for child. Instruct them not to use powder in diaper area *to avoid caking and subsequent skin breakdown.*

Evaluations for expected outcomes
• Child regains normal elimination pattern.
• Child maintains balanced intake and output within normal limits for age.
• Auscultation reveals normal bowel sounds.
• Child remains afebrile.

• Child's urine specific gravity remains between 1.010 and 1.015.
• Child's skin remains intact, without signs of redness or irritation.
• Caregivers demonstrate appropriate skin care techniques.

Documentation
• Frequency and characteristics of stool
• Appearance of skin
• Intake and output
• Weight (recorded daily)
• Evidence of caregivers' knowledge of dietary management and skin care techniques
• Evaluations for expected outcomes

■ Diversional activity deficit

related to prolonged illness and separation from friends and family

Definition
Restriction or decrease in child's ability to use unoccupied time to advantage or satisfaction

Assessment
• Level of comfort, including mobility and activity tolerance
• Cardiovascular status
• Respiratory status
• Neurologic status, including level of consciousness, orientation, mood, behavior, memory, and coordination
• Psychosocial status, including presence of family members, social interaction, cultural and ethnic background, hobbies, interests, and changes or adaptations needed to carry out activities
• Environment, including isolation and availability of diversional activities

• Developmental level (physical, cognitive, psychosocial, and linguistic) and learning needs

Defining characteristics
• Environmental limitations (such as hospitalization) or physical limitations affecting participation in usual activities
• Statements of boredom or wishing for something to do

Associated medical diagnoses (selected)
This diagnosis can occur in any child hospitalized for a prolonged period. Associated conditions include bone marrow transplantation, burns, chemotherapy, cystic fibrosis, and fractures.

Expected outcomes
• Child will select and participate in age-appropriate play.
• Child will express enjoyment in selected play activity.
• Child will achieve developmental tasks appropriate to age.

Interventions and rationales
• Provide various toys, supplies, and activities for child's use. Make sure items are appropriate to child's age, developmental level, and environment. *Ready access to diversional activities entices child to make use of time alone. Age-appropriate items are geared to child's cognitive, motor, and safety needs.*
• Encourage family members to bring child's favorite toys, family pictures, or other objects from home. Provide space in child's room for cards and gifts from family and friends. Encourage parents to tape-record stories for their child and provide tape player so child can listen *to maintain sense of attachment to family and provide sense of security.*

• Encourage child to visit playroom and participate in individual and group activities. *Participating in play activities helps child meet developmental needs.*
• Discuss child's diversional activity deficit with play therapist *to enable play therapist to better address child's special needs.*
• Schedule time to personally engage child in therapeutic or developmental play. Schedule play periods for both day and evening shifts. *This ensures that child has ample opportunity for diversional activity and prevents child from being isolated for prolonged periods. Participation in play will also strengthen your relationship with child.*
• For child confined to bed, provide creative, challenging games. For example, make fishing pole with large safe hook and challenge child to pick up items around room; glue Velcro on soft balls and create "dart board" on wall; or make string-and-paper-cup "telephones" to use with other patients in room. *Creative play encourages age-appropriate behavior, helps make environment more enjoyable and challenging, and gives child greater control and independence.*
• Provide opportunities for therapeutic play. For example, encourage child to play with safe hospital equipment, play nurse or doctor, play house, pound clay, or perform "procedures" on doll. *Therapeutic play offers child opportunity to express fears, fantasies, sadness, and misconceptions; to learn more about his illness and its treatment; and to release pent-up feelings safely. This helps child develop better sense of control and enhances ability to cope with hospitalization and treatment.*
• Provide art and craft supplies for preschool or school-age child *to en-hance child's creativity, provide emotional outlet, and encourage development of initiative and industry.*

Evaluations for expected outcomes
• Child voluntarily participates in age-appropriate activities.
• Child expresses contentment with activities.
• Child achieves age-appropriate developmental tasks.

Documentation
• Child's expressions of boredom and desire for activity
• Assessment of child's physical, cognitive, and psychosocial developmental abilities
• Evaluation of child's physical, educational, and psychosocial need for activity
• Nursing interventions directed at providing diversional activity
• Child's response to play
• Evaluations for expected outcomes

■ Fear

related to separation from familiar environment and people

Definition
Feelings of threat or danger arising from an identifiable source

Assessment
• Age
• Psychosocial factors, including child's understanding of his illness and treatment plan, verbal and nonverbal indicators of fear, and availability of family and friends
• Changes in behavior, eating, or sleeping patterns
• Physiologic manifestations of fear, including temperature, pulse rate,

blood pressure, respiratory rate, and skin color and temperature

Defining characteristics
• Aggression
• Bedwetting
• Expressed feelings of alarm, apprehension, dread, horror, panic, or terror
• Identification of and concentration on object of fear
• Immediate response to object of fear
• Impulsive behavior
• Increased alertness
• Increased tension, worrying, and wariness
• Jitteriness
• Wide-eyed appearance

Associated medical diagnoses (selected)
This diagnosis can occur in any hospitalized child.

Expected outcomes
• Child will identify sources of fear.
• Child will demonstrate effective use of coping mechanisms.
• Child will seek comfort from parents.
• Child will express understanding of medical procedures.
• Child's vital signs will remain within normal limits for age.
• Child will exhibit fewer physiologic or behavioral manifestations of fear.

Interventions and rationales
• Acknowledge child's fear. *Bringing feelings out allows for discussion and identification of coping strategies.*
• Don't dismiss fear or blithely reassure child that "everything will be all right." *Refusing to acknowledge fear or giving false reassurance impairs coping.*
• Spend as much time as possible talking with child. For infants and toddlers, use nonverbal communication such as holding and rocking. *Es-*

tablishing rapport encourages child to express feelings and provides comfort.
• Help child identify sources of fear *to enable child to put emotions into perspective.*
• Provide child with accurate information about condition and scheduled procedures and treatments. Orient child to facility's sights and sounds. *Accurate information dispels misconceptions that can fuel fear.*
• Encourage parents and family members to stay with child as much as possible and participate in care, as appropriate, *to enhance child's ability to cope and decrease fear caused by separation.*

Evaluations for expected outcomes
• Child verbalizes known sources of fear.
• Child demonstrates effective use of coping mechanisms.
• Child expresses feelings of comfort.
• Child expresses understanding of medical procedures.
• Child's vital signs remain within normal limits for age.
• Child exhibits marked decrease in physiologic and behavioral manifestations of fear.

Documentation
• Child's verbal and behavioral expressions of fear
• Physiologic manifestations of fear
• Interventions performed to reduce fear
• Child's response to interventions
• Family's involvement in child's care
• Child's response to family involvement
• Evaluations for expected outcomes

■ Fluid volume deficit

related to excessive loss of fluids and electrolytes

Definition
Excessive loss of fluids and electrolytes caused by diarrhea and vomiting

Assessment
- Age
- Height and weight
- History of diarrhea or vomiting
- GI status, including usual bowel patterns, changes in bowel patterns, stool characteristics (color, amount, size, consistency, and frequency), auscultation of bowel sounds, and inspection of abdomen
- Stool culture, ova, and parasites
- Nutritional status, including dietary intake, changes from usual pattern, appetite, current weight, and recent weight changes
- Fluid and electrolyte status, including intake and output, urine specific gravity, skin turgor, mucous membranes, and serum sodium and potassium, blood urea nitrogen, and hematocrit levels
- Medication use, including laxatives, enemas, and antibiotics
- Neurologic status, including level of consciousness
- Presence of sick children or adults at home, school, or day care
- Respiratory status, including increased respiratory rate
- Child's and family members' knowledge of factors that cause vomiting or diarrhea

Defining characteristics
- Changes in mental status
- Decreased pulse volume and pressure
- Decreased urine output
- Dry skin and mucous membranes
- Increased body temperature
- Increased hematocrit
- Increased pulse rate
- Increased urine concentration
- Low blood pressure
- Poor turgor of skin or tongue
- Sudden weight loss
- Thirst
- Weakness

Associated medical diagnoses (selected)
Colitis, Crohn's disease, cystic fibrosis, diabetes insipidus, diarrhea, diverticulitis, failure to thrive, gastroenteritis

Expected outcomes
- Child will maintain normal weight.
- Child's intake and output will be balanced and within normal limits for age.
- Child's electrolyte values will remain within normal limits for age.
- Child will maintain urine specific gravity of 1.010 to 1.015.
- Child will exhibit moist mucous membranes, good skin turgor, and flat fontanels (in infant).
- Child will exhibit normal elimination patterns for age.
- Child will retain feedings and won't experience emesis.

Interventions and rationales
- Record intake and output every shift. Include urine, stool, vomitus, nasogastric or chest tube drainage, and any other output *to obtain fluid status. Increased output and decreased intake indicate fluid deficit.*
- Weigh child each morning before first feeding. *Weight loss of 5% per day indicates fluid deficit.*
- Assess skin turgor, mucous membranes, and fontanels (in infant) every shift. *Fluid loss occurs first in extra-*

cellular spaces, resulting in poor skin turgor, dry mucous membranes, and sunken fontanels.
• Monitor vital signs every 4 hours or more frequently if needed. *Fever and increased respiratory rate contribute to fluid loss. Weak, thready pulse and drop in blood pressure indicate dehydration.*
• Check urine specific gravity every voiding. *Increased specific gravity indicates lack of fluids to dilute urine.*
• Monitor laboratory study results (electrolytes, pH, and hematocrit). *During fluid loss, electrolytes are excreted, which may lead to electrolyte imbalance.*
• Assess child's behavior and activity level every shift. *Children with dehydration may develop anorexia, decreased activity level, and general malaise.*
• After diarrhea and vomiting have decreased, offer small amounts (5 to 15 ml) of clear fluids frequently *to replace fluid loss without causing further GI irritation.*
• If child can have nothing by mouth, provide mouth care every 4 hours and as needed *to help keep mucous membranes moist. In infants, oral care and pacifier help meet developmental need for sucking.*
• Monitor I.V. fluid infusion every hour. *Because fluid balance is less stable in young children, an infusion rate that is too fast or too slow can lead to fluid imbalance more rapidly than in adults.*
• Secure I.V. site by wrapping it in Kling bandage *to protect site and allow child free movement of extremity.*

Evaluations for expected outcomes
• Child maintains normal weight.
• Child exhibits balance of intake and output within normal limits for age

• Child's electrolyte levels, pH, and hematocrit remain within age-appropriate ranges.
• Child's urine specific gravity remains between 1.010 and 1.015.
• Child exhibits moist mucous membranes, good skin turgor, and flat fontanels (in infant).
• Child experiences normal elimination patterns for age.
• Child retains feedings without emesis.

Documentation
• Intake and output
• Weight (recorded daily)
• Skin turgor, mucous membranes, vital signs, and other physical findings
• Urine specific gravity and other laboratory values
• Interventions and child's response
• Evaluations for expected outcomes

■ Fluid volume deficit, risk for

related to presence of risk factors for fluid and electrolyte imbalance

Definition
Presence of risk factors that could lead to excessive fluid and electrolyte loss

Assessment
• Age
• History of problems that can cause excessive fluid loss, such as vomiting, diarrhea, hemorrhage, and ketoacidosis
• Vital signs
• Level of consciousness
• Fluid and electrolyte status, including intake and output, urine specific gravity, skin turgor, mucous membranes, fontanels (in infant), elec-

trolyte levels, and blood urea nitrogen levels
• GI status, including usual bowel patterns, changes in bowel patterns, stool characteristics (color, amount, consistency, and frequency), auscultation of bowel sounds, and inspection of abdomen
• Nutritional status, including dietary intake, changes from usual pattern, appetite, current weight, and recent weight changes
• Psychosocial status, including developmental level, stressors (such as school, disease process, family discord, or separation from family), and coping mechanisms
• Respiratory status, including increased respiratory rate
• Child's and family members' knowledge of factors that cause vomiting or diarrhea

Risk factors
• Conditions that influence fluid needs (such as a hypermetabolic state)
• Excessive loss of fluid from normal routes (such as from diarrhea)
• Extremes of age or weight
• Factors that affect intake of, absorption of, or access to fluids (such as immobility)
• Knowledge deficit related to fluid volume
• Loss of fluid through abnormal routes (such as a drainage tube)
• Medications that cause fluid loss

Associated medical diagnoses (selected)
Acoustic neuroma, Crohn's disease, cystic fibrosis, diabetes insipidus, diabetes mellitus, failure to thrive, gastroenteritis, head injury

Expected outcomes
• Child will maintain weight.
• Child's urine specific gravity will remain between 1.010 and 1.015.

• Child's intake and output will be balanced and within normal limits for age.
• Child will exhibit good skin turgor, moist mucous membranes, and flat fontanels (in infant).
• Child will exhibit appropriate elimination patterns for age.
• Child won't show signs of fluid and electrolyte imbalance.
• Child will retain feedings without experiencing emesis.

Interventions and rationales
• Record intake and output every shift. Include urine, stool, vomitus, nasogastric or chest tube drainage, and any other output *to obtain fluid status. Increased output and decreased intake result in fluid deficits.*
• Weigh child each morning before first feeding. *Weight loss of 5% per day indicates fluid deficit.*
• Assess skin turgor, mucous membranes, and fontanels (in infant) every shift. *Fluid loss first occurs in extracellular spaces, resulting in poor skin turgor, dry mucous membranes, and sunken fontanels.*
• Monitor vital signs at least every 4 hours or more frequently if needed. *Increased temperature and increased respiratory rate contribute to fluid loss. A weak, thready pulse and drop in blood pressure indicate dehydration.*
• Check urine specific gravity every voiding. *Increased specific gravity indicates lack of fluids to dilute urine.*
• Monitor laboratory studies (electrolytes, pH, and hematocrit). *During fluid loss, electrolytes are excreted, which may lead to electrolyte imbalance.*
• Assess child's behavior and activity level every shift. *Children with dehydration may develop anorexia, de-*

creased activity level, and general malaise.
• When diarrhea and vomiting have decreased, offer small amounts (5 to 15 ml) of clear fluids *to replace fluid loss without causing further GI irritation.*
• If child can take nothing by mouth, provide mouth care every 4 hours and as needed *to help keep mucous membranes moist. In infants, oral care and pacifier help meet developmental need for sucking.*
• Monitor I.V. fluid infusion every hour. *Because fluid balance is less stable in young children, too rapid or too slow infusion rate can lead to fluid imbalance more quickly than in adults.*
• Secure I.V. site by wrapping it in Kling bandage *to protect site and allow child to move hand or arm freely.*

Evaluations for expected outcomes
• Child maintains weight.
• Child's urine specific gravity remains between 1.010 and 1.015.
• Child exhibits balanced intake and output within normal limits for age.
• Child exhibits good skin turgor, moist mucous membranes, and flat fontanels (in infant).
• Child has appropriate elimination pattern for age.
• Child's electrolyte values, pH, and hematocrit remain within age-appropriate ranges.
• Child retains feedings without experiencing emesis.

Documentation
• Intake and output
• Weight (recorded daily)
• Skin turgor, mucous membranes, vital signs, and other physical findings
• Urine specific gravity and other laboratory values
• Interventions and child's response

• Evaluations for expected outcomes

■ Grieving, anticipatory
related to chronic or terminal illness

Definition
Grief response in anticipation of loss of a significant person, ideal, material object, or body part

Assessment
• Child's state of grief and mourning
• Child's developmental level
• Perceived value of loss
• Usual patterns of coping with loss
• Behavioral manifestations of grieving
• Somatic problems associated with grieving process, including changes in appetite, sleep pattern, and activity level
• Available support systems

Defining characteristics
• Altered activity level
• Altered communication pattern
• Anger
• Changes in eating habits
• Changes in sleep or dream patterns
• Denial of significance of potential loss
• Difficulty taking on new or different roles
• Expressions of distress at potential loss
• Expressed feelings of guilt or bargaining with a higher power
• Resolution of grief before occurrence of loss
• Sorrow

Associated medical diagnoses (selected)
This diagnosis may occur in newly diagnosed chronic or terminal dis-

eases, such as acquired immunodeficiency syndrome, cancer, diabetes mellitus, juvenile rheumatoid arthritis, and leukemia.

Expected outcomes

• Child will express feelings in nondestructive manner.
• Child will seek emotional support from family members to help cope with loss.
• Child will take advantage of available resources, such as participation in play therapy, to help cope with loss.
• Parents will express understanding of grieving process.
• Parents will participate in care of child and interact positively with child.

Interventions and rationales

• Encourage child to express feelings through drawing, puppetry, or gross motor play *to provide safe outlet for pent-up emotions. Children don't have verbal and cognitive skills to express feelings and need alternative means of expression. Allow child to express grief in own way; intervene only to prevent physically destructive behavior.*
• Plan to spend time each shift with child. If child doesn't wish to talk, spend the time in silence *to convey concern, understanding, and support.*
• Reassure child that it's all right to be angry or sad. Assess whether child feels responsible for loss, and clear up misconceptions *to help alleviate guilt feelings.*
• Reassure family that grief is normal reaction to loss; explain stages of grieving process and normal responses. Help parents understand that child's feelings and behavior are normal under present circumstances. *Un-*

derstanding grieving process will enhance family's ability to cope.
• Encourage parents and siblings to participate in care of child. Remind them of child's need for emotional support at this time. *Child may fear he'll no longer be loved or cared for after loss. It's crucial that child receives emotional reassurance.*
• Offer child simple choices related to care issues *to give child sense of control and to meet developmental needs for initiative and industry.*
• Encourage child and family members to develop coping strategies for dealing with loss, such as participating in diversional activities, reminiscing, or seeking out support groups *to facilitate grieving process.*
• Provide positive feedback for effective coping behavior *to help child and family members regain self-confidence.*

Evaluations for expected outcomes

• Child expresses feelings in nondestructive manner.
• Child's verbal expressions and behavior indicate that he knows he will receive emotional support from family and won't be blamed, punished, or abandoned because of loss.
• Child uses available resources to help cope with loss.
• Parents express understanding of grieving process.
• Parents participate in care of child and interact positively with child.

Documentation

• Child's verbal expressions and behavior
• Child's eating, sleeping, and activity patterns
• Observation of emotional responses
• Child's attempts to gain control, such as making decisions and using support systems

• Interaction between parents and child
• Nursing interventions and child's response to them
• Evaluations for expected outcomes

■ Growth, altered, risk for

Definition
Presence of risk factors that may cause child to deviate from growth norms for age

Assessment
• Age
• Sex
• Physiologic status, including basal metabolic rate, temperature, motor development, sleep patterns (time and quality of sleep), activity level, and vision and hearing screening
• Growth history, including changes in child's size and form, current height and weight, percentile on pediatric growth grid, body proportions, bone development (determined through X-ray examination), tooth development, organ systems development, neuroendocrine function (growth hormone, thyroid hormone, and androgen levels), genetic abnormalities that may affect growth, prenatal influences (fetal exposure to alcohol or illicit drugs, maternal smoking or malnutrition), birth trauma (possible oxygen deprivation or nerve injuries), and breast-feeding or bottle-feeding
• Environmental factors, including chemical or radiation exposure, lead exposure, passive inhalation of tobacco smoke, and exposure to water, air, or food contaminants
• Nutritional status, including dietary intake, appetite, ability to feed self or availability of feeding assistance, and consumption of adequate calories and appropriate number and size of servings for child's age and sex (based on the U.S. Department of Agriculture's Food Guide Pyramid)
• Social status, including family structure, type and quality of parents' or guardian's interactions with child, peer relationships (if age-appropriate), and socioeconomic status
• Cultural information, including nationality, ethnicity, religious affiliation, and beliefs and practices regarding health and child rearing
• Health history, including psychiatric or medical diagnoses and use of over-the-counter or prescription medications

Risk factors
• Altered nutritional status
• Any disease that persists over time, especially during critical periods of development
• Environmental hazards, such as chemical or radiation exposure, lead exposure, passive inhalation of tobacco smoke, and exposure to water, air, or food contaminants
• Genetic abnormalities
• Inability to digest and absorb nutrients
• Neuroendocrine factors, such as altered levels of growth or thyroid hormones or androgens
• Prenatal influences, such as maternal exposure to drugs or alcohol, severe maternal malnutrition, and maternal smoking
• Financial or socioeconomic hardship

Associated medical diagnoses (selected)
Adrenocortical insufficiency, chromosomal abnormalities, congenital heart disease, cystic fibrosis, dwarfism, endocrine disorders, fetal alcohol syndrome, growth hormone deficiency,

hypopituitarism, hypothyroidism, Marfan syndrome, maternal substance abuse or alcoholism, metabolic disturbances, musculoskeletal disorders, respiratory disorders, Turner's syndrome

Expected outcomes
• Child will grow and gain weight as expected based on growth-chart norms for age and sex.
• Child will consume _____ calories and _____ ml of fluids representing ____ servings (specify for each food group).
• Child will sleep _____ hours daily.
• Child will maintain age-appropriate activity level.
• Child and parents or guardian will identify risk factors that may lead to altered growth.
• Child and parents or guardian will state understanding of preventive measures to reduce risk for altered growth.

Interventions and rationales
• Weigh and measure child and review growth-chart curve *to establish current height and weight values and compare results with growth history.*
• Collaborate with dietary department to establish a meal program that meets child's nutritional needs. Educate child and parents or guardian on nutritional requirements for child's age and sex. Discuss the various meals available to child at home *to promote growth.*
• Establish a routine sleep schedule for child. Provide a comfortable environment that promotes rest *to ensure adequate duration and quality of sleep and to initiate a routine sleep pattern that may be continued when child returns home.* Naps may be recommended, depending on age of child.

• Identify age-appropriate activities and exercises for child *to stimulate bone growth and muscle development and to promote cardiovascular health.*
• Teach child and parents or guardian about risk factors associated with altered growth, such as poor nutrition, lack of regular sleep, environmental hazards, or lack of age-appropriate activities. Help them identify preventive measures to be taken in the home *to promote continuity of care.*
• Encourage healthy, loving interactions between child and family. Model healthy, positive interactions with child for parents. *Altered growth may be associated with emotional deprivation.*
• If a medical or psychiatric illness places child at risk for altered growth, make sure child gets adequate follow-up medical care *to ensure appropriate, professional care.* If parents or guardian cannot afford care, assist with obtaining access to community resources *to promote continuity of care.*
• If financial hardship interferes with family's ability to provide for child, offer referral to social worker *to improve family's access to community resources.*

Evaluations for expected outcomes
• Child continues to grow and gain weight as expected based on growth-chart norms for age and sex.
• Child consumes _____ calories and _____ ml of fluids representing ____ servings (specify for each food group).
• Child sleeps _____ hours daily.
• Child maintains activity level appropriate for age.
• Child and parents or guardian identify risk factors that may lead to altered growth.

• Child and parents or guardian express understanding of preventive measures to reduce risk for altered growth.

Documentation
• Child's age, sex, height, and weight
• Growth history
• Presence of risk factors for altered growth
• Input and output
• Daily appetite level
• Duration of sleep (including any disruptions in sleep cycle)
• Child's level of participation in activities and the type of activities
• Teaching provided to child and parents or guardian regarding altered growth
• Parents' or guardian's response to teaching, including statements indicating understanding of altered growth, ability to identify risk factors for altered growth, and understanding of need to make alterations in child's environment and daily schedule
• Follow-up care plan and referrals
• Evaluations for expected outcomes

■ Growth and development alteration

related to physical disability or environmental deprivation

Definition
State in which a child deviates from developmental norms for age

Assessment
• Child's age, both chronological and developmental
• Nature of physical disability
• Past experience with hospitalization
• Family history, including parents' educational level and knowledge of child development, family member roles and support systems, and resources and home environment
• Child's capabilities, including communication skills, motor skills, socialization skills, and cognitive abilities

Defining characteristics
• Altered physical growth
• Delay or difficulty in performing motor, social, or expressive skills typical of age-group
• Flat affect
• Listlessness and decreased responses
• Inability to perform self-care activities or maintain self-control at age-appropriate level

Associated medical diagnoses (selected)
Cerebral palsy, Down syndrome, encephalitis, failure to thrive, fetal alcohol syndrome, head injury, Reye's syndrome, seizure disorders, spinal cord defects

Expected outcomes
• Child will demonstrate skills appropriate for age.
• Child will participate in developmental stimulation program to increase skill levels.
• Parents will express understanding of norms for growth and development.
• Parents will use community resources to promote child's development.
• Parents will provide play activities to promote child's development.

Interventions and rationales
• Monitor child's height, weight, nutritional intake, and cardiovascular and pulmonary status *to ensure child is healthy enough to participate in activity.*
• Provide appropriate play activities, such as building blocks, dolls,

crayons, or games, *to promote development*. Select play activities and related materials according to child's abilities rather than chronological age *to promote use of existing skills as basis for mastering higher skill levels.*
• Teach selected activities to parents and family members, and encourage frequent play with child. *Parents need to reinforce learning at home.*
• Monitor developmental progress at regular intervals *to detect changes in level of functioning and, as appropriate, adapt activity program.*
• Provide parents with referrals to appropriate community resources, including sources of financial assistance, child care, and suppliers of adaptive equipment, *to ensure child's right to receive remedial and educational care in accordance with his disability, as guaranteed by federal law.*

Evaluations for expected outcomes
• Child demonstrates skills appropriate for age.
• Child participates in developmental stimulation program to increase skill level.
• Parents express understanding of developmental norms and means to promote child's development.
• Parents use community resources to obtain adaptive equipment and appropriate educational opportunities for child.
• Parents provide play activities that offer developmental stimulation for child.

Documentation
• Assessment of child's developmental level
• Evidence of parents' knowledge of child's abilities and motivation to promote development

• Interventions performed to stimulate development
• Child's response to nursing interventions
• Evaluations for expected outcomes

■ Hyperthermia
related to infection

Definition
Elevation of body temperature above normal range

Assessment
• History of present illness
• History of exposure to communicable disease
• Age, gestational age at birth
• Health history, including chronic disease or disability, pathologic conditions known to cause dehydration, recent traumatic event, exposure to sources of infection (intrauterine or extrauterine), exposure to communicable diseases, and other related events
• Medications
• Physiologic manifestations of fever, including vital signs, skin temperature, and skin color
• Fluid and electrolyte status, including skin turgor, intake and output, mucous membranes, serum electrolyte levels, and urine specific gravity
• Laboratory studies, including white blood cell count and culture and sensitivity findings
• Neurologic status, including level of consciousness and history of seizures
• Skin integrity, including presence of open lesions and rashes

Defining characteristics
• Body temperature above 99.5° F (37.5° C)
• Flushed, warm skin
• Increased respiratory and heart rates
• Mild to severe dehydration
• Possible seizures

Associated medical diagnoses (selected)
Bacterial, mycotic, rickettsial, viral, and other infections

Expected outcomes
• Child will remain afebrile.
• Child will maintain adequate hydration, with balanced intake and output within normal limits for age, urine specific gravity between 1.010 and 1.015, and moist mucous membranes, good skin turgor, and flat fontanels (in infant).
• Child will remain alert and responsive and won't show evidence of seizure activity or decreased level of consciousness.
• Parents will identify risk factors for infection and state measures to prevent infection.
• Parents will demonstrate correct technique for assessing temperature.
• Parents will identify appropriate measures to reduce fever and prevent dehydration.

Interventions and rationales
• Take axillary or oral temperature every 1 to 4 hours and 1 hour after administration of antipyretics. Record measurements and identify route *to obtain accurate core temperature.*
• Administer antipyretic medication, as ordered, and record effectiveness. *Antipyretics act on hypothalamus to regulate temperature.* Avoid using aspirin. *Aspirin use in children with viral symptoms, especially with flulike symptoms or varicella (chickenpox), has been linked to Reye's syndrome.*

• Use nonpharmacologic measures to reduce high fever, such as removing sheets, blankets, and most clothing (except diapers and underwear); placing cool cloths on axillae and groin; and sponging with tepid water. Explain these measures to child and family members. *Nonpharmacologic measures lower body temperature and promote comfort. Sponging reduces body temperature by increasing evaporation from skin. Tepid water is used because cold water increases shivering, thereby increasing metabolic rate and causing temperature to rise.*
• Use hypothermia blanket if child's temperature rises above 103° F (39.4° C). Monitor vital signs every 15 minutes for 1 hour and then as indicated. *Too-rapid reduction of fever can cause vascular collapse in young children.* Turn off blanket if shivering occurs. *Because shivering increases metabolic rate, it's counterproductive to cooling therapy.*
• Monitor heart rate and rhythm, blood pressure, respiratory rate, level of consciousness and responsiveness, and capillary refill time every 1 to 4 hours *to evaluate effectiveness of interventions and monitor for complications such as seizures.*
• Determine child's preferences for oral fluids and encourage child to drink as much as possible, unless contraindicated. Monitor and record intake and output, and administer I.V. fluids if indicated. *Because insensible fluid loss increases by 10% for every 1° C increase in temperature, child must increase fluid intake to prevent dehydration.*
• Discuss precipitating factors with parents or primary caregiver. Teach parents:
– how to take a temperature correctly
– measures to prevent fever, such as increased fluid intake

– not to overdress young child.
Effective teaching will help prevent future episodes of hyperthermia.
• Describe complications of fever to parents and explain which signs and symptoms they need to report to doctor. *Early recognition and treatment of fever reduces risk of complications, such as dehydration and febrile seizures.*

Evaluations for expected outcomes
• Child remains afebrile.
• Child maintains adequate hydration.
• Child remains alert and responsive and doesn't exhibit evidence of seizure activity.
• Parents identify risk factors for infection and state measures to prevent infection.
• Parents demonstrate correct technique for assessing temperature.
• Parents identify appropriate measures to reduce fever and prevent dehydration.

Documentation
• Observations of physical findings
• Nursing interventions, including administration of medications
• Child's response (behavioral, cognitive, and physiologic) to interventions, including administration of antipyretics
• Evaluations for expected outcomes

■ Incontinence, total

related to neuropathy, trauma, or disease affecting spinal nerves

Definition
Involuntary, continuous, and unpredictable passage of urine or stool

Assessment
• History of trauma, surgery, congenital anomalies, and disease
• History of sensory or neuromuscular impairment
• Vital signs
• Age
• Sex
• Bowel elimination status, including usual bowel pattern, frequency, awareness of need, presence or absence of anal sphincter reflex, and bowel sounds
• Genitourinary status, including palpation of bladder, previous bladder elimination procedures, urinalysis, urine characteristics, use of urinary assistive devices, and voiding pattern
• Fluid and electrolyte status, including fluid intake and output, mucous membranes, skin turgor, serum electrolyte levels, and urine specific gravity
• Neuromuscular status, including degree of neuromuscular function, motor ability to start or stop urine stream, and sensory ability to perceive bladder fullness and urge to defecate
• Nutritional status, including usual dietary pattern, appetite, tolerance or intolerance of foods, and current weight
• Activity status, including usual play patterns
• Appearance of skin

Defining characteristics
• Constant flow of urine occurring at unpredictable times without distention or uninhibited bladder contractions or spasms
• Lack of awareness of incontinence, perineal fullness, or bladder filling
• Nocturia
• Unsuccessful incontinence treatments

Associated medical diagnoses (selected)

Brain tumor, cerebral palsy, cerebrovascular accident, neuromuscular disease, spinal cord defects, spinal cord injury

Expected outcomes

• Child will maintain fluid balance, with intake equal to output.
• Child will experience bowel movement when placed on commode or toilet at specified time.
• Child's skin will remain clean and intact.
• Parents will express understanding of bowel and bladder care.
• Parents will express understanding of need to regulate food and fluid intake to promote continence.
• Parents and child will demonstrate correct catheterization technique.

Interventions and rationales

• Monitor and document child's voiding pattern and intake and output. *Careful monitoring allows you to identify problems and individualize interventions.*
• Assist with specific bladder elimination procedures, as ordered, such as:
– external catheterization. Apply catheter according to established procedure. Maintain patency and avoid constriction. Clean penis or vagina with soap and water at least twice daily. *External catheter keeps skin dry and protected from contact with urine. Clean skin helps prevent skin breakdown and infection.*
– insertion of indwelling urinary catheter. Insert according to established procedure and monitor patency; keep tubing free of kinks *to avoid drainage pooling and ensure effective drainage.* Keep drainage bag below bladder level *to prevent urine reflux into bladder.* Maintain closed drainage *to prevent bacteria from in-*

filtrating into bladder. Secure catheter to leg (in females) or abdomen (in males) *to avoid tension on bladder and urinary sphincter.*
– insertion of suprapubic catheter. Monitor patency, change dressing, and perform catheter care according to established protocols *to help prevent skin irritation and breakdown.* Maintain closed drainage *to prevent bacterial infiltration.*
– use of incontinence aids, including diapers, pads and pants, drip collector, linen protector, or absorbent pouch to cover penis. Use as alternatives to indwelling devices. *Incontinence aids prevent soiling of clothes and linen, reduce embarrassment, and draw urine away from skin. Compared to indwelling devices, incontinence aids allow for greater mobility and carry decreased risk of infection.*
– intermittent self-catheterization. Assess child's readiness to learn self-catheterization. Instruct child or family member in technique and request return demonstration *to evaluate understanding and ability;* maintain sterile technique in hospital and clean technique at home *to prevent infection.*
• Establish regular pattern for bowel care; for example, after breakfast each morning, place child on toilet or commode for 1 hour after inserting glycerin suppository; allow child to remain upright for 30 minutes, then clean anal area. *Regular bowel care encourages adaptation and routine physiologic function.*
• Teach parents bowel care routine *to foster continuity of care.*
• Teach parents need to regulate child's consumption of foods or fluids that cause diarrhea or constipation *to promote helpful nutritional patterns.*

• Maintain diet log *to identify irritant foods that need to be eliminated from child's diet.*
• Teach parents to regulate child's fluid intake according to specific schedule *to encourage voiding at appropriate time.* Limit fluid intake after dinner *to reduce need to void at night.*
• Clean and dry perianal area after each incontinent episode *to prevent skin breakdown and promote comfort.*

Evaluations for expected outcomes
• Child maintains adequate fluid balance, as evidenced by intake and output, urine specific gravity, and skin turgor.
• Child has normal bowel movements when placed on commode or toilet.
• Child's skin remains clean, dry, and intact.
• Parents express understanding of bowel and bladder care.
• Parents express understanding of need to regulate food and fluid intake to maintain continence and plan appropriate diet for child.
• Parents and child demonstrate correct catheterization technique.

Documentation
• Observations of incontinence and child's response to treatment
• Nursing interventions performed and child's response to them
• Instructions given to child and family members and their demonstrated ability to perform bowel and bladder program
• Observations of skin integrity
• Evaluations for expected outcomes

■ Injury, risk for
related to developmental factors

Definition
Risk of tissue injury in a child with physiologic, mental, or emotional disabilities

Assessment
• Age
• Environmental factors, including toxic substances within reach of child, stairs not blocked, and unsafe play equipment
• Developmental status, including cognitive abilities (language and reasoning), sensory perception, response to stimuli (pain, touch, and warmth), level of independence, and motor skills
• Child's and family members' understanding of safety practices
• Behavior
• Laboratory studies, including toxicology screening

Risk factors
• Age (independence-seeking toddlers especially vulnerable)
• Child's inability to understand safe use of medication or equipment
• Child's lack of knowledge about safety hazards (such as electric sockets or matches)
• Decreased level of consciousness
• Decreased or absent sensory perception, including blindness or deafness
• Environmental hazards (such as steep steps, unsteady chairs, clutter, lack of childproofing in home, or toxic substances within child's reach)
• Family members' lack of knowledge about or indifference toward safety practices
• High bed without side rails
• Hyperactivity

Associated medical diagnoses (selected)
Burns, depression, developmental disorders, learning disabilities

Expected outcomes
• Child will remain free from physical injury.
• During hospitalization, staff members will keep toxic substances out of child's reach, have equipment inspected for safety, and remove unsafe equipment.
• Child and family members will express understanding of safety measures.
• Family members will take action to eliminate household safety hazards.

Interventions and rationales
• Assess and document any motor, mental, or sensory deficits *to identify specific safety needs.*
• Keep frequently used items within child's easy reach *to help prevent falls.*
• Encourage use of necessary assistive devices, such as hearing aids, glasses, and leg braces, *to enhance safety and help prevent injury.*
• Orient child to immediate environment, as necessary, *to promote mobility and improve safety.*
• Assess amount of supervision child needs to ensure safety. *Maintaining supervision is especially important if child is hyperactive, disoriented, or unconscious.*
• Keep bed side rails up at all times *to prevent falls.*
• Keep bed in low position except when providing direct care *to ease getting in and out of bed and to reduce danger of falling.*
• Use locks on wheelchairs, stretchers, and beds when appropriate *to immobilize equipment and enhance safety.*

• Ensure that all equipment, medical supplies, and toys in child's room are appropriate for his developmental age. Make sure infant's or toddler's room doesn't contain small objects, sharp instruments, or sharp furniture corners *to reduce risk of injury.*
• Promote electrical safety. Apply electrical outlet covers to all unused outlets. Inspect all electrical appliances brought from home and have them approved by safety officer before use. Don't place liquids, jellies, or creams on electrical appliances. Finally, test all electrical equipment before using on child. *Electrical appliances pose potential hazards for both child and staff members.*
• Instruct child and family members in standard safety practices, including:
– wiping up all spills immediately
– providing nonslip surfaces in hallways, on stairs, and in bathtubs and shower stalls
– draining all water from bathtubs immediately after bath
– placing toxic substances in locked cabinets or out of reach of child.
Teaching promotes household safety.

Evaluations for expected outcomes
• Child remains free from physical injury.
• During hospitalization, staff members keep toxic substances out of child's reach, have equipment inspected for safety, and remove unsafe equipment.
• Child and family members express understanding of safety measures.
• Family members eliminate safety hazards from home.

Documentation
• Statements by child or family members that indicate high risk for injury
• Assessment of home environment

- Observation of physical findings
- Child's and family members' knowledge of safety practices
- Nursing interventions to reduce the risk of injury
- Child's and family members' responses to interventions
- Evaluations for expected outcomes

■ Knowledge deficit

related to lack of exposure

Definition
Inadequate understanding of information needed to practice health-related behaviors

Assessment
- Age
- Developmental status, including learning ability (affective, cognitive, and psychomotor domains), decision-making ability, and developmental stage
- Psychosocial status, including family's resources, health beliefs and attitudes, interest in learning, knowledge and skill regarding current health problem, obstacles to learning, support systems (willingness and capability of others to help child), and usual coping pattern
- Neurologic status, including level of consciousness, memory, mental status, and orientation
- Parents' understanding of child's illness, including severity, prescribed treatment, and overall health needs

Defining characteristics
- Inability to follow through with instruction
- Inability to perform well on test

- Inappropriate or exaggerated behaviors (hysteria, hostility, agitation, apathy)
- Verbalization of problem

Associated medical diagnoses (selected)
This diagnosis can occur in association with any medical diagnosis.

Expected outcomes
- Child and family members will communicate need to gain knowledge and establish realistic learning goals.
- Child and family members will demonstrate understanding of what they have been taught.
- Child and family members will demonstrate ability to perform recently learned health-related behaviors.
- Child and family members will verbalize their intention to make needed changes in lifestyle.

Interventions and rationales
- Establish environment of mutual trust and respect to enhance learning. Communicate openly and honestly with child and encourage parents and others to visit regularly *to enhance child's feelings of trust in staff and comfort within hospital environment.*
- Identify child's level of cognitive, physical, linguistic, and perceptual development *to establish appropriate learning goals.*
- Select teaching methods appropriate to child's developmental level:
– For preschooler or early school-age child, use stuffed animals or puppets. *Children in this age-group use their senses and manipulation of objects to learn.*
– For older school-age child, use demonstration techniques, role-playing, and illustrations. Relate new terms and concepts to child's experiences. For example, to explain ventricular septal defect you might say

"your heart is like a house with four rooms and a door to one of the rooms isn't working right." *Children at this age think concretely and best understand explanations if related to past experiences.*
• Limit number of new skills taught each day according to child's age and ability. *Limiting daily teaching helps to avoid overloading child with new information.* Keep in mind that young children who successfully learn single concepts may still have difficulty determining when to apply learned rules.
• Develop daily schedule for child while in hospital with plans for rest, meals, play, and performing learned skills. *Establishing routines provides more controlled, pleasant environment for child and thereby fosters learning. Play is a valuable component of any child's life.*
• Encourage family members to participate in planning child's daily schedule, making it as similar as possible to typical day at home. *Involving child's family helps reinforce skills necessary for home care after discharge.*
• Regularly discuss progress toward goal achievement with child and family members. Make changes in plan of care as necessary. *Evaluation helps to reinforce effective learning techniques and identify ineffective techniques. It allows analysis of progress and redirection of activities as necessary.*
• Have child and family members demonstrate learned skills. *Return demonstration allows you to evaluate learning and helps child and family members gain confidence in new skills.*

Evaluations for expected outcomes
• Child and family members communicate need to gain knowledge and establish realistic learning goals.
• Child and family members express understanding of material being taught.
• Child and family members demonstrate ability to perform new health-related behaviors correctly.
• Child and family members express intention to institute needed changes in child's lifestyle.

Documentation
• Child's and family members' knowledge and skills
• Child's and family members' statements that indicate knowledge deficit
• Child's and family members' expressions that indicate motivation to learn
• Learning objectives
• Teaching methods used
• Information taught
• Skills demonstrated
• Responses to teaching
• Evaluations for expected outcomes

■ Nutrition alteration: Less than body requirements

related to inability to absorb nutrients or insufficient intake

Definition
Insufficient intake or absorption of nutrients that results in changed body weight and inability to meet metabolic needs

Assessment
• Age
• Developmental level
• GI status, including usual bowel patterns, change in bowel habits, stool

characteristics (color, amount, size, and consistency), pain or discomfort, nausea and vomiting, history of GI disorder or surgery, presence of colic, inspection of abdomen, palpation for masses and tenderness, percussion for tympany and dullness, auscultation of bowel sounds, and sucking and swallowing ability of infant
• Medication history, including antibiotic therapy
• Nutritional status, including dietary history, change in type of food tolerated, height, weight, physical growth percentile (from pediatric growth grid), meal preparation, sociocultural influences, usual dietary pattern, weight fluctuations in the past year, and weight maintenance as height increases
• Change in intrapersonal or interpersonal factors, including desire to eat and rate of food consumption
• Psychosocial status, including body image (perception of observer and self-perception), level of attachment with primary caregiver, and family's financial resources
• Laboratory studies, including hemoglobin and hematocrit
• Health status, including heart rate, respiratory status, integumentary status, and oral mucosa
• Presence and type of tube feedings
• Activity level and mood

Defining characteristics
• Abdominal pain or cramping, with or without pathology
• Aversion to or lack of interest in eating
• Body weight 20% or more under ideal weight
• Diarrhea and steatorrhea
• Hyperactive bowel sounds
• Inadequate food intake (less than recommended daily allowances)

• Loss of body weight despite adequate food intake
• Pale conjunctivae and mucous membranes
• Perceived inability to ingest food
• Poor muscle tone
• Satiety immediately after eating
• Sore, inflamed buccal cavity

Associated medical diagnoses (selected)
Colitis, Crohn's disease, cystic fibrosis, eating disorders, failure to thrive, gastric ulcer, intestinal obstruction, pyloric stenosis, tracheoesophageal fistula

Expected outcomes
• Child will exhibit no further weight loss and, if malnourished, will gain 2.2 lb (1 kg)/week.
• Child will take in ____ calories/day and will retain feedings without emesis.
• Child and family members will express understanding of total parenteral nutrition (TPN), if appropriate, or demonstrate understanding of other feeding techniques essential to daily nutritional requirements.
• Family members will express willingness to continue feeding regimen at home.

Interventions and rationales
• Provide diet meeting child's daily caloric requirements. Daily caloric intake depends on age, metabolic status, and activity level. General guidelines include:
– under age 6 months — 108 kcal/kg/day
– ages 6 to 12 months — 98 kcal/kg/day
– ages 1 to 3 — 1,300 kcal/day
– ages 4 to 6 — 1,800 kcal/day
– ages 7 to 10 — 2,000 kcal/day
– ages 11 to 14 — 2,500 kcal/day
– ages 15 to 18 — 3,000 kcal/day.

Diet meeting child's caloric requirements helps meet child's maintenance and growth needs.
• Provide small, frequent feedings *to reduce fatigue and improve intake.*
• For infants over age 6 months, offer solid foods before formula or breast milk. Place solid foods in center of tongue, using small spoon to press downward slightly *to facilitate swallowing. Older infants and young toddlers may resist solid foods, preferring milk or formula.*
• Record and describe food intake. Refer family members to dietitian or nutritional support team for dietary management. *Dietitian or nutritional support team can individualize child's diet within prescribed restrictions.*
• Promote adequate rest *to reduce fatigue and improve child's ability and desire to eat.*
• Obtain and record child's weight each morning before first feeding *to accurately monitor response to therapy.*
• Provide parenteral fluids as ordered *to ensure adequate fluid and electrolyte levels.*
• Monitor electrolyte values and report abnormalities. *Poor nutritional status may cause electrolyte imbalances.*
• Monitor and record amount, color, consistency, and presence of occult blood in emesis and stool. *Characteristics of vomitus and stool provide clues to nutrient absorption.*
• If child is receiving tube feedings:
– Use continuous infusion pump, if possible, *to help prevent diarrhea, fatigue, and stimulation of vagal response. Continuous infusion pump also helps prevent reduction in cough or gag reflex and overstimulation of stomach.*
– Provide infant with opportunities to suck on pacifier *to satisfy oral needs.*

– Check feeding tube placement before each feeding *to verify tube placement in GI tract rather than in lung.*
– Begin regimen with small amounts and diluted concentrations *to decrease diarrhea and improve absorption.* Increase volume and concentration as tolerated.
– Keep head of bed elevated during feedings *to reduce risk of aspiration.*
– Teach parents correct technique for tube feeding *to ensure compliance with feeding regimen at home.*
• If child is receiving TPN:
– Carefully monitor delivery of TPN *to promote effective therapy and prevent circulatory overload.*
– Monitor blood glucose level, urine specific gravity, and urine glucose, protein, and metabolite levels at least every shift *to detect metabolic complications, osmotic diuresis, hypoglycemia, and pulmonary edema.*
– Provide or assist with oral hygiene *to enhance child's comfort and improve appetite.*
– Teach parents correct technique for maintaining TPN infusion at home *to ensure parents continue feeding regimen after discharge.*

Evaluations for expected outcomes
• Child's weight stabilizes or increases.
• Child takes in enough calories and essential nutrients and retains feedings.
• Child and family members demonstrate understanding of nutritional principles and requirements, feeding techniques, and special needs.
• Family members express willingness to provide nutritional care at home.

Documentation
• Child's weight (recorded daily)
• Child's sucking and swallowing reflexes

- Intake and output
- Incidence of emesis or diarrhea
- Characteristics of emesis or stool
- Presence of complications
- Statements by child and family members that indicate understanding of feeding protocol
- Evaluations for expected outcomes

■ Pain

related to physical, biological, or chemical agents

Definition

An unpleasant sensory and emotional experience arising from actual or potential tissue damage or described in terms of such damage; pain may be of sudden or slow onset, vary in intensity from mild to severe, and be constant or recurring; duration of pain is less than 6 months; and period of pain has an anticipated or predictable end

Assessment

- Age
- Sex
- Descriptive characteristics of pain, including location, quality, intensity rated on a pictorial assessment scale, temporal factors, and sources of relief
- Physiologic variables, including pain tolerance
- Psychological variables, such as body image, personality, previous experience with pain, anxiety, and secondary gain
- Sociocultural variables, including cognitive style, culture, ethnicity, attitude, values, and birth order
- Environmental variables, such as setting and time

Defining characteristics

- Alteration in muscle tone (may range from listless to rigid)
- Autonomic responses (diaphoresis; blood pressure, pulse rate, and respiratory rate changes; and dilated pupils)
- Changes in appetite and eating
- Communication (verbal or coded) of pain
- Distracting behavior (such as pacing, seeking out other people, or performing repetitive activities)
- Expressions of pain (such as moaning and crying)
- Facial mask of pain (grimacing)
- Guarding or protective behavior
- Narrowed focus (including altered time perception, withdrawal from social contacts, and impaired thought processes)
- Self-focusing
- Sleep disturbance

Associated medical diagnoses (selected)

This diagnosis may be associated with most medical diagnoses.

Expected outcomes

- Child will express feeling of improved comfort or demonstrate pain relief through playful, smiling, responsive behavior.
- Child will identify measures effective in relieving pain.
- Parents will express awareness of child's pain and will perform measures to comfort child.

Interventions and rationales

- Assess child's physical symptoms and behavioral cues. If appropriate, encourage child to describe pain on pictorial scale depicting happy face (no pain) and series of grimacing faces gradually increasing to sad face with tears (worst pain possible). *Young children lack verbal skills to* describe variations in pain sensation. *Pain scales and observation of nonverbal behavior provide alternative means to assess pain in young children.*

• Administer analgesics as ordered and document effectiveness and adverse effects. *Analgesics depress central nervous system, thereby reducing pain.*

• Using pain flow chart, record time of medication administration and results of pain assessment every hour until next dose *to monitor effectiveness of therapy.*

• Demonstrate acceptance when child reveals pain. *This helps establish trusting relationship with child and encourages open expression of feelings. Children may deny pain to appear "good."*

• Provide comfort measures, such as massage, repositioning, and instruction in deep breathing and relaxation techniques. *Nonpharmacologic techniques decrease focus on pain and may enhance effectiveness of analgesics by reducing muscle tension.*

• Apply heat or cold, as appropriate, to pain site. *Applying heat relaxes muscles and decreases pain. Applying cold results in vasoconstriction, decreasing inflammatory response and reducing pain.*

• Provide diversional activities, such as books, toys, and arts and crafts. *Because of their immature cognitive functioning and short attention span, young children may be distracted from pain by diversional activities. Older children are less easily distracted.*

• Provide honest information to child before potentially painful procedures. Tell child reasons for pain and how long it should last. *Honest information builds trust and fosters sense of control over pain.*

• Help child obtain uninterrupted periods of rest. *Adequate rest promotes child's well-being and enhances effectiveness of pain medication.*

• Discuss child's pain with parents or primary caregiver and enlist their help in pain assessment and management. Ascertain parents' usual means of providing comfort to child. *Because parents are most familiar with child's usual behavior, they can offer valuable information to assist pain assessment and management.*

• Try to anticipate onset of pain. Provide prescribed medication before painful procedures such as dressing changes or activities such as deep breathing. *Careful pain management can improve relief and may enable child to cope better with procedures.*

• Encourage child to report which pain-relief measures prove most effective *to give child sense of control and promote effective modification of therapy.*

Evaluations for expected outcomes

• Child demonstrates reduced pain, as evidenced by verbal reports of pain relief, absence of behavioral signs of pain, and resumption of activities of daily living (age-appropriate diversional activities, social interaction, and adequate nutritional intake and rest).

• Child identifies most effective pain relief measures.

• Parents respond to child's expression of pain and provide comfort to child.

Documentation

• Child's description of pain, feelings about pain, and statements about pain relief

• Observations of child's physical and psychological responses to pain

• Comfort measures and medications provided to reduce pain
• Effectiveness of interventions
• Information taught to child and family members about pain and pain relief
• Additional interventions provided to assist child with pain control
• Evaluations for expected outcomes

■ Parent-infant attachment, altered, risk for

Definition
Disrupted interaction between parents and an infant that interferes with the development of a protective, nurturing relationship

Assessment
• Family status, including marital status, composition of family, ages of family members, ability of family to meet physical and emotional needs of its members, evidence of abuse, and health history
• Parental status, including level of education, knowledge of normal growth and development, stability of relationship, and available support systems
• Parents' psychological status, including energy level, motivation, recent life changes, psychiatric history, maternal history of drug abuse, and alcohol or antidepressant use by either partner
• Infant's neurologic status, including muscle tone and reflexes; infant lethargy, irritability, seizures, or tremors; and Brazelton Neonatal Behavioral Assessment, Dubowitz Gestational Age Assessment, and Bayley Scales of Infant Development
• Infant's sensory status, including vision or hearing loss, visual and

auditory-evoked potentials, and audiometric tests
• Sleep pattern, including infant's usual hours of sleep

Risk factors
• Anxiety over parental role
• Illness in infant that doesn't allow initiation of contact with parents
• Inability of parents to meet their personal needs
• Lack of privacy
• Physical barriers
• Prematurity of infant
• Separation
• Substance abuse

Associated medical diagnoses (selected)
Blindness, child abuse, deafness, persistent pervasive developmental disorder, prematurity

Expected outcomes
• Parents will initiate positive interaction with infant, as evidenced by mutual responsiveness and eye contact.
• Parents will touch infant appropriately, call him by name, and speak to him.
• Parents will express confidence in their ability to respond to infant's needs.
• Parents will respond appropriately to infant.
• Parents will express positive feelings about infant.
• Parents will express confidence in their ability to care for infant at home.
• Parents will recognize when they need assistance.
• Infant will respond positively to parents, show interest in their faces, and become calm when soothed by them.

Interventions and rationales
• Perform ongoing assessment of parent and infant interaction *to evaluate*

whether parent-infant attachment is proceeding normally.
• Speak positively about infant in parents' presence *to encourage parents to develop positive view of infant.*
• Maintain eye contact with infant when caring for him, talk to him, and touch him appropriately *to demonstrate healthy interactions with infant.*
• Help parents learn to understand behavioral cues from infant. For example, infant may become fussy when he's ready for nap or may pull his ear if he has an earache. *Developing better understanding of their infant's behavior will decrease parents' frustration and help them to care more effectively for infant.*
• Provide parents and infant with privacy *to promote attachment.*
• Assess parents' knowledge of infant care and development *to develop appropriate teaching plan.*
• Teach parents to provide physical care for infant *to increase their sense of competence and self-confidence.*
• Encourage parents to make eye contact with infant, caress and talk to him in soothing tone, call him by name, and make positive remarks about him *to foster healthy parent-child attachment and to help ensure infant's well-being.*
• Observe parents; note whether their responses to infant are appropriate. Compliment them when they exhibit successful parenting skills *to increase their confidence.*
• Discuss life changes precipitated by birth *to help parents express their frustrations and feelings about role changes.* Topics may include altered finances, changes in living space, caretaking arrangements, and new roles and responsibilities for parents and siblings.

• Provide parents with sources of ongoing support and care *to ensure adequate follow-up.*
• Assess the home environment. Discuss adaptations parents need to make. *Adaptations in the home environment may be needed to help the parents properly care for their infant.*

Evaluations for expected outcomes
• Parents initiate positive interactions with infant.
• Parents make eye contact with infant, caress and talk to him, and call him by name.
• Parents express confidence in their ability to meet infant's needs.
• Parents respond appropriately to infant's behavioral cues, provide stimulation when he is alert and ready, don't overstimulate him, and recognize when he needs to nap.
• Parents express positive feelings about infant.
• Parents express confidence in ability to care for infant at home.
• Parents recognize when they need assistance and make plans to contact appropriate resources.
• Infant responds positively to parents, shows interest in their faces, and becomes calm when soothed by them.

Documentation
• Description of parent and infant interactions
• Nursing interventions to promote attachment
• Parents' responses to nursing interventions
• Infant's responses to modifications in parents' behavior
• Evaluations for expected outcomes

■ Parental role conflict

related to child's hospitalization

Definition

State in which one or both parents experience role confusion and conflict in response to crisis

Assessment

• Parental status, including age and maturity; apprehension, fear, and guilt; coping mechanisms employed; developmental state of family and other children; knowledge of normal growth and development of children; past response to crises; understanding of child's present condition; previous parent-child relationship; spiritual practices of parents and family; stability of parental relationship; and support systems available to parent

• Parent-child interaction, including eye contact, response to appearance (such as bandages, deformities, and hospital equipment), smiling, touching, and verbalization

• Child's health status, including severity of illness and health care needs

• Child's level of development

Defining characteristics

• Disruption in caretaking routines

• Expressed concern about changes in parental role and family functioning, communication, and health

• Expressed feeling of inadequacy to provide for child's needs

• Expressed loss of control over decisions relating to child

• Expressed or demonstrated feelings of guilt, anger, fear, anxiety, and frustration about effect of child's illness on family

• Reluctance to participate in usual caregiving activities, even with support

Associated medical diagnoses (selected)

This diagnosis can be associated with any disease or condition, short-term or long-term, that results in child's hospitalization. Examples include cystic fibrosis and prematurity.

Expected outcomes

• Parents will communicate feelings about present situation.

• Parents will participate in daily care of their child.

• Parents will express feelings of greater control and ability to contribute more to child's well-being.

• Parents will express knowledge of child's developmental needs.

• Parents will hold, touch, and convey warmth and affection to child.

• Parents will use available support systems or agencies to assist in coping.

Interventions and rationales

• Orient parents or primary caregivers to hospital environment, visiting procedures, medical equipment, and staff. *Familiarity decreases anxiety.*

• Provide family-centered care by obtaining parents' input for child's care. *Parents can meet many of child's needs better than staff.* Involve parents in child's care conferences and in physical care of child. *Participation may decrease parents' feelings of helplessness.*

• Teach parents normal childhood physical and psychological development *to prepare parents to deal with changes.*

• Encourage parental involvement in appropriate support groups or agencies when necessary or ordered. *Such groups can provide emotional support and help reduce feelings of being overwhelmed.*

• Ask parents if they have questions about child's status and provide information as requested *to reduce feelings of helplessness.*

• Provide for needs of parents as appropriate. Offer facilities for showering, sleeping, and eating. Be available to care for child if parents need opportunity to rest. *Helping parents to meet their needs will empower them to meet child care demands.*

Evaluations for expected outcomes

• Parents communicate feelings about present situation.

• Parents participate in daily care of their child.

• Parents express feelings of control in present situation.

• Parents communicate knowledge of child's developmental needs.

• Parents hold, touch, and express warmth and affection to child.

• Parents contact support systems or community agencies to assist in coping.

Documentation

• Observations of parents' ability to cope and their level of involvement in child's hospital care and daily needs

• Interventions performed to help parents lower stress and cope with situation

• Referrals to outside agencies or support groups

• Child's medical and emotional state

• Evaluations for expected outcomes

■ Parental role conflict

related to home care of a child with special needs

Definition

State in which one or both parents experience role confusion and crisis in response to the special needs of a child at home

Assessment

• Extent of child's special needs

• Parental status, including age and maturity, developmental state of family, authority within family, employment status, financial needs, marital status, stability of parental relationship, knowledge of normal growth and development, understanding of child's condition and prognosis, expectations regarding child, participation in community, past response to crises, and coping mechanisms

• Available support systems, including other family members, friends, visiting nurses, and community resources

• Parent-child interaction

• Parent-child relationship before development of special needs and any changes that have occurred

• Religious practices of parents and family

• Presence of conflict between family's lifestyle and child's needs

• Home environment

Defining characteristics

• Disruption in caretaking routines

• Expressed concern about changes in parental role and family functioning, communication, and health

• Expressed feeling of inadequacy to provide for child's needs

• Expressed loss of control over decisions relating to child

- Expressed or demonstrated feelings of guilt, anger, fear, anxiety, and frustration about effect of child's illness on family
- Reluctance to participate in usual caregiving activities, even with support

Associated medical diagnoses (selected)
This diagnosis may be associated with any condition requiring long-term home care. Examples include acquired immunodeficiency syndrome, cystic fibrosis, developmental disorders, Down syndrome, and hemophilia.

Expected outcomes
- Parents will seek out and accept external support, education, and assistance in caring for their child at home.
- Parents will demonstrate knowledge of child's developmental needs.
- Parents will begin to provide physical, emotional, and developmental care to their child at home.
- Parents will seek assistance in meeting their own emotional and developmental needs.
- Parents will express feelings of greater control and capability in meeting their child's needs.
- Siblings will voice their emotional needs.

Interventions and rationales
- Provide family-centered care by involving parents in their child's care. Explain their rights as primary caregivers. Provide information to help them make informed decisions. Give them opportunity to support child during painful procedures. *Parents can better meet needs of their child than staff members. Parents need to receive proper information and have*

their own needs met before they can meet child's needs.
- Promote emotional well-being of parents by providing respite care, encouraging parents to spend time away from child to enhance their marital relationship, and providing information about additional sources of support. *Encouraging parents to pay attention to their own emotional needs will enhance their ability to care for their child.*
- Listen to parents, child, and siblings openly and without passing judgment *to gain their trust.*
- Help parents develop realistic expectations of their child and formulate achievable short-term goals based on child's needs and abilities *to reduce frustration and feelings of helplessness.*
- Ensure attention to all of child's normal health needs, including dental care, immunizations, safety, and educational and nutritional needs. *Chronically ill child needs total health care, not just illness-related interventions.*
- Pay attention to needs of siblings at home. Devote time to discussing their feelings about having brother or sister with special needs. How do their friends react? Contact their school nurse for assistance. Encourage them to help care for their brother or sister, but make sure activities are age-appropriate. *Becoming involved will help siblings achieve greater self-esteem and enhance their sense of control.*
- Advocate normal growth and development for child with special needs. Encourage visits by friends and discourage overprotective behavior *to help child obtain social acceptance. Increased social interaction will encourage parents, siblings, and others to view child as unique individual in-*

stead of burden. This, in turn, will help promote child's self-esteem.

• Act as liaison between family and multidisciplinary health care team, equipment vendors, community agencies, and third-party payers. *Organized approach with one central coordinator decreases stress for family and enhances continuity of care.*

Evaluations for expected outcomes
• Parents seek out and use community resources to assist in meeting child's physical, psychological, and educational needs.
• Parents express increased knowledge of their child's needs and demonstrate comfort in caring for child at home.
• Parents provide appropriate physical, emotional, and developmental care to their child at home.
• Parents seek help to meet their own emotional and developmental needs.
• Parents express feelings of greater control and capability in meeting child's needs.
• Siblings come to terms with having brother or sister with special needs.

Documentation
• Family members' expressions of feelings about their role in caring for child at home
• Observations of parent-child interaction
• Physical and psychological status of child with special needs
• Nursing interventions to resolve parental role conflict in home
• Parents', child's, and siblings' responses to interventions
• Evaluations for expected outcomes

■ Parenting alteration
related to lack of knowledge

Definition
Inability of a nurturing figure to promote optimum growth and development in an infant or child

Assessment
• Parental status, including age, degree of apprehension, developmental state, family roles, and relationship with spouse or significant other
• Sex and health status of other children
• Parents' knowledge of child care and normal growth and development
• Previous bonding history
• Interaction of parent and infant or child, including care practices, eye contact, smiling, touching, verbalization, visual and voice responses, and response to appearance, handicaps, and sex of child
• Psychosocial status, including financial stressors and previous experience, work demands, and support of family, friends, and significant other

Defining characteristics
• Child: behavioral disorders, failure to thrive, frequent accidents and illness, history of trauma or abuse, lack of attachment, no separation anxiety, poor academic performance, poor cognitive development, poor social competence, tendency to run away
• Parents: evidence of inflexibility in meeting child's needs; evidence of neglectful behavior toward or abandonment of child; expressed frustration over inability to fulfill role; expressed inability to control child; expressed inability to meet child's needs; expressed negative feeling about child; inadequate child health

maintenance; inappropriate child care arrangements; inappropriate visual, tactile, or auditory stimulation for child; inconsistent caregiving; inconsistent management of child's behavior; poor or inappropriate caregiving skills; poor parent-child interaction, with little cuddling; punitive or abusive behavior toward child; rejection of or hostility toward child; unsafe home environment; weak or no attachment to child

Associated medical diagnoses (selected)
Burns, child abuse, failure to thrive, fractures, head injury, prolonged hospitalization, shaken baby syndrome, soft-tissue injuries

Expected outcomes
• Parents will establish eye, physical, and verbal contact with infant or child.
• Parents will voice satisfaction with infant or child.
• Parents will demonstrate correct feeding, bathing, and dressing techniques.
• Parents will express willingness to work to maintain relationship with each other.
• Parents will state plans for well-child care.
• Parents will express knowledge of developmental norms.
• Parents will provide play activities for child.
• Parents will identify ways to express anger and frustration that don't harm child.

Interventions and rationales
• Involve parents in care of infant or child immediately *to promote attachment to child.*
• Provide opportunities for caretaking by allowing parents to share room with infant or child or by extending visitation periods. *Participation in care increases parent's feeling of self-esteem and self-worth.*
• Educate parents in:
– normal growth and development
– breast-feeding or bottle-feeding techniques
– infant care, such as bathing and dressing
– routine well-child care
– signs and symptoms of illness
– child's need for tactile and sensory stimulation.
Knowledge of normal growth and development may decrease unrealistic expectations and increase chances of successful parenting.
• When caring for child in parents' presence, act as role model for effective parenting skills. *Lack of knowledge of routine child care practices and growth and developmental norms significantly contributes to child abuse. Demonstration is more effective means of teaching parenting skills than lecturing.*
• Encourage questions about caretaking and provide appropriate information *to allay anxiety and monitor knowledge retention.*
• Praise parents when they display appropriate parenting skills *to provide positive reinforcement.*
• Refer parents to family support group and other community resources such as Parents Anonymous. *Battering parents typically lack support system and have sense of being alone. Support group may help ease isolation.*
• Encourage verbalization of infant's or child's impact on family life. *Ventilation of feelings assists parents to deal more effectively with stress of child care.*
• Be alert for symptoms of child abuse, including neglect, uncleanliness, and frequent accidents or with-

drawn, fearful behavior on part of child. Report actual or suspected child abuse to appropriate authorities. *Reporting child abuse is your professional duty. The United States legally requires nurses to report abuse.*

Evaluations for expected outcomes
• Parents make appropriate physical, verbal, and eye contact when interacting with infant or child.
• Parents make statements indicating satisfaction with infant or child.
• Parents demonstrate correct feeding, bathing, and dressing techniques.
• Parents express willingness to maintain their relationship with each other.
• Parents bring infant for routine well-child care.
• Parents verbalize knowledge of developmental norms.
• Parents provide play activities for child.
• Parents identify ways to express anger and frustration that don't harm child.

Documentation
• Parents' expressions of feelings about child
• Parents' expressions of concern about their performance as parents
• Observation of parental visits, bonding, caretaking, and knowledge level
• Instructions given to parents and parents' understanding of their responsibilities
• Infant's weight
• Evaluations for expected outcomes

■ Parenting alteration, risk for
related to lack of knowledge or ineffective role model

Definition
Presence of risk factors that may interfere with primary caregiver's ability to promote optimum growth and development in an infant or child

Assessment
• Ages of caregiver and child
• Caregiver's psychosocial status, including developmental state, educational level, family roles, presence or absence of spouse or significant other, financial stressors, previous parenting experience, work demands, and support of family, friends, or significant other
• Interaction between caregiver and infant or child, including care practices, eye contact, response to appearance and sex of infant, smiling, touching, verbalization, and visual and voice responses

Risk factors
• Lack of prenatal care
• Lack of proper role model
• Parent of young age
• Physical or developmental disability
• Role strain
• Single parent

Associated medical diagnoses (selected)
Burns, child abuse, failure to thrive, fractures, head injury, nutritional deficiencies, prolonged hospitalization, shaken baby syndrome, soft-tissue injuries

Expected outcomes

• Caregiver will establish eye, physical, and verbal contact with infant or child.
• Caregiver will demonstrate correct feeding, bathing, and dressing techniques.
• Caregiver will state plans to bring infant or child to clinic for routine physical and psychological examinations.
• Caregiver will express understanding of developmental norms.
• Caregiver will provide play activities appropriate to child's age.

Interventions and rationales

• Assess amount of developmental stimulation provided by caregiver. For example, use Caldwell Home Inventory Measure on home visit *to assess whether home environment is developmentally stimulating.*
• Instruct caregiver in basics of infant and child care. *Research shows that primary source of information about parenting is caregiver's own parents. If caregiver lacks effective role model, you may need to supply basic information about parenting.*
• When caring for child in caregiver's presence, act as role model for effective parenting skills. Demonstrate comfort measures, such as rocking infant, and show caregiver how to hold infant in an en face position *to familiarize caregiver with routine child care practices.*
• Teach caregiver about normal growth and development, and identify ages at which child should master developmental tasks such as rolling over, crawling, and walking. *This will help caregiver monitor child's growth and development and practice appropriate safety precautions, such as blocking stairways, securing crib side rails, and preventing other accidents.*

Also discuss problem behaviors associated with specific ages, such as colic, temper tantrums, and sleeping difficulties, *to further enhance caregiver's understanding of developmental norms.*
• Discuss child's need for tactile and sensory stimulation. Demonstrate play activities that promote developmental skills, such as shaking rattle in front of infant to build eye-and-hand coordination or placing mobile above infant to encourage visual tracking and trunk and head control. *Sensory experiences promote cognitive development.*
• Familiarize caregiver with techniques for detecting symptoms of illness in infant or child, including:
– taking temperatures and reading thermometers
– assessing child's respiratory status
– observing for behavioral cues of illness, such as increased crying, rubbing ears, or drawing legs to abdomen.
Knowledge of how to monitor child's health status will assist in diagnosis and early treatment of problems.
• Encourage caregiver to ask questions about infant and child care. Identify questions parents commonly ask about infant care, such as cord care, feeding techniques, and bathing. Reassure caregiver that other parents also need to ask basic questions. *Caregiver who lacks effective parenting role models may not know what questions to ask or may hesitate to ask questions because of embarrassment.*
• Praise caregiver for display of appropriate parenting skills *to provide positive reinforcement.*
• Emphasize importance of making regular visits to health care professional, even when child appears healthy. *Routine visits allow early de-*

tection of developmental delays and provision of preventive care, such as immunizations.

• As necessary, refer caregiver and family to doctor, nurse practitioner, or social services for follow-up *to ensure continuity of care.*

Evaluations for expected outcomes

• Caregiver makes appropriate eye, physical, and verbal contact with infant or child.
• Caregiver demonstrates correct feeding, bathing, and dressing techniques.
• Caregiver brings infant or child to clinic for routine examinations.
• Caregiver expresses understanding of developmental norms.
• Caregiver accurately assesses child's developmental status and needs.
• Caregiver provides play activities appropriate to child's age.

Documentation

• Evidence of neglect of infant or child
• Observations of caregiver's skills and knowledge level
• Presence or absence of caregiver-child bonding behaviors
• Questions asked by caregiver about care of infant or child
• Instructions given to caregiver and caregiver's response
• Evaluations for expected outcomes

■ Self-care deficit: Bathing and hygiene

related to developmental delay

Definition

Inability to carry out aspects of self-care, such as bathing and personal hygiene

Assessment

• Age
• History of neurologic, sensory, or developmental impairment
• Self-care abilities, including knowledge and use of adaptive equipment, preparation of equipment and supplies, and technical or mechanical skills
• Musculoskeletal status, including range of motion, muscle tone, gait, muscle size and strength, functional capabilities, and mechanical restrictions (such as splints, casts, or traction)
• Neurologic status, including cognition, communication ability, insight or judgment, level of consciousness, memory, motor ability, orientation, and sensory ability
• Psychosocial status, including child's affective reaction to imbalances between motor abilities and cognitive reasoning abilities, usual lifestyle, and parents' perception of developmental delay

Defining characteristics

• Impaired ability to get into and out of bathroom
• Impaired ability to obtain bath supplies
• Impaired ability to obtain or get to water source
• Impaired ability to regulate water temperature or flow
• Impaired ability to wash or dry body

Associated medical diagnoses (selected)

This diagnosis can occur with any musculoskeletal, cognitive, or perceptual impairment.

Expected outcomes

• Child's skin will remain clean, dry, and intact.
• Child and family members will voice feelings about self-care deficit.

• Child or family member will demonstrate ability to perform bathing and hygiene.
• Child or family member will perform self-care program daily.

Interventions and rationales

• Assess child's functional, cognitive, and perceptual level at established intervals. Document and report any changes. *Ongoing assessment allows you to identify changing needs and adjust interventions accordingly.*
• Provide prescribed treatment for child's underlying condition. Monitor and report progress *to provide basis for plan of care.*
• Monitor completion of bathing and hygiene *to evaluate self-care abilities and identify areas of need.* Provide help only when child has difficulty.
• Teach child and family members bathing and hygiene techniques. Have them perform return demonstrations *to identify problem areas and build self-confidence.*
• Allow ample time to perform self-care. Encourage child to complete each task. Provide constructive feedback. *Rushing creates unnecessary stress and promotes failure. Completing task without assistance promotes self-confidence. Positive feedback encourages progress.*
• Provide privacy for self-care activities. *Modesty becomes important to children around age 6.*
• Provide safety equipment *to promote safety.*
• Refer child and family to support groups or community services *to provide continued assistance for efforts to promote self-care independence.*

Evaluations for expected outcomes

• Child's skin remains clean, dry, and intact.

• Child and family members voice feelings about self-care deficit.
• Child or family member displays competence in performing bathing and hygiene through return demonstration.
• Child or family member performs self-care program daily.

Documentation

• Child's expressions of frustration or feelings of inadequacy
• Family members' expressions of concern regarding child's inability to carry out bathing and hygiene
• Child's response to treatment for underlying condition
• Child's motor and sensory status
• Observations of child's impaired self-care ability
• Interventions to promote self-care skills and provide supportive care
• Instructions to child and family members, their understanding of instructions, and their demonstrated ability to carry out bathing and hygiene
• Child's and family members' responses to nursing interventions
• Evaluations for expected outcomes

■ Self-care deficit: Dressing and grooming

related to developmental delay

Definition

Inability to carry out activities associated with dressing and grooming

Assessment

• Age
• History of neurologic, sensory, or developmental impairment
• Self-care abilities, including knowledge and use of adaptive equipment,

preparation of equipment and supplies, and technical or mechanical skills
• Musculoskeletal status, including range of motion, muscle tone, gait, muscle size and strength, functional capabilities, and mechanical restrictions (such as splints, casts, or traction)
• Neurologic status, including cognition, communication ability, insight or judgment, level of consciousness, memory, motor ability, orientation, and sensory ability
• Psychosocial status, including child's affective reaction to imbalances between motor abilities and cognitive reasoning abilities, usual lifestyle, and parents' perception of developmental delay

Defining characteristics
• Impaired ability to clothe part or all of body
• Impaired ability to fasten clothing (such as inability to use zippers)
• Impaired ability to obtain or replace items of clothing
• Impaired ability to put on or take off specific articles of clothing (such as socks or shoes)
• Inability to choose clothing
• Inability to maintain appearance at satisfactory level
• Inability to pick up clothing
• Inability to use assistive devices

Associated medical diagnoses (selected)
This diagnosis can occur with any musculoskeletal, cognitive, or perceptual impairment.

Expected outcomes
• Child will be dressed and well groomed each day.
• Child and family members will express feelings and concerns regarding child's self-care deficit.

• Child or family member will display competence in performing dressing and grooming skills through return demonstration.
• Child or family member will perform self-care program daily.

Interventions and rationales
• Assess child's functional, cognitive, and perceptual level at periodic intervals. Document and report any changes. *Ongoing assessment allows you to identify changing needs and adjust interventions accordingly.*
• Provide prescribed treatment for child's underlying condition. Monitor and report progress *to provide basis for plan of care.*
• Monitor completion of dressing and grooming *to evaluate self-care abilities and identify areas of need.* Provide help only when child has difficulty. *Appropriate assistance provides an opportunity to teach self-care and promote good habits.*
• Suggest clothing that child can manage easily, such as clothing slightly larger than regular size or pants and shoes with Velcro fasteners *to foster independence and improve self-esteem.*
• Instruct child and family members in dressing and grooming techniques. Have them perform return demonstrations *to identify problem areas and build self-confidence.*
• Allow ample time to perform self-care. Encourage child to complete each task. Provide constructive feedback. *Rushing creates unnecessary stress and promotes failure. Completing task without help promotes self-confidence. Positive feedback encourages progress.*
• Provide privacy for dressing and grooming. *Modesty becomes important to children around age 6.*

• Refer child and family to support groups or community services *to provide ongoing assistance.*

Evaluations for expected outcomes
• Child is dressed and well groomed each day.
• Child and family members voice feelings regarding deficit in grooming and dressing skills.
• Child or family member displays competence in performing dressing and grooming skills through return demonstration.
• Child or family member performs self-care program daily.

Documentation
• Child's expressions of frustration or feelings of inadequacy
• Family members' expressions of feelings and concerns regarding child's inability to carry out dressing and grooming
• Child's response to treatment for underlying condition
• Child's motor and sensory status
• Interventions to promote self-care skills and provide supportive care
• Instructions provided to child and family members, their understanding of instructions, and their demonstrated ability to carry out dressing and grooming
• Child's and family members' responses to nursing interventions
• Evaluations for expected outcomes

■ Self-care deficit: Feeding
related to developmental delay

Definition
Inability to carry out feeding routine

Assessment
• Age
• History of injury or disease associated with musculoskeletal impairment
• Self-care abilities, including knowledge and use of adaptive equipment, preparation of equipment and supplies, and technical and mechanical skills
• Musculoskeletal status, including coordination, functional ability, muscle tone and strength, range of motion, and mechanical restrictions (such as cast, splint, or traction)
• Neurologic status, including cognition, communication ability, level of consciousness, motor ability, and sensory status
• Nutritional status, including weight and food preferences
• Psychosocial status, including child's affective reaction to imbalances between motor abilities and cognitive reasoning abilities, usual lifestyle, and parents' perception of developmental delay

Defining characteristics
• Inability to prepare food
• Inability to open containers
• Inability to use assistive devices
• Inability to handle utensils
• Inability to handle cup or glass
• Inability to get food onto utensil
• Inability to bring food from receptacle to mouth
• Inability to chew food
• Inability to swallow food
• Inability to ingest food safely and in socially acceptable manner
• Inability to ingest sufficient food
• Inability to complete meals

Associated medical diagnoses (selected)
This diagnosis can occur with any musculoskeletal, cognitive, or perceptual impairment.

Expected outcomes
• Child will consume adequate calories and maintain desired weight.
• Auscultation will reveal clear chest sounds.
• Child and family members will express feelings and concerns.
• Child or family member will demonstrate correct feeding technique.

Interventions and rationales
• Assess child's functional, cognitive, and perceptual level at periodic intervals. Document and report any changes. *Ongoing assessment allows you to identify changing needs and adjust interventions accordingly.*
• Provide prescribed treatment for child's underlying condition. Monitor and report progress *to provide basis for plan of care.*
• Weigh child daily and record results *to assess nutritional status.*
• Determine type of food child handles most and tolerates best (finger foods, soft or liquid diet) *to enhance self-feeding ability.*
• Monitor and record breath sounds every 4 hours. Report any evidence of crackles, wheezing, or rhonchi *to detect aspiration.*
• Monitor feeding routine *to evaluate self-care abilities and identify areas of need.* Assist only if necessary; for example, cut food into bite-size portions. *Appropriate assistance provides an opportunity to teach self-care and promote good habits.*
• Instruct child and family members in feeding routine. Have them perform return demonstrations *to build self-confidence.*
• Allow ample time to perform self-care activities. *Rushing creates unnecessary stress and promotes failure.* Encourage child to complete each task. *Completing task without assistance promotes self-confidence.* Provide constructive feedback.
• Position child in upright sitting position. Use supportive devices as needed to maintain child's posture. Sit at eye level with child. *These measures will help decrease risk of aspiration. Sitting at eye level will help prevent child from hyperextending his neck, which may increase risk of aspiration.*
• Teach specific tasks (such as grasping spoon, opening mouth, closing lips around utensil, or swallowing) rather than total feeding skill. Use behavior modification techniques of praise and reward to mark accomplishments. *Children may not have cognitive or motor abilities to complete total skill. Breaking down behavior into smaller units increases likelihood of success.*

Evaluations for expected outcomes
• Child maintains weight above 5th percentile on pediatric growth charts.
• Aspiration doesn't occur as evidenced by clear breath sounds heard during auscultation.
• Child and family members voice feelings regarding feeding routine.
• Child or family member demonstrates correct feeding technique.

Documentation
• Child's expressions of frustration or feelings of inadequacy
• Family members' expressions of concern
• Child's response to treatment for underlying condition
• Child's motor and sensory status
• Interventions performed to promote self-care skills and provide supportive care
• Instructions provided to child and family members, their understanding of instructions, and their demonstrated ability to carry out feeding routine

• Child's and family members' responses to nursing interventions
• Evaluations for expected outcomes

■ Self-care deficit: Toileting

related to developmental delay

Definition
Inability to carry out aspects of self-care associated with bowel and urine elimination

Assessment
• Developmental factors, including age, maturity, and smooth muscle control
• History of neurologic, sensory, or developmental impairment
• Self-care abilities, including knowledge and use of adaptive equipment, preparation of equipment and supplies, and technical or mechanical skills
• Musculoskeletal status, including range of motion, muscle tone, gait, muscle size and strength, functional capabilities, and mechanical restrictions (such as splints, casts, or traction)
• Neurologic status, including cognition, communication ability, insight or judgment, level of consciousness, memory, motor ability, orientation, and sensory ability
• Psychosocial status, including child's affective reaction to imbalances between motor abilities and cognitive reasoning abilities, usual lifestyle, and parents' perception of developmental delay

Defining characteristics
• Inability to carry out proper toilet hygiene

• Inability to get to toilet or commode
• Inability to manipulate clothing for toileting
• Inability to sit on or rise from toilet or commode
• Inability to flush toilet or empty commode

Associated medical diagnoses (selected)
This diagnosis can occur with any musculoskeletal, cognitive, or perceptual impairment.

Expected outcomes
• Child will maintain normal urine and bowel elimination patterns for age.
• Child and family members will voice feelings about impaired toileting ability.
• Child and family members will demonstrate correct toileting activities.
• Child's skin will remain clean, dry, and intact.

Interventions and rationales
• Observe child's functional, cognitive, and perceptual level. Document and report any changes. *Ongoing assessment allows you to identify changing needs and adjust interventions.*
• Provide prescribed treatment for child's underlying condition. Monitor and report progress *to provide basis for plan of care.*
• Monitor intake and output *to detect fluid and electrolyte imbalances.*
• Assess skin condition, especially in perianal area, *to detect evidence of skin breakdown.*
• Assist with toileting when necessary. As much as possible, allow child to perform toilet routine independently *to enhance toileting ability and promote feelings of control.*

• Teach child and family members toileting routine. Have child and family members demonstrate toileting routine under supervision. *Return demonstration allows you to evaluate learning and increases child's and family members' confidence.*
• Provide privacy for toileting activities. *Beginning around age 6, modesty becomes important to children.*
• Assist with specific bladder elimination procedures, such as intermittent self-catheterization, as prescribed. Assess child's readiness to learn self-catheterization. Instruct child or family members in technique and request return demonstration *to evaluate understanding and ability.* Maintain sterile technique in hospital and clean technique at home *to prevent infection.*
• Assist with use of incontinence aids, such as diapers, pads, and pants, which may be prescribed as an alternative to indwelling devices. *Incontinence aids prevent soiling of clothes and linen, reduce embarrassment, and draw urine away from skin.*
• Establish regular pattern for bowel care. For example, after breakfast, place child on toilet or commode for 1 hour after inserting glycerin suppository; allow child to remain upright for 30 minutes, and then clean anal area. *Regular bowel care encourages routine physiologic function.*
• Teach parents bowel care routine *to foster compliance.*
• Maintain diet log *to identify irritant foods,* and then eliminate such foods from child's diet *to promote regular bowel function.* Teach parents need to regulate child's intake of foods and fluids that cause diarrhea or constipation *to encourage healthful nutritional patterns.*
• Teach parents to regulate child's fluid intake according to specific schedule and to limit fluid intake after dinner *to encourage voiding at appropriate time.*

Evaluations for expected outcomes
• Child maintains normal elimination patterns for age.
• Child and family members express feelings associated with child's toileting routine.
• Child and family members demonstrate correct toileting activities.
• Child's skin remains intact with no evidence of breakdown.

Documentation
• Child's expressions of feelings of inadequacy or depression
• Family members' concerns about child's inability to carry out toileting activities
• Child's response to treatment for underlying condition
• Child's motor and sensory status
• Interventions to promote self-care skills and to provide supportive care
• Child's and family members' responses to nursing interventions
• Instructions to child and family members, their understanding of instructions, and demonstrated ability to carry out toileting routine
• Evaluations for expected outcomes

■ Thermoregulation, ineffective
related to child's illness or trauma

Definition
Potentially extreme fluctuations in body temperature

Assessment
• Age

• History of illness or injury, including related events, such as exposure to infection (intrauterine or extrauterine)
• Perinatal history, including asphyxia
• Health history, including chronic disease or disability
• Medication history
• Vital signs, including temperature, pulse rate, blood pressure, and respirations
• Skin color and temperature
• Fluid and electrolyte status, including skin turgor, intake and output, mucous membranes, serum electrolyte levels, and urine specific gravity
• Neurologic status, including level of consciousness
• Nutritional status, including willingness and ability to eat, current weight, and weight gain pattern (on growth chart)

Defining characteristics
• Cyanotic nail beds
• Increased capillary refill time
• Fluctuations in body temperature above or below normal range
• Flushed skin
• Hypertension
• Increased respiratory or heart rate
• Mild shivering
• Moderate pallor
• Piloerection
• Seizures
• Warm or cool skin

Associated medical diagnoses (selected)
Brain tumors (especially if located in hypothalamus, pituitary, or medulla), cerebral edema, chemical toxicity (including reactions to drugs or anesthesia), dehydration, heart failure, infection, near-drowning, smoke inhalation or other anoxic events

Expected outcomes
• Child will maintain body temperature at normal levels (96.8° to 99° F [36° to 37.2° C]).
• Child's fluid intake and output will remain balanced and within normal limits for age.
• Child will maintain adequate glucose intake and will consume ___ calories per day.
• Child and family members will identify risk factors and describe measures to prevent dehydration.
• Family members will demonstrate procedure for assessing axillary or oral temperature accurately.
• Family members will demonstrate measures to care for child with fever.

Interventions and rationales
• Take axillary or oral temperature every 1 to 4 hours. Avoid taking rectal temperatures. Record temperature and route. *Physically and psychologically safer than rectal thermometers, axillary and oral thermometers provide accurate core temperature.*
• If child has fever, remove sheets, blankets, and most clothing (except diapers and underwear). Place cool cloths on axilla and groin. Perform tepid sponging procedure. Use hypothermia blanket for temperature above 103° F (39.4° C). Set blanket temperature at 41° F (5° C). Discontinue if shivering occurs *because shivering increases metabolic rate and supports fever.* Monitor vital signs every 15 minutes for 1 hour and as indicated *because decreasing body temperature too rapidly can cause vascular collapse. These steps reduce excessive fever.*
• Monitor heart rate, rhythm, and respiratory rate. *Careful monitoring determines need for more aggressive intervention.*

• Calculate child's fluid, glucose, and electrolyte requirements. Administer I.V. fluids as indicated. Monitor and record intake and output *to compensate for increase in metabolic rate and to prevent dehydration. Insensible fluid losses increase by 10% for every 1° C rise in temperature.*
• If child has body temperature below 96.8° F (36° C), use warming blanket. Set blanket temperature at 100.4° F (38° C). Keep child wrapped in blankets and cover child's head. *Body surface area, particularly head, is proportionately larger in young children; adequate covering will prevent heat loss. These steps combat hypothermia.*
• Teach parents how to take accurate temperature and have parents provide return demonstration *to ensure accurate monitoring after discharge.*
• Determine child's preferences for oral fluids. Push fluids in manner appropriate to child's age and level of development. *Well-hydrated child's temperature returns to normal range more quickly.*
• Discuss factors that precipitate neurogenic temperature drift with family members *to prevent future episodes.*

Evaluations for expected outcomes
• Child's temperature remains within normal limits.
• Child maintains balanced fluid intake and output within normal limits for age.
• Child maintains adequate glucose and caloric intake.
• Child and family members identify risk factors and describe measures to prevent dehydration.
• Family members demonstrate ability to measure axillary or oral temperature accurately.
• Family members demonstrate measures to care for child with fever.

Documentation
• Observations of physical findings
• Nursing interventions performed
• Medications administered
• Child's response to nursing interventions
• Evaluations for expected outcomes

■ Verbal communication impairment
related to developmental factors

Definition
Decreased ability to speak, understand, or use words appropriately

Assessment
• Age
• Health history, including past respiratory, neurologic, or musculoskeletal disorders or surgery
• Respiratory status, including dyspnea, use of accessory muscles, and respiratory pattern
• Neurologic status, including mental status and speech (pattern, signing, and such communication aids as artificial larynx, computer-assisted speech device, pen and pencil, picture board, and alphabet board)
• Musculoskeletal status, including range of motion and manual dexterity
• Parental status, including understanding of normal speech development, level of frustration with child's speech impairment, and coping skills

Defining characteristics
• Disorientation
• Difficulty expressing thought verbally (aphasia, dysphasia, apraxia, dyslexia)
• Difficulty comprehending and maintaining usual communication pattern

• Difficulty forming words or sentences (aphonia, dyslalia, dysarthria)
• Difficulty using or inability to use facial expressions or body language
• Dyspnea
• Impaired articulation
• Inability or lack of desire to speak
• Inability to speak dominant language
• Inappropriate verbalizations
• Lack of eye contact or poor selective attention
• Visual deficit (partial or total)

Associated medical diagnoses (selected)

This diagnosis may be associated with any disorder that alters child's ability to speak. Examples include cleft lip or palate, deafness, head injury, prematurity, and respiratory distress syndrome.

Expected outcomes

• Family members will express desire to better understand child's communication impairment.
• Family members will demonstrate understanding of verbal development in children and alternative communication techniques.
• Child will communicate needs.

Interventions and rationales

• Teach parents to:
– talk to, read to, and play music for child
– repeat sound child makes
– point to objects and name them
– use generative speech ("What would you like to wear today?") rather than directive speech ("Do you want to wear the red shirt?").
These measures stimulate language development. Generative speech requires child to generate words rather than simply responding with yes or no.

• Describe to family members alternative methods of assessing needs of speech-delayed children. Toddlers and preschoolers may communicate their needs through role-playing with dolls and stuffed animals. Preschoolers and school-age children may communicate through drawing. Parents may use pictoral (faces) pain scale to assess ill child's level of discomfort. *These techniques will enable family to better understand their speech-delayed child.*
• Assess family members' level of understanding of speech development process. Tell them that toddler has limited receptive language skills and should be given one direction at a time. Preschooler has limited vocabulary and may communicate through gestures and symbols. Further explain that children develop speech at different rates. *These measures increase family members' understanding of child's speech impairment.*

Evaluations for expected outcomes

• Family members describe stages of speech development.
• Family members demonstrate alternative methods of assessing needs of speech-delayed child.
• Child communicates needs.

Documentation

• Family members' understanding of speech development process
• Family members' demonstration of alternative methods of assessing needs of speech-delayed child
• Family members' understanding of alternative methods of communicating with child
• Nursing interventions and family's and child's response to them
• Evaluations for expected outcomes

MATERNAL-NEONATAL HEALTH

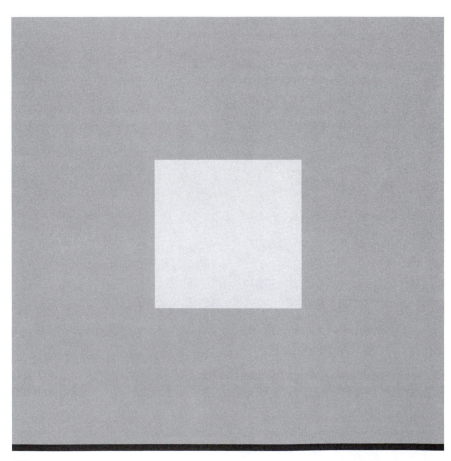

INTRODUCTION

This section covers maternal, fetal, and neonatal care, with an emphasis on meeting the changing needs of the mother, child, and family. Because of the dynamic nature of pregnancy and childbirth, you'll need to be flexible in your care planning. Expect to form new nursing diagnoses continually during the time that you're providing care.

During pregnancy, you'll assess maternal factors, such as age, past experience with pregnancy and delivery, health history, reaction to fetal movement, and nutritional status. Keep in mind that the mother's health status directly affects the fetus's well-being.

After birth, you'll assess neonatal factors, such as Apgar scores, gestational age, weight in relation to gestational age, vital signs, feeding patterns, muscle tone, condition of fontanels, and characteristics of the neonate's cry.

Throughout your assessment, maintain a family-centered, holistic approach. Assess family status. Be aware of how pregnancy and the neonate's arrival affect parents, siblings, and the rest of the family. Evaluate how well the mother, father, siblings, and other family members bond with the neonate.

Use information gathered during assessment to develop appropriate nursing diagnoses. In this section, you'll find nursing diagnoses and related etiologies for the prenatal period, labor and delivery, and the postpartum period. Neonatal health is covered as well. These nursing diagnoses state actual or potential health problems of the developing family, focusing on the physiologic and psychosocial needs of its members.

When implementing your plan of care, reinforce your interventions with thorough patient teaching. Encourage family members to become involved in the planning and implementation of care. Stay attuned to their changing educational needs, and remain sensitive to the new mother and supportive of her emotional concerns.

Inform other members of the health care team of your nursing goals, and enlist their support as needed. Keep colleagues informed about the family's progress in attaining goals.

Evaluate the plan of care frequently. This will allow you to determine the need for revisions promptly, thereby ensuring that the plan of care accurately reflects the developing family's current needs.

■ Anxiety

related to hospitalization and birth process

Definition

Feeling of threat or danger to self related to pregnancy or birth

Assessment

• History of stress-related signs or symptoms
• Current worries, fears, and concerns
• Expectations of labor experience, including knowledge and past experience
• Behavior, including reaction to fetal movement and uterine activity, motor activity, excessive or extraneous movements, and interactions with nurse and significant others
• Cognitive status, including ability to concentrate, learn, and remember
• Physiologic status
• Usual coping methods
• Mood
• Personality
• Progress of labor

Defining characteristics

• Excessive attention to fetal movement or uterine activity
• Excessive or uncontrolled reaction to labor contractions
• Expressed concern about pregnancy or birth
• Expressed fear of unspecified negative outcome
• Expressed feelings of helplessness or incapacity
• Fear, apprehension, and wariness
• Inability to concentrate, understand, or remember
• Increased muscle tension in body or face
• Perspiration
• Rapid pulse rate

• Restlessness, shakiness, trembling, jittery behavior, and extraneous movements

Associated medical diagnoses (selected)

Maternal psychological stress, multiple births, pregnancy, premature labor

Expected outcomes

• Patient will express feelings of anxiety.
• Patient will identify causes of anxiety.
• Patient will make use of available emotional support.
• Patient will show fewer signs of anxiety.
• Patient will identify positive aspects of her efforts to cope during childbirth.
• Patient will acquire increased knowledge about childbirth and will be better prepared to cope with future births.

Interventions and rationales

• Assess patient's knowledge, experience, and expectations of labor *to learn precise source of anxiety and increase effectiveness of interventions.*
• Discuss normal labor progression with patient and explain what to expect during labor *to increase patient's knowledge about normal progression of labor and understanding of her own experience.*
• Involve patient in making decisions about care *to reduce sense of powerlessness that some women experience during labor.*
• Share information on labor progression, vital signs, and neonate's condition with patient *to provide reassurance of normality and increase her sense of participation.*
• Interpret environmental sights and sounds (electronic fetal monitor strip, fetal monitor sounds, and activities in

unit) for patient *to make environment seem less threatening.*
• Attend to patient's comfort needs *to increase trust and reduce anxiety.*
• Encourage patient to employ coping skills used successfully in past *to enhance her sense of control.*
• Teach new coping skills (relaxation, breathing techniques, and positioning) *to diminish anxiety by increasing patient's sense of power and control.* Review skills with patient periodically *because anxiety impairs recall.*
• Organize work to spend as much time as possible with patient *to provide comfort and assistance, thereby promoting patient's sense of security.*
• Allow family members to participate in care *to provide comfort and help patient cope with labor.*

Evaluations for expected outcomes
• Patient expresses feelings of anxiety about pregnancy or birth.
• Patient identifies causes of anxiety.
• Patient communicates with nurse or family members to gain reassurance, information, or emotional support.
• Patient's physiologic or behavioral signs return to normal.
• Patient, verbally or nonverbally, indicates that giving birth was positive experience and expresses satisfaction with her behavior while giving birth.
• Patient verbalizes increased knowledge about childbirth and displays confidence in her ability to cope with future births.

Documentation
• Patient's expressions of anxiety
• Patient's statements of reasons for anxiety
• Observation of physical or behavioral signs of anxiety
• Interventions to assist patient with coping

• Patient's response to interventions
• Evaluations for expected outcomes

■ Aspiration, risk for

related to neonate's immature cough or gag reflex

Definition
Entry of GI secretions, oropharyngeal secretions, or exogenous fluids into neonate's tracheobronchial passages

Assessment
• Gestational age
• Neonate's weight in relation to gestational age
• Maternal sedation before delivery and effects of maternal sedation on labor
• Neonate's health status, including preexisting conditions, anomalies, intrauterine environment, urologic status, cardiovascular status, respiratory status, and GI status
• Laboratory studies of neonate, including fluid, electrolyte, and arterial blood gas levels
• Neonate's vital signs
• Neonate's nutritional status, including continuous or intermittent gavage feeding

Risk factors
• Decreased GI motility
• Delayed gastric emptying
• Depressed cough and gag reflexes
• Feeding or GI tubes
• Impaired swallowing
• Incompetent lower esophageal sphincter
• Increased gastric residual contents
• Increased intragastric pressure
• Medication administration
• Reduced level of consciousness

• Situations hindering elevation of upper body
• Surgery or trauma to face, mouth, or neck
• Tracheostomy or endotracheal tube

Associated medical diagnoses (selected)
Esophageal atresia, neonatal asphyxia, prematurity, pyloric stenosis

Expected outcomes
• Neonate will receive suctioning as needed and will maintain clear airway.
• Neonate won't exhibit gastric distention.
• Neonate will demonstrate minimal to moderate quantity of nasopharyngeal and oropharyngeal secretions.
• Neonate will tolerate initial feeding.
• Neonate won't demonstrate any color changes during feeding.
• Neonate will demonstrate appropriate suck and swallow reflex.
• Neonate will have no adventitious breath sounds.
• Neonate won't exhibit signs and symptoms of aspiration.

Interventions and rationales
• Regularly assess neonate's respiratory status until stable *to evaluate respiratory system transition to extrauterine life.*
• Monitor vital signs, according to facility protocol, and report changes *to determine multisystem adjustment to extrauterine existence.*
• Suction as needed *to keep upper and lower airways clear.* If neonate aspirates meconium, assist doctor with laryngoscopy to suction below vocal cords. If in delivery room, suction oropharynx and nasopharynx with bulb syringe, DeLee catheter, or suction catheter attached to wall suction. *These measures may prevent additional respiratory compromise.*

• Perform head-to-toe physical assessment *to detect abnormalities in other body systems that may affect respiratory effort.*
• Withhold oral feedings if signs of respiratory distress occur. Provide I.V. fluids as ordered. *Sucking may place additional stress on neonate in respiratory distress and may lead to aspiration.*
• When offering initial feeding, observe for suck and swallow reflex, gag and cough reflex, and color changes. Have suction equipment available and ready to use. *Early detection of difficulty may prevent neonatal morbidity and mortality.*
• If neonate is receiving gavage feeding:
– Keep head of bed elevated during and after feedings unless contraindicated.
– Ensure proper positioning of neonate before feeding or administering medication.
– Monitor residual gastric contents and follow parameters for withholding feedings.
– Once per shift, measure abdominal girth to check for distention and stop gavage feeding immediately if you suspect aspiration. Keep suction apparatus at bedside and suction as needed. Turn neonate on side. *Preventive measures reduce risk of aspiration.*
• Review laboratory results and report abnormalities. *Early identification of abnormal laboratory values reduces risk of aspiration.*
• Explain to parents reasons for interventions *to gain parental understanding and cooperation, which contributes to positive outcome.*
• Instruct parents in feeding techniques that will help prevent distended abdomen leading to aspiration. Tell them to avoid overfeeding and to burp

neonate at frequent intervals (after intake of ½ to 1 oz). Instruct parents to position neonate on right side with head of bed elevated for 30 to 60 minutes after feeding. *Providing instructions encourages parental understanding and cooperation.*

Evaluations for expected outcomes
• Neonate receives suctioning as needed and maintains patent airway.
• Neonate doesn't have gastric distention.
• Neonate has minimal to moderate nasopharyngeal and oropharyngeal secretions.
• Neonate tolerates initial feeding.
• Neonate doesn't demonstrate color changes during feeding.
• Neonate has appropriate suck and swallow reflex.
• Neonate has no adventitious breath sounds.
• Neonate shows no signs or symptoms of aspiration.

Documentation
• Neonate's tolerance of initial feeding and of gavage feedings
• Residual gastric contents after gavage feeding
• Incidents of vomiting, aspiration, or both
• Breath sounds
• Observations of physical findings
• Interventions performed to prevent aspiration
• Evaluations for expected outcomes

■ Breast-feeding, effective

Definition
State in which mother, neonate, and family exhibit proficiency and satisfaction with breast-feeding process

Assessment
• Maternal status, including age and maturity, parity, level of prenatal breast-feeding preparation, past breast-feeding experience, previous postpartum history, physical condition (actual or perceived inadequate milk supply and comfort level), and psychosocial factors (apprehension level, body image, stress from family and career, sociocultural views of breast-feeding, and emotional support from significant others)
• Neonatal status, including satisfaction and contentment, growth rate, age-weight relationship, urine output, quantity and characteristics of stools, and ability to latch onto breasts

Defining characteristics
• Ability to position infant at breast to promote successful latching on (mother)
• Adequate elimination pattern for age (infant)
• Appropriate weight pattern for age (infant)
• Eagerness to nurse (infant)
• Effective communication pattern (mother and infant)
• Evidence of contentment after feeding (infant)
• Expressed satisfaction with breast-feeding process (mother)
• Regular and sustained sucking and swallowing at breast (infant)
• Signs and symptoms of oxytocin release (mother)

Associated medical diagnoses (selected)
Vaginal or cesarean section delivery of term or preterm neonate

Expected outcomes
• Mother will breast-feed neonate successfully and will experience satisfaction with breast-feeding process.

• Neonate will feed successfully on both breasts and appear satisfied.
• Neonate will grow and develop in pace with accepted standards.
• Mother will continue breast-feeding neonate after early postpartum period.

Interventions and rationales
• Assess mother's knowledge and experience of breast-feeding *to focus teaching on specific learning needs.*
• Educate mother and selected support person about breast-feeding techniques:
– Clean hands and breasts before nursing.
– Position neonate for feeding (neonate should be able to grasp most of areola).
– Change positions to decrease nipple tenderness and use both breasts at each feeding.
– Remove neonate from breast by breaking suction; avoiding setting time limits in early stage.
Greater understanding of techniques improves chances for success.
• Teach mother how to use warm showers and compresses, relaxation and guided imagery, infant suckling, holding infant close to breasts, and listening to infant cry *to stimulate let-down.*
• Educate mother about her nutritional needs. She requires well-balanced diet plus an additional 500 calories and two extra glasses of fluid each day *to maintain adequate milk supply.* She should limit caffeine and avoid foods that make her uncomfortable.
• Teach mother what to expect from breast-feeding neonate *to prepare mother for care of neonate at home.* Neonate should pass one to six stools and wet six to eight diapers per day. Stools should be soft to liquid and nonodorous. Neonate should feed

every 2 to 3 hours, be quiet after feeding, and appear generally well. Explain that neonate also requires non-nutritive sucking.
• Assist mother and family in planning for home care. Mother needs to rest when neonate sleeps, practice self-care, learn techniques for expressing and storing breast milk, and recognize signs of engorgement and infection. Family members should understand importance of helping. *Mothers often stop breast-feeding once they return home and resume work, usually because of fatigue.*
• Provide quiet and privacy *to enhance development of breast-feeding skills.*
• Encourage mother to express concerns about breast-feeding *to reduce anxiety.*
• Offer information about breast-feeding support groups *to help meet emotional and learning needs.*

Evaluations for expected outcomes
• Mother demonstrates successful breast-feeding of neonate and expresses satisfaction with breast-feeding.
• Neonate feeds on both breasts and appears satisfied.
• Neonate's weight and length remain consistent and within 10th and 90th percentiles on pediatric growth grid.
• Mother continues to breast-feed infant after discharge from hospital.

Documentation
• Mother's expressions about breast-feeding experience
• Observations of breast-feeding techniques and mother-infant interaction during breast-feeding
• Teaching and instructions given
• Neonate's growth and weight
• Referrals to support groups

• Mother's plans for breast-feeding after discharge
• Evaluations for expected outcomes

■ Breast-feeding, ineffective

related to dissatisfaction with breast-feeding process

Definition
State in which mother, neonate, or family experience dissatisfaction or difficulty with breast-feeding process

Assessment
• Maternal status, including age and maturity, relationships with significant others, previous bonding history, parity, level of prenatal breast-feeding preparation, knowledge or previous breast-feeding experience, physical condition (actual or perceived inadequate milk supply, nipple shape, and comfort level), and psychosocial factors (apprehension level, body image and perceptions, stress from family and career, sociocultural views of breast-feeding, and emotional support from significant others)
• Neonatal status, including satisfaction and contentment, growth rate, and age-weight relationship

Defining characteristics
• Actual or perceived inadequate milk supply (mother)
• Arching and crying when at breast (infant)
• Inability to latch on to nipple correctly (infant)
• Evidence of inadequate intake (infant)
• Fussiness and crying within first hour after feeding (infant)

• Insufficient emptying of each breast (mother)
• Inadequate opportunity for suckling (infant)
• Lack of observable signs of oxytocin release (mother)
• Lack of response to other comfort measures (infant)
• Lack of sustained suckling at breast (infant)
• Persistently sore nipples after first week of breast-feeding (mother)
• Resistance to latching on (infant)
• Unsatisfactory breast-feeding process (mother and infant)

Associated medical diagnoses (selected)
Maternal nipple anomaly, maternal psychological stress, neonatal anomaly, prematurity

Expected outcomes
• Mother will express physical and psychological comfort with breast-feeding techniques and practice.
• Mother will show decreased anxiety and apprehension.
• Neonate will feed successfully on both breasts and appear satisfied for at least 2 hours after feeding.
• Neonate will grow and thrive.
• Mother will state at least one resource for breast-feeding support.

Interventions and rationales
• Educate mother in breast care and breast-feeding techniques. *This reduces anxiety and enhances proper nutrition of neonate.*
• Be available yet discreet during breast-feeding. *Assessment of mother's technique can reveal problem areas.* Encourage mother's questions *to increase understanding and reduce anxiety.*
• Teach techniques for encouraging let-down reflex:
– warm shower

– breast massage
– physically caring for neonate
– holding neonate close to breasts.
These measures reduce anxiety and promote let-down reflex.
• Provide mother and infant with quiet, private, comfortable environment with decreased external stressors *to promote successful breast-feeding.*
• Encourage expression of fears and anxieties between mother and significant other *to reduce anxiety and increase mother's sense of control.*
• Offer written information, reading list, or information about breast-feeding support groups *to help meet mother's emotional and learning needs.*

Evaluations for expected outcomes
• Mother expresses physical and psychological comfort with breast-feeding techniques and practice.
• Mother displays decreased anxiety and apprehension.
• Neonate feeds successfully on both breasts and appears satisfied for at least 2 hours after feeding.
• Neonate grows and thrives.
• Mother states at least one available resource for breast-feeding support.

Documentation
• Mother's expressions of feelings of comfort with breast-feeding ability
• Observations of bonding and breast-feeding processes
• Teaching and instructions given
• Referrals to support groups
• Neonate growth and weight
• Evaluations for expected outcomes

■ Breast-feeding, ineffective

related to limited maternal experience

Definition
State in which mother, neonate, or family experiences dissatisfaction or difficulty with breast-feeding process

Assessment
• Maternal status, including age and maturity, relationships with significant others, previous bonding history, parity, level of prenatal breast-feeding preparation, knowledge or previous breast-feeding experience, and physical condition (actual or perceived inadequate milk supply, nipple shape, and comfort level)
• Psychosocial status, including apprehension level, body image and perceptions, stressors such as family and career, sociocultural views of breast-feeding, and emotional support from significant others
• Neonatal status, including satisfaction and contentment, growth rate, age-weight relationship, neurologic status, respiratory status, suck reflex, presence of factors that interfere with proper sucking (cleft lip or palate), and previous feedings with artificial nipples

Defining characteristics
• Actual or perceived inadequate milk supply (mother)
• Arching and crying when at breast (infant)
• Inability to latch on to nipple correctly (infant)
• Evidence of inadequate intake (infant)
• Fussiness and crying within first hour after feeding (infant)

• Insufficient emptying of each breast (mother)
• Inadequate opportunity for suckling (infant)
• Lack of observable signs of oxytocin release (mother)
• Lack of response to other comfort measures (infant)
• Lack of sustained suckling at breast (infant)
• Persistently sore nipples after first week of breast-feeding (mother)
• Resistance to latching on (infant)
• Unsatisfactory breast-feeding process (mother and infant)

Associated medical diagnoses (selected)
Maternal: Breast engorgement, inverted nipples, mammaplasty, maternal psychological stress
Neonatal: Cleft lip or palate, prematurity

Expected outcomes
• Mother will express understanding of breast-feeding techniques and practice.
• Mother will display decreased anxiety and apprehension.
• Mother and neonate will experience successful breast-feeding.
• Neonate's initial weight loss will be within accepted norms.
• Neonate's nutritional needs will be met.

Interventions and rationales
• Assess mother's knowledge *to help direct your interventions.*
• Educate mother in breast care and breast-feeding techniques *to reduce anxiety and help ensure proper nutrition of neonate.*
• Provide appropriate pamphlets and audiovisual aids *to help meet mother's learning needs. Mother can review written material at her own pace; audiovisual materials illustrate proper technique.*
• Determine mother's level of anxiety or ambivalence related to breast-feeding. *Anxiety and ambivalence can interfere with mother's ability to learn and with let-down reflex.*
• Teach techniques for encouraging let-down reflex:
– warm shower
– breast massage
– relaxation and guided imagery
– infant suckling
– holding neonate close to breasts.
These measures reduce anxiety and facilitate let-down reflex.
• Remain with mother and neonate during several feedings *to pinpoint problem areas.* Encourage mother to ask questions *to increase understanding and reduce anxiety.*
• Evaluate position of neonate's tongue during breast-feeding. *To produce proper sucking motion, neonate's tongue must be down during breast-feeding, with nipple directly on top.*
• Instruct mother to offer breast as soon as possible after neonate awakens and not to wait until neonate is crying vigorously. *Getting an extremely upset neonate to breast-feed effectively is difficult.*
• Evaluate need for nipple shield and instruct mother in its use. *Nipple shields help draw out partially inverted nipples.*
• Make sure neonate is awake and alert when feeding; unwrap as needed. *A tightly wrapped, sleepy neonate won't be alert enough to suckle sufficiently.*
• Sprinkle glucose water on nipples before feeding if needed. *When making preliminary attempts at breast-feeding, neonate may open his mouth on tasting glucose water. Mother can then direct and attach neonate's open mouth to nipple.*

• Evaluate neonate for anomalies that may interfere with breast-feeding ability *to plan comprehensive treatment and teaching.*

• Instruct mother in proper breast care techniques, such as wearing supportive bra, using cream, washing, and air drying. *Proper breast care helps prevent nipple drying, cracking, soreness, and bleeding, which can interfere with effective breast-feeding.*

• Instruct mother on ways to alleviate breast engorgement. *Breast engorgement can prevent neonate from effectively latching on to nipple.*

• Review principles of milk production and identify factors that can alter production or quality of breast milk, such as emotional upset and intake of alcohol, drugs, and certain foods. *Any substance mother ingests passes through to breast milk. Mother must be aware of possible dangerous adverse effects.*

• Provide positive reinforcement for mother's efforts *to decrease anxiety and enhance feelings of self-esteem and success.*

• Provide mother with information about breast-feeding support groups. *Participation in support group after discharge can help meet mother's emotional and learning needs.*

Evaluations for expected outcomes

• Mother properly positions neonate during breast-feeding, uses appropriate techniques to encourage attachment to nipple, and (if applicable) correctly uses supplemental devices.

• Mother expresses decreased anxiety and continued enthusiasm for breast-feeding.

• Neonate feeds successfully on both breasts and appears satisfied for at least 2 hours after feeding.

• Neonate's initial weight loss remains within accepted norms.

• Neonate's nutritional needs are met.

Documentation

• Mother's level of knowledge related to breast-feeding

• Mother's expressions of dissatisfaction with breast-feeding ability

• Mother's emotional response to breast-feeding

• Mother's breast care practices

• Maternal conditions that may interfere with breast-feeding, such as inverted nipples or mammaplasty

• Mother's and neonate's behavior during and after breast-feeding, including positioning of neonate, neonate's response to being put to breast, and neonate's level of satisfaction

• Mother's use of such devices as nipple shield

• Frequency and duration of feedings

• Neonate's growth, weight, output, and any supplemental feedings administered

• Teaching and instructions given and mother's response to instructions

• Goals established by mother

• Referrals to support groups

• Mother's and neonate's responses to nursing interventions

• Evaluations for expected outcomes

■ Breast-feeding, interrupted

related to a contraindicating condition

Definition

Break in the continuity of breast-feeding resulting from a maternal or neonatal problem

Assessment

• Maternal status, including age and maturity, employment hours, relationship with significant other, parity, level of prenatal breast-feeding knowledge or experience, and physical condition (comfort level, nipple shape, presence of infection, and use of medication)
• Neonatal status, including age-weight relationship, growth rate, neurologic status, respiratory status, suck reflex, and factors that interfere with proper sucking (such as cleft lip or palate)

Defining characteristics

• Continued desire to maintain lactation and provide breast milk for infant's nutritional needs (mother)
• Failure to receive nourishment at breast for some or all feedings (infant)
• Lack of knowledge about expressing and storing breast milk (mother)
• Separation of mother and infant

Associated medical diagnoses (selected)

Maternal or infant illness, maternal nipple anomaly, maternal psychological stress, neonatal anomaly, neonatal hyperbilirubinemia, prematurity

Expected outcomes

• Mother will express her understanding of factors that necessitate interruption in breast-feeding.
• Mother will express comfort with her decision whether or not to resume breast-feeding.
• Mother will express and store breast milk appropriately.
• Mother will resume breast-feeding when interfering factors cease.
• Mother will have adequate milk supply when breast-feeding resumes.
• Mother will obtain relief from discomfort associated with engorgement.
• Infant's nutritional needs will be met.

Interventions and rationales

• Assess mother's understanding of reasons for interrupting breast-feeding *to evaluate need for additional instruction.*
• Reassure mother that neonate's nutritional needs will be met through other methods *to allay her anxiety.*
• Assess mother's desire to resume breast-feeding *to help plan interventions.*
• Provide appropriate educational materials, including audiovisual aids and written materials. *Audiovisual aids demonstrate proper expressing and storing techniques; written material allows mother to review information at her own pace.*
• Instruct mother in techniques for expressing and storing breast milk *to ensure adequate milk supply.*
• Recommend use of breast pump according to following guidelines *to provide maximum stimulation and prolactin production:*
– Initiate pumping 24 to 48 hours after delivery.
– Pump minimum of five times per day.
– Pump minimum of 100 minutes per day.
– Pump long enough to soften breasts each time, regardless of duration.
• Encourage mother to save her breast milk in sterile container and store it in refrigerator or freezer for future feedings. *Preserving breast milk ensures that neonate receives maternal antibodies and helps to encourage maternal involvement in neonatal care.*
• If mother must pump for prolonged period, encourage her to use piston-style electric pump. *Using electric*

pump rather than hand pump produces milk with higher fat content.
• If mother intends to resume breast-feeding, instruct her in ways to relieve breast engorgement *to prevent discomfort that may keep neonate from sucking effectively.*
• If appropriate, instruct mother in use of devices such as nipple shield, *which is designed to alter flat or inverted nipples, a condition that may interfere with successful breast-feeding.*
• Review mother's daily routine *to advise her how to incorporate breast-feeding into her schedule.*
• Provide mother with information about breast-feeding support groups. *Support group can help mother obtain needed emotional support and continue learning.*
• If mother doesn't intend to resume breast-feeding, advise her to wear a supportive bra, apply ice, and take a mild analgesic, such as acetaminophen, *to alleviate discomfort associated with engorgement.*

Evaluations for expected outcomes
• Mother describes factors that necessitate interruption in breast-feeding.
• Mother expresses comfort with her decision whether or not to resume breast-feeding.
• Mother demonstrates proper milk expression and storage techniques.
• Mother resumes breast-feeding when interrupting factors are eliminated.
• Mother has adequate milk supply when breast-feeding resumes.
• Mother obtains relief from discomfort associated with engorgement.
• Infant's nutritional needs are met, as evidenced by appropriate weight gain (for example, 1 oz per day for first 6 months of life).

Documentation
• Factors that necessitated interruption in breast-feeding (reassessed periodically to determine status)
• Mother's expression of feelings about need to interrupt breast-feeding
• Mother's decision whether to continue breast-feeding when possible
• Mother's efforts to ensure adequate milk supply
• Mother's responses to nursing interventions
• Neonate's growth, weight, and output
• Referrals to support groups
• Evaluations for expected outcomes

■ Breathing pattern, ineffective

related to adjustment to extrauterine existence

Definition
State in which a neonate's breathing pattern doesn't provide adequate pulmonary inflation or deflation to promote successful transition to extrauterine life

Assessment
• Gestational age
• Weight in relation to gestational age
• Maternal sedation before delivery
• Preexisting conditions, including anomalies, adverse intrauterine environment, and prematurity
• Health assessment, including laboratory studies and neurologic, cardiovascular, respiratory, integumentary, GI, and fluid and electrolyte status

Defining characteristics
• Accessory muscle use
• Altered chest excursion

• Altered respiratory rate or depth or both
• Decreased inspiratory/expiratory pressure
• Decreased minute ventilation
• Decreased vital capacity
• Dyspnea
• Nasal flaring
• Retractions
• Shortness of breath

Associated medical diagnoses (selected)
Meconium aspiration, neonatal asphyxia, perinatal asphyxia, prematurity

Expected outcomes
• Neonate will establish normal respiratory rate (40 to 60 breaths/minute) within 1 hour of birth.
• Neonate will have no signs of respiratory distress 1 hour after birth.
• Neonate won't require assisted ventilation or supplemental oxygen.
• Neonate will have Apgar score of 8 to 10 at 5 minutes after birth.
• Neonate will make successful transition to extrauterine life with adequate respiratory function.

Interventions and rationales
• Immediately after delivery:
– Vigorously dry neonate and place under radiant warmer.
– Suction oropharynx and nasopharynx as needed with bulb syringe, DeLee catheter, or suction catheter connected to wall suction.
– Obtain 1-minute and 5-minute Apgar scores.
– Provide whiffs of oxygen, if indicated.
– Remove wet blankets and replace with dry ones.
– Observe for signs of respiratory distress (nasal flaring, tachypnea, retractions, grunting, and use of accessory muscles for breathing).

– Provide or assist with resuscitative measures, as indicated, including bag and mask; naloxone (Narcan) administration, as ordered, if respiratory distress is secondary to maternal sedation; intubation; and suctioning below vocal cords under direct visualization. *Respiratory difficulties are responsible for most morbidity and mortality during neonatal period. Accurate assessment and prompt intervention at delivery are critical to sustaining life.*
• Transfer to nursery when neonate is stable or if neonate needs more extensive resuscitation measures *to help improve transition to extrauterine life.*
• On admission to nursery:
– Obtain neonate's vital signs. Observe central and peripheral color. Note signs of respiratory distress.
– Perform physical assessment, noting anomalies or other abnormal findings.
– Maintain neutral thermal environment.
– Obtain brief obstetric history, including course of labor and delivery and condition of neonate before arrival in nursery. Note presence of risk factors.
– Obtain laboratory studies as ordered.
– Provide resuscitative measures if needed.
– Continue monitoring vital signs until stable, then routinely or as ordered. *Obtaining baseline data and identifying risk factors will help direct interventions.*
• Perform chest physiotherapy as indicated *to clear lungs of fluid.*
• Continually assess need to repeat suctioning to maintain patent airway. *Repeated pharyngeal suctioning can prevent aspiration caused by neonate's immature glottal reflex.*

Evaluations for expected outcomes
• Neonate establishes respiratory rate of 40 to 60 breaths/minute within 1 hour of birth.
• Neonate has no signs of respiratory distress 1 hour after birth.
• Neonate doesn't require assisted ventilation or supplemental oxygen.
• Neonate has Apgar score of 8 to 10 at 5 minutes after birth.
• Neonate makes successful transition to extrauterine life with adequate respiratory function.

Documentation
• Vital signs
• Physical findings
• Interventions performed to enhance neonate's ability to breathe effectively
• Neonate's responses to nursing interventions
• Evaluations for expected outcomes

■ Coping, ineffective family: Compromised

related to neonatal health problems

Definition
Inability of family to use adaptive behaviors in dealing with neonatal health problems

Assessment
• Family process, including normal pattern of interaction among family members; family's understanding and knowledge of neonate's condition; support systems available (financial, social, and spiritual); family's response to past crises, including coping behaviors and problem-solving techniques; recreational activities; and communication patterns used to express anger, affection, and confrontation

• Neonate's health status
• Family's perception of present situation
• Degree of difficulty imposed by care of neonate
• Possible impact of neonate on family's future structure and lifestyle

Defining characteristics
• Attempts to care for neonate that meet with unsatisfactory results
• Display of excessive or inadequate protective behavior
• Inadequate understanding or knowledge base that interferes with ability to care for neonate
• Preoccupation with personal reaction to neonate's health problem
• Withdrawal from neonate at time of need

Associated medical diagnoses (selected)
This nursing diagnosis may be associated with any disorder that severely compromises a neonate, including cleft lip or palate, fetal alcohol syndrome, neonatal asphyxia, neonatal neurologic impairment, perinatal asphyxia, and prematurity.

Expected outcomes
• Family members will communicate feelings about neonate's condition.
• Family members will engage in healthy coping behaviors.
• Family members will become involved in planning for and providing neonate's care.
• Family members will identify and use available support systems.
• Family members will set realistic goals for neonate.
• Family members will express feeling of having greater control over their situation.

Interventions and rationales

• Encourage family members to voice feelings about neonate's condition *to decrease tension by clearing up misunderstandings and misconceptions.*

• Identify and reduce unnecessary environmental stimuli *to enhance family members' ability to focus on caring for neonate.*

• Assess family members' understanding of neonate's condition. Help them view situation realistically and understand its future implications. *Setting realistic goals helps family plan for future and avoid unnecessary disappointment.*

• Actively involve family members in learning to care for neonate *to decrease feelings of helplessness and isolation from neonate.*

• Explain rationale for all treatments and procedures to family members *to help reduce anxiety and enhance cooperation.*

• Involve family members in decision-making when possible *to increase their feelings of involvement and control.*

• Provide positive feedback when family members care for neonate *to increase self-esteem and reinforce ability to care for neonate successfully.*

• Encourage family members to identify and contact support systems and resources, such as extended family, friends, clergy, and community groups, *to decrease sense of being overwhelmed.*

• Help family members identify and use appropriate coping behaviors *to reduce anxiety and tension.*

• Coordinate referrals to other health care professionals, such as social worker or physical therapist, *to ensure clear communication among health care providers, which enables neonate to receive appropriate comprehensive care.*

• Provide family members with up-to-date reports on neonate's condition *to ease anxiety and help family plan for future needs.*

Evaluations for expected outcomes

• Family members voice their feelings about neonate's condition.

• Family members identify and use at least two healthy coping behaviors.

• Family members demonstrate ability to plan for and provide neonate's care.

• Family members identify and use available support systems.

• Family members set realistic goals for neonate.

• Family members express feeling of increased control over their situation.

Documentation

• Family members' perceptions of neonate's health and long-term implications

• Observations of family members' behaviors, including interactions with neonate

• Family members' statements indicating their feelings toward neonate

• Teaching and referrals given to family members

• Family members' abilities to meet neonate's physical and emotional needs

• Consultations with other health team members

• Interventions to help family members cope

• Family members' responses to nursing interventions

• Evaluations for expected outcomes

■ Coping, ineffective individual

related to labor and delivery

Definition

Inability to use adaptive behaviors in response to labor and delivery

Assessment

• Psychosocial status, including age, developmental stage, health beliefs and attitudes, feelings about pregnancy, decision-making ability, usual coping patterns, support systems, income, ability to learn (cognitive, affective, and psychomotor domains), motivation to learn, and obstacles to learning
• Neurologic status, including level of consciousness, orientation, memory, and mental status
• Pain threshold, perception of pain, and response to analgesia or anesthesia
• Labor, including stage and length of labor, complications, patient's ability to concentrate, patient's ability to use breathing techniques, and presence and effectiveness of support person
• Circumstances surrounding delivery, including method of delivery (vaginal [complicated or uncomplicated], cesarean section [elective or nonelective], or vaginal birth after previous cesarean section), analgesia or anesthesia, presence and effectiveness of support person, and outcome (actual and perceived)
• Previous experience with pregnancy, labor, and delivery and knowledge of birth process
• Medical history, including preexisting and pregnancy-induced conditions

Defining characteristics

• Change in communication pattern
• Decreased use of social support
• Destructive behavior toward self or others
• Expressed inability to cope
• Fatigue
• Inability to meet basic needs and role expectations
• Lack of goal-directed behavior, such as inability to attend, difficulty organizing information, poor concentration, and poor problem-solving abilities

Associated medical diagnoses (selected)

This diagnosis can occur in any condition associated with labor and delivery. Examples include complicated or uncomplicated vaginal delivery, elective or nonelective cesarean section delivery, and multiple births.

Expected outcomes

• Patient will express need to develop better coping behaviors.
• Patient will set realistic learning goals.
• Patient will demonstrate ability to use newly learned coping skills.
• Patient will communicate feelings about pregnancy, labor, and delivery.
• Patient will maintain appropriate sense of control throughout course of labor and delivery.
• Patient will enlist help from support person and nurses to obtain physical and psychological comfort.
• Patient will demonstrate ability to cope with unexpected change.

Interventions and rationales

• Establish environment of mutual trust and respect *to enhance patient's learning.*
• Negotiate with patient to develop learning goals *to promote cooperation and foster sense of control.*
• Select teaching strategies (discussion, demonstration, role-playing, and

visual materials) appropriate for patient's learning style *to encourage compliance.*

• Teach skills that patient can use during labor and delivery. Have her give return demonstration of each new skill. *Patient must thoroughly understand skills before labor begins because painful contractions will reduce her attention span.*

• During first (latent) phase of labor (dilation 1 to 4 cm), take these steps:

– Encourage patient to ventilate her feelings and to participate in her own care. Offer diversions such as reading materials. Review breathing techniques she can use during labor. *These measures help allay patient's fears and help her achieve sense of control.*

– Involve support person in care and comfort measures *to allay patient's fears.*

– Provide continuous monitoring *to identify deviations from normal.*

• During active phase of labor (dilation 4 to 8 cm), take these steps:

– Encourage patient to assume comfortable position *to promote relaxation between contractions.*

– Assist patient with breathing techniques *to reduce anxiety and prevent hyperventilation.*

– Encourage support person to participate in patient care — for example, by changing soiled linen, offering ice chips to suck on, and providing sacral pressure, back support, or back rub — *to provide continuity of care and encourage therapeutic relationship.*

– Provide encouragement and instruction between contractions *to foster sense of control.*

– Administer analgesia as ordered *to reduce pain.*

– Provide opportunities for rest between contractions when appropriate.

Reassure patient about fetal status. *These measures reinforce patient's ability to cope.*

• During transitional phase of labor (dilation 8 to 10 cm), take these steps:

– Assist patient with breathing during contractions. Advise her not to push until complete dilation occurs.

– Encourage rest between contractions.

– Identify and reduce unnecessary stimuli in environment.

– Explain all treatments and procedures and answer patient's questions. *These measures help allay fear and reduce sensory overload.*

• During delivery, provide these measures:

– Instruct patient in effective pushing techniques *to promote effectiveness of her bearing-down efforts.*

– Continue to reassure patient and provide encouragement. Explain physiologic changes and procedures being performed *to prepare patient psychologically for delivery.*

– Escort support person to delivery room. Explain each step of process. Instruct support person in how to effectively coach patient *to provide further support for patient and strengthen her ability to cope.*

• During delivery of placenta, take these steps:

– Enlist patient's cooperation in maintaining position *to facilitate delivery of placenta.*

– Show neonate to patient and explain care being provided. Reassure patient about neonate's condition *to provide emotional support.*

– If permitted, allow patient and support person to hold neonate. If patient desires, allow her to breast-feed neonate *to promote bonding.*

• In cesarean delivery, allow patient to express feelings. Explain procedure and care being provided. Allow support person to be present before and during delivery, if permitted. *Failure to provide patient with source of support and opportunity to express negative feelings may interfere with her ability to cope with impending tasks of motherhood.*

Evaluations for expected outcomes
• Patient states need for better coping behaviors.
• Patient participates in establishing learning goals.
• Patient successfully uses breathing and relaxation techniques during labor and delivery.
• Patient becomes more comfortable with expressing feelings about pregnancy, labor, and delivery.
• Patient maintains appropriate sense of control during labor and delivery.
• Support person and nurses provide effective comfort to patient during labor and delivery.
• Patient demonstrates ability to cope with unexpected change.

Documentation
• Patient's previous knowledge of labor and delivery
• Patient's expressions indicating her motivation to learn
• Patient's learning objectives
• Methods used to teach patient
• Information taught and skills demonstrated to patient
• Patient's responses to nursing interventions
• Patient's and support person's level of satisfaction with delivery
• Patient's expressions of comfort, discomfort, or both
• Evaluations for expected outcomes

■ Family process alteration
related to impending birth

Definition
Altered role functions within the family resulting from pregnancy and pending change in family structure

Assessment
• Age of pregnant woman and partner
• Availability of family members or friends to help
• Planned or unplanned pregnancy
• Family status, including number and ages of other children, usual patterns of interaction among family members, family members' assumed or expected roles, communication patterns, support systems, financial resources, past responses to change, spiritual resources, and living conditions
• Perceived impact of pregnancy on family unit
• Presence of obstetric or fetal complications or other medical conditions

Defining characteristics
Changes in:
• assigned tasks and effectiveness in completing those tasks
• availability for affective responsiveness and intimacy
• availability for emotional support
• communication patterns
• expressions of conflict with or isolation from community resources
• expressions of conflict within family
• mutual support
• participation in problem solving and decision making
• patterns and rituals
• power alliances
• satisfaction with family
• somatic complaints

• stress-reduction behaviors

Associated medical diagnoses (selected)
This diagnosis can occur in any pregnancy, whether complicated or uncomplicated, planned or unplanned.

Expected outcomes
• Family members will take on portion of duties carried out by pregnant woman, such as housecleaning, heavy lifting, and meal preparation.
• Patient and family members will voice realistic expectations about pregnancy's impact on their future.
• Patient and family members will share their feelings about pregnancy with each other.
• Family members will identify and contact appropriate support systems.
• Family will welcome new member.

Interventions and rationales
• Encourage family members to express their feelings about pregnancy. Tell them that wide range of emotions, ranging from fear to excitement, may accompany diagnosis of pregnancy. *Pent-up feelings can lead to misunderstanding and resentment.*
• Provide emotional support to patient and family members *to help them come to terms with altered roles and responsibilities.*
• Encourage pregnant woman to voice her concerns about pregnancy's potential impact on family structure and finances *to identify unrealistic fears and decrease anxiety.*
• Arrange and participate in family conferences as needed. *Some families may require help to improve interpersonal communication.*
• Refer family members to classes in prepared childbirth or parenting, psychological counseling, or social service and health care agencies, as ap-

propriate, *to provide additional information and support.*
• Periodically assess woman's acceptance of pregnancy *to determine need for further interventions. Mother normally grows to accept the pregnancy as uterus develops and she feels fetus kick. She may also fantasize about what neonate will look like and begin preparing for birth.*

Evaluations for expected outcomes
• Family members take on portion of patient's duties.
• Patient and family members voice realistic expectations about emotional and financial impact of pregnancy on family structure.
• Patient and family members honestly communicate feelings about pregnancy.
• Patient and family members identify and contact potential support groups or organizations.
• Neonate is successfully integrated into family.

Documentation
• Reactions of pregnant woman and partner to diagnosis of pregnancy
• Referrals to outside agencies
• Pregnant woman's adherence to prescribed medical practices
• Observations of pregnant woman's acceptance of and interest in pregnancy as it progresses
• Interventions to assist pregnant woman and family
• Woman's and family's responses to nursing interventions
• Evaluations for expected outcomes

■ Family process alteration

related to inclusion of new member

Definition
Disruption in expected role functions within the family after the birth of a child

Assessment
• Family status, including assumed or expected roles, communication patterns, developmental stage of family members, number and ages of children, financial resources, past responses to change, available support systems, significant others, and spiritual practices
• Family members' perceptions of impact of birth on their assumed roles

Defining characteristics
Changes in:
• assigned tasks and effectiveness in completing those tasks
• availability for affective responsiveness and intimacy
• availability for emotional support
• communication patterns
• expressions of conflict with or isolation from community resources
• expressions of conflict within family
• mutual support
• participation in problem solving and decision making
• patterns and rituals
• power alliances
• satisfaction with family
• somatic complaints
• stress-reduction behaviors

Associated medical diagnoses (selected)
Childbirth

Expected outcomes
• Family members will voice feelings about neonate.
• Family members will express need to assume new or altered roles and adapt to changes within family structure.
• Family members will contact support groups for help if needed.
• Neonate will be successfully assimilated into family structure.

Interventions and rationales
• Encourage family members to express feelings about arrival of neonate and altered roles and responsibilities *to help clear up misunderstandings and misconceptions.*
• Explore with family members ways neonate will affect family structure and functioning. Topics may include changes in finances and living space, caretaking arrangements, and new roles or responsibilities for parents and siblings. *Discussing legitimate concerns may improve family members' attitudes toward neonate.*
• Discuss with family members degree of sibling preparation and possibility of sibling rivalry. *Siblings must be reassured that they're still vital members of family.* Encourage siblings to visit neonate at hospital *to decrease separation anxiety, foster sense of family, and facilitate bonding.*
• Assess measures taken to prepare home for arrival of neonate. *Lack of preparation may indicate limited financial resources or difficulty accepting neonate.*
• Assess need for help from social services or community agencies and coordinate referrals *to ensure ongoing comprehensive care.*

Evaluations for expected outcomes
• Family members share feelings about neonate with each other.
• Family members assume new or additional responsibilities as needed, such as preparing meals, assisting with transportation, shopping, cleaning, and providing child care.
• Family members contact community agencies or support group for assistance if needed.
• Family members come to terms with arrival of neonate.

Documentation
• Observations of family members' reactions to neonate
• Family members' statements indicating attitude toward neonate
• Interventions performed to help family cope with new arrival
• Family members' responses to nursing interventions
• Referrals to outside agencies
• Evaluations for expected outcomes

■ Fluid volume deficit

related to altered intake during labor

Definition
Excessive loss of body fluids and electrolytes during labor

Assessment
• Vital signs, including temperature, pulse rate, blood pressure, and respirations
• Fluid and electrolyte status, including weight, intake and output, urine specific gravity, skin turgor, mucous membranes, and electrolyte and blood urea nitrogen levels

Defining characteristics
• Changes in mental status
• Decreased pulse volume and pressure
• Decreased urine output
• Decreased venous filling
• Dry skin and mucous membranes
• Increased body temperature
• Increased hematocrit
• Increased pulse rate
• Increased urine concentration
• Low blood pressure
• Poor turgor of skin or tongue
• Sudden weight loss (except in third-space fluid shifting)
• Thirst
• Weakness

Associated medical diagnoses (selected)
Diabetes mellitus, hemorrhage, pregnancy-induced hypertension (PIH), premature rupture of membranes, shock

Expected outcomes
• Patient will maintain fluid balance.
• Patient will demonstrate optimal hydration.
• Patient will show no signs of dehydration.

Interventions and rationales
• Monitor vital signs as often as policy dictates. *Decreased blood pressure and increased pulse rate may be late signs of fluid volume loss. With PIH, increased blood pressure may occur.*
• Assess skin turgor and examine oral mucous membranes for dryness. *Dehydration can cause dry mucous membranes, skin tenting, and dry, cracked lips.*
• Continuously monitor intake and output. Administer and monitor parenteral fluids. Maintain intake according to order or protocol (usually 125 to 175 ml/hour). Output should approximate intake. *These measures help ensure adequate hydration.*

• Monitor electrolyte values and report abnormalities. *Hypernatremia may indicate dehydration, requiring I.V. volume replacement. Hypernatremia may be related to excessive insensible water loss.*

• Provide patient with ice chips or cool, damp, 4" × 4" gauze compress *to increase patient comfort and decrease mouth dryness, especially if patient breathes through mouth.*

• Measure amount and character of vomitus to assess need for antiemetic. *When labor begins, blood is rerouted to serve energy needs of contracting uterus and blood flow to GI tract decreases. GI motility and absorption also decrease so that food may remain in stomach for up to 12 hours. These factors predispose patient to nausea and vomiting, especially during transition phase of labor.*

• As ordered, administer antiemetic if needed and evaluate its effectiveness *to help control emesis and prevent excessive fluid loss.*

• Keep patient cool and comfortable. Change gown as indicated and apply cool compresses to face and body *to reduce discomfort caused by diaphoresis.*

• Position patient on her left side *to aid kidney perfusion and increase cardiac and urine output.*

• If urine output is reduced, carefully assess patient for peripheral edema, hyperreflexia, increased blood pressure, and presence of urine protein. *Decreased urine output, increased blood pressure, hyperreflexia, and peripheral edema may indicate intrapartal PIH. Proteinuria may result from dehydration, exhaustion, or preeclampsia.*

Evaluations for expected outcomes
• Patient maintains fluid balance, with intake approximately equaling output.
• Patient maintains optimal hydration.
• Patient has no signs of dehydration; her mucous membranes remain pink and moist, skin turgor remains optimal, vital signs stay within normal limits, and urine output is at least 30 ml/hour or 100 ml in 4 hours.

Documentation
• Patient's vital signs
• Observation of patient's fluid volume status
• Intake and output
• Nursing interventions performed to maintain adequate fluid intake
• Patient's response to nursing interventions
• Evaluations for expected outcomes

■ Fluid volume deficit
related to postpartum hemorrhage

Definition
Excessive fluid and electrolyte loss resulting from excessive postpartum bleeding

Assessment
• History of problems that can cause fluid loss, such as hemorrhage, vomiting, diarrhea, and indwelling catheters
• Vital signs
• Fluid and electrolyte status, including weight, intake and output, urine specific gravity, skin turgor, mucous membranes, and serum electrolyte and blood urea nitrogen levels
• Laboratory studies, including hemoglobin (Hb) and hematocrit (HCT)

• Factors that place patient at high risk for postpartum hemorrhage, including grand multipara, overdistended uterus, prolonged labor, previous history of postpartum hemorrhage, traumatic delivery, uterine fibroids, overstimulation with oxytocin, and bleeding disorders

Defining characteristics
• Changes in mental status
• Decreased pulse volume and pressure
• Decreased urine output
• Decreased venous filling
• Dry skin and mucous membranes
• Increased body temperature
• Increased HCT
• Increased pulse rate
• Increased urine concentration
• Low blood pressure
• Poor turgor of skin or tongue
• Sudden weight loss (except in third-space fluid shifting)
• Thirst
• Weakness

Associated medical diagnoses (selected)
Abnormal rupture of membranes, hemorrhage, postpartum hemorrhage, retained placental fragments

Expected outcomes
• Patient's vital signs will remain stable.
• Patient's hematology studies will be within normal range.
• Patient's uterus will remain firm.
• Medical personnel will quickly identify signs of possible shock and initiate treatment.
• Patient's bladder won't become distended.
• Patient's blood volume will return to normal.

Interventions and rationales
• Immediately after delivery, monitor color, amount, and consistency of lochia every 15 minutes for 1 hour, then every 4 hours for 24 hours, then every shift until discharge. Weigh or count sanitary pads if lochia is excessive. *Hemorrhage is the most common cause of mortality during childbirth.*
• Monitor and record vital signs every 15 minutes for 1 hour, then every 4 hours for 24 hours, then every shift until discharge *to detect signs of hemorrhage and shock, such as increased pulse and respiratory rates and decreased blood pressure.*
• Immediately after delivery, palpate fundus every 15 minutes for 1 hour, then every 4 hours for 24 hours, then every shift until discharge. Note location and tone. *Palpation of fundus will enable you to detect uterine atony (lack of normal uterine muscle tone or strength), the most common cause of postpartum hemorrhage.*
• Gently massage boggy fundus; avoid overstimulation. *Gentle stimulation can help fundus to become firm; overstimulation can cause relaxation.*
• Explain to patient process of involution and need to palpate fundus. Teach patient to assess and gently massage fundus and to notify you if bogginess persists. *Explaining normal postpartum physiologic adjustments can decrease patient's anxiety and increase cooperation.*
• Evaluate postpartum hematology studies and report abnormal results. Consider whether patient needs typing and crossmatching for transfusion. *Comparison of postdelivery Hb and HCT with previous results provides information about amount of blood loss and allows time to plan interventions, such as requesting blood from blood bank.*

• Administer fluids, blood or blood products, or plasma expanders, as ordered, *to replace lost blood volume.* Monitor for adverse reactions.

• Monitor patient's intake and output every shift. Note bladder distention and catheterize as ordered. *Distended bladder interferes with involution of uterus.*

• Administer oxytocic agents, such as oxytocin (Pitocin), methylergonovine (Methergine), and ergonovine (Ergotrate), as ordered, and evaluate effectiveness. *Oxytocic agents stimulate uterine musculature, controlling postpartum hemorrhage and atony.*

• Regularly assess patient for signs and symptoms of shock, including rapid, thready pulse; increased respiratory rate; decreased blood pressure and urine output; and cold, clammy, pale skin. *Prompt recognition and treatment of shock limits amount of fluid lost and impact on other body systems.*

Evaluations for expected outcomes

• Patient's vital signs remain stable.

• Results of patient's hematology studies are within normal range.

• Patient's uterus remains firm.

• If patient develops shock, medical personnel identify it quickly and promptly start treatment.

• Patient doesn't develop distended bladder.

• Patient's blood loss after delivery is less than 500 ml and fluid volume is replenished.

Documentation

• Estimation of blood loss

• Signs of possible shock

• Location and tone of fundus

• Laboratory results

• Replacement of lost fluid

• Nursing interventions to control active blood loss

• Patient's response to nursing interventions

• Evaluations for expected outcomes

■ Growth and development alteration

related to perinatal insult or injury

Definition

State in which neonate deviates from growth and development norms for age

Assessment

• Maternal history, including age, use of controlled substances, trauma, and anesthesia or analgesia during labor

• Labor and delivery record

• Neonate status, including gestational age, Apgar scores, vital signs, feeding patterns, muscle tone, condition of fontanels, and characteristics of cry

• Neonate's neurologic status, including reflexes, responsiveness, activity level, and presence of seizures

• Diagnostic tests, including laboratory studies and ultrasound examinations

Defining characteristics

• Altered physical growth

• Diminished or absent reflexes

• Flat affect

• Listlessness and decreased responses

Associated medical diagnoses (selected)

Cerebral palsy, neonatal asphyxia, perinatal asphyxia, perinatal trauma, prematurity, sepsis

Expected outcomes

• Neonate's alteration in growth and development will be evaluated, and supportive measures will be initiated.

• Family members will express realistic expectations for neonate's growth.

• Neonate will receive appropriate physical therapy on regular basis.
• Family members will demonstrate understanding of neonate's special needs.
• Family members will accept referrals to available community resources.

Interventions and rationales
• Reposition hypotonic neonate every 2 hours *to prevent skin breakdown and pulmonary complications of immobility.*
• Measure neonate's head circumference every shift. *Increasing head circumference indicates increased intracranial pressure (ICP).*
• Evaluate and record activity level every shift. *Altered activity level may indicate such conditions as sepsis, hyperbilirubinemia, increased ICP, or intraventricular hemorrhage.*
• Monitor and report changes in neonate's neurologic status *to detect exacerbation or lessening of danger signs.*
• Refer neonate to appropriate health care specialist, such as physical therapist, social worker, developmental specialist, or neurologist. Provide parents or other family members with information on community resources *to ensure comprehensive care for neonate.*
• Provide emotional support to family members who have difficulty accepting neonate's condition. Assess their goals for neonate's development. *By offering support and identifying unrealistic goals, you can help family members come to terms with neonate's condition.*
• Involve family members in neonate's daily care and keep them abreast of neonate's condition. *Personal involvement promotes bonding, decreases anxiety, and helps prepare for discharge.*

• Assess neonate's ability to suck on an ongoing basis. *A weak suck reflex may indicate neurologic defect or need for nutritional supplementation.*
• Monitor neonate's temperature every 4 hours or as ordered. Maintain neutral thermal environment *to minimize oxygen consumption, prevent cold stress, and promote growth by decreasing unnecessary caloric use.*

Evaluations for expected outcomes
• Neonate's alteration in growth and development is evaluated and his nutritional, physical, and safety needs are met.
• Family members express realistic understanding of neonate's present condition and potential for improvement.
• Neonate receives appropriate physical therapy on regular basis.
• Family members demonstrate ability to meet neonate's physical and emotional needs.
• Family members agree to seek help and support from appropriate community resources.

Documentation
• Observed characteristics of neonate, including seizure activity, characteristics of cry, hypoactive or hyperactive muscle activity, condition of fontanels, presence or absence of reflexes, feeding ability, and vital signs
• Use of respiratory support
• Family members' responses to neonate's condition
• Consultations with other health team members
• Referrals to outside agencies
• Nursing interventions and neonate's response
• Evaluations for expected outcomes

■ Hypothermia

related to cold, stress, or sepsis

Definition
State in which neonate's body temperature is below normal range

Assessment
• History of present illness
• Gestational age
• Prenatal and intrapartal history
• Presence of maternal risk factors, such as fever, diabetes mellitus, drug use, dystocia, and history of perinatal asphyxia
• Neurologic status, including level of consciousness and sensory status
• Cardiovascular status, including core temperature, heart rate and rhythm, blood pressure, and capillary refill time
• Respiratory status, including rate, rhythm, and depth; breath sounds; and arterial blood gas values
• Integumentary status, including temperature, color (central versus peripheral), and turgor
• Nutritional status, including dietary pattern, birth weight, current weight, and recent weight changes
• Fluid and electrolyte status, including intake and output, serum glucose and electrolyte levels, and urine specific gravity
• Psychosocial status, including behavior, parental stressors, parental coping skills, and financial resources

Defining characteristics
• Body temperature below normal range
• Cool, pale skin
• Cyanotic nail beds
• Increased blood pressure and heart rate
• Piloerection
• Shivering
• Slow capillary refill

Associated medical diagnoses (selected)
Neonatal asphyxia, perinatal asphyxia, perinatal trauma, prematurity, sepsis

Expected outcomes
• Neonate will exhibit normal body temperature.
• Neonate will have warm, dry skin and normal capillary refill time.
• Neonate's cardiovascular status will be normal.
• Neonate won't develop complications of hypothermia.
• Neonate won't shiver.
• Neonate won't develop signs of hyperthermia related to radiant heat source.
• Neonate will be weaned from Isolette or radiant warmer bed as tolerated.
• Family members will verbalize knowledge of how hypothermia develops and will state measures to prevent recurrent hypothermia.
• Family members will demonstrate ability to measure neonate's temperature accurately.
• Family members will demonstrate willingness to provide adequate home care for neonate.

Interventions and rationales
• Monitor body temperature every 1 to 3 hours by axillary or inguinal route (avoid rectal measurement). Record temperature and route. *Monitoring body temperature helps to detect developing complications.* If using electronic heat source such as radiant warmer, monitor device's temperature reading hourly and compare it with neonate's body temperature *to evaluate effectiveness of interventions.*

• Monitor and record neurologic status every 1 to 4 hours. *Falling body temperature and slowed metabolic rate may cause decreased level of consciousness.*

• Monitor and record vital signs every 1 to 4 hours. As ordered, initiate and maintain continuous electronic cardiorespiratory monitoring. *These measures help avert metabolic acidosis and respiratory arrest.*

• Provide supportive measures:

– Maintain neutral thermal environment, a narrow range of environmental temperature that maintains stable core temperature with minimal caloric and oxygen expenditure. Determination of neutral thermal environment depends on neonate's age and weight.

– If indicated, place neonate in open crib. For mild hypothermia, dress with undershirt, diaper, and knitted or stockinette cap and cover with double blankets.

– Avoid overheating neonate.

– Keep diaper area dry.

– Cover all metal or plastic surfaces that could come in contact with neonate.

– Maintain room temperature between 75° and 78° F (23.9° and 25.6° C).

– Perform all procedures under radiant warmer, if possible. Postpone bath.

These measures protect neonate from heat loss.

• For severe hypothermia, place neonate in Isolette or overhead radiant warmer bed. Provide these supportive measures:

– Keep neonate undressed.

– Set mechanism to desired skin temperature (96.8° to 97.8° F [36° to 36.6° C]).

– If neonate is under radiant warmer, use plastic wrap placed like blanket to prevent heat and fluid loss. Use sheet large enough to cover only neonate. Border with tape.

– Attach skin probe to right upper quadrant of abdomen. Don't place over bone or rib cage.

– Use heat shield for very unstable neonate inside Isolette.

– Monitor carefully for evaporative loss and insensible fluid loss. Keep in mind that radiant warmer and Isolette therapy increase fluid maintenance needs.

These measures help ensure safe use of radiant warmer or Isolette.

• Follow prescribed treatment regimen for hypothermia, which may include administering antibiotic in cases of sepsis, administering I.V. fluids, and feeding neonate (small, frequent portions, if appropriate). *Prescribed treatment helps eliminate infection and meet neonate's fluid and nutrient needs.*

• Discuss precipitating factors with family members *to help prevent recurrence.*

• Instruct family members in preventive measures, such as dressing neonate appropriately and providing adequate nutrition for neonate's growth needs. If family requires financial help, refer them to appropriate social service agency. *These precautions may help protect neonate from future cold stress episodes.*

Evaluations for expected outcomes

• Neonate's temperature returns to normal range.

• Neonate exhibits warm, dry skin and normal capillary refill time.

• Neonate has normal cardiovascular assessment findings.

• Neonate doesn't develop complications of hypothermia.

• Neonate doesn't begin shivering.

• Neonate doesn't demonstrate signs of hyperthermia related to radiant heat source.
• Neonate is successfully weaned from Isolette or radiant warmer bed.
• Family members verbalize understanding of causes of hypothermia and preventive measures.
• Family members demonstrate proper axillary or inguinal temperature measurement technique.
• Family members demonstrate willingness to provide adequate home care for neonate.

Documentation
• Neonate's physical findings, including cardiovascular status, temperature, and shivering
• Nursing interventions and neonate's response to them
• Family members' willingness and abilities to provide adequate home care
• Evaluations for expected outcomes

■ Infant behavior, disorganized

related to pain, prematurity, oral problems, motor problems, feeding intolerance, environmental overstimulation, or lack of stimulation

Definition
A disturbance in infant behavior, such as inappropriate responses to stimuli, problems regulating physiologic function, or apparent inability to interact with the environment.

Assessment
• Cardiovascular status, including pulse and respirations

• GI status, including feeding pattern, food tolerance, defecation pattern, ability to maintain adequate weight, and abdominal bloating and distention
• Neurologic status, including muscle tone, newborn reflexes, excessive crying, lethargy, irritability, seizures, tremors, and assessments such as Brazelton Neonatal Behavioral Assessment and Dubowitz Gestational Age Assessment
• Sensory status, including responsiveness to visual, tactile, and auditory stimuli and experience with pain
• Parental status, including knowledge of normal growth and development
• Sleep status, including sleep patterns and usual hours of sleep
• Parents' psychological status, including energy level, motivation, self-image, competence, recent life changes, experience with children, and eye contact and interaction with infant

Defining characteristics
• Evidence of problems in behavioral and neurologic development, such as deficient response to visual and auditory stimuli; excessive crying; hyperextension of arms and legs; irregular sleep pattern or difficulty obtaining adequate sleep; tremors, startles, and twitches; excessive yawning; and apnea

Associated medical diagnoses (selected)
Colic, failure to thrive, prematurity

Expected outcomes
• Parents will learn to identify and understand infant's behavioral cues.
• Parents will identify their own emotional responses to infant's behavior.
• Parents will identify means to help infant overcome his behavioral disturbance.

• Parents will identify ways to improve their ability to cope with infant's responses.
• Infant will begin to show appropriate signs of maturation.
• Parents will express positive feelings about their ability to care for infant.
• Parents will identify resources for help with infant.

Interventions and rationales

• Explain to parents that infant maturation is developmental process and that their participation is crucial *to help them understand importance of nurturing infant.*
• Explain to parents that their actions can help modify some of their infant's behavior. However, make it clear that infant maturation isn't completely within their control. *This explanation may help decrease parents' feelings of incompetence.*
• Explain to parents that infants give behavioral cues that indicate their needs. Discuss appropriate ways to respond to these behavioral cues — for example, providing stimulation that doesn't overwhelm infant, stopping stimulation when infant gives behavioral cues (such as yawning, looking away, or becoming agitated), and finding methods to calm infant if he becomes agitated (such as swaddling, gentle rocking, and quiet vocalizations). Help parents to identify and cope with their responses to infant's behavioral disturbance *to help them recognize and adjust their response patterns. When infant doesn't respond positively to them, parents may feel inadequate or become frustrated. They need to understand that these reactions are normal.*
• Demonstrate appropriate ways of interacting with infant *to show parents how to identify and interpret infant's behavioral cues and how to respond appropriately. For example, if infant becomes agitated, it may be because of overstimulation. At this point, parents should stop stimulating infant and allow him to rest.*
• Explore with parents ways to cope with stress imposed by infant's behavior *to help them develop better coping skills.*
• Praise parents when they demonstrate appropriate methods of interacting with infant *to provide positive reinforcement.*
• Provide parents with information on sources of support and special infant services *to help them cope with infant's long-term needs.*

Evaluations for expected outcomes

• Parents state their understanding of infant's behavioral cues.
• Parents discuss appropriate ways of responding to infant's behavior.
• Parents exhibit decreased frustration with infant's behavior.
• Parents identify ways to help infant overcome his behavioral disturbance by recognizing infant's needs and responding appropriately.
• Parents report improved ability to cope with stress of caring for infant.
• Infant begins to show appropriate signs of maturation, such as longer periods of sleep, shorter periods of crying, longer periods of being awake and alert, smoother transitions between behavioral states, and positive responses to parents' interventions.
• Parents express positive feelings about their ability to care for infant.
• Parents identify resources for help with infant.

Documentation
• Assessment of factors that may enhance or retard infant behavioral development
• Parents' expressed feelings about caring for infant
• Nursing interventions and infant's response to them
• Evaluations for expected outcomes

■ Infant behavior, potential for enhanced organization

Definition
State in which an infant's behavioral development is satisfactory but can be improved

Assessment
• Cardiovascular status, including pulse and respirations
• GI status, including feeding and defecation patterns, food tolerance, ability to maintain adequate weight, and abdominal distention and bloating
• Neurologic status, including excessive crying, poor sleep patterns, lethargy, irritability, seizures, tremors, muscle tone, newborn reflexes, and such assessments as Brazelton Neonatal Behavioral Assessment and Dubowitz Gestational Age Assessment
• Sensory status, including responsiveness to visual, tactile, and auditory stimuli and experience with pain
• Sleep status, including usual hours of sleep
• Parental status, including knowledge of normal growth and development
• Parents' psychological status, including energy level, motivation, experience with children, eye contact and interaction with infant, and Home Observation Measurement of the Environment results

Defining characteristics
• Ability to use some self-regulatory behaviors
• Definite sleep-wake states
• Responsiveness to visual and auditory stimuli
• Stable physiologic measures

Associated medical diagnoses (selected)
This nursing diagnosis may apply to any infant.

Expected outcomes
• Parents will express understanding of their role in infant's behavioral development.
• Parents will express confidence in their ability to interpret infant's behavioral cues.
• Parents will identify means to promote infant's behavioral development.
• Parents will express positive feelings about their ability to care for infant.
• Parents will identify resources for help with infant.

Interventions and rationales
• Explain to parents that infant maturation is developmental process. Further explain that infants exhibit three behavioral states: sleeping, crying, and being awake and alert. Also explain that infants provide behavioral cues that indicate their needs. *Education will help parents understand importance of nurturing infant and prepare them to respond to infant's behavioral cues.*
• Explain to parents that their actions can help promote infant development. Make it clear, however, that infant maturation isn't completely within their control. *This explanation may decrease feelings of anxiety and incompetence and help to prevent unrealistic expectations.*

• Demonstrate appropriate ways of interacting with infant, such as moderate stimulation, gentle rocking, and quiet vocalizations, *to help parents identify most effective methods of interacting with their child.*

• Help parents interpret behavioral cues from their infant *to foster healthy parent-child interaction.* For example, help them recognize when infant is awake and alert, and point out to them that this is a good time to provide stimulation.

• Help parents to identify ways they can promote infant's development, such as providing stimulation by shaking rattle in front of infant, talking to infant in gentle voice, and looking at infant when feeding him, *to encourage practices that promote infant's development. Sensory experiences promote cognitive development.*

• Explore with parents ways to cope with stress caused by infant's behavior *to increase their coping skills.*

• Praise parents for their attempts to enhance their interaction with infant *to provide positive reinforcement.*

• Provide parents with information on sources of support and special infant services *to encourage them to continue to foster their infant's development.*

Evaluations for expected outcomes

• Parents express understanding of their role in infant's behavioral development.

• Parents express confidence in their ability to recognize infant's behavioral cues.

• Parents identify activities that foster positive responses from infant and provide appropriate sensory and tactile stimulation.

• Parents express positive feelings about their ability to care for infant.

• Parents identify resources for help with infant.

Documentation

• Assessment of factors that may enhance infant's behavioral development

• Parents' expressed feelings about caring for their infant

• Nursing interventions and infant's response to them

• Evaluations for expected outcomes

■ Infant behavior, disorganized, risk for

related to pain, prematurity, oral problems, motor problems, feeding intolerance, environmental overstimulation, or lack of stimulation

Definition

Risk for behavioral disturbance in an infant

Assessment

• Cardiovascular status, including pulse and respirations

• GI status, including feeding and defecation patterns, food tolerance, ability to maintain adequate weight, and abdominal bloating and distention

• Neurologic status, including muscle tone, newborn reflexes, excessive crying, lethargy, irritability, seizures, tremors, and such assessments as Brazelton Neonatal Behavioral Assessment and Dubowitz Gestational Age Assessment

• Sensory status, including infant's responsiveness to visual, tactile, and auditory stimuli and experience with pain

• Sleep status, including sleep pattern and usual hours of sleep

• Parental status, including knowledge of normal growth and development
• Parents' psychological status, including energy level, motivation, experience with children, and eye contact and interaction with infant

Risk factors
• Environmental overstimulation
• Invasive or painful procedures
• Lack of containment or boundaries
• Oral or motor problems
• Pain
• Prematurity

Associated medical diagnoses (selected)
Colic, failure to thrive, prematurity

Expected outcomes
• Parents will identify factors that place infant at risk for behavioral disturbance.
• Parents will identify potential signs of behavioral disturbance in infant.
• Parents will identify appropriate ways to interact with infant.
• Parents will identify their reactions to infant (including ways of coping with occasional frustration and anger).
• Parents will express positive feelings about their ability to care for infant.
• Parents will identify resources for help with infant.

Interventions and rationales
• Explain to parents that infant maturation is developmental process and that their participation is crucial *to help them understand importance of nurturing infant.*
• Explain to parents that their actions can help modify some of their infant's behavior. However, make it clear that infant maturation isn't completely within their control. *This explanation*

may decrease parents' feelings of incompetence.
• Explain to parents that certain risk factors may interfere with infant's ability to achieve optimal development. These risk factors include overstimulation, lack of stimulation, lack of physical contact, and painful medical procedures. *Educating parents will help them understand their role in interpreting infant's behavioral cues and providing appropriate stimulation.*
• Describe for parents potential signs of behavioral disturbance in infant: inappropriate responses to stimuli, such as failure to respond to human contact or tendency to become agitated with human contact; physiologic regulatory problems, such as breathing disturbance in premature infant; and apparent inability to interact with environment. *Education will help parents recognize if infant has problem in behavioral development.*
• Demonstrate appropriate ways of interacting with infant *to help parents to identify and interpret infant's behavioral cues and respond appropriately.* For example, help them recognize when infant is awake and alert, and help them understand when infant needs more stimulation, such as being spoken to or held.
• Explore with parents ways to cope with stress imposed by infant's behavior *to increase their coping skills.* Help them identify their emotional responses to infant's behavior *to help them recognize and adjust their response patterns.* Explain that it's normal for parents to experience feelings of inadequacy, frustration, or anger if infant doesn't respond positively to them.
• Praise parents when they demonstrate appropriate methods of interact-

ing with infant *to provide positive reinforcement.*

• Provide parents with information on sources of support and special infant services *to help them cope with infant's long-term needs.*

Evaluations for expected outcomes

• Parents identify risk factors for behavioral disturbance.

• Parents identify potential signs of behavioral disturbance in infant.

• Parents identify actions that promote their infant's development.

• Parents report improvement in their ability to cope with the stress of raising an infant.

• Parents express positive feelings about their ability to care for infant.

• Parents identify resources for help with infant.

Documentation

• Assessment of factors that could disturb infant's behavioral development

• Parents' expression of feelings about caring for infant

• Nursing interventions and infant's response to them

• Evaluations for expected outcomes

■ Infant feeding pattern, ineffective

related to neurologic impairment or developmental delay

Definition

Impaired ability of an infant to suck or coordinate the suck and swallow response

Assessment

• Perinatal history, including gestational age and Apgar score

• Suck and swallow reflex, including condition of lip and palate

• Nutritional status, including intake (type, amount, and frequency of feedings), output (frequency, amount, and characteristics of urine), current weight, weight change since birth, skin turgor, and signs of dehydration

• Laboratory studies, including glucose and bilirubin levels

• Parental assessment, including age, maturity level, and previous experience with infant feeding

Defining characteristics

• Inability to coordinate sucking, swallowing, and breathing

• Inability to initiate or sustain effective suck

Associated medical diagnoses (selected)

Cleft lip or palate, microcephaly, neonatal anomaly, neonatal neurologic impairment, prematurity

Expected outcomes

• Neonate won't lose more than 10% of birth weight within first week of life.

• Neonate will gain 4 to 7 oz (113.4 to 198.5 g)/week after first week of life.

• Parents or caregivers will identify factors that interfere with neonate establishing effective feeding pattern.

• Parents will express increased confidence in their ability to perform appropriate feeding techniques.

• Neonate won't become dehydrated.

• Neonate will receive adequate supplemental nutrition until able to suckle sufficiently.

• Neonate will establish effective suck and swallow reflexes that allow for adequate intake of nutrients.

Interventions and rationales
• Weigh neonate at same time each day on same scale *to detect excessive weight loss early.*
• Continuously assess neonate's sucking pattern *to monitor for ineffective patterns.*
• Assess parents' knowledge of feeding techniques *to help identify and clear up misconceptions.*
• Assess parents' level of anxiety about neonate's feeding difficulty. *Anxiety may interfere with parents' ability to learn new techniques.*
• Remain with parents and neonate during feeding *to identify problem areas and direct interventions.*
• Teach parents to place neonate in upright position during feeding *to prevent aspiration.*
• Teach parents to unwrap and position sleepy neonate before feeding *to ensure that neonate is awake and alert enough to suckle sufficiently.*
• Provide positive reinforcement for parents' efforts to improve feeding technique *to decrease anxiety and enhance feelings of success.*
• For bottle-feeding, record amount ingested at each feeding; for breast-feeding, record number of minutes neonate nurses at each breast and amount of any supplement ingested *to monitor for inadequate caloric and fluid intake.*
• Provide alternative nipple, such as preemie nipple. *Preemie nipple has larger hole and softer texture, which make it easier for neonate to obtain formula.*
• For breast-feeding, ensure neonate's tongue is properly positioned under mother's nipple *to promote adequate sucking.*
• Monitor neonate for poor skin turgor, dry mucous membranes, decreased or concentrated urine, and sunken fontanels and eyeballs *to detect possible dehydration and allow for immediate intervention.*
• Record number of stools and amount of urine voided each shift. *Altered bowel elimination pattern may indicate decreased food intake; decreased amounts of concentrated urine may indicate dehydration.*
• Assess need for gavage feeding. *Neonate may temporarily require alternative means of obtaining adequate fluids and calories.*
• Alternate oral and gavage feeding *to conserve neonate's energy.*
• If neonate requires I.V. nourishment, assess insertion site, amount infused, and infusion rate every hour *to monitor fluid intake and identify possible complications, such as infiltration and phlebitis.*
• Assess neonate for neurologic deficits or other pathophysiologic causes of ineffective sucking *to identify need for more extensive evaluation.*

Evaluations for expected outcomes
• Neonate doesn't lose more than 10% of birth weight within first week of life.
• Neonate gains 4 to 7 oz/week after first week of life.
• Parents identify factors that interfere with effective feeding.
• Parents demonstrate competence when feeding neonate.
• Neonate maintains urine output of 1 ml/kg/day, urine specific gravity of 1.003 to 1.013, good skin turgor, moist mucous membranes, and soft, flat fontanels.
• Neonate receives adequate nutrition.
• Neonate establishes effective sucking reflex and coordinated suck and swallow response.

Documentation
• Frequency, amount, and type of fluid ingested by neonate
• Effectiveness of suck reflex
• Neonate's daily weight
• Parents' knowledge of feeding techniques, involvement with caregiving, and bonding with neonate
• Frequency of neonate's bowel elimination and urination
• Signs of dehydration
• Nursing interventions
• Use of special feeding techniques and equipment
• Parents' and neonate's responses to nursing interventions
• Evidence of neurologic or other physical impairment in neonate
• Evaluations for expected outcomes

■ Infection, risk for

related to altered primary defenses during the postpartum period

Definition
Presence of internal or external hazards that threaten maternal well-being

Assessment
• Laboratory studies, including white blood cell (WBC) and platelet count, clotting factors, hemoglobin and hematocrit, serum albumin level, and cultures of blood, body fluid, sputum, urine, and wound drainage
• Labor and delivery record, including episiotomy; presence of invasive devices, such as I.V. and urinary catheters; and premature rupture of membranes
• Presence of medical conditions such as diabetes mellitus that may increase incidence of infection

• Signs and symptoms of infection, including pallor, fatigue, malaise, anorexia, chills, foul-smelling lochia, calf tenderness, elevated temperature, dysuria, marked abdominal tenderness, and tender, reddened breasts that are warm to the touch

Risk factors
• Altered immune function
• Chronic illness
• Environmental exposure to pathogens
• Inadequate primary defenses (such as broken skin) or secondary defenses (such as suppressed inflammatory response)
• Invasive procedures
• Lack of knowledge about causes of infection
• Malnutrition
• Premature membrane rupture
• Tissue destruction
• Trauma
• Medication use

Associated medical diagnoses (selected)
Diabetes mellitus, endometritis, gestational diabetes, premature rupture of membranes, pneumonia, urinary tract infection

Expected outcomes
• Patient's vital signs will remain within normal range.
• Results of laboratory studies won't indicate infection.
• Patient's respiratory secretions and urine won't show evidence of infection.
• Patient's episiotomy or abdominal incision site will remain free from infection.
• Patient's I.V. sites won't become inflamed.
• Patient will maintain good personal hygiene.

• Patient will state risk factors that can lead to infection.
• Patient will remain free from signs and symptoms of infection.

Interventions and rationales
• Minimize patient's risk of infection by:
– washing hands before and after providing care. *Hand washing is single best way to avoid spreading pathogens.*
– wearing gloves to maintain asepsis when providing direct care and when in contact with blood or body secretions. *Gloves reduce possibility of transmitting disease.*
• After delivery, monitor vital signs every 15 minutes for 1 hour, then every 4 hours for 24 hours, then every shift until discharge. Report abnormal readings. *Elevated temperature, pulse or respiratory rates, or blood pressure may indicate infection. Temperature greater than 100.4° F (38° C) on two consecutive readings after first 24 hours postdelivery may indicate puerperal sepsis, urinary tract infection, endometritis, mastitis, or other infection.*
• Monitor WBC count, as ordered, and promptly report abnormal values. *Total WBC count above 11,000/μl indicates increased production of leukocytes by bone marrow, usually in response to bacterial pathogens.*
• As ordered, culture urine, respiratory secretions, wound drainage, or blood *to identify pathogens and guide antibiotic therapy.*
• Instruct patient in proper personal hygiene, such as use of sitz bath and perineal irrigation bottle, hand washing, and breast care, *to reduce risk of infection.* Explain to patient that most common site of localized postpartum infection is episiotomy site. Tell patient how to apply sanitary pads (front

to back) and how to remove them (back to front). Tell her to wipe perineum after elimination and to clean perineum from front to back. *These measures decrease bacterial concentration and help prevent genitourinary infections.*
• Follow facility's infection-control policy *to minimize risk of nosocomial infection.*
• Use strict aseptic technique when performing invasive procedures, such as urinary catheterization or I.V. line insertion, *to minimize risk of introducing pathogens into body.*
• Assess I.V. site every 4 hours, noting presence of redness or warmth. Change I.V. tubing and site every 72 hours or as dictated by facility policy. *These measures keep pathogens from entering the body.*
• Instruct postoperative patient to deep-breathe and cough *to help remove secretions and prevent respiratory complications.*
• Ensure adequate nutritional intake. *Diet high in protein, iron, and vitamin C helps promote healing.*
• Assess patient for generalized signs and symptoms of infection (pallor, fatigue, malaise, anorexia, and chills) every shift, and instruct her to report danger signs immediately. These include foul-smelling lochia, calf tenderness, elevated temperature, dysuria, marked abdominal tenderness, and tender, reddened breasts that feel warm to touch. *Prompt detection of infection helps minimize complications.*

Evaluations for expected outcomes
• Patient's vital signs remain within normal limits.
• Patient's WBC count and differential remain within normal range, and cultures don't indicate any pathogens.

- Patient's respiratory secretions are clear and odorless, and urine is clear yellow, odorless, and sediment-free.
- Patient's episiotomy or abdominal incision site remains free from infection.
- Patient's I.V. sites don't become inflamed.
- Patient performs proper personal hygiene on regular basis.
- Patient states risk factors that can lead to infection.
- Patient remains free from infection.

Documentation
- Vital signs
- Appearance of episiotomy or abdominal incision site
- Date, time, and sites of cultures
- Date, time, and sites of catheter insertions
- Appearance of invasive catheter and I.V. sites
- Patient teaching about infection control
- Interventions performed to reduce risk of infection
- Patient's response to nursing interventions
- Evaluations for expected outcomes

■ Infection, risk for

related to labor and delivery

Definition
Presence of internal or external hazards that threaten maternal and neonatal well-being

Assessment
- Vital signs, including fetal heart rate
- Health history, including previous infections
- Rupture of membranes, including time of rupture and characteristics of amniotic fluid (amount, color [blood tinged or meconium stained], and odor)
- Laboratory studies, including white blood cell (WBC) and platelet count, clotting factors, hemoglobin and hematocrit, serum albumin level, and cultures of blood or body fluid, sputum, urine, and wound drainage
- Signs and symptoms of chorioamnionitis, including maternal pulse rate over 160 beats/minute, malodorous amniotic fluid, increasing uterine tenderness, and fetal tachycardia

Risk factors
- Altered immune function
- Amniotic membrane rupture
- Chronic illness
- Environmental exposure to pathogens
- Inadequate primary defenses (such as broken skin) or secondary defenses (such as suppressed inflammatory response)
- Invasive procedures
- Lack of knowledge about causes of infection
- Malnutrition
- Tissue destruction
- Trauma
- Medication use

Associated medical diagnoses (selected)
Abnormal rupture of membranes, peritonitis, premature labor, pyelonephritis, urinary tract infection

Expected outcomes
- Patient will maintain good hygiene.
- Patient will remain free from infection.
- Patient's temperature will remain within normal range.

Interventions and rationales

• Monitor and record temperature every 4 hours before rupture of membranes and every 2 hours after rupture. *Temperature elevations are an early sign of infection.*

• Use continuous fetal monitoring to assess fetal heart rate and variability. Report rates over 160 beats/minute and variability under 3 to 5 beats/minute. *Fetal heart rates over 160 beats/ minute and minimal variability may indicate maternal fever.*

• Wash hands thoroughly, using proper technique, before and after providing care *to prevent spread of infection.*

• Maintain universal precautions. Wear gloves if you might come into contact with patient's blood and body secretions. *Universal precautions protect you and patient from transfer of microorganisms.*

• Use strict aseptic technique when suctioning lower airway, applying scalp electrodes, or inserting urinary catheters, pressure catheters, or I.V. lines *to reduce likelihood of nosocomial infections.*

• After spontaneous or artificial rupture of membranes, assess color, amount, and odor of amniotic fluid and presence of blood or meconium. *Alterations in color, amount, and odor of amniotic fluid may indicate infection. Meconium may indicate predisposition to intrauterine infection and fetal distress.*

• After rupture of membranes, minimize vaginal examinations and always use sterile gloves *to decrease risk of chorioamnionitis or other uterine infection.*

• Maintain good patient hygiene. Clean perineal area from front to back and keep area dry *to reduce risk of infection.*

• Carefully monitor intake and output *to assess for dehydration. Signs and symptoms of infection (tachycardia, dry mucous membranes, and poor skin turgor) may resemble those of dehydration.*

Evaluations for expected outcomes

• Patient maintains good hygiene.

• Patient remains free from infetion, as evidenced by clear, odorless, sediment-free urine; WBC count within acceptable limits for labor and delivery (up to 20,000/µl); and cultures free from pathogens.

• Patient's temperature ranges from 97° F to 99° F (36.1° to 37.2° C).

Documentation

• Maternal vital signs

• Fetal heart rate and variability

• Date, time, and sites of cultures

• Date, time, and sites of catheter insertions

• Appearance of all invasive catheter and tube sites and wounds

• Nursing interventions performed to reduce risk of infection

• Patient's response to nursing interventions

• Evaluations for expected outcomes

■ Infection, risk for

related to neonate's immature immune system

Definition

Presence of internal or external hazards that threaten neonate's physical well-being

Assessment

• Gestational age

• Neonate's temperature and vital signs

• Labor and delivery record, including premature rupture of membranes, characteristics of amniotic fluid (odorous or foul-smelling), and maternal temperature
• Maternal infections (recent or current), maternal disease or infection during pregnancy, and maternal pathogens passed on during birth process
• Condition of umbilical cord and skin at base of cord, including redness, odor, and discharge
• Signs and symptoms of neonatal infection, including lethargy, poor weight gain, restlessness, jaundice, visible lesions, thrush, temperature elevations or unstable low temperature, hypoglycemia, altered feeding patterns, diarrhea, vomiting, and subtle color changes such as cyanosis, mottling, or grayish skin tones
• Signs of respiratory distress, including grunting, retractions, nasal flaring, and cyanosis
• Evidence of chronic intrauterine infections, including growth retardation, microcephaly, and hepatosplenomegaly

Risk factors

• Altered immune function
• Amniotic membrane rupture
• Environmental exposure to pathogens
• Inadequate primary defenses (such as broken skin) or secondary defenses (such as suppressed inflammatory response)
• Invasive procedures
• Malnutrition
• Tissue destruction
• Trauma
• Medication use

Associated medical diagnoses (selected)

This diagnosis may be associated with maternal disease during pregnancy or maternal pathogens passed on to neonate during the birth process. Examples of associated diagnoses include acquired immunodeficiency syndrome, chlamydia, gonorrhea, infant respiratory distress syndrome, and syphilis.

Expected outcomes

• Neonate's vital signs will remain within normal range.
• Neonate will be alert and active.
• Neonate will remain free from signs and symptoms of infection.
• Neonate's umbilical cord will heal properly and remain free from infection.
• Family members will demonstrate good hand-washing technique before handling neonate.

Interventions and rationales

• Review maternal chart and delivery record *to detect risk factors that predispose neonate to infection.*
• Assess neonate's gestational age. *Passive immunity of neonate via placenta increases significantly in last trimester, making premature neonate much more susceptible to infection.*
• Follow aseptic technique. Remove all rings, bracelets, and wristwatches before handling neonate. Scrub hands and arms with antimicrobial preparation before entering nursery and after contact with contaminated material. Wash hands again after handling neonate. Instruct parents and siblings in hand-washing techniques and procedures. *These measures help prevent spread of pathogens.*
• Monitor all hospital personnel, parents, and visitors for potential infection *to prevent spreading infection to neonate.*
• Organize nursery. Make sure aisles are 36″ (1 m) wide and cribs are 18″

(45 cm) apart. Keep individual supplies separate for each neonate. *These measures help prevent cross-contamination.*

• Provide cover gowns for nonnursing personnel who enter nursery *to prevent spread of pathogens.*

• Provide eye prophylaxis as facility policy dictates *to prevent ophthalmia neonatorum or gonococcal or chlamydia infections.*

• Perform umbilical cord care with each diaper change, as facility policy dictates, *to promote healing, remove urine and stool, and facilitate desiccation process.*

• Assess respirations, pulse, and blood pressure every 15 minutes for 1 hour, then every hour for 4 hours, then once per shift or more frequently as indicated. Assess temperature every 4 hours for 24 hours, then every 8 hours or as indicated. *Unstable vital signs, persistent elevations in temperature, or hypothermia may indicate neonatal infection.*

• Observe neonate for signs and symptoms of infection. Notify doctor immediately if signs and symptoms of infection appear *to ensure rapid identification and early treatment.*

• Observe universal precautions. Wear gloves before neonate's first bath and when in contact with blood and body secretions. *Following universal precautions prevents cross-contamination and transmission of pathogens, including human immunodeficiency virus.*

• Encourage mother to begin breast-feeding early. *Colostrum and breast milk contain high amounts of immunoglobulin A, which provides passive immunity to neonate and helps reduce infection.*

• As ordered, monitor laboratory studies, including white blood cell (WBC) count, serum levels of immunoglobulin M (IgM), and blood cultures. Culture any lesions, pustules, or drainage. *Decreased WBC count commonly indicates infection in neonate; elevated IgM levels indicate that infectious process has occurred in utero. Cultures identify pathogens and help guide antibiotic therapy.*

• Administer topical, oral, and parenteral antibiotics, as ordered, *to eradicate pathogenic organisms.*

• Observe circumcision site for color, healing, and presence of drainage. *Fresh, healing circumcision site is port of entry for bacteria.*

Evaluations for expected outcomes

• Neonate's vital signs remain within normal range.

• Neonate is alert and active.

• Neonate is free from signs and symptoms of infection.

• Umbilical cord is clean, dry, and healing.

• Family members demonstrate proper hand-washing technique before handling neonate.

Documentation

• Vital signs
• Appearance of umbilical cord
• Date, time, and sites of cultures
• Feeding patterns and weight gain
• Bowel elimination patterns
• Condition of oral mucosa
• Skin color and rashes
• Activity pattern
• Interventions performed to reduce risk of infection
• Neonate's response to nursing interventions
• Evaluations for expected outcomes

■ Injury, risk for

related to labor

Definition

Increased risk to maternal or fetal well-being resulting from oxytocin stimulation

Assessment

• Previous pregnancies
• Prenatal history, including prenatal laboratory studies, pelvic measurements, allergies, weight gain, last menstrual period, and estimated date of confinement
• Physical examination, including maternal vital signs, Leopold's maneuvers (to determine fetal position), palpation of uterus (to assess frequency, intensity, and duration of contractions), sterile vaginal examination (to assess ripeness of cervix [Bishop score]), presentation, estimation of maternal pelvis, and fetal heart rate
• Diagnostic studies, including ultrasound test to determine gestational age and fetal size, and nonstress test or contraction stress test to assess fetal-placental function
• Laboratory studies, including complete blood count, blood type and Rh factor, platelets, Nitrazine test (to confirm rupture of membranes), and urine protein and glucose levels
• Contraindications to oxytocin stimulation, such as absolute cephalopelvic disproportion, fetal distress, grand multipara, overdistention of uterus from multiple gestation or polyhydramnios, vaginal bleeding, and unfavorable fetal presentation or position

Risk factors

• Dysfunctional labor
• Home far from hospital
• Hypotonic contractions
• Postmaturity
• Previous precipitous delivery
• Prolonged rupture of membranes

Associated medical diagnoses (selected)

Cyanotic maternal cardiac disease, labor, multiple births

Expected outcomes

• Patient will have uterine contractions every 2 to 3 minutes, with intensity of 40 to 60 mm Hg (by internal monitoring).
• Continuous fetal monitoring will show fetal heart rate maintains variability of 6 to 10 beats/minute, with reassuring pattern.
• Patient will achieve good labor pattern, and neonate will be delivered without complications.
• Medical personnel will monitor patient closely for adverse reactions to oxytocin stimulation and will initiate appropriate interventions.
• Patient will maintain fluid balance.
• Patient and fetus will maintain optimal well-being.

Interventions and rationales

• Explain oxytocin protocol to patient and her support person. Describe how oxytocin-induced contractions may peak more quickly and last longer than spontaneous contractions *to allay apprehension and encourage patient participation.*
• Before applying fetal monitor or administering oxytocin, encourage patient to void. Palpate bladder every 2 hours for distention. *Full bladder causes discomfort, especially when equipment is placed on patient's abdomen.*
• Monitor intake and output, and measure urine specific gravity. *Decreased output with increased specific gravity*

may indicate urine retention, which may impede fetal descent.

• Place patient in as comfortable a position as possible. Left lateral tilt relieves pressure of gravid uterus on inferior vena cava and promotes blood flow to placenta. *Correct positioning enhances patient comfort and may help you obtain clearer fetal monitoring strip.*

• Apply fetal monitor and obtain a 15- to 20-minute baseline strip *to ensure adequate assessment of fetal heart rate and contraction pattern.*

• Use an 18G or 20G catheter when starting primary I.V. line *to prepare for possible emergency interventions, such as cesarean section or blood administration.*

• Prepare oxytocin as ordered. Add drug to dextrose 5% injection or normal saline solution (initially, 10 units to 1,000 ml of solution). Label bottle with patient's name, amount of oxytocin, date and time prepared, and your name. Note that doctor must be present in facility during oxytocin infusion. *Strict procedure ensures uniform administration and accurate assessment of uterine response.*

• Piggyback oxytocin solution to primary I.V. line at site most proximal to patient. Use I.V. infusion pump to control flow rate. *Insertion at most proximal site to patient prevents bolus infusion if oxytocin is stopped and flow rate of primary I.V. solution is increased. Infusion pump guarantees exact dose administration.*

• Begin infusion at rate of 0.5 to 1 mU/minute. Remain with patient during first 20 minutes. *Initiating oxytocin at this rate enables you to evaluate patient's individual response to stimulation.*

• Increase oxytocin infusion by increments of 1 to 2 mU/minute, as ordered, every 30 to 60 minutes until desired contraction pattern is achieved and cervix is dilated 5 to 6 cm. Monitor blood pressure before and after each increase in dosage. *Increasing oxytocin slowly avoids hyperstimulation, which can cause fetal distress and uterine hypoxia.*

• If you increase to infusion rate of 20 mU/minute without patient achieving desired contraction pattern, notify doctor. *Increments above 20 mU/ minute increase risk of hyperstimulation and water intoxication.*

• Monitor maternal vital signs every 15 to 30 minutes, as indicated by facility policy, *to assess for oxytocin-induced hypertension.*

• Monitor contractile pattern and fetal heart rate every 15 minutes. Assess contractions by palpation or intrauterine pressure catheter. At least every 30 minutes, document heart rate, variability, and fetal monitor strip changes. *Assessment of fetal heart rate and variability allows you to detect nonreassuring fetal heart patterns. Palpation of contractions or intrauterine catheter monitoring allows you to monitor uterine activity.*

• If patient responds poorly to oxytocin infusion, take these steps:
– Check I.V. mixture.
– Check lines for patency.
– Increase oxytocin flow rate, according to facility policy.
– Palpate uterine fundus for quality, duration, and relaxation of contractions.

Errors in oxytocin mixture and I.V. administration can cause poor uterine response. An unripe cervix or uterus will also diminish desired response. If patient's response doesn't improve, the infusion may have to be discontinued after 8 to 12 hours and restarted next day.

• Observe for hypertonicity — contractions lasting longer than 90 seconds and occurring less than 2 minutes apart. When using intrauterine pressure catheter, reading greater than 75 mm Hg indicates hypertonicity. *Because hypertonicity is unpredictable, patient must be monitored carefully.*
• If you detect hypertonicity, discontinue infusion immediately. Check maternal vital signs and notify doctor. Increase flow rate of primary I.V. solution and position patient on left side. *These measures will help arrest hypertonicity.*
• Monitor continuously for loss of variability, late decelerations, or persistent bradycardia *to detect fetal distress. Fetal distress may result from impaired uteroplacental perfusion caused by increased tonicity of contractions.*
• If you detect signs of fetal distress, take these steps:
– Discontinue oxytocin infusion *to minimize risk to fetus.*
– Administer 8 to 12 L of oxygen via tight rebreathing mask *to increase oxygen supply to the fetus.*
– Increase flow rate of primary I.V. line *to increase fluids.*
– Reposition patient on left or opposite side *to increase placental blood flow.*
– Notify doctor *to expedite medical evaluation of maternal and fetal status.*
– Assess maternal vital signs *to monitor for early signs of distress.*
– Perform or assist with sterile vaginal examination *to rule out possibility of umbilical cord prolapse.*
– Make sure patient isn't left unattended *to promote safety.*
• Assess patient's intake and output, and monitor amount of oxytocin administered over course of stimulation.

Total fluid intake shouldn't exceed 125 ml/hour. *Over time, antidiuretic effects of oxytocin combined with administration of large volumes of electrolyte-free solutions can lead to water intoxication.*

Evaluations for expected outcomes
• Patient has contractions every 2 to 3 minutes that last 30 to 60 seconds and are of moderate intensity with adequate resting tonus.
• Continuous fetal monitoring shows fetal heart rate maintains variability of 6 to 10 beats/minute, with reassuring pattern.
• Patient achieves good labor pattern and delivers neonate without complications.
• Medical personnel monitor patient closely for adverse reactions to oxytocin stimulation and initiate appropriate interventions.
• Patient maintains fluid balance.
• Patient and fetus maintain optimal well-being during labor and delivery.

Documentation
• Patient's vital signs on admission and every 15 to 30 minutes, according to facility policy
• Baseline assessment of uterine activity (frequency, intensity, interval, duration, and tonus) before oxytocin stimulation and every 30 minutes thereafter via continuous electronic fetal monitoring
• Assessment of fetal heart rate, including baseline rate, long-term variability, short-term variability (with internal monitoring), accelerations, and periodic changes
• Patient's physical and emotional response to induction or augmentation of labor or both

• Nursing interventions to reduce risk of injury to patient or fetus from oxytocin stimulation
• Patient's response to nursing interventions
• Evaluations for expected outcomes

■ Injury, risk for

related to internal and external neonatal risk factors

Definition
Accentuated risk of accidental tissue damage ·

Assessment
• Ability of parents to care for neonate
• Apgar scores
• Developmental stage (neonate and parents or caregivers)
• Environment, including air temperature, water temperature, and stability of equipment
• Labor and delivery record
• Laboratory studies, including blood glucose and bilirubin levels, white blood cell count, clotting factors, platelet count, hemoglobin and hematocrit, and maternal and neonatal blood types
• Neonatal health history, including traumatic delivery, blood dyscrasia, hypothermia, and hyperthermia
• Neurologic status (neonate and parents or caregivers)
• Prenatal history

Risk factors
• Extremes in environmental temperature
• Hyperbilirubinemia
• Improperly functioning radiant warmer and temperature probe

• Improper padding of cold surfaces
• Litter or liquid spills on floor
• Malfunctioning equipment
• Parents' or caregiver's cognitive, emotional, or motor difficulties
• Parents' or caregiver's lack of familiarity with information resources
• Placement of neonate near drafts
• Requests for information by parents or family members
• Unsafe handling of neonate
• Water temperature at improper setting for washing neonate

Associated medical diagnoses (selected)
Amniotic fluid embolism, congenital heart disease, hyperbilirubinemia, meconium aspiration syndrome, neonatal asphyxia, perinatal asphyxia, perinatal trauma

Expected outcomes
• Neonate will have physical and safety needs met.
• Family members will provide safe environment for neonate after discharge.
• Family members will recognize and report dangerous or potentially dangerous situations.
• Neonate won't experience injury.

Interventions and rationales
• Assess family members' baseline knowledge of neonatal safety. Instruct them as needed. *Education in safety techniques minimizes risk of injury.* Consider which teaching methods (pamphlets, videotapes, or demonstrations) best suit each family member's individual learning style *to facilitate learning.*
• Immediately report malfunctioning equipment to appropriate personnel for replacement or repair *to help prevent accidents.*

• Keep one hand 1″ to 2″ (2.5 to 5 cm) above neonate when measuring weight *to prevent neonate from accidentally slipping off scale.*
• When transporting neonates from nursery, take one bassinet at a time, if possible, *to improve safety.*
• Discourage family members from walking in hall while holding neonate *to avoid falls caused by wet or slippery floors.*
• Discourage mother from sleeping in bed with neonate. *While sleeping, she may accidentally turn over onto, or lose her grip on, neonate.*
• Monitor neonate's skin color for signs of jaundice every shift. *Hyperbilirubinemia occurs in approximately 50% of all neonates. Elevated bilirubin levels can lead to neurologic and developmental difficulties.*
• Test water temperature before washing neonate. Temperature shouldn't exceed 100° F (37.8° C). *Neonates' fragile skin can't tolerate high temperatures.*
• Don't allow ill staff members or visitors to approach neonate *to prevent transfer of pathogens.*
• Assess neonate's potential for injury based on prenatal and labor and delivery records. *Early detection and treatment can minimize injury from intrauterine or perinatal insults.*
• Never leave neonate unattended in unprotected area. *Neonates are totally dependent on others for their physical, emotional, and safety needs.*
• Monitor respiratory and neurologic status as well as laboratory test results. Promptly report abnormal findings *to ensure immediate intervention and prevent complications.*
• Avoid heat loss to neonate from evaporation. *Cold stress leads to increased metabolic rate, which can result in oxygen consumption and hypoglycemia.*

• Review with family members state regulations regarding car seats before discharge *to decrease risk of automobile injury or fatality.*

Evaluations for expected outcomes
• Parents meet neonate's physical and safety needs.
• Family members express understanding of techniques to ensure neonate's safety and practice safety techniques during neonate's stay in hospital.
• Family members express understanding of potentially dangerous situations.
• Neonate doesn't experience injury.

Documentation
• Neonate's skin color
• Temperature of radiant warmer and presence of functioning temperature probe
• Laboratory results
• Observations of physical findings
• Observations or knowledge of unsafe practices
• Instructions given to family members and their responses
• Interventions performed to prevent injury
• Neonate's response to nursing interventions
• Evaluations for expected outcomes

■ Knowledge deficit

related to lack of information about birth process

Definition
Inadequate understanding of, or inability to perform, skills needed to cope effectively with the process of labor

Assessment
• Age
• Psychosocial status, including developmental stage, previous experience with childbearing, expectations of the birth process, interest in learning, and current level of knowledge about pregnancy, birth, and recovery
• Ability to learn, including cognitive domain, intellectual and conceptual skills, and attention span
• Support systems, including presence of support person and support person's interest in helping patient and ability to participate in doing so

Defining characteristics
• Inability to follow through with instruction
• Inappropriate or exaggerated behaviors (hysteria, hostility, agitation, apathy)
• Poor performance on test of knowledge
• Verbalization of problem

Associated medical diagnoses (selected)
Labor, multiple births, pregnancy, premature labor

Expected outcomes
• Patient will recognize that increased knowledge and skill will help her cope better with birth process.
• Patient will demonstrate understanding of what she is taught.
• Patient will demonstrate ability to perform skills needed for coping with labor.
• Patient will express realistic expectations about birth process.
• Patient's level of anxiety about giving birth will be realistic.
• Patient will express satisfaction with her increased knowledge.

Interventions and rationales
• Find quiet, private environment for teaching patient and support person. *Freed of distractions, patient and support person will learn more effectively.*
• Establish trusting relationship with patient. Develop mutual goals for learning. *These measures will enhance learning.*
• Select teaching strategies appropriate to material and patient's learning style (lecture, discussion, demonstration, practice, or audiovisual materials). *Careful selection of teaching strategies will enable you to better meet patient's needs.*
• Teach information and skills needed for understanding and coping during birth *to decrease patient's anxiety and increase her sense of competence.* Evaluate patient's level of understanding and ability to use knowledge during birth process.

Evaluations for expected outcomes
• Patient expresses intention to put knowledge to use during labor.
• Patient describes birth process in her own words.
• Patient correctly performs labor skills.
• Patient expresses realistic expectations of labor.
• Patient responds to labor without undue anxiety, using breathing, relaxation, and position changes to cope.
• Patient voices satisfaction with newly acquired knowledge and skills.

Documentation
• Patient's current understanding about birth process
• Patient's expression of need for better understanding or skills
• Learning goals established in cooperation with patient

• Information and skills taught to patient
• Teaching method used
• Patient's response to teaching
• Patient's mastery of information, including demonstration of new skills
• Evaluations for expected outcomes

■ Knowledge deficit

related to neonatal care

Definition
Inadequate understanding of, or inability to perform, skills needed to provide neonatal care

Assessment
• Psychosocial status, including age, learning ability (affective, cognitive, and psychomotor domains), decision-making ability, developmental stage, financial resources, health beliefs and attitudes, interest in learning, knowledge and skills regarding neonatal care, obstacles to learning, support systems (willingness and capability of others to help), and usual coping pattern
• Neurologic status, including level of consciousness, memory, mental status, and orientation

Defining characteristics
• Inability to follow through with instruction
• Inappropriate or exaggerated behaviors (hysteria, hostility, agitation, apathy)
• Poor performance on test of knowledge
• Verbalization of problem

Associated medical diagnoses (selected)
Childbirth

Expected outcomes
• Patient will express need to improve her understanding of neonatal care.
• Patient will set realistic learning goals for developing competence in caring for neonate.
• Patient will express understanding of neonatal care.
• Patient will demonstrate ability to care for neonate independently or with minimal assistance.
• Patient will identify specific learning goals and target dates for mastering new skills.
• Patient will express intention to adjust lifestyle to accommodate arrival of neonate.
• Patient or family member will contact community resources when necessary.
• Family members will take active role in caring for neonate.

Interventions and rationales
• Establish environment of mutual trust and respect *to enhance learning. Achieving rapport is especially important in light of maternity patient's short length of stay.*
• Assess patient's level of knowledge. Does she have other children? Has she had recent experience caring for a neonate? *Answering these questions will determine whether patient requires basic information or reinforcement of previous learning.*
• Negotiate with patient to develop goals for learning. *Allowing patient to participate in decision making enhances learning.*
• Select teaching strategies appropriate for patient's individual learning style, such as one-on-one discussion and demonstration, attending unit-based neonatal care class, or viewing audiovisual materials. *Choosing approach that best serves patient increases chance for successful learning.*

• Teach skills that patient must incorporate into daily life *to ensure relevance of learning experience.* Have patient give return demonstration of each new skill, such as feeding, diapering, and bathing neonate, *to increase comfort level and identify areas of misunderstanding.*

• Have patient incorporate learned skills into daily routine during hospital stay. Encourage patient to care for neonate in hospital and allow for rooming-in if possible. *Practicing skills leads to proficiency.* Acknowledge positive efforts *to increase patient's self-esteem.*

• Provide patient with names and telephone numbers of resources (such as local breast-feeding association or child welfare service) to contact with questions. *Patient may benefit from additional sources of support during her hospital stay as well as after discharge.*

• Encourage family members to become involved in care of neonate *to promote family unity and bonding with neonate.*

Evaluations for expected outcomes

• Patient expresses need to improve her understanding of neonatal care.

• Patient sets realistic learning goals.

• Patient expresses understanding of neonatal care.

• Patient demonstrates ability to care for neonate, including comfortably holding and playing with neonate, bottle-feeding or breast-feeding and burping neonate at appropriate intervals, caring for circumcision (when applicable) and umbilical cord site, providing scalp care, and bathing and diapering neonate.

• Patient sets specific learning goals and target dates for mastering new skills.

• Patient adjusts lifestyle to accommodate arrival of neonate.

• Patient or family members express willingness to follow up on referrals to community resources.

• Family members demonstrate willingness to take active role in neonatal care.

Documentation

• Patient's current level of knowledge and skills

• Patient's expressions indicating her motivation to learn

• Patient's learning objectives

• Methods used to teach patient

• Teaching provided

• Skills demonstrated

• Patient's response to teaching

• Evaluations for expected outcomes

■ Knowledge deficit

related to postpartum self-care

Definition

Inadequate understanding of postpartum self-care activities or inability to perform skills needed to practice health-related behaviors

Assessment

• Psychosocial status, including age, learning ability (affective, cognitive, and psychomotor domains), decision-making ability, developmental stage, financial resources, health beliefs and attitudes, interest in learning, knowledge and skill regarding postpartum self-care, obstacles to learning, support systems (willingness and capability of others to help patient), and usual coping pattern

• Neurologic status, including level of consciousness, memory, mental status, and orientation

• Physical ability to perform self-care activities

Defining characteristics
• Inability to follow through with instruction
• Inappropriate or exaggerated behaviors (hysteria, hostility, agitation, apathy)
• Poor performance on test of knowledge
• Verbalization of problem

Associated medical diagnoses (selected)
Cesarean section, pregnancy, vaginal delivery, with or without complications

Expected outcomes
• Patient will communicate desire to learn how to care for herself after delivery.
• Patient will establish realistic learning goals.
• Patient will verbalize or demonstrate understanding of what she has learned about self-care.
• Patient will incorporate newly learned skills into daily routine.
• Patient will make changes in postpartum routine, including seeking help from health care professional if necessary.

Interventions and rationales
• Establish environment of mutual trust and respect *to enhance patient's learning. Establishing rapport is especially important in light of maternity patient's short length of stay.*
• Assess patient's level of understanding of postpartum self-care activities *to establish baseline for learning and provide direction for goal development.*
• Negotiate with patient target dates for mastering postpartum self-care skills.

Having patient participate in decision making will promote learning.
• Select teaching strategies (discussion, demonstration, role-playing, or visual materials) best suited for patient's individual learning style *to enhance learning.*
• Teach skills that patient must incorporate into daily postpartum routine, including perineal care, use of sitz bath, use of witch hazel compresses, application and removal of perineal pads, and breast care. *Relevant topics enhance patient's motivation to learn.*
• Have patient give return demonstration of each new skill *to reinforce learning.*
• Teach patient about process of involution *to help her understand postpartum occurrences.*
• Teach patient importance of adequate nutrition and hydration *to ensure proper urinary and bowel elimination.*
• Discuss importance of adequate rest *to promote emotional and physical stability.*
• Have patient incorporate learned skills into daily routine during hospitalization. Acknowledge her efforts. *Practicing learned skills will help patient gain proficiency.*
• Provide patient with names and telephone numbers of appropriate resource people and community service agencies *to provide further resources to help with problem solving, both during patient's stay and after discharge.*

Evaluations for expected outcomes
• Patient expresses motivation to learn.
• Patient establishes realistic goals.
• Patient expresses or demonstrates understanding of what she has learned, including process of involution and

deviations from normal that she should report, ability to use sitz bath, and knowledge of hemorrhoidal care.
• Patient incorporates skills into her daily routine, including performing breast and perineal care, resuming normal bowel and bladder elimination, and obtaining adequate rest and sleep.
• Patient states intention of making changes in daily routine and seeking help from health care professional if necessary.

Documentation
• Patient's understanding of and skill in postpartum self-care (including insight into her own abilities)
• Patient's expressions that indicate her motivation to learn
• Learning objectives
• Methods used to teach patient
• Information imparted to patient
• Skills demonstrated to patient
• Patient's responses to teaching
• Evaluations for expected outcomes

■ Knowledge deficit

related to premature labor

Definition
Inadequate understanding of, or inability to perform, skills needed to cope with premature labor

Assessment
• Age
• Psychosocial status, including decision-making ability, developmental stage, financial resources, health beliefs and attitudes, interest in learning, knowledge and skill regarding pregnancy and birth process, learning ability (affective, cognitive, and psychomotor domains), obsta-

cles to learning, previous experience with premature labor, support systems (willingness and capability of others to help patient), and usual coping pattern
• Neurologic status, including level of consciousness, memory, mental status, and orientation

Defining characteristics
• Inability to follow through with instruction
• Inappropriate or exaggerated behaviors (hysteria, hostility, agitation, apathy)
• Poor performance on test of knowledge
• Verbalization of problem

Associated medical diagnoses (selected)
Premature labor

Expected outcomes
• Patient will communicate desire to learn about premature labor and will set realistic learning goals.
• Patient will express understanding of causes, signs and symptoms, and management of premature labor.
• Patient will identify and immediately report danger signals during and after hospitalization.
• Patient will voice emotional response to premature labor.
• Patient will use available support systems.
• Patient will cope successfully with premature labor.
• Pregnancy will result in positive outcome.

Interventions and rationales
• Introduce yourself to patient and support person, and orient them to surroundings. Explain all procedures beforehand. *These measures reduce patient's anxiety.*

• Establish environment of mutual trust and respect *to calm patient, decreasing uterine stimulation from stress, and to provide atmosphere conducive to learning.*

• Work with patient to develop realistic learning goals. *Unrealistic goals will frustrate you and patient. Failure to achieve goals may reduce patient's interest in learning.*

• Select teaching strategy most appropriate for patient and support person *to enhance learning.*

• Assess patient's understanding of pregnancy and premature labor *to establish basis for nursing plan of care and help guide future interventions.*

• Explain causes, signs and symptoms, and treatment of premature labor to patient and support person *to prepare them to actively participate in care.* Avoid information overload. *Anxiety may limit patient's ability to assimilate information.*

• Project warm, caring attitude and convey willingness to listen *to encourage patient to ask questions and voice feelings.*

• Don't place unrealistic demands on patient *to avoid exacerbating feelings of inadequacy and anxiety.*

• Remain with patient for uninterrupted periods. Assure patient and support person that they can rely on staff for emotional support *to ease anxiety and establish therapeutic relationship.*

• Include patient in decision-making process when possible *to give her sense of participation and control.*

• Provide positive feedback to patient *to strengthen her self-esteem.*

• Provide patient with information related to her health status and condition of fetus. Inform support person as well. *Continued knowledge of maternal and fetal health status helps relieve anxiety.*

• Teach patient danger signs to report immediately, such as contractions occurring every 10 minutes or less for 1 hour, fluid leaking from vagina, or lack of or altered fetal movement. *Promptly identifying and reporting danger signs helps avoid premature labor.*

• If patient is discharged to home before delivery, review discharge instructions. Emphasize taking prescribed medications, limiting activities as instructed, and reporting danger signs. *If patient understands her needs and limitations, she may be able to avoid recurrence of premature labor.*

Evaluations for expected outcomes

• Patient expresses desire to learn about premature labor and sets realistic learning goals.

• Patient identifies possible causes and signs and symptoms of premature labor and expresses understanding of methods of managing it.

• Patient promptly reports danger signs and receives appropriate interventions.

• Patient expresses emotional response to premature labor.

• Patient uses available support systems.

• Patient successfully copes with premature labor as demonstrated by verbal and nonverbal behaviors.

• Pregnancy results in positive outcome.

Documentation

• Patient's statements indicating her understanding of premature labor

• Patient's expressions indicating her motivation to learn

• Learning objectives

• Methods used to teach patient and support person

• Information discussed with patient and support person

• Patient's and support person's responses to teaching
• Maternal and fetal physical status
• Evaluations for expected outcomes

■ Knowledge deficit

related to self-care activities during pregnancy

Definition
Inadequate understanding of information needed to practice health-related behaviors during pregnancy

Assessment
• Age
• Psychosocial status, including decision-making ability, developmental stage, financial resources, health beliefs and attitudes, interest in learning, knowledge and skill regarding pregnancy, learning ability (affective, cognitive, and psychomotor domains), obstacles to learning, previous obstetric history, support systems (willingness and capability of others to help patient), and usual coping pattern
• Neurologic status, including level of consciousness, memory, mental status, and orientation

Defining characteristics
• Inability to follow through with instruction
• Inappropriate or exaggerated behaviors (hysteria, hostility, agitation, apathy)
• Poor performance on test of knowledge
• Verbalization of problem

Associated medical diagnoses (selected)
Pregnancy

Expected outcomes
• Patient will communicate need for more information about self-care and will set realistic learning goals.
• Patient will demonstrate understanding of material taught.
• Patient will demonstrate ability to perform new health-related behaviors she has learned.
• Patient will continue to practice appropriate health-related behaviors after pregnancy.

Interventions and rationales
• Establish environment of mutual trust and respect *to help patient relax and be receptive to learning.*
• Negotiate realistic learning goals with patient. *Unrealistic goals will frustrate you and patient. Failure to achieve goals may reduce patient's interest in learning.*
• Using open-ended questions, assess patient's knowledge of pregnancy-related health practices *to establish basis for nursing plan of care and help guide future interventions.*
• Adapt teaching strategies (discussion, demonstration, role-playing, or use of visual materials) to patient's individual learning style. *Tailoring teaching and content to patient's learning style helps enhance learning.*
• Refer patient to appropriate resource people, agencies, and organizations *to ensure comprehensive care.*
• Discuss appropriate dental care and instruct patient to visit dentist early in pregnancy. *Poor oral hygiene and caries may result from nausea, vomiting, heartburn, and gum hyperemia associated with pregnancy.*
• Review possible effects of caffeine, alcohol, addicting drugs, and tobacco on developing fetus *to help ensure fetal well-being.* Tell patient that any substance she ingests during pregnan-

cy can affect fetus. Explain that alcohol may cause developmental anomalies, marijuana and tobacco may cause intrauterine growth retardation and prematurity, and cocaine may cause abruptio placentae in mother and prematurity, poor feeding patterns, irritability, neural tube defects, and increased respiratory and cardiac rates in neonate.

• Urge patient to consult her doctor or nurse-midwife before taking any medications *to avoid possible teratogenic effects on fetus.*

• Review exercise routines designed for pregnant women and, if appropriate, refer patient to organized exercise group. *Regular exercise program during pregnancy enhances well-being and helps improve muscle tone in preparation for childbirth.*

• Review dietary intake for 1 week and instruct patient in proper nutrition during pregnancy. Explain to patient that she needs extra 300 calories each day, for total of 2,100 to 2,400 calories per day. Refer patient to dietitian if appropriate. *Patient needs more calories to maintain optimal use of protein, allow for fetal and maternal tissue synthesis, and meet increased basal metabolic needs.*

• Discourage patient from wearing constrictive clothing and shoes or high-heeled shoes. *High-heeled shoes increase likelihood of developing low back strain, backache, and poor balance. Constrictive clothing and shoes can alter venous circulation.*

• Discuss exposure to possible sources of toxic chemicals or gases *to avoid possible teratogenic effects on developing fetus.*

• Review patient's daily routine at home and at work. *Patient may need to alter her routine during pregnancy. For example, if she holds sedentary job, she should walk about periodically to increase circulation to her legs. If she stands for long periods, she may need to adopt less physically demanding posture.*

• Instruct patient to contact doctor or nurse-midwife immediately if she experiences any danger signs or symptoms, including severe vomiting, frequent and severe headaches, epigastric pain, visual disturbances, swelling of fingers or face, altered or absent fetal movements after quickening, signs of vaginal or urinary tract infection, unusual or severe abdominal pain, or fluid discharge from vagina. *Prompt identification of danger signs reduces risk of abnormal pregnancy.*

Evaluations for expected outcomes

• Patient communicates need for more information about self-care and establishes realistic learning goals.

• Patient demonstrates understanding of material taught, including importance of:
– maintaining appropriate diet
– following appropriate exercise regimen
– limiting or stopping smoking (if applicable)
– not consuming illicit drugs or alcohol
– checking with doctor or nurse-midwife before taking any medication
– limiting caffeine intake
– obtaining sufficient rest
– avoiding areas that may contain toxic chemicals or gases
– not wearing constrictive clothing and shoes or high-heeled shoes
– reporting danger signals to doctor or nurse-midwife
– visiting dentist early in pregnancy
– taking prenatal vitamins as prescribed.

• Patient demonstrates ability to perform health-related behaviors she has learned during pregnancy.
• Patient continues to practice appropriate health-related behaviors after pregnancy.

Documentation
• Patient's knowledge of self-care activities during pregnancy
• Expressions indicating patient's motivation to learn
• Learning objectives
• Teaching methods
• Subject matter discussed in teaching session
• Record of dietary intake for 1 week
• Demonstration and return demonstration of skills
• Patient's response to teaching
• Written and audiovisual materials given to patient
• Evaluations for expected outcomes

■ Nutrition alteration: Less than body requirements

related to ineffective suck reflex

Definition
Inability to ingest sufficient fluids and nutrients resulting from an ineffective suck reflex

Assessment
• Gestational age
• Perinatal history
• Apgar score
• Suck and swallow reflex, including intactness of lips and palate
• GI assessment, including vomiting and regurgitation, stool characteristics (color, amount, consistency, and frequency), inspection of abdomen, auscultation of bowel sounds, palpation for masses, and percussion for tympany or dullness
• Nutritional status, including intake and output, current weight, weight change since delivery, skin turgor, urine characteristics (frequency and amount), signs of dehydration, and feedings (type, amount, and frequency)
• Laboratory studies, including urine glucose levels, urine bilirubin levels, and urine specific gravity
• Maternal assessment, including anesthetic used during labor and delivery, parity, knowledge level, and breast-feeding (condition of nipples and positioning of neonate)

Defining characteristics
• Aversion to or lack of interest in feeding
• Body weight 20% or more under ideal weight
• Diarrhea and steatorrhea
• Evidence of lack of food intake
• Fragile capillaries
• Hyperactive bowel sounds
• Inadequate intake
• Pale conjunctivae and mucous membranes
• Poor muscle tone
• Satiety immediately after feeding
• Signs of abdominal pain or cramping, with or without pathology
• Weakness of muscles required for sucking

Associated medical diagnoses (selected)
Cleft lip or palate, esophageal fistula, hyperbilirubinemia, prematurity

Expected outcomes
• Mother will demonstrate effective feeding techniques.
• Neonate won't lose more than 10% of birth weight.
• Neonate will retain entire feeding without vomiting or regurgitating.

• Neonate will ingest 130 to 200 oz/kg and 95 to 145 calories/kg per day.
• Neonate will establish effective suck and swallow reflexes, allowing for adequate nutritional intake.
• Neonate will maintain good (elastic) skin turgor, moist mucous membranes, urine specific gravity between 1.005 and 1.015, and flat, soft fontanels.
• Infant will gain at least 1 oz (28.4 g) each day for first 6 months after birth.

Interventions and rationales
• Obtain neonate's weight at same time each day, using same scale, *to ensure early recognition of excessive weight loss.*
• If bottle-feeding, record amount ingested at each feeding. If breastfeeding, record number of minutes neonate nurses at each feeding as well as ingestion of any supplement *to aid in early recognition of inadequate caloric and fluid intake.*
• Assess parents' knowledge of feeding techniques. As needed, teach parents how much and how often to feed neonate and how to prepare formula, position neonate during and after feeding, and burp neonate. *Early detection of knowledge deficits and appropriate instruction help eliminate misconceptions.*
• Regularly assess neonate's sucking pattern. Try to correct ineffective sucking patterns *to help eliminate ongoing difficulties.*
• Provide preemie nipple or breast shell, as appropriate. *Preemie nipple's larger hole and softer texture make it easier for neonate to obtain formula. Breast shell helps draw out inverted nipple.*
• Make sure neonate's tongue is properly positioned under nipple *to enable neonate to suck adequately.*

• Make sure neonate is awake before feeding. Unwrap blanket and tap soles of feet. *Tightly wrapped, drowsy neonate is less likely to be interested in feeding. Neonate must be fully awake and stimulated to suck effectively.*
• Record number of stools and amount of urine voided each shift. *Decreased amounts of concentrated urine may indicate dehydration; altered bowel elimination pattern may indicate decreased food intake.*
• Monitor neonate for signs of dehydration, such as poor (inelastic) skin turgor, dry mucous membranes, decreased or concentrated urine, and sunken fontanels and eyeballs, *to establish need for immediate medical intervention.*
• Assess neonate for neurologic or other physical causes of ineffective sucking *to identify need for more extensive evaluation.*
• Assess need for gavage feeding. *Neonate may temporarily require alternative means of obtaining adequate fluids and calories.*

Evaluations for expected outcomes
• Mother demonstrates competence when feeding neonate.
• Neonate returns to birth weight by 10 days after delivery.
• Neonate retains entire feeding.
• Neonate ingests 130 to 200 oz/kg and 95 to 145 calories/kg each day.
• Neonate establishes effective suck and swallow reflexes.
• Neonate maintains good skin turgor, moist mucous membranes, urine specific gravity between 1.005 and 1.015, and flat, soft fontanels.
• Infant gains at least 1 oz each day for first 6 months after birth.

Documentation
• Frequency, amount, and type of fluid ingested
• Incidence of vomiting and regurgitation
• Effectiveness of suck reflex
• Neonate's daily weight
• Parent's knowledge, level of caregiving, and bonding with neonate
• Frequency of bowel elimination and urination
• Signs of dehydration
• Nursing interventions and neonate's response
• Use of special nipple (such as preemie nipple)
• Results of laboratory studies
• Presence of physical or neurologic impairment
• Evaluations for expected outcomes

■ Pain

related to physiologic changes of pregnancy

Definition
An unpleasant sensory and emotional experience arising from actual or potential tissue damage or described in terms of such damage; pain may be of sudden or slow onset, vary in intensity from mild to severe, and be constant or recurring; pain lasts less than 6 months; and period of pain has an anticipated or predictable end

Assessment
• Characteristics of pain, including location, quality, intensity on a scale of 1 to 10, temporal factors, and sources of relief
• Physiologic variables, such as age and pain tolerance

• Psychological variables, such as body image, personality, previous experience with pain, anxiety, and secondary gain from symptoms
• Sociocultural variables, such as cognitive style, culture or ethnicity, and attitude and values
• Environmental variables, such as setting and time
• Understanding of pregnancy and birth process

Defining characteristics
• Alteration in muscle tone (may range from listless to rigid)
• Autonomic responses (diaphoresis; blood pressure, pulse rate, and respiratory rate changes; and dilated pupils)
• Changes in appetite and eating
• Communication (verbal or coded) of pain
• Distracting behavior (such as pacing, seeking out other people, and performing repetitive activities)
• Expressions of pain (such as moaning and crying)
• Facial mask of pain (grimacing)
• Guarding or protective behavior
• Narrowed focus (including altered time perception, withdrawal from social contact, and impaired thought processes)
• Self-focusing
• Sleep disturbance

Associated medical diagnoses (selected)
Abdominal infections, appendicitis, backache, Braxton Hicks contractions, breast masses or infection, cervical disk abnormality, cholecystitis, constipation, eclampsia, gastric ulcer, gallbladder disease, headache, heartburn, hemorrhoids, hiatal hernia, hydatidiform mole, hyperemesis gravidarum, intestinal flu, labor, leg cramps, pleurisy, preeclamptic

headache, pregnancy-induced hypertension, pulmonary emboli, round ligament pain, thrombosed veins, thrombophlebitis, urinary frequency, urinary tract infection, varicosities

Expected outcomes
• Patient will identify characteristics of pain.
• Patient will articulate factors that intensify pain and will modify behavior accordingly.
• Patient will carry out appropriate interventions for pain relief.

Interventions and rationales
• Provide care for patient experiencing nausea and vomiting:
– Assess and document extent of nausea and vomiting *to create database for nursing interventions and patient teaching.*
– Reassure patient that nausea will usually subside by 4th month of pregnancy *to reduce patient's anxiety level and enhance compliance with nursing interventions.*
– Instruct patient to eat dry, unsalted crackers before rising in morning *to prevent nausea resulting from empty stomach.*
– Tell patient to avoid greasy or spicy foods. *Spicy foods irritate stomach. Fats with meals depress gastric motility and digestive enzyme secretion and slow intestinal peristalsis. These effects may lead to gastroesophageal reflux.*
– Tell patient to avoid cooking odors that predispose her to nausea and to use electric fan while cooking *to help avoid nausea. Air circulation dilutes odors.*
– Advise patient to eat six small meals per day instead of three large ones *to avoid overloading stomach.*

– Advise patient to eat foods high in carbohydrates. *Such foods are easier to digest.*
– Tell patient to take iron pills and vitamins after meals *to avoid irritating stomach.*
– Advise patient to take frequent walks outdoors. *Walking in fresh air reduces nausea and helps reinforce positive outlook.*
– Tell patient to separate food and fluid intake by ½ hour. *Drinking excessive fluids with meals distends stomach, predisposing patient to nausea. Taking fluids between meals also prevents dehydration.*
– Advise patient to avoid very cold fluids and foods at mealtimes. *Cold fluids and foods may cause nausea and abdominal cramping.*
– Caution patient to consult doctor before taking over-the-counter medications to treat nausea and vomiting *to avoid harmful effects on fetus.*
• Provide care for patient experiencing urinary frequency:
– Assess patient for frequency and dysuria *to rule out possible urinary tract infection (UTI).*
– Reassure patient that urinary frequency is normal in early and late stages of pregnancy because enlarging uterus places pressure on bladder. *Reassurance may reduce patient's confusion and anxiety.*
– Tell patient to avoid drinking large amounts of liquids within 2 to 3 hours of bedtime *to prevent frequent nocturnal urination and sleep loss.*
– Instruct patient to ingest required amount of liquids early in day *to reduce need for evening liquids.*
– Instruct patient to void when urge occurs *to prevent bladder distention and urinary stasis, which may predispose patient to UTI.*

– Teach patient signs and symptoms of UTI. Urge her to report signs and symptoms promptly. *Early detection of UTI allows early treatment and helps prevent complications, such as pyelonephritis and premature labor.*

• Provide care for patient experiencing breast fullness and tingling:

– Assess patient's breast discomfort *to obtain database for further interventions.*

– Assure patient that breast changes and discomfort are natural. Tell her that fullness will last entire pregnancy but that tenderness will resolve after first trimester. *Reassurance decreases patient's anxiety level and promotes compliance.*

– Advise patient to wear supportive bra with wide, adjustable straps and smooth lining *to decrease irritation and provide support for enlarging breasts.*

– Instruct patient to avoid tight bras and clothing that may confine breasts. *Pressure increases tenderness, tingling sensations, and discomfort.*

– Teach patient anatomy and physiology of breast changes during pregnancy. If indicated, begin preparation for breast-feeding at end of third trimester *to enhance breast-feeding experience.*

• Provide care for pregnant patient who develops headache:

– Assess type and location of headache and associated signs and symptoms. *Assessment provides information for selection of interventions and clues to patient's discomfort. Presence of associated factors, such as proteinuria, weight gain, edema, elevated blood pressure, and hyperreflexia, may indicate occurrence of pregnancy-induced hypertension.*

– Advise patient to sleep 8 hours each night and to nap or rest for 2 hours in afternoon *to alleviate fatigue.*

– Advise patient to drink 6 to 8 glasses (1,500 to 2,000 ml) of fluid per day *to prevent or alleviate headache resulting from dehydration. Increasing fluids may eliminate headache by increasing vascular space and dilating cerebral veins.*

– Instruct patient to apply cool, wet compresses to forehead and back of neck and to massage neck, shoulders, face, and scalp. *Cool compresses may eliminate headaches resulting from emotional tension and spasms of sternocleidomastoid muscles of neck and back.*

– Instruct patient to take two acetaminophen tablets every 4 to 6 hours, as ordered. Tell her to avoid aspirin because of its anticoagulant action. Remind her to consult doctor before taking over-the-counter medications. *Acetaminophen effectively relieves minor headaches of pregnancy.*

• Provide care to patient experiencing heartburn:

– Assess patient's nutritional habits *to obtain clues to patient's discomfort and information for selection of interventions.*

– Reassure patient that normal pregnancy changes can cause heartburn *to decrease anxiety and increase compliance with nursing interventions.*

– Advise patient to eliminate greasy and spicy foods from her diet and to avoid fats. *Such foods decrease stomach motility and increase secretion of stomach acids and gastric acidity.*

– Instruct patient to reduce fluid intake with meals. *Liquids tend to inhibit gastric juices.*

– Instruct patient to avoid very cold foods. *Very cold foods promote gastric reflux.*

– Instruct patient to drink cultured milk such as buttermilk rather than regular whole milk. *Cultured milk has less fat than regular milk.*

– Instruct patient in good posture. *Good posture gives patient's stomach more room to function.*

– Instruct patient to take small, frequent meals to avoid overloading stomach and to remain upright for 3 to 4 hours after each meal *to decrease possibility of reflux.*

– Advise patient to use antacids that are low in sodium *to reduce risk of tissue edema.* Tell her to take antacids that contain both aluminum and magnesium (such as Maalox and Riopan). *Aluminum-based antacids (such as Amphojel) may cause constipation. Magnesium-based antacids (such as Milk of Magnesia) have laxative effects. Aluminum-magnesium combinations tend to balance these effects.* Tell patient to avoid antacids that contain sodium bicarbonate *to prevent hypokalemia, metabolic alkalosis, and hypernatremia.*

• Provide care for patient with round ligament pain:

– Assess onset and site of round ligament discomfort and associated uterine activity *to rule out possibility of premature labor activity.*

– Reassure patient that round ligament pain is normal during pregnancy and results from stretching of ligaments that support expanding uterus. *Reassurance will decrease anxiety and promote cooperation.*

– Instruct patient to avoid sudden jerky movement, to rise slowly from recumbent positions, and to avoid excessive exercise, standing, or walking. *Sudden, jerky movements or twisting of torso pulls on round ligaments, causing unilateral or bilateral pain. Excessive exercise, standing, or walking can also strain abdominal muscles.*

• Provide care to patient who experiences backache:

– Assess patient's posture, lifting techniques, and footwear *to pinpoint causes of pain.*

– Instruct patient to wear low-heeled shoes, maintain good posture, and hold shoulders back *to increase spinal curvature, which may reduce backache.*

– Instruct patient in proper body mechanics *to help her avoid stress to lower back.*

– Tell patient to rest in recumbent position or with her legs bent and elevated on bed or chair *to relieve strain on lower back.*

– Instruct patient to perform moderate daily exercise *to tone and maintain muscle strength in lower back.*

– Discuss benefits of massaging and applying warm, moist heat to lower back. *These measures will help relax and soothe tight muscles.*

• Provide care for patient with hemorrhoids:

– Assess patient's diet for fiber, fluids, and iron intake *to plan appropriate diet that will enhance bowel function.*

– Assess prepregnancy bowel habits and history of hemorrhoids *to provide database for planning interventions.*

– Instruct patient to avoid constipation by increasing intake of dietary fiber, bran cereals, and fluids. She should also drink warm water when she arises in morning. *Avoiding constipation helps prevent straining at stool and lessens risk of hemorrhoids. Dietary fiber, bran cereals, and fluids increase intestinal peristalsis and facilitate bowel function.*

– Encourage patient to take sitz baths and to use witch hazel and Epsom salt

compresses. *Warm sitz baths cause tissue dilation, increased blood flow, and healing. Witch hazel pads (such as Tucks) and Epsom salt compresses reduce tissue swelling.*
– According to doctor's recommendation, encourage use of analgesic ointments and topical preparations *to reduce pain.*
– Administer stool softeners, as ordered, *to allow normal evacuation without straining.*
• Provide care for the pregnant patient with varicosities:
– Assess for degree of pain, family history, level of exercise, extent of varicosities, and history of varicosities before pregnancy. *Assessing pain helps rule out thrombophlebitis. Assessing extent of varicosities and patient's level of exercise helps plan for nursing interventions.*
– Reassure patient about cause and usual duration of her discomfort *to decrease anxiety and promote compliance.*
– Tell patient to rest in recumbent position, with her legs elevated above body level, twice per day *to promote venous return and avoid stagnation and pooling of venous blood.*
– Instruct patient to put on supportive stockings before arising in morning and to raise her legs when putting them on. *Supportive stockings promote venous return and increase comfort.*
– Tell patient to avoid garters and tight knee-high stockings and not to cross her legs *to reduce risk of venous pooling and thrombus formation.*
– Advise patient to perform regular exercise, take frequent walks, and avoid sitting for long periods *to increase blood flow and retard stasis and pooling.*
• Provide care for patient suffering from leg cramps:

– Assess patient's diet for excessive soft drink intake or inadequate dairy protein. *Inadequate dairy protein or excessive intake of soft drinks, which contain large amounts of phosphorus, can disrupt body's calcium-phosphorus ratio, thereby leading to leg cramps.*
– Instruct patient to limit intake of soft drinks *to reduce consumption of phosphorus.*
– Reassure patient that leg cramps are normal during pregnancy *to reduce anxiety and promote compliance.*
– Tell patient to consult with doctor about supplementing milk intake with aluminum hydroxide (Amphojel). *Taken with milk, aluminum hydroxide helps to remove dietary phosphorus from intestinal tract.*
– Instruct patient to elevate legs periodically and to avoid lying prone with toes pointed. *Lying prone with toes pointed predisposes patient to blood vessel occlusion and subsequent cramping.*
– Tell patient to exercise and use good body mechanics *to prevent leg cramping by increasing general circulation.*
– Advise patient to take warm baths at bedtime *to relax muscle fibers and increase blood flow circulation to the muscles.*
– If cramping occurs, tell patient to straighten affected leg and dorsiflex foot. *These measures pull contracted muscle taut, thus relieving cramp caused by contraction.*
– Caution patient not to rub affected calf *to avoid risk of dislodging undetected thrombus.*
• Provide care for patient who experiences Braxton Hicks contractions:
– Assess patient for frequency, strength, and regularity of contractions *to rule out preterm or true labor.*

– Reassure patient that Braxton Hicks contractions are normal in pregnancy *to reduce anxiety.*
– Instruct patient to walk. *Walking may cause Braxton Hicks contractions to cease and can help distinguish them from true labor.*
– Advise patient to assume left lateral position when at rest *to increase blood flow to uterus, which may decrease intensity and frequency of contractions.*

Evaluations for expected outcomes
• Patient identifies characteristics of pain.
• Patient lists factors that intensify pain and modifies behavior accordingly.
• Patient carries out appropriate interventions for pain relief.

Documentation
• Patient's description of pain and expression of feelings about pain
• Observations about patient's physical, psychological, and sociocultural responses to pain
• Comfort measures and medications provided to reduce pain
• Effectiveness of pain relief interventions
• Patient teaching about pain and pain relief
• Additional nursing interventions performed to assist patient with pain control
• Evaluations for expected outcomes

■ Pain
related to physiologic response to labor

Definition
An unpleasant sensory and emotional experience arising from actual or potential tissue damage or described in terms of such damage; pain may be of sudden or slow onset, vary in intensity from mild to severe, and be constant or recurring; pain lasts less than 6 months; and period of pain has an anticipated or predictable end.

Assessment
• Descriptive characteristics of pain, including location, quality, intensity on scale of 1 to 10, temporal factors, and sources of relief
• Physiologic variables, including age and pain tolerance
• Psychological variables, including body image, personality, previous experience with pain, anxiety, and secondary gain from symptoms
• Sociocultural variables, including cognitive style, culture or ethnicity, and attitude and values
• Environmental variables, including setting and time
• Understanding and expectations of labor and delivery

Defining characteristics
• Alteration in muscle tone (may range from listless to rigid)
• Autonomic responses (diaphoresis; blood pressure, pulse rate, and respiratory rate changes; and dilated pupils)
• Changes in appetite and eating
• Communication (verbal or coded) of pain

• Distracting behavior (such as pacing, seeking out other people, and performing repetitive activities)
• Expressions of pain (such as moaning and crying)
• Facial mask of pain (grimacing)
• Guarding or protective behavior
• Narrowed focus (including altered time perception, withdrawal from social contact, and impaired thought processes)
• Self-focusing
• Sleep disturbance

Associated medical diagnoses (selected)
Abruptio placentae, hydatidiform mole, labor, pregnancy-induced hypertension

Expected outcomes
• Patient will identify characteristics of pain and will describe factors that intensify it.
• Patient will modify behavior to decrease pain.
• Patient will express decrease in intensity of discomfort.
• Patient will experience satisfaction with her performance during labor and delivery.

Interventions and rationales
• Orient patient on admission to labor and delivery suite. Show patient her room and explain operations of her bed and call light. Explain admission protocol and labor process. *These measures will allay patient's initial anxiety.*
• Assess patient's knowledge of labor process and her current anxiety level *to plan supportive strategies.*
• Explain available analgesics and anesthesia to patient and support person. *Awareness that medications are available reduces anxiety.*

• Encourage support person to remain with patient in labor. *Woman in labor will respond more readily to supportive measures offered by familiar, caring person.*
• Instruct patient and support person in techniques to decrease discomfort of labor:
– Discuss techniques of conscious relaxation. *During labor, relaxation enables patient to use coping techniques.*
– Tell patient to concentrate on internal or external focal point. *Focal point allows controlled thought while breathing.*
– Instruct patient in basic deep chest breathing, which is similar to normal breathing but slower and deeper. *Deep chest breathing creates sense of relaxation during contractions.*
– Instruct patient in shallow chest breathing. Tell her to take slow, pantinglike breaths. *Slow breathing avoids hyperventilation. Shallow chest breathing lifts diaphragm from uterus during contractions, decreasing intensity of contractions.*
– Instruct patient in effleurage —
• In early labor, provide patient with diversional activities, such as watching television, *to decrease anxiety.*
• As labor progresses, modify environment to reduce distractions (close door, turn off television, and close curtains). *These measure help patient to concentrate during active phase of labor.*
• Apply sacral pressure to patient if needed *to decrease back pain.*
• Help patient to change positions and use pillows *to make herself more comfortable.* Make sure all body parts are supported, with joints slightly flexed. *Frequent position changes reduce stiffness, prevent pressure sores, and promote comfort.*

• Assess bladder for distention and encourage patient to void every 2 hours. *Distended bladder increases patient's discomfort during contractions and interferes with fetal descent.*
• Provide frequent mouth care. According to protocol, provide ice chips, water-based jelly, or a wet 4″ × 4″ gauze swab for dry lips *to relieve dry mouth and lips caused by breathing techniques and nothing-by-mouth status.*
• Apply cool, damp cloth to patient's forehead *to relieve diaphoresis.*
• Change patient's gown and bed linens as needed. *Diaphoresis and vaginal discharge can dampen gown and bed and cause discomfort.*
• Encourage patient to rest and relax between contractions *to decrease fatigue. Fatigue worsens pain perception and decreases patient's ability to cope with contractions.*
• Discuss with patient and support person which pain medications are available if alternative pain control methods prove inadequate. *Patient may need prescribed analgesics to cope with labor process.*

Evaluations for expected outcomes
• Patient identifies characteristics of pain and describes factors that intensify it.
• Patient modifies behavior to decrease pain, including using breathing techniques, asking for analgesia when needed, and assuming more comfortable position.
• Patient reports decrease in intensity of discomfort.
• Patient expresses satisfaction with her performance during childbirth.

Documentation
• Patient's childbirth preparation and plans for giving birth

• Patient's description of pain
• Observation of patient's response to labor
• Nursing interventions to decrease discomfort
• Patient's response to nursing interventions
• Evaluations for expected outcomes

■ Pain

related to postpartum physiologic changes

Definition
An unpleasant sensory and emotional experience arising from actual or potential tissue damage or described in terms of such damage; pain may be of sudden or slow onset, vary in intensity from mild to severe, and be constant or recurring; pain lasts less than 6 months; and period of pain has an anticipated or predictable end

Assessment
• Descriptive characteristics of pain, including location, quality, intensity on scale of 1 to 10, temporal factors, and sources of relief
• Physiologic variables, such as age and pain tolerance
• Psychological variables, such as body image, personality, previous experience with pain, anxiety, and secondary gain from symptoms
• Sociocultural variables, including cognitive style, culture or ethnicity, attitude and values, and birth order
• Environmental variables, such as setting and time
• Physical factors, including perineal pain, sulcus tears, hemorrhoids, hematomas, uterine discomfort, breast fullness and engorgement, nipple

soreness or cracking, and episiotomy (type, extension, redness, edema, ecchymosis, discharge, and approximation)

Defining characteristics
• Alteration in muscle tone (may range from listless to rigid)
• Autonomic responses (diaphoresis; blood pressure, pulse rate, and respiratory rate changes; and dilated pupils)
• Changes in appetite and eating
• Communication (verbal or coded) of pain
• Distracting behavior (such as pacing, seeking out other people, and performing repetitive activities)
• Expressions of pain (such as moaning and crying)
• Facial mask of pain (grimacing)
• Guarding or protective behavior
• Narrowed focus (including altered time perception, withdrawal from social contact, and impaired thought processes)
• Self-focusing
• Sleep disturbance

Associated medical diagnoses (selected)
Mastitis, pelvic thrombophlebitis, perineal lacerations and extensions, puerperal infections, septicemia, vulval or vaginal hematoma

Expected outcomes
• Patient will identify characteristics of pain and will describe factors that intensify it.
• Patient will understand and carry out appropriate interventions for pain relief.
• Patient will expresses comfort and relief from pain.

Interventions and rationales
• Assess patient's pain symptoms *to obtain information and plan appropriate nursing interventions.*
• As ordered, administer pain medications *to provide pain relief.*
• Discuss with patient reasons for her discomfort and its expected duration *to decrease anxiety and increase compliance.*
• Examine episiotomy site for redness, edema, ecchymosis, drainage, and approximation *to detect trauma to perineal tissues or developing complications.*
• Inspect rectum for hemorrhoids. Provide instruction on hemorrhoidal care, as appropriate. Tell patient to apply ice for 20 minutes every 4 hours, apply witch hazel compress, and use sitz baths. *Hemorrhoidal care will help decrease patient discomfort. Ice aids in regression of hemorrhoids and vulval irritation by promoting localized vasoconstriction.*
• Apply ice packs to episiotomy site for first 24 hours *to increase vasoconstriction and reduce edema and discomfort.*
• Encourage use of sitz baths. Baths should be cool to cold for first day and warm (100° to 105° F [37.8° to 40.6° C]) thereafter. Patient should take sitz baths three or four times per day, with each lasting about 20 minutes. *Sitz baths with cold water decrease edema and promote comfort. After 24 hours, moist heat increases circulation to perineum, reduces edema, promotes healing, and enhances oxygenation and nutrition of tissues.*
• As ordered, teach patient how to use sprays, creams, and ointments for perineal area. *These products penetrate sensory nerve endings, providing depressant effect on peripheral nerves, thereby reducing response to sensory*

stimulation. Astringents such as witch hazel shrink tissues and reduce swelling.

• Assess for uterine tenderness and presence and frequency of after-birth pains every hour for first 24 hours, then every shift as indicated. *In first 12 hours after birth, uterine contractions are strong and regular. Factors that may intensify contractions include multiparity, breast-feeding, and oxytocin administration.*

• Encourage patient to tighten buttocks before sitting and to sit on flat, padded surface. She should avoid foam donuts or soft pillows. *Tightening gluteal muscles before sitting reduces stress and direct pressure on perineum. Because foam donuts separate buttocks, they may decrease venous blood flow to affected area, thereby increasing discomfort.*

• Inspect breast and nipple tissue for engorgement or cracked nipples *to ensure selection of appropriate nursing interventions.*

• Encourage breast-feeding mother to wear supportive bra *to increase comfort* and to position neonate properly during feedings. She shouldn't use same position every time. *This will help prevent sore nipples.*

• If breast-feeding patient is engorged, instruct her to use warm compresses or take warm shower before breast-feeding and to breast-feed more often *to relieve discomfort. Warm compresses and showers help stimulate flow of milk and may help relieve stasis and engorgement.*

• If breast-feeding mother's nipples become sore, instruct her to air dry nipples for 20 to 30 minutes after feedings *to help toughen nipples* and to apply breast creams as ordered *to soften nipples and relieve irritation.* If only one nipple is sore or cracked, instruct her to offer nontender nipple first for several feedings *to reduce potential trauma on sore nipple.*

• Tell non-breast-feeding patient to wear tight supportive bra or breast binder and apply ice packs as needed *to prevent or reduce lactation.*

• Assess for bladder distention. Implement measures to facilitate voiding and provide appropriate patient teaching. *Bladder fullness can cause discomfort.*

• After epidural or spinal anesthesia, assess patient for spinal headache. Pain is primarily located behind eyes but may radiate to temples and occipital area. Supine position decreases pain; sitting or standing increases pain. Don't give pain medications before medical evaluation of source of headache. Increase oral fluids, and notify doctor or anesthesiologist, as indicated. *Epidural or spinal anesthesia may lead to leakage of cerebrospinal fluid and subsequent headache. Increasing oral fluids helps to compensate for loss of cerebrospinal fluid.*

• After cesarean section, provide abdominal pillow and teach patient to splint incision site when moving or coughing *to provide support for abdominal muscles.*

Evaluations for expected outcomes

• Patient identifies characteristics of pain and describes factors that intensify it.

• Patient understands and carries out appropriate interventions for pain relief, including taking sitz baths and prescribed medications.

• Patient expresses comfort and relief from it.

Documentation
• Patient's description of physical pain, pain relief, and feelings about pain
• Nurse's observations about patient's physical, psychological, and sociocultural responses to pain
• Comfort measures and medications provided to reduce pain
• Effectiveness of pain relief interventions
• Information provided to patient about pain and pain relief
• Additional nursing interventions performed to help patient control pain
• Evaluations for expected outcomes

■ Parenting alteration

related to inadequate attachment to high-risk neonate

Definition
Inability of a nurturing figure to promote optimum growth and development of a high-risk neonate

Assessment
• Parental status, including age and maturity, apprehension, parental role models during childhood, knowledge of child care and normal growth and development, previous bonding history, available support systems, coping mechanisms, and feelings about pregnancy and neonate
• Family status, including age, sex, status, and developmental stage of other children and parents' relationship with each other and with other children
• Mother's medical condition
• Neonatal status, including medical condition, separation from parents, and presence of medical equipment
• Psychosocial status, including financial stressors and work demands

Defining characteristics
• *Neonate:*
– failure to thrive
– frequent illness
– history of trauma or abuse
– no evidence of attachment
– no separation anxiety
• *Parents:*
– evidence of inflexibility in meeting neonate's needs
– evidence of neglectful behavior toward or abandonment of neonate
– expressed frustration of inability to fulfill role
– expressed inability to meet neonate's needs
– expressed negative feelings about neonate
– inadequate child health maintenance
– inappropriate child care arrangements
– inappropriate visual, tactile, or auditory stimulation for neonate
– inconsistent caregiving
– poor or inappropriate caregiving skills
– poor interaction with neonate, with little cuddling
– punitive or abusive behavior toward neonate
– rejection of or hostility toward neonate
– unsafe home environment
– weak or no attachment to neonate

Associated medical diagnoses (selected)
This diagnosis can be associated with any condition associated with high-risk neonates, such as multiple births or premature labor.

Expected outcomes
• Parents will establish contact with neonate.

• Parents will communicate feelings and anxieties about neonate's condition and their parenting skills.
• Parents will express willingness to care for neonate and will demonstrate competent parenting skills.
• Parents will demonstrate knowledge of neonate's developmental needs.
• Parents will become involved in planning and providing neonate's care.
• Parents will use available support systems to assist with care of neonate.

Interventions and rationales

• Before parents' first visit to neonatal intensive care unit (NICU), explain appearance of neonate and presence of supportive devices *to prepare parents for sights and sounds that may otherwise upset them.*
• Encourage mother to visit NICU. Assess whether mother is physically able to go, and offer assistance if necessary. *Mother may hesitate to ask for help or may be unsure of physical surroundings.*
• Provide parents with picture of neonate *to help them accept reality of birth.*
• If neonate must be transferred to another facility, arrange for parents to meet transfer team and visit with neonate beforehand. *Seeing neonate and meeting transfer team will increase parents' feelings of involvement and help them come to terms with neonate's condition.*
• Encourage father or other family member to visit neonate soon after admittance to NICU or transfer to other facility, especially if mother can't visit. *Firsthand reports from family member about neonate's condition and physical surroundings will help allay fears of rest of family.*

• Assess parents' level of understanding of neonate's condition and their expectations *to clear up misunderstandings, allow for prompt intervention, and promote realistic planning.*
• Encourage parents to express anxieties related to neonate's condition and their parenting skills *to identify and clarify misconceptions.*
• Make sure parents are informed of neonate's ongoing condition *to help decrease their anxiety and help them plan for future.*
• Encourage parents to touch and talk to neonate and call neonate by name. Reassure them that touching infant won't cause any harm. *This will stimulate bonding between parents and infant.*
• Allow time for parents to care for neonate within secure environment of hospital. Provide positive feedback for parent's efforts to care for neonate *to increase parents' self-confidence.*
• Provide parents with NICU telephone number and encourage phone calls at any time *to make information about neonate readily available.*
• Refer parents to social services, as needed, *to help ensure comprehensive care.*
• Encourage parents to bring in personal items for neonate, such as small stuffed animals or pictures of family members, *to encourage emotional bonding with neonate.*

Evaluations for expected outcomes

• Parents initiate regular contact with neonate.
• Parents voice their anxieties about neonate's condition and their ability to provide care.
• Parents express willingness to meet neonate's basic needs and, if appropriate, special care needs and display appropriate caregiving and attach-

ment behaviors, including providing appropriate verbal, tactile, and auditory stimulation for neonate.
• Parents demonstrate knowledge of neonate's developmental needs.
• Parents take part in planning and providing neonate's care.
• Parents express awareness of and willingness to contact available sources of support.

Documentation
• Observations of parents' behavior
• Parents' statements concerning neonate
• Information provided to parents and their level of understanding
• Parents' interactions with neonate
• Parents' willingness to meet neonate's physical and emotional needs
• Consultations with health team members
• Parents' and neonate's responses to nursing interventions
• Evaluations for expected outcomes

■ Self-esteem disturbance

related to behavior during labor and delivery

Definition
Negative perception of behavior that disturbs healthy functioning

Assessment
• Availability of support
• Patient's and support person's perception of labor and delivery
• Patient history, including past labor and delivery experience, ethnic and cultural background, and usual pattern of coping with stress

• Physiologic and behavioral changes during labor and delivery

Defining characteristics
• Expressions of self-negating thoughts
• Expressed shame or guilt
• Hypersensitivity to slights or criticism
• Perception of self as unable to deal with events
• Projection of blame or responsibility for problems onto others
• Rationalization of personal failures
• Rejection of positive feedback and exaggeration of negative feedback about self

Associated medical diagnoses (selected)
Vaginal or cesarean section delivery of term, postterm, or preterm infant

Expected outcomes
• Patient will express feelings about labor and delivery.
• Patient will set realistic goals for her behavior during labor and delivery.
• Patient will receive adequate emotional and physical support during labor and delivery.
• Patient will project positive self-concept through behavior and verbal expression.

Interventions and rationales
• Encourage patient and support person to articulate their expectations of labor and delivery experience *to identify and correct misconceptions early in the couple's experience.*
• Provide positive feedback about patient's behavior on an ongoing basis *to clear up misconceptions and increase feelings of self-esteem.*
• Emphasize realistic goals for behavior during labor and delivery. *Placing unrealistic demands on patient can*

lead to feelings of inadequacy and poor self-esteem.

• Encourage support person to express feelings about labor and delivery. *Patient may misunderstand how support person viewed her behavior during labor.*

• Encourage patient to take active role in self-care activities after delivery *to reinforce patient's ability to care for self and increase self-esteem.*

Evaluations for expected outcomes

• Patient expresses feelings about labor and delivery.

• Patient expresses realistic understanding of what to expect from her own behavior during labor and delivery.

• Patient expresses satisfaction with emotional and physical support received during labor and delivery.

• Patient's behavior and remarks reflect positive self-image.

Documentation

• Patient's behaviors and expressions that indicate lowered self-esteem

• Nurse's perceptions of patient's readiness for decision making

• Nursing interventions to improve patient's self-concept

• Patient's response to nursing interventions

• Patient's willingness to perform self-care activities

• Patient's expressions of well-being

• Evaluations for expected outcomes

■ Skin integrity impairment

related to episiotomy or abdominal incision

Definition
Interruption in skin integrity after delivery

Assessment
• Age
• Vital signs
• Integumentary status, including color, elasticity, hygiene, lesions, moisture, quantity and distribution of hair, sensation, temperature, texture, and turgor
• Musculoskeletal status, including area affected by anesthetic procedure, joint mobility, muscle strength and mass, paralysis, and range of motion
• Health history, including past skin problems, trauma, surgery, chronic debilitating disease, and immobility
• Nutritional status, including appetite, dietary intake, hydration, present weight, and change from normal
• Laboratory studies, including hemoglobin and hematocrit and serum albumin levels
• Psychosocial status, including coping patterns, family or significant other, mental status, occupation, self-concept, and body image
• Knowledge, including patient's current understanding of her physical condition and physical, mental, and emotional readiness to learn
• Presence of medical condition that may interfere with healing
• Extent of interruption in skin integrity because of delivery

Defining characteristics
• Destruction of skin layers surrounding episiotomy or abdominal incision

• Disruption of skin surfaces
• Invasion by pathogens

Associated medical diagnoses (selected)
Cesarean delivery, perineal lacerations
(first-, second-, third-, and fourth-
degree), tubal ligation, vaginal delivery

Expected outcomes
• Patient will demonstrate understanding of self-care activities.
• Patient will perform skin care routine.
• Patient will identify possible danger
signs and report them immediately to
doctor.
• Patient will regain skin integrity.
• Patient's episiotomy or abdominal
incision will heal without infection.
• Patient and partner will express feelings about possible change in body
image.

Interventions and rationales
• Inspect incision every shift using
REEDA (redness, edema, ecchymosis, discharge, and approximation)
method. Document findings. *Frequent
assessment can detect signs and
symptoms of possible infection.*
• Perform prescribed treatment regimen. Monitor progress and report favorable and adverse responses. *Periodic cleaning decreases bacterial
concentrations, thus aiding healing
process. Monitoring response to treatment can help identify possible need
for alternative interventions.*
• Instruct and assist patient with general hygiene, including hand-washing
and toileting practices. *Proper hand
washing is the most effective method
of disease prevention. Bacteria from
hands can easily contaminate other
areas.*
• Instruct and assist patient in use of
sitz baths (three to four times daily)

and perineal irrigation bottle (after
each elimination). *Sitz baths aid healing process by increasing circulation
to perineum and decreasing edema.
Perineal irrigation bottles maintain
cleanliness, thus decreasing bacterial
concentration.*
• Teach patient how to apply and remove maternity perineal pad. Tell her
to apply clean pad from front to back
and to remove soiled pad from back
to front *to decrease risk of contami-
nating vaginal area with stool.*
• Maintain infection control standards
*to help minimize risk of nosocomial
infections.*
• Provide splinting pillow for patient
with abdominal incision. *Splinting
provides support to area, minimizing
discomfort and encouraging patient
to move and cough.*
• Help patient assume comfortable
position *to minimize incidence of
pain-induced immobility.*
• Inform patient of purpose of self-
care practices *to increase compliance.*
• Encourage patient and partner to
discuss impact of altered skin integrity. Patient's self-esteem may be lowered because of scar from abdominal
incision. Patient or partner may be
concerned about effect episiotomy
will have on sexual relations. *Open
communication increases understanding between partners.*
• Instruct patient and partner in possible danger signs and symptoms that
should be reported to doctor immediately. These include:
– temperature above 100.4° F (38° C)
on two consecutive readings
– incisional drainage
– increased discomfort at episiotomy
or incision site
– reddened or warm skin surrounding
episiotomy or incision site.

Prompt reporting of danger signs and symptoms may help prevent major complications.

Evaluations for expected outcomes
• Patient demonstrates correct self-care practices.
• Patient performs skin care routine.
• Patient identifies possible danger signs and reports them immediately to doctor.
• Patient regains skin integrity.
• Patient's episiotomy or abdominal incision site shows no redness, edema, ecchymosis, or discharge, and edges are approximated.
• Patient and partner communicate feelings about possibly altered body image or sexuality.

Documentation
• Patient's concerns about change in skin integrity
• Patient's willingness and ability to perform self-care practices
• Observations of episiotomy or abdominal incision site and response to treatment regimen
• Presence and type of skin closure method
• Instructions regarding treatment regimen and patient's understanding of instructions
• Prescribed treatment
• Interventions to provide supportive care
• Patient's response to nursing interventions
• Self-care practices performed by patient
• Evaluations for expected outcomes

■ Thermoregulation, ineffective

related to immaturity

Definition
Fluctuations in body temperature caused by thermoregulatory disturbances in neonate

Assessment
• Gestational age
• Weight in relation to gestational age
• Neurologic status, including level of consciousness and motor and sensory status
• Cardiovascular status, including blood pressure, capillary refill time, electrocardiogram results, heart rate and rhythm, pulses (apical and peripheral), and temperature
• Respiratory status, including arterial blood gas measurements, breath sounds, and rate, depth, and character of respirations
• Integumentary status, including color, temperature, and turgor
• Fluid and electrolyte status, including blood urea nitrogen levels, intake and output, serum electrolyte levels, and urine specific gravity
• Laboratory studies, including clotting factors, hemoglobin and hematocrit, and platelet and white blood cell counts
• Environmental factors that contribute to heat loss, including radiation (loss of heat to objects not in direct contact with neonate), conduction (loss of heat through direct contact with cooler objects), convection (loss of heat from body surface to cooler surrounding air), and evaporation (changing of liquid to vapor)
• Coexisting conditions and diagnoses
• Maternal sedation before delivery

Defining characteristics
- Cyanotic nail beds
- Increased capillary refill time
- Fluctuations in body temperature above or below normal range
- Flushed or mottled skin
- Hypertension
- Increased respiratory or heart rate
- Mild shivering
- Moderate pallor
- Piloerection
- Seizures
- Warm or cool skin

Associated medical diagnoses (selected)
Infant respiratory distress syndrome, postmaturity, prematurity

Expected outcomes
- Neonate will maintain body temperature at normal levels.
- Neonate will have warm, dry skin.
- Neonate will maintain heart rate, respiratory rate, and blood pressure within normal range.
- Neonate won't exhibit signs of compromised neurologic status.
- Staff members will take steps to maintain neonate's body temperature at normal level.
- Parents will recognize and avoid possible sources of heat loss.
- Parents will express understanding of neonate's thermoregulatory disturbance and thermoregulation.

Interventions and rationales
- Monitor neonate's body temperature after delivery *to obtain baseline.* According to facility protocol, continue routine monitoring of neonate's body temperature until discharge *to determine need for intervention and effectiveness of therapy. Timely intervention prevents complications related to prolonged cold stress.*

- Monitor and record heart rate, respiratory rate, and blood pressure after delivery and routinely thereafter until discharge *to help ensure prompt diagnosis and treatment of conditions that may affect thermoregulation.*
- Monitor results of laboratory studies for indications of sepsis or of metabolic or respiratory disorders. *Difficulty maintaining normal body temperature may indicate underlying disorder. Conditions resulting from cold stress may further interfere with effective thermoregulation. For example, hypoxia, central nervous system trauma, and hypoglycemia may impair neonate's ability to maintain normal body temperature.*
- Place neonate under radiant warmer device, with temperature probe. When temperature is stable, transfer healthy neonate to regular open crib. Transfer sick neonate to servo-controlled open warmer bed or incubator. *These measures will help minimize oxygen consumption and metabolic rate, cause sweat gland activity to cease, and maintain deep body temperature at appropriate level.*
- Closely monitor neonate's temperature and compare with temperature of warming device. Be aware of potential hazards:
– Make sure temperature probe doesn't become detached from neonate's skin *to prevent hyperthermia. Overheating increases metabolic rate and, subsequently, oxygen consumption and may lead to apneic spells, particularly in premature neonate.*
– Don't place temperature probe between neonate and mattress. *This can result in falsely high reading, causing warming device to decrease heat output, thus leading to hypothermia.*
– Maintain accurate record of environmental and core temperatures. Ob-

serve for variations in heater output. *Consistent variations in heater output may be symptomatic of sepsis.*

– Monitor neonate for signs of dehydration, including inelastic skin turgor, increased urine specific gravity, and dry mucous membranes. *Warming devices may contribute to insensible water loss.*

• Provide fluids based on neonate's age, size, and condition. Monitor intake and output, and administer parenteral fluids as ordered. *Neonate may need increase in fluids to compensate for water loss caused by increase in metabolic rate.*

• Maintain environmental temperature at comfortable setting. Take these steps:

– Dry neonate thoroughly after delivery.

– Provide bath only when neonate's temperature is stable. After bath, return neonate to incubator or warmer device until temperature returns to normal range.

– Monitor nursery temperature and humidity.

– Provide heated, nebulized oxygen when ordered.

– Use overhead warmer during procedures and extensive examinations.

– Keep incubator or radiant warmer away from windows and cold walls.

– Ensure that linen and clothing are clean and dry.

– Warm hands before performing examinations and procedures.

– Warm examination table and instruments, such as scales and stethoscope, when possible, before exposure to neonate.

Maintaining temperature of external environment reduces effects of heat loss from body surface to environment.

• Teach family members about:

– signs and symptoms of altered body temperature, such as cool extremities

– factors in home that contribute to neonatal heat loss and ways to minimize heat loss

– signs of prolonged heat loss, including poor weight gain

– importance of contacting health care provider when problems related to temperature regulation arise.

Careful teaching allows family members to take active role in maintaining neonate's health.

Evaluations for expected outcomes

• Neonate's temperature is stable at 96.8° to 98.6° F (36° to 37° C) within 4 hours of birth.

• Neonate has warm, dry skin.

• Neonate maintains heart rate, respiratory rate, and blood pressure within normal limits.

• Neonate exhibits no signs of compromised neurologic status.

• Staff members keep neonate in neutral thermal environment throughout hospitalization.

• Parents minimize or eliminate potential for heat loss in home environment and incorporate precautions against ineffective thermoregulation into routine care of neonate.

• Parents express understanding of neonate's thermoregulatory disturbance and thermoregulation.

Documentation

• Physical findings
• Intake and output
• Laboratory results
• Vital signs, including blood pressure
• Environmental temperature
• Teaching provided to parents regarding thermoregulation
• Parents' expressions indicating understanding of problems related to thermoregulation

- Nursing interventions
- Neonate's response to interventions
- Evaluations for expected outcomes

■ Urinary elimination alteration

related to sensory impairment during labor

Definition
Alteration or impairment in urinary function

Assessment
- Vital signs
- History of sensory or neuromuscular impairment, urinary tract trauma, surgery, or infection
- Genitourinary status, including palpation of the bladder, voiding pattern, urine characteristics, and presence of pain or discomfort
- Labor and delivery, including anesthesia (regional or local) and oxytocin induction or augmentation
- Fluid and electrolyte status, including skin turgor, intake and output, urine specific gravity, and inspection of mucous membranes
- Neuromuscular status, including ability to perceive bladder fullness

Defining characteristics
- Frequency
- Hesitancy
- Incontinence
- Retention
- Urgency

Associated medical diagnoses (selected)
Episiotomy, hemorrhage, severe intrapartal pregnancy-induced hypertension, vaginal laceration

Expected outcomes
- Patient's vital signs will remain within normal limits.
- Patient will empty bladder regularly, as confirmed by abdominal palpation.
- Patient's intake and output will remain roughly equivalent.
- Patient's urinary function will remain normal and free from complications.

Interventions and rationales
- Review patient's intake and output before and during labor. Note amount, color, concentration, and urine specific gravity. *Decreased output may indicate dehydration, hemorrhage, pregnancy-induced hypertension, and excessive oxytocin stimulation. Urine specific gravity reflects kidneys' ability to concentrate urine and patient's hydration status.*
- Assess for dehydration (poor skin turgor; flushed, dry skin; confusion; dry mucous membranes; fever; and rapid, thready pulse). *Dehydration leads to decreased circulatory blood volume and decreased urine output.*
- Palpate abdomen above symphysis pubis every 2 hours *to detect bladder distention and degree of fullness.*
- Encourage patient to void every 2 hours *to promote optimum bladder tone, prevent distention, and assist in promoting fetal descent.*
- To facilitate voiding, help patient to relax by:
– having her sit in upright position. Assist her to bathroom, if appropriate. *Upright or squatting position promotes contraction of pelvis and intra-abdominal muscles, thereby assisting in sphincter control and bladder contraction.*
– providing privacy *to promote relaxation.*

– pouring warm water over perineum *to stimulate urge to void.*
– providing audible sound of slow running water. *This technique helps many patients void through power of suggestion.*
• As ordered, catheterize patient if she can't void independently. *Overdistended bladder can cause atony and impede fetal descent or can become traumatized by presenting part of fetus during delivery.*

Evaluations for expected outcomes
• Patient's vital signs remain within normal range.
• Patient empties her bladder adequately at least every 2 hours.
• Patient's intake roughly equals output.
• Patient's urinary function remains normal and free of complications.

Documentation
• Intake and output
• Vital signs
• Results of bladder assessment
• Nursing interventions performed to promote voiding
• Patient's response to nursing interventions
• Evaluations for expected outcomes

GERIATRIC HEALTH

INTRODUCTION

This section focuses on nursing diagnoses and plans of care for patients age 65 and older — an age-group that makes up approximately 12.8% of the North American population and is growing twice as fast as younger age-groups.

Traditionally, our culture has valued youth over old age. In keeping with this cultural prejudice, our health care system emphasizes cure over care, acute intervention over long-term rehabilitation, and highly specialized technology over nurturing and support. Not surprisingly, such a system frequently fails to adequately meet the needs of elderly patients. With the older population growing so rapidly, nurses and other health care providers face the challenge of finding newer and better approaches to geriatric care. Nursing diagnoses and associated plans of care offer an important alternative framework for meeting the needs of elderly patients.

Holistic geriatric care involves not only helping the patient cope with the effects of aging and chronic illness but also supporting his efforts to maintain self-reliance and autonomy. Your assessment should therefore take into account the patient's psychosocial functioning as well as his physiologic status. Don't neglect to consider such factors as the amount and quality of contact with family and friends, the opportunity to perform meaningful life roles, access to transportation, and available financial resources. Such factors have a tremendous influence on older patients' well-being.

Because older people now lead longer and more productive lives, geriatric care is increasingly focused on health promotion. Your interventions may include encouraging the patient to make lifestyle changes, such as seeking and maintaining social support, moving to a more healthful environment, and exercising and eating properly. If the patient becomes ill, your task may be to help restore optimal functioning. If recovery is unlikely, your task may be to help the patient adjust to his condition and make sure he receives necessary assistance.

Always keep in mind that interventions must be tailored to the individual patient's needs. Although aging is common to all, each person ages differently. Factors that influence aging include genetics, culture, nutrition, environment, stress, and lifestyle, among others. Modifying your plan of care to meet the patient's individual needs not only leads to better nursing practice but also demonstrates respect for the patient's rich life experiences.

■ Activity intolerance

related to functional changes accompanying the aging process

Definition
Insufficient physical or psychological energy to endure or complete required or desired daily activities

Assessment
• Usual activity level, including self-care (dressing, feeding self, toileting), transfer, walking, stair climbing, and aids for ambulation
• Pain
• Cardiovascular status, including blood pressure, heart rate and rhythm (at rest and with activity), skin temperature and color, edema, and chest pain or discomfort
• Respiratory status, including arterial blood gas results, auscultation of breath sounds, and rate, rhythm, depth, and pattern of respiration at rest and with activity
• Musculoskeletal status, including range of motion and muscle size, strength, tone, and functional mobility grades as follows:
0 = completely independent
1 = requires use of equipment or device
2 = requires help, supervision, or teaching from another person
3 = requires help from another person and equipment or device
4 = dependent; doesn't participate in activity
• Laboratory studies, including complete blood count
• Environmental factors, including safety hazards
• History of chronic illnesses (cardiopulmonary, cardiovascular, musculoskeletal, and neuromuscular)
• Sensory deficits, including hearing, vision, and tactile
• Psychosocial status, including cognitive and mental status, mood, affect, behavior, family support, and coping style
• Economic status
• Medication history, including prescription and over-the-counter medications

Defining characteristics
• Abnormal heart rate or blood pressure in response to activity, arrhythmia or ischemic changes on electrocardiogram, and exertional discomfort or dyspnea
• Verbal report of fatigue or weakness

Associated medical diagnoses (selected)
Chronic obstructive pulmonary disease, dementia, macular degeneration, osteoarthritis, Parkinson's disease

Expected outcomes
• Patient's pulse, respirations, and blood pressure will remain within established parameters.
• Patient will use assistive devices to carry out activities.
• Patient will modify activities to adjust to decreased activity tolerance.
• Patient will seek help in performing activities of daily living (ADLs) as needed.
• Patient will demonstrate willingness to perform activities needed to follow prescribed plan of care.
• Patient will verbalize acceptance of decreased activity level.
• Patient will experience less discomfort when ambulating, transferring, or performing other activities.
• Patient will state plan to use support services.

Interventions and rationales

• Establish realistic goals for improving patient's activity level, taking into account patient's physical limitations and energy level *to help improve patient's quality of life. Keep in mind that in some older patients with chronic conditions, even minimal improvements in activity level are noteworthy.*

• Demonstrate use of assistive devices, such as cane or walker, shopping cart on wheels, or trapeze, *to teach methods of conserving energy and maintaining independence.*

• Establish progressive goals to increase ambulation, for example:
– ambulate 20′ (6 m) three times per day for 1 week
– ambulate 40′ (12 m) three times per day for 1 week
– ambulate 60′ (18 m) three times per day for 1 week.
Older patients may tire easily; therefore, activity level should be increased gradually. Monitor vital signs before and after ambulation *to detect cardiovascular insufficiency.*

• Provide encouragement if patient achieves even small improvements in activity level *to help restore self-confidence.*

• Coordinate activities of interdisciplinary team when developing activity regimen for patient. For example, doctor can prescribe treatment for medical condition, physical therapist can design exercise program, dietitian can design nutrition plan, and social worker can locate community resources, such as Meals On Wheels or home health services, *to address patient's physical and psychosocial needs.*

• Refer depressed patient to mental health practitioner *to address psychosocial problems that may be causing impairment in activity.*

• Encourage patient to express feelings about decreased energy levels that may accompany advanced age *to enhance acceptance.*

• Teach patient about good nutrition and importance of getting adequate rest *to improve poor health practices.*

• Monitor patient's medication regimen regularly *to identify drugs that may cause gait, posture, or ambulatory problems.*

• Help patient identify activities that are personally meaningful and develop realistic plan to incorporate meaningful activities into daily routine *to heighten satisfaction with energy expenditure.*

• Encourage patient to take part in exercise and social activities as tolerated *to increase stamina and decrease social isolation.*

• Modify environment *to maximize independent activity.* For example, place bed on first floor of home with easy access to bathroom and instruct patient to obtain and use energy-saving devices, such as elevated toilet seat, trapeze bar on bed, and chair with arms and seat that raises patient to standing position, *to promote independence.*

• Perform periodic health assessments and monitor for complaints of weakness or fatigue *to assess whether acute illness or exacerbation of chronic condition is causing activity intolerance.*

• Refer to home health agency for follow-up care. Discuss impact on self-esteem of incorporating help from attendants or using assistive devices. Encourage patient to interview and select home health personnel *to foster patient's sense of independence.*

Evaluations for expected outcomes
• Patient's pulse, respirations, and blood pressure are within established parameters.
• Patient uses assistive devices to carry out activities.
• Patient demonstrates necessary skills for modifying activity level to adjust to activity intolerance.
• Patient requests help to complete ADLs when necessary.
• Patient demonstrates willingness to perform activities needed to follow plan of care, including maintaining balanced diet, getting adequate rest, and participating in modified exercise program.
• Patient's verbal statements indicate that he is learning to accept decreased energy level and to come to terms with the fact that he may not regain former level of activity.
• Patient reports experiencing less discomfort and pain when ambulating, transferring, and performing ADLs.
• Patient states that acceptance of support services won't damage self-esteem or alter independent living efforts.

Documentation
• Observations of patient's activity level, both deficits and improvements
• Patient's compliance with treatment regimen and response to multidisciplinary approach
• Teaching provided to patient and family members and their responses
• Modification of home or facility environment to ease patient's activity level
• Evaluations for expected outcomes

■ Adult failure to thrive

related to illness, disability, or environmental deprivation

Definition
Impaired health or interrupted rehabilitation resulting from illness, disability, lack of resources, or environmental deprivation

Assessment
• Age
• Weight and fluctuations in weight
• Condition of hair, skin, and nails
• Nutritional status, including daily food intake, meal preparation, and use of supplements or vitamins
• Sleep patterns
• Mobility status
• Socioeconomic status, including ethnic background, education, financial resources, family support system, religious affiliation, activity and exercise patterns, involvement in social activities, and access to transportation
• Health habits and beliefs, including participation in fad diets, excessive concern with preventing obesity, and recent immigration to this country with little experience in selecting appropriate foods in American markets
• Mental status, including orientation to time, person, and place; insight regarding current situation; judgment; abstract thinking; mood; affect; recent and remote memory; thought processes; and thought content

Defining characteristics
• Apathy
• Inadequate nutrition
• Lack of eye contact
• Memory problems
• Pallor
• Poor hygiene
• Recent acute illness

- Weight loss
- Withdrawn behavior

Associated medical diagnoses (selected)

Alzheimer's disease, amyotrophic lateral sclerosis, anemia, chemical dependency, cancer, chronic obstructive pulmonary disease, depression, heart failure, organic brain syndrome, vitamin or mineral deficiency

Expected outcomes

- Patient will express understanding of causes underlying failure to thrive.
- Patient will express realization that he is depressed.
- Patient will consume sufficient amounts of food and nutrients.
- Patient will sleep for ___ hours without interruption.
- Family members will demonstrate understanding of measures necessary to meet patient's needs.
- Patient will gain weight.
- Patient will report feeling safe.
- Patient will follow up on referrals for social service assistance.
- Patient will follow up on referrals for psychiatric evaluation.
- Patient and family members will use community resources to enhance patient's health.

Interventions and rationales

- Spend uninterrupted time with patient *to learn his perception of problems related to failure to thrive; for example, difficulty maintaining independence in activities.*
- Encourage patient and family members to establish a plan for addressing patient's failure to thrive *to encourage patient and family members to assume responsibility for meeting patient's needs to the extent that they are physically, mentally, and emotionally able.*
- Create a pleasant mealtime environment for patient. Provide unlimited

access to nourishing foods and nutritional supplements. Attempt to accommodate ethnic food preferences. *These measures help promote weight gain.*
- Measure and record patient's weight at the same time every day *to ensure accuracy and monitor patient's progress.*
- Monitor fluid intake and output. *A decrease in body weight may result from fluid loss.*
- Monitor electrolyte levels and report abnormal values. *Poor nutritional status can cause electrolyte imbalance.*
- Urge participation in exercise and activities consistent with capabilities. *Mild exercise and socialization may improve self-esteem.*
- Teach patient, family members, or caregiver how to maintain progress in reversing failure to thrive without direct supervision by nurse. *Education helps prepare patient to live as independently as possible and helps family to understand how best to support patient.*
- Refer patient and family members to appropriate agencies in the community, such as Meals On Wheels, that can help meet patient's needs *to ensure continuity of care.*
- Refer patient and family members to appropriate resources if patient has additional needs, such as the need for financial assistance, psychiatric help, or more in-depth nutritional counseling. *This will help ensure adherence to a comprehensive care plan.*

Evaluations for expected outcomes

- Patient expresses understanding of causes underlying failure to thrive.
- Patient expresses realization that he is depressed.
- Patient consumes sufficient amounts of food and nutrients.

• Patient sleeps for ___ hours without interruption.
• Family members demonstrate understanding of measures necessary to meet patient's needs.
• Patient gains weight.
• Patient reports feeling safe.
• Patient follows up on referrals for social service assistance.
• Patient follows up on referrals for psychiatric evaluation.
• Patient and family members use community resources to enhance patient's health.

Documentation
• Description of patient's physical condition
• Daily weight
• Fluid intake and output
• Patient's mental and emotional status
• Teaching provided to patient and family
• Patient's and family members' expressions indicating understanding of patient's problem
• Referrals to community agencies and response from these agencies
• Patient's response to nursing interventions
• Evaluations for expected outcomes

■ Body image disturbance

related to negative self-image

Definition
Disruption in self-perception that results from normal physical changes associated with aging

Assessment
• Sensory acuity, including vision and hearing

• Skin changes, including discoloration (for example, age spots), thinning, sagging, dryness associated with diminished sebaceous gland production, and wrinkling associated with diminished underlying connective structures
• Hair, including thinning and loss of color
• Musculature, including diminished muscle mass, alterations in body shape, and sagging skin
• Mental status, including denial, depression, discouragement, fear, and grief
• Activity level, including activities of daily living and physical exercise

Defining characteristics
• Excessive or inappropriate use of cosmetics to cover signs of aging
• Excessive or inappropriate use of hair-coloring products
• Frequent disparaging remarks about aging and its physical manifestations
• Hypersensitivity to remarks about advancing age
• Inappropriate dress for safety and comfort needs
• Indulgence in dangerous physical activities with intent of demonstrating youthful capabilities
• Personal rigidity or unwillingness to change
• Reluctance or refusal to wear corrective lenses or hearing aids
• Use of cosmetic surgery to reverse signs of aging
• Unwillingness to acknowledge physical changes associated with aging
• Unwillingness or inability to view aging in positive light

Associated medical diagnoses (selected)
Cataracts, osteoarthritis, osteoporosis, presbycusis, presbyopia, psoriasis

Expected outcomes

• Patient will alter skin care routine to reflect age-related changes and will use cosmetics appropriately.

• Patient will identify physical changes caused by aging without disparaging comments.

• Patient will identify at least one positive aspect of aging.

• Patient will use vision and hearing aids appropriately.

• Patient will dress appropriately with regard to safety, comfort, and personal taste.

• Patient will clean and style hair appropriately, without excessive coloring.

• Patient will demonstrate increased flexibility and willingness to consider lifestyle changes.

• Patient will participate in at least one social activity or group regularly.

• Patient will exercise and engage in other physical activity at level consistent with desire, ability, and safety.

Interventions and rationales

• Encourage patient to express feelings about physical changes associated with aging. *Active listening conveys caring and accepting attitude.*

• Provide information on appropriate self-care activities, such as:

– maintaining proper diet

– bathing less frequently

– using skin lotions to combat dryness

– exercising appropriately to maintain muscle mass, bone strength, and cardiorespiratory health

– avoiding fractures related to osteoporosis.

Providing accurate self-care information helps patient establish realistic goals.

• Encourage patient to consider new grooming styles or to seek advice from barber or cosmetologist on "updating" hair and makeup styles. *At-tractive, tasteful grooming may help older patient achieve sense of control over aging process.*

• Provide patient with referrals for corrective eyewear and hearing aids *to address sensory deficits.*

• Provide patient with positive role models. For example, offer to share literature that emphasizes accomplishments, capabilities, and contributions of older adults *to promote positive self-image and more positive view of elderly population.*

• During conversations with patient, focus on patient's strengths and what patient can do; emphasize positive aspects of aging *to increase patient's self-esteem.*

• Encourage patient to engage in social activities with people from all age-groups *to increase opportunities for human interaction, positive feedback, and development of new interests.*

Evaluations for expected outcomes

• Patient has clean, well-cared-for skin and uses cosmetics appropriately.

• Patient identifies age-related physical changes and comments on them positively.

• Patient identifies at least one personal advantage to growing older and one aspect of his life or personality that is better than it was 10 years ago.

• Patient uses vision and hearing aids comfortably.

• Patient dresses appropriately.

• Patient's hair appears clean and well groomed.

• Patient demonstrates increased flexibility and willingness to consider lifestyle changes.

• Patient participates in at least one social activity or group regularly.

• Patient engages in regular, appropriate exercise or activity.

Documentation
• Patient's statements about appearance, ability, and age
• Mental status assessment (baseline and ongoing)
• Physical assessment
• Interventions directed toward improving patient's body image
• Patient's response to nursing interventions
• Evaluations for expected outcomes

■ Body temperature alteration, risk for

related to decreased sensitivity of thermoreceptors

Definition
State of being at risk for failure to maintain body temperature within normal range

Assessment
• Age
• History of present illness
• Medical history, especially endocrine or nervous system illness
• Environmental temperature
• Medication history
• Neurologic status, including level of consciousness, knowledge level, and sensory, motor, and mental status
• Cardiovascular status, including heart rate and rhythm, blood pressure, pulses, capillary refill time, and electrocardiogram results
• Respiratory status, including breath sounds, arterial blood gas results, and respiratory rate, depth, and character
• Integumentary status, including temperature, color, and turgor
• GI status, including evidence of enema or laxative abuse, inspection of abdomen, and auscultation of bowel sounds

• Support systems, including family, friends, volunteer organizations, and clergy

Risk factors
• Advanced age
• Altered metabolic rate
• Dehydration
• Exposure to cold or hot environment
• Illness or trauma that affects temperature regulation
• Inactivity or vigorous activity
• Inappropriate clothing for temperature
• Extremes of weight (overweight or underweight)
• Sedation
• Use of medication that causes vasoconstriction or vasodilation

Associated medical diagnoses (selected)
Any disease, injury, or degenerative change may affect thermoreceptors in the elderly patient. Examples include adrenal insufficiency, Cushing's syndrome, diabetes insipidus, diabetes mellitus, diabetic ketoacidosis, hyperparathyroidism, hyperthyroidism, hypothyroidism, leukemia, and lung abscess.

Expected outcomes
• Patient's body temperature will remain normal.
• Patient's skin will remain warm and dry.
• Patient will state feelings of comfort.
• Patient won't exhibit signs of hypothermia or hyperthermia.
• Patient or family member will identify warning signs of hypothermia and hyperthermia.
• Patient or family member will express understanding of factors that cause hypothermia and hyperthermia.

• Patient or family member will describe ways to prevent altered body temperature.

Interventions and rationales

• Monitor patient's body temperature every 8 hours or more frequently, as indicated, *to ensure temperature doesn't vary more than 1° F from average normal (98.6° F [37° C] oral).* If it does, monitor more frequently.
• Assess patient's knowledge and lifestyle before teaching about hypothermia and hyperthermia *to gear teaching plan to patient's needs.*
• Using large black type, provide patient with list of signs and symptoms of altered body temperature:
– *Hypothermia:* shallow respirations; slow, weak pulse; decreased body temperature; low blood pressure; and pallor
– *Hyperthermia:* shivering, shaking chill; feeling hot; thirst; elevated body temperature; and high blood pressure. *Listing signs and symptoms helps patient to learn and identify warning signals of altered body temperature. Large black type is easier for older patient to read.*
• Encourage patient to remain active when in cool environment *to keep warm and maintain normal metabolism.*
• Explain to patient or family member why patient needs warm clothing in cool climates, even indoors. Suggest socks, nonslip house shoes, and leg warmers *to provide warmth to vulnerable lower extremities, where vascular changes may cause decreased temperature sensation.*
• Instruct patient or family member to label home thermostats with large numbers and to use black or bright contrasting colors to indicate appropriate temperature settings. *Easy-to-read labels will help patient maintain room temperature.*
• Teach patient or family member about dangers of too much direct sunlight on warm days *to prevent overheating in older patient with faulty thermoreceptors.*
• Discuss appropriate clothing for warm and cool climates. Suggest wearing clothes in layers, which can be removed or added as needed, *to accommodate increased susceptibility to temperature variations caused by aging vasculature.*
• Suggest that friend, family member, or volunteer from local community organization visit patient daily *to help ensure patient's safety.*

Evaluations for expected outcomes

• Patient's body temperature remains within normal limits.
• Patient's skin remains warm and dry.
• Patient reports absence of pain.
• Patient doesn't exhibit or report signs or symptoms of hypothermia or hyperthermia.
• Patient or family member identifies warning signs of hypothermia and hyperthermia.
• Patient or family member correctly identifies factors that may cause hypothermia or hyperthermia.
• Patient or family member describes changes to lifestyle that will prevent recurrence of altered body temperature.

Documentation

• Patient's or family member's perception of problem, including reports of excessive cold or heat
• Patient's temperature
• Observations of risk factors for altered body temperature
• Instructions regarding preventive measures

• Patient's or family member's statements of understanding of instructions
• Evaluations for expected outcomes

■ Cardiac output, decreased

related to reduced myocardial perfusion

Definition
Cardiovascular or respiratory symptoms resulting from insufficient blood being pumped by the heart

Assessment
• Mental status, especially sudden mental deterioration accompanied by confusion, agitation, and restlessness
• Cardiovascular status, including history of arrhythmias and syncope; skin color, temperature, and turgor; jugular vein distention; hepatojugular reflux; heart rate and rhythm; heart sounds; blood pressure; peripheral pulses; electrocardiogram (ECG), echocardiogram, and phonocardiogram results; serum digitalis level; and aspartate aminotransferase, lactate dehydrogenase, and creatine kinase isoenzyme levels.
• Respiratory status, including respiratory rate and depth, breath sounds, chest X-ray, and arterial blood gas results
• Renal status, including weight, intake and output, urine specific gravity, and serum electrolyte levels

Defining characteristics
• Abnormal chest X-ray and cardiac enzyme levels
• Accessory muscle use
• Altered mental state
• Arrhythmias, ECG changes, and increased heart rate

• Audible S_3 or S_4 heart sounds
• Chest pain, coughing and wheezing, fatigue, restlessness, and cold, clammy skin
• Crackles
• Decreased cardiac output and peripheral pulses
• Dyspnea, increased respiratory rate, orthopnea, and paroxysmal nocturnal dyspnea
• Edema
• Ejection fraction less than 40%
• Elevated pulmonary artery pressure
• Jugular vein distention
• Mixed venous oxygen
• Oliguria
• Skin color changes
• Variations in blood pressure readings
• Weight gain

Associated medical diagnoses (selected)
Anemia, cardiac arrhythmias, cor pulmonale, digitalis toxicity, heart failure, myocardial infarction (MI)

Expected outcomes
• Patient won't experience tachypnea, restlessness, anxiety, dyspnea, confusion, fainting, dizzy spells, lightheadedness, nausea, fatigue, or weakness.
• Patient will tolerate exercise and activities at usual level, taking into account any cardiac damage.
• Patient will maintain respiratory status within established parameters.
• Patient's cardiac status will stabilize, with no evidence of arrhythmias.
• Patient and family members will understand and comply with prescribed therapeutic regimen.

Interventions and rationales
• Administer medications as ordered, monitor intake and output, and observe for adverse reactions. *In older patients, decreased renal and liver function may lead to rapid development of toxicity.*

• Monitor for dyspnea or breathlessness every 2 to 4 hours, and report changes from baseline. *Older patients with silent or painless MI frequently develop dyspnea related to left-sided heart failure.*

• Monitor mental status every 2 to 4 hours and report deviations from baseline. *Dizziness, confusion, lightheadedness, and restlessness may indicate decreased cerebral blood flow caused by slow carotid sinus reflex.*

• Administer diuretics cautiously to patient. Monitor closely for cardiac overload by taking frequent vital signs and documenting intake and output accurately. Report signs and symptoms of cardiac overload, such as elevated central venous pressure, fluid intake above output, and increased pulmonary artery pressure. *When fluid in lungs and lower extremities is mobilized and returns to circulation, it may overtax patient's weakened myocardium.*

• Assess apical and radial pulses every 2 to 4 hours and report deviations from baseline *to monitor for arrhythmias, impending cardiac arrest, hypertension, or shock.*

• Administer oxygen to patient, as ordered, especially after patient eats or during increased activity, *to increase oxygenation of brain and heart.*

• Make sure patient gets adequate rest and doesn't exceed activity tolerance level *to ease dyspnea, decrease oxygen demand on myocardium, and prevent hydrostatic pneumonia, venous thrombosis, and cardiovascular deconditioning.*

• Teach patient or family member symptoms of possible cardiac problems:
– dizziness
– indigestion
– nausea
– retrosternal pain
– shortness of breath
– unusual fatigue and weakness.
Knowing symptoms of decreased cardiac functioning helps patient to feel greater control over situation and encourages compliance with treatment plan.

• Reduce stressful elements, such as excessive noise or light in patient's environment, *to help decrease arrhythmias, anxiety, and restlessness.*

• Encourage patient to increase fluid intake and dietary fiber and to take natural stool softeners *to avoid Valsalva's maneuver during defecation, which can increase heart rate and blood pressure, cause reflex bradycardia, and decrease cardiac output.*

Evaluations for expected outcomes

• Patient experiences fewer dyspneic episodes, with no syncope or dizzy spells.

• Patient returns to normal activity and exercise levels, taking into account extent of cardiac damage.

• Patient maintains normal respiratory status.

• Physical examination reveals that arrhythmias are absent.

• Patient and family members understand and comply with prescribed therapeutic regimen.

Documentation

• Patient's chief complaint
• Signs or symptoms of decreased cardiac output
• Therapeutic interventions and patient's responses
• Activity and exercise tolerance
• Diet and sleep patterns
• Teaching provided to patient and family member
• Evaluations for expected outcomes

■ Constipation

related to diet, fluid intake, activity level, and personal bowel habits

Definition

Change in normal bowel habits characterized by decreased frequency, difficult or incomplete passage of stool, or passage of dry, hard stool

Assessment

• History of bowel disorder or surgery
• GI status, including nausea and vomiting, usual bowel habits, tenesmus, distention, flatulence, laxative or enema use, and medications
• Oral status, including inspection of oral cavity (gums, tongue, and dentition), pain or discomfort, and salivation
• Activity status, including type, duration, and frequency of exercise; lifestyle; and access to toilet facilities during work and recreation
• Nutritional status, including appetite, dietary intake, amount and type of dietary fiber, fluid intake, food likes and dislikes, meal pattern, access to food supply and storage facilities, access to shopping and transportation, and financial resources available for food
• Drug history, including use of constipating agents (such as aluminum-based antacids, anticholinergics, antidepressants, iron supplements, laxatives, and narcotics) and history of laxative abuse

Defining characteristics

• Abdominal tenderness or pain and feeling of rectal fullness or pressure
• Borborygmi, hypoactive or hyperactive bowel sounds, or abdominal dullness on percussion
• Bright red blood with stool; bark-colored or black, tarry stool; or hard, dry stool
• Change in bowel pattern
• Changes in mental status, urinary incontinence, unexplained falls, or elevated body temperature
• Decreased frequency and stool volume
• Distended abdomen and increased abdominal pressure
• Inability to pass stool
• General fatigue, anorexia, headache, indigestion, nausea, or vomiting
• Oozing liquid stool
• Palpable rectal or abdominal mass
• Severe flatus
• Soft, pastelike stool in rectum
• Straining and possibly pain during defecation

Associated medical diagnoses (selected)

Anxiety disorder, cerebrovascular accident, depression, diabetes mellitus, diverticulitis, hypothyroidism

Expected outcomes

• Patient will participate in development of bowel program.
• Patient will report urge to defecate, as appropriate.
• Patient will increase fluid and fiber intake.
• Patient will report easy and complete evacuation of stool.
• Patient will increase activity level.
• Patient will have elimination pattern within normal limits.
• Patient will describe changes in personal habits that will help maintain normal elimination.

Interventions and rationales

• Monitor frequency and characteristics of patient's stool. *Careful monitoring forms basis of effective treatment plan.*

• Monitor and record patient's fluid intake and output. *Inadequate fluid intake contributes to dry feces and constipation. Monitoring fluid balance ensures adequate fluid intake and promotes elimination.*

• Provide privacy for elimination *to promote physiologic functioning.*

• Encourage patient to use bedside commode or walk to toilet facilities. Avoid use of bedpan *because such use may inhibit normal positioning for evacuation, thereby exacerbating constipation.*

• Work with patient to plan and implement individualized bowel regimen *to establish regular elimination schedule.*

• Emphasize to patient importance of responding to urge to defecate. Be alert for any mental status changes that may impair patient's ability to recognize or attend to need to defecate or to report need to caregiver. *Timely response to urge to defecate is necessary to maintain normal physiologic functioning and to avoid pressure and discomfort in lower GI tract.*

• Teach patient to locate public restrooms and to wear easily removable clothing on outings *to promote normal bowel functioning.*

• Teach patient to massage his abdomen once per day. Show him how to locate and gently massage along transverse and descending colon. *In older patient, neural centers in lower intestinal wall may be impaired, making it more difficult for body to evacuate feces. Massage may help stimulate peristalsis and urge to defecate.*

• If abdominal pressure is inadequate to complete defecation, encourage patient to perform rocking motion of upper body *to aid in elimination.*

• Plan and implement exercise routine, such as walking, leg raising, abdominal muscle strengthening, and Kegel exercises. *Exercise promotes abdominal and pelvic muscle tone necessary for normal elimination.*

• Encourage intake of high-fiber foods. *Many older patients have reduced intestinal muscle tone and decreased strength in abdominal muscles, resulting in slower peristalsis, dry feces, and decreased ability to exert pressure for evacuation. High-fiber foods supply bulk for normal elimination and improve intestinal muscle tone.*

• Unless contraindicated, encourage fluid intake of 6 to 8 glasses daily *to maintain normal metabolic processes and prevent excessive reabsorption of fluid from GI contents.*

• Teach patient sensible use of laxatives and enemas *to avoid laxative dependency. Overuse of laxatives and enemas may cause fluid and electrolyte loss and damage to intestinal mucosa.*

• Help patient understand diet modification plan. If appropriate, have patient consult with dietitian *to encourage compliance with prescribed diet.*

Evaluations for expected outcomes

• Patient participates in planning and implementing bowel program.

• Patient reports urge to defecate, as appropriate.

• Patient's daily diet includes high-fiber foods and adequate fluids.

• Patient reports easy and complete evacuation of stool.

• Patient increases activity level.

• Patient achieves routine bowel function without excessive use of laxatives, enemas, straining, or discomfort.

• Patient makes adaptations to lifestyle to ensure maintenance of bowel function.

Documentation
• Patient's expressions of concern regarding constipation, dietary changes, laxative use, and bowel pattern
• Physical findings
• Intake and output
• Observations of diet, characteristics of stool, and activity level
• Teaching provided and patient's response
• Patient's expressions indicating understanding of bowel program
• Evaluations for expected outcomes

■ Coping, ineffective family: Compromised

related to caring for dependent, aging family member

Definition
State in which a normally functioning family provides insufficient, ineffective, or compromised support, comfort, assistance, or encouragement to patient

Assessment
• Patient status, including age, medical history, self-concept, physical disabilities or limitations, present living arrangements, and role in family
• Family assessment, including communication style, family coping style, perceptions of the aging process (myths vs. realities), health problems of other members, financial status, support systems, and additional stressors
• Patient's current health crisis (emotional or physical)

Defining characteristics
• Attempts to assist or support patient with unsatisfactory results (family member)

• Displays of protective behavior disproportionate to patient's abilities or need for autonomy (family member)
• Expressed concern about family's response to health problem (patient)
• Expressed inadequate understanding or knowledge base that interferes with effective assistive or supportive behaviors (family member)
• Reported preoccupation with personal reaction to patient's health problem (family member)
• Withdrawal from or limited communication with patient at time of need (family member)

Associated medical diagnoses (selected)
This nursing diagnosis can be associated with any condition that results in temporary or permanent dependence on family members, such as adrenal insufficiency, Alzheimer's disease, cerebrovascular accident, hip fracture, joint replacement, osteoarthritis, and Parkinson's disease.

Expected outcomes
• As appropriate, family members will assume responsibilities formerly held by patient.
• Family members will express feelings about responsibilities in caring for an older relative.
• Patient and family members will express understanding of maturational and developmental issues that contributed to crisis.
• Patient and family members will identify and make use of appropriate community services.
• Family members will demonstrate improved capacity to plan care for older relative.
• Patient and family members will express satisfaction with their improved ability to cope with current crisis.

Interventions and rationales

• Identify primary caregiver in the family and assess roles of other family members *to establish family hierarchy and plan interventions.*

• Educate patient and family members about aging process. Discuss how changes in patient have affected family *to assess needs of patient and family members.*

• Avoid becoming involved in power struggle among family members. *Patient may no longer be able to fulfill his family role, and sudden shift in roles may lead to power struggle among family members. Patient or family members may try to manipulate you as part of this power struggle. Maintaining neutral, objective approach will help family members to adjust to role changes.*

• As appropriate, arrange and conduct conference for family members; include patient when possible. *Long-established communication patterns may interfere with family members' ability to resolve conflicts and make decisions. Your presence may help family members to express feelings, identify needs and resources, and develop more healthy ways of interacting.*

• Encourage family members to express their feelings about caring for older family member. *Nonjudgmental attitude promotes effective communication.*

• Encourage family members to identify strengths and weaknesses in family system. Help them explore values, beliefs, perceived changes, and actual role changes related to older patient's altered physical or emotional condition *to enhance insight.*

• Assist patient and family members in developing short-term and long-term goals and contingency plans *to increase sense of control and direction for future.*

• Help patient and family members identify appropriate community services, such as adult day-care, respite care, and geriatric outreach services, *to provide access to additional sources of support.*

• Suggest using care manager to help with ongoing coordination of patient's needs. Help family identify care manager they can relate to. *Care manager may help simplify decision making and limit family conflict.*

• Help family members explore coping strategies used effectively during past crises and discuss how to apply these strategies to present situation *to make family members aware of their demonstrated ability to adapt to change.*

• Provide emotional support for primary caregiver. *Family member who takes on the most responsibility for patient has double burden of caring for older adult and adjusting to new role in the family.*

• Maintain nonjudgmental attitude while working with family members. Some families may hesitate to accept outside help. Other families may be unwilling to make even small sacrifices to care for older relative. Remember that, if family members haven't been supportive or close to patient before, you're unlikely to change their attitudes. *Nonjudgmental outlook benefits both patient and family members. Learning to accept your limitations will help you avoid burnout.*

• Remain supportive and understanding if patient or family members are reluctant to use needed community resources, such as adult day-care, respite care, and home health services. *Older patient may feel that using outside resources means sacrificing independence; family members may feel that asking for help indicates lack of caring.*

Evaluations for expected outcomes
• As appropriate, family members assume responsibilities formerly held by patient.
• Patient and family members share feelings about current crisis.
• Patient and family members express understanding of maturational and developmental issues that led to crisis.
• Patient and family members acknowledge need for outside help to cope with crisis and identify and contact community resources.
• Family members demonstrate improved capacity for short-term and long-term planning.
• Patient and family members express satisfaction with their improved ability to cope with current crisis.

Documentation
• Patient's and family members' understanding of aging process and current health crisis
• Observations of patient's and family members' reactions to crisis
• Family members' willingness to become involved in patient care
• Nursing interventions
• Teaching provided
• Patient's and family members' responses to interventions and instructions
• Referrals to community agencies
• Evaluations for expected outcomes

■ Coping, ineffective individual

related to inability to solve problems or adapt to demands of daily living

Definition
Impaired ability to adapt behavior to meet life's demands and role expectations

Assessment
• Age
• Lifestyle changes necessitated by disease or illness
• Role changes caused by retirement, relocation, or death of spouse, family members, or friends
• Changes associated with normal aging, such as decreased vision, hearing, and physical endurance
• Perceived coping ability
• Usual coping mechanisms
• Support systems, including family, friends, church, and community organizations

Defining characteristics
• Change in communication patterns
• Decreased use of social support
• Destructive behavior toward self or others
• Difficulty asking for help
• Fatigue
• High illness rate
• Inability to meet basic needs and role expectations
• Lack of goal-directed behavior, such as inability to attend, difficulty organizing information, poor concentration, and poor problem-solving abilities
• Maladaptive coping behaviors
• Risk-taking behaviors
• Sleep disturbance

• Statements indicating inability to cope
• Substance abuse

Associated medical diagnoses (selected)

Alzheimer's disease, cataracts, deafness, end-stage disease (renal or cardiac), paralysis, Parkinson's disease, rheumatoid arthritis

Expected outcomes

• Patient will verbalize increased ability to cope.
• Patient will expand support network to meet social and emotional needs.
• Patient will locate and use appropriate resources for help in problem solving.
• Patient will report increased ability to meet demands of daily living.
• Patient will make changes to environment to ensure enhanced coping or move into long-term care facility as needed.

Interventions and rationales

• Refer patient to social service agencies, such as geriatric assessment centers, adult day-care programs, and home health care agencies, as appropriate, *to expand his support network and help him cope with physical, psychosocial, and economic stressors.*
• Assist patient in becoming involved with informal community programs, such as volunteer, foster grandparent, church, or synagogue groups, *to provide peer and social contact and decrease patient's loneliness and isolation.*
• Encourage patient to reminisce about past *to help him recall past challenges and successful coping strategies.*
• Provide patient with information about aging process, methods of coping with stress, and techniques used by other older adults to meet demands of daily living *to assist patient in implementing coping strategies.*
• If patient must enter long-term care facility or undergo lengthy home-based convalescence, help him put situation in perspective. Explain to patient that extreme stress can overwhelm anyone, even well-adapted individuals with strong support systems. When stress becomes overwhelming, rehabilitation in secure environment may be best option. Entering long-term care facility isn't "the beginning of the end," as many people think, but rather an additional mechanism for ensuring optimal recovery. *Taking time to provide carefully worded explanation may help patient come to terms with his situation.*
• If patient requires treatment in long-term care facility, provide least restrictive environment possible *to reduce patient's fear and anxiety, help him retain sense of control, and encourage him to use his abilities to maximum.*
• Discuss with patient possibility of making lifestyle changes, such as moving closer to relatives, moving to retirement community, or hiring someone to help with housework, *to improve ability to cope.*

Evaluations for expected outcomes

• Patient states understanding of strategies to improve coping ability.
• Patient reports success in developing support network to meet social and emotional needs.
• Patient contacts resources to help with problem solving.
• Patient reports increased ability to meet demands of daily living.
• Patient identifies lifestyle changes that will improve his ability to cope

or states that he understands and accepts need to move to long-term care facility or retirement community.

Documentation
• Patient's expression of feelings about present life situation and difficulty coping
• Formal and informal sources of support identified by patient or family members
• Observations of patient's behavior in response to stressful situations
• Teaching provided and patient's response
• Use of outside support services
• Evaluations for expected outcomes

■ Denial

related to fear or anxiety about aging

Definition
Attempt to disavow knowledge or meaning of an event to reduce fear of growing older

Assessment
• Age
• Appearance
• Activity patterns, including sudden interest or participation in activities that may be dangerous
• Self-concept, including self-esteem, body image, and perception of self in life continuum
• Coping behaviors
• Mental status, including affect, communication, memory, mood, orientation, perception, abstract thinking, judgment, and insight

Defining characteristics
• Delay in seeking medical attention or refusal of medical attention to detriment of health
• Inability to admit impact of aging on life pattern
• Inappropriate affect
• Minimization of signs and symptoms of aging
• Refusal to admit fear of death or invalidism
• Use of dismissive gestures or comments when speaking of distressing events
• Use of self-treatment to relieve symptoms

Associated medical diagnoses (selected)
This diagnosis may be associated with any disorder that causes physical disability or limitations. Examples include angina pectoris, chronic obstructive pulmonary disease, chronic renal failure, coronary artery disease, hip fracture, hypertension, macular degeneration, osteoporosis, presbycusis, presbyopia, renal calculi, and rheumatoid arthritis.

Expected outcomes
• Patient will discuss aging process and impact on ability to participate in hobbies and other activities.
• Patient will express interest in age-appropriate community activities.
• Patient will set aside time for reminiscing as part of daily routine.
• Patient will express more positive view of growing older.
• Patient will adapt activities to avoid unnecessary physical stress on body.

Interventions and rationales
• Discuss challenge of being older adult in today's youth-oriented society *to encourage patient to express feelings and help him recognize that*

he doesn't have to accept society's prejudices about aging.
• Discuss with patient and family members changes that normally occur as part of aging process *to correct misconceptions.*
• Discuss how to adapt activities and hobbies to accommodate physical changes that occur with aging *to avoid excess physical stress.*
• Discuss advantages of growing older, such as having more time to pursue hobbies and other interests, *to help patient develop positive view of aging.*
• Emphasize variety of activities that patient can continue to do well *to enhance self-esteem.*
• Encourage patient to set aside time for reminiscing as part of daily routine. *Reminiscing helps patient to affirm past and promotes self-esteem.*
• Provide information about senior volunteer groups and part-time work or volunteer opportunities *to help patient maintain physical and mental functioning and promote social interaction.*
• Invite active member of senior citizens club, social group, senior sports league, or advocacy group to visit patient *to provide positive role model.*

Evaluations for expected outcomes
• Patient expresses positive and negative feelings about aging.
• Patient states intention to engage in age-appropriate community activity.
• Patient expresses willingness to set aside time for reminiscing.
• Patient expresses more positive view of growing older.
• Patient adapts activities to avoid unnecessary physical stress on body.

Documentation
• Evidence of patient's difficulty adjusting to the aging process

• Nursing interventions
• Referrals provided
• Patient's response to nursing interventions
• Patient's statements that indicate more positive attitude toward growing older
• Evaluations for expected outcomes

■ Gas exchange impairment

related to carbon dioxide retention or excess mucus production

Definition
Interference in cellular respiration caused by inadequate exchange or transport of oxygen and carbon dioxide

Assessment
• Age
• Sex
• Smoking history
• Occupational or environmental risk factors, such as exposure to asbestos, smog, and pollutants
• Respiratory status, including history of respiratory disorders, breath sounds, sputum characteristics, accessory muscle use, cyanosis, and arterial blood gas (ABG) levels
• Cardiovascular status, including skin color and temperature, heart rate and rhythm, heart sounds, blood pressure, hemoglobin and hematocrit, red and white blood cell and platelet counts, prothrombin and partial thromboplastin times, and serum iron concentrations
• Psychosocial status, including mental status, knowledge level, lifestyle, and support systems

• Activity status, including ability to perform activities of daily living (ADLs)

Defining characteristics
• Abnormal arterial pH and ABG levels
• Abnormal respiratory rate, rhythm, and depth
• Confusion
• Diaphoresis
• Dyspnea
• Headache on awakening
• Hypoxia and hypoxemia
• Irritability
• Nasal flaring
• Pale, dusky skin
• Restlessness or somnolence
• Tachycardia
• Vision disturbances

Associated medical diagnoses (selected)
Chronic bronchitis, chronic obstructive pulmonary disease, emphysema, heart failure

Expected outcomes
• Patient will exercise and perform ADLs without experiencing dyspnea or excessive fatigue.
• Patient will maintain adequate fluid intake.
• Patient will maintain adequate ventilation and have clear breath sounds on auscultation.
• Patient or family members will state understanding of causes for impaired gas exchange and behaviors to prevent it.

Interventions and rationales
• Establish baseline values for respiratory assessment *to distinguish age-related changes that may mimic disease states from disease. Older adults take shorter breaths. This decreases maximum breathing capacity, vital capacity, residual volume, and functional capacity.*
• Auscultate lungs every 4 hours, taking into account anatomic changes that may occur in older patients, such as kyphosis, deviated trachea, and dowager's hump, *to detect abnormal breath sounds.* Report abnormalities.
• Administer and monitor oxygen therapy, as ordered, *to enhance oxygenation and detect signs of decompensation. Older patients have high incidence of chronic cardiac and chronic pulmonary disorders. Detecting early changes in condition allows for early intervention.*
• Teach patient relaxation techniques and ask for return demonstration. *Using relaxation techniques may help reduce tissue oxygen demand.*
• Incorporate patient's past experiences into teaching plan when conveying information about disease, medications, and lifestyle changes. *Information becomes more meaningful when related to previous experiences.*
• Help patient schedule ADLs to allow for rest periods. *Older patients have more fibrous, less elastic alveoli that contain fewer functional capillaries, which decreases exertional capacity. Patient needs rest periods to conserve respiratory effort.*
• Help patient identify positions that maximize ventilatory capacity, such as leaning over bedside table when sitting or using large wedge pillow under shoulders. *In older patient, accessory muscles of pharynx and larynx may atrophy, making it necessary for patient to assume breathing positions that maximize ventilation, perfusion, and thoracic expansion.*
• Encourage adequate fluid intake. *Older adults may have diminished sense of thirst, which may lead to dry mucous membranes. Dry mucous membranes*

in turn may impede removal of secretions and promote respiratory infection. Consuming adequate fluids helps to liquefy secretions, reducing energy required to mobilize them. Record intake and output *to monitor fluid status.*
• Perform bronchial hygiene, such as positioning, coughing, deep breathing, percussion, postural drainage, and suctioning, *to promote and maintain patent airway.*
• Evaluate home environment and recommend changes, such as moving patient's bedroom to first floor, *to reduce exertion.*

Evaluations for expected outcomes
• Patient performs exercise and ADLs with minimum fatigue and increased endurance.
• Patient maintains adequate fluid intake.
• Patient maintains adequate ventilation and has clear breath sounds on auscultation.
• Patient or family members state understanding of causes for impaired gas exchange and behaviors to prevent it.

Documentation
• Patient's complaints of dyspnea or fatigue
• Observations of patient's condition
• Patient's response to nursing interventions
• Teaching provided and patient's response
• Patient's expressions indicating understanding of plan of care
• Evaluations for expected outcomes

■ Grieving, anticipatory

related to perceived potential loss of life

Definition
Intellectual and emotional responses through which an individual attempts to adjust self-concept based on a perceived personal loss. The concept of anticipatory grieving can be applied to families and communities as well.

Assessment
• Age
• Developmental stage
• Presence of living will, durable power of attorney for health care, and other advance directives
• History of chronic illness or terminal diagnosis
• Mental status, including level of consciousness and orientation
• Emotional status, including evidence of anger, apathy, depression, or hostility
• Support systems, including family members, significant other, friends, and clergy
• Spiritual practices, including religious affiliation and use of spiritual support systems
• Customs and beliefs related to illness, death, and suffering

Defining characteristics
• Altered communication patterns
• Change in eating habits, sleep and dream patterns, activity level, or libido
• Denial of potential loss of life
• Difficulty taking on different roles
• Expressions of distress over potential loss of life
• Expressed guilt, anger, sorrow, and bargaining

• Resolution of grief before loss of life

Associated medical diagnoses (selected)

Brain tumors, cor pulmonale, end-stage disease (cardiac or renal), Hodgkin's disease, hydatidiform mole, leukemia, multiple myeloma, multiple sclerosis, pemphigus

Expected outcomes

• Patient will express and accept feelings about anticipated death.
• Patient will progress through stages of grieving process in his own way.
• Patient will practice religious rituals and use other coping mechanisms appropriate to end of life.
• Family members or significant other will participate in providing supportive care and comfort to patient.

Interventions and rationales

• Provide time for patient to express feelings about death or terminal illness. *Active listening helps patient to lessen feelings of loneliness and isolation.* Don't approach patient with busy, hurried attitude, *which can block communication.*
• Establish relationship that encourages patient to express concerns about death. *Basic nursing care combined with genuine interest in patient fosters trust and understanding.*
• Guide patient in life review. Encourage him to write or tape record life history as lasting gift to family members. *Life review allows patient to survey events from his past and give them meaningful interpretation.*
• Involve interdisciplinary team (including psychologist, nurse, patient, nutritionist, doctor, physical therapist, and chaplain) in providing care for dying patient. *Each team member offers unique expertise for meeting dying patient's needs.*

• Encourage family members to become involved in care of dying patient. Communicate with patient and family members honestly and compassionately. *Giving family members role in patient care helps to relieve anxiety and lessen feelings of regret and guilt. Honest communication is important because family members need opportunity to acknowledge loss and say farewell.*
• Demonstrate acceptance of patient's response to anticipated death, whatever that response may be: crying, sadness, anger, fear, or denial. *Each patient responds to dying in his own way. Helping him express his feelings freely will enhance his ability to cope.*
• Help patient progress through psychological stages associated with anticipated death, including shock and denial, anger, bargaining, depression, and acceptance, *to help you anticipate dying patient's psychological needs. Keep in mind, however, that not all dying patients go through each stage.*
• Support patient's spiritual coping behaviors. For example, arrange for patient to have at bedside objects that provide spiritual comfort (such as Bible, prayer shawl, pictures, statues, or rosary beads). *Even patients for whom religious practice hasn't been dominant part of life frequently turn to religion when confronted by death or serious illness.*
• Inform patient about hospice services. Hospice services emphasize symptomatic relief and caring, with aim of improving patient and family comfort until death occurs, instead of prolonging life for its own sake. *Hospice care is appropriate alternative for patient with incurable illness.*
• Provide referrals for home health assistance if patient will be cared for at home *to support patient's decision to remain at home.*

Evaluations for expected outcomes
• Patient expresses and accepts feelings brought about by anticipated death.
• Patient progresses through stages of grief in his own way.
• Patient participates in religious rituals and uses other appropriate coping mechanisms.
• Patient receives adequate support during end of life from family members, friends, and members of health care team.

Documentation
• Patient's verbal expressions indicating feelings about anticipated death
• Observations of emotional responses, such as crying, anger, and withdrawal
• Interventions to help patient cope with anticipated death
• Patient's requests for assistance in achieving spiritual comfort (spiritual objects and visits from minister, priest, or rabbi)
• Patient's responses to interventions
• Evaluations for expected outcomes

■ Home maintenance management impairment

related to impaired cognitive, emotional, or psychomotor functioning

Definition
Disruption in patient's ability to meet household maintenance needs adequately

Assessment
• Age
• Sex
• Home environment

• Financial resources
• Patient's psychosocial status, including perception of reality, communication patterns, role responsibilities, degree of awareness and concern, history of psychiatric-related illness, support systems, and cognitive, memory, and motor abilities
• Caregiver's psychosocial status, including stressors, support systems, and understanding of patient's care requirements

Defining characteristics
• Description of outstanding debts or financial crisis
• Expressed difficulty in maintaining comfortable home
• Household in disrepair, marked by excessive clutter, unwashed clothing and cooking equipment, offensive odors, presence of rodents and insects, accumulation of dirt and food wastes, and inappropriate temperature
• Lack of necessary equipment or aids
• Requests for assistance with home maintenance
• Expressed sense of being overtaxed, marked by exhaustion and anxiety

Associated medical diagnoses (selected)
This diagnosis can be associated with any acute or chronic alteration in patient's health status, such as osteoarthritis and Parkinson's disease.

Expected outcomes
• Patient and caregiver will express concern about poor home maintenance and verbalize plans to correct health and safety hazards in the home.
• Patient and caregiver will identify community organizations that can help ease transition from hospital to home or long-term care facility.
• Patient and caregiver will develop schedule for doing household tasks.

Interventions and rationales

• Help patient and caregiver identify strengths and weaknesses in current home maintenance practices *to provide focus for interventions.*

• Discuss with patient and caregiver obstacles to meeting home maintenance needs *to provide basis for program to meet health and safety requirements.*

• Determine patient's capability and motivation to achieve higher level of home maintenance. *Self-motivation is necessary to ensure change.*

• Help patient and caregiver explore community resources, such as Meals On Wheels, senior centers, home health care agencies, homemaker services, cleaning services, self-help groups, church programs, and retired senior volunteer programs, *to ease transition from hospital to home.*

• Allow caregiver to express feelings about responsibility for patient's health care regimen and household upkeep. When appropriate, discuss opportunities for caregiver to assign responsibility to other family members or make use of community resources. Encourage caregiver to ask questions, seek help, and make decisions *to enhance communication and help caregiver and family members form realistic expectations.*

• Conduct home visit or evaluate patient's description of home *to assess safety needs and make recommendations for structural alterations. For example, patient may benefit from installing ramps, enlarging doorways, or moving second-floor bedroom to first-floor family room.*

• Discuss alternative housing opportunities with patient and caregiver, such as moving patient to life care community, *to provide necessary information to make appropriate decisions regarding patient's future.*

• Based on assessment of patient's health and home environment, determine need for assistive devices, including:
– hearing aids
– hand-held or table-stand magnifying glasses
– hospital bed
– large-print items
– telephones for hearing impaired
– telephone dial covers with large numbers
– telephones with programmed dialing
– wheelchair
– amplifiers for phone receivers
– clocks that chime or recite time
– canes
– walkers
– handrails
– safety bars for toilet and bath
– automatic chair lifts
– commode chairs
– shower chairs
– orthotics.

Using assistive devices helps patient remain independent and improves self-confidence and self-esteem.

• Help patient develop written daily and weekly schedules for performing household tasks *to provide structure and consistency and set standards for measuring progress.*

• Involve patient in decision-making process by providing choice of where, when, and how to carry out appropriate home maintenance activities *to increase patient's feelings of independence and self-esteem.*

• If patient can't perform certain tasks without assistance, teach caregiver or others how to provide help *to ensure patient's needs are met.*

Evaluations for expected outcomes

• Patient and caregiver express understanding of changes needed to promote maximum health and safety in home.

• Patient and caregiver list community resources to assist with home maintenance deficits.
• Patient and caregiver establish and follow daily and weekly schedules for home maintenance activities.

Documentation
• Patient's perception of problems in home maintenance
• Observations regarding magnitude of home maintenance deficits
• Interventions to alleviate home maintenance deficits
• Responses of caregiver and others asked to assist patient with home maintenance
• Evaluations for expected outcomes

■ Incontinence, stress

Definition
Involuntary passage of urine, which occurs when intravesical pressure exceeds the maximum ureteral pressure and detrusor function is insufficient or absent

Assessment
• History of incontinence symptoms, including onset and pattern
• Physical observations, including personal and perineal hygiene and complete bladder assessment
• Mental status, including cognition and affect
• Mobility status
• Emotional status, including evidence of social withdrawal
• Current medication regimen

Defining characteristics
• Dribbling with increased abdominal pressure
• Frequency
• Urgency

Associated medical diagnoses (selected)
Alzheimer's disease, atrophic senile vaginitis, cerebrovascular accident, cirrhosis, depression, diabetes mellitus, obesity, urinary incontinence, urinary tract infections, uterine prolapse

Expected outcomes
• Patient will understand causes of stress incontinence.
• Patient will establish plan compatible with lifestyle to manage symptoms.
• Patient will resume normal social activities.
• Patient will maintain continence with the aid of incontinence pads or frequent toileting.
• Patient will perform Kegel exercises.

Interventions and rationales
• Discuss stress incontinence and associated social stigma with patient in nonjudgmental manner. Tell patient many people experience incontinence. *Patient may be reluctant to discuss incontinence, which can have negative effect on self-image. Nonjudgmental approach may help to ease embarrassment and encourage open discussion of problem.*
• Assist patient in obtaining appropriate evaluation and care for underlying causes of stress incontinence *to ensure prompt diagnosis and treatment.*
• Review current medication regimen for drugs that can contribute to stress incontinence, including diuretics, central nervous system depressants, and anticholinergics. Discuss with doctor possibility of changing medications or medication schedule *to relieve symptoms.*
• Develop individualized toileting schedule, increasing intervals by 30 minutes until patient achieves 2- to 3-hour pattern. *Bladder retraining may help alleviate symptoms.*

• Teach patient to do Kegel exercises to strengthen pelvic floor muscles. Instruct patient to tighten muscles of pelvic floor to stop flow of urine while urinating and then to release muscles to restart flow *to strengthen urinary sphincter muscle and restore control.*
• Discuss benefits and costs of adult incontinence pads with patient. *Pads, although costly, are nonintrusive, easy to manage, and easily removed.*
• Encourage patient to take short trips outside home when symptoms are under control *to enhance patient's confidence and reduce social embarrassment.*
• When mobility is problem, help patient obtain bedside commode *to reduce need for adult incontinence pads, which can adversely affect patient's self-image.*

Evaluations for expected outcomes
• Patient expresses, without embarrassment, understanding of causes of stress incontinence.
• Patient manages symptoms successfully.
• Patient begins to resume social activity.
• Patient maintains continence with aid of incontinence pads or frequent toileting.
• Patient performs Kegel exercises.

Documentation
• Patient's symptoms of stress incontinence, including onset and pattern
• Patient teaching, including Kegel exercises, use of incontinence pads, and other control strategies
• Patient's responses to nursing interventions
• Evaluations for expected outcomes

■ Incontinence, urinary urge, risk for

Definition
Potential for involuntary passage of urine occurring shortly after a strong sense of urgency to void

Assessment
• Age and sex
• Vital signs
• Drug history
• History of illness that may cause neuromuscular dysfunction, including cerebrovascular accident, spinal cord injury, head injury, urinary tract disease, and infection
• Genitourinary status, including pain or discomfort, urinalysis, urine specific gravity, use of urinary assistive devices, voiding pattern, and cystometrogram results
• Fluid and electrolyte status, including intake and output, mucous membranes, postvoiding residual volume, skin turgor, and serum electrolyte, blood urea nitrogen, and creatinine levels
• Neuromuscular status, including ambulation ability, cognitive status, sensory ability, and degree of neuromuscular function
• Sexuality status, including patient's or partner's expressions of concern
• Psychosocial status, including coping skills, self-concept, stressors (finances, family, job), patient's and family members' perceptions of health problem, and patient's motivation to meet self-care needs

Risk factors
• Bladder contraction or spasms
• Dysuria
• Frequency
• Hesitancy
• Incontinence

- Loss of urine regardless of position
- Mobility impairment
- Nocturia
- Sensory or neuromuscular impairment
- Urgency

Associated medical diagnoses (selected)

Brain abscess, cerebral aneurysm, cerebrovascular accident, cystitis, Guillain-Barré syndrome, head injury, multiple sclerosis, muscular dystrophy, myasthenia gravis, Parkinson's disease, spinal cord injury or tumor, urinary tract infection

Expected outcomes

- Patient will state if he can anticipate when episodes of incontinence are likely to occur.
- Patient will state understanding of potential causes of urge incontinence and its treatment.
- Patient will avoid complications of urge incontinence or such complications will be minimized.
- Patient will discuss potential effects of urologic dysfunction on self and family members.
- Patient or family members will demonstrate skill in managing incontinence.
- Patient and family members will identify community resources to help them cope with alterations in urinary status.

Interventions and rationales

- Observe voiding pattern, and document intake and output *to ensure correct fluid replacement therapy and provide information about patient's ability to void adequately.*
- Determine patient's premorbid elimination status *to ensure that interventions are realistic and based on the patient's health status and goals.*

- Use an interdisciplinary approach to caring for incontinence. Incorporate recommendations from urologist, urology nurse specialist, other health care providers, and patient. Monitor progress and report patient's response to interventions. *Interdisciplinary approach helps to ensure that patient receives adequate care. Encouraging patient participation on team will help foster motivation.*
- Assess patient's ability to sense and communicate elimination needs *to maximize self-care.*
- Make sure patient's toilet environment is warm, clean, and free from odor *to promote continence.*
- Place a commode beside bed. *A bedside commode requires less energy expenditure than using a bedpan or ambulating to a bathroom.*
- Keep bed and commode at same level *to facilitate easy access.*
- Provide good lighting from bed to bathroom *to reduce confusion and risk of falls.*
- Remove all obstacles between bed and bathroom *to reduce risk of falls.*
- Provide a clock *to promote patient's orientation to time.*
- Unless contraindicated, provide 2½ to 3 qt (2,500 to 3,000 ml) of fluid daily *to moisten mucous membranes and ensure adequate hydration.* Space out fluid intake through day and limit to 150 ml after supper *to reduce need to void at night.*
- Have patient wear easily removed clothes (gown instead of pajamas, Velcro fasteners instead of buttons or zippers) *to facilitate removal of clothing and foster independence.*
- Instruct patient to stop and take a deep breath if he experiences intense urge to urinate before he is able to reach bathroom. *Anxiety and rushing may increase bladder contraction.*

• Have patient keep diary recording episodes of incontinence. Use information from diary as basis for planning interventions. Possible bladder training interventions may include voiding every 2 hours, avoiding high fluid intake, maintaining proper hygiene, or notifying a health care professional if urge incontinence occurs with frequency. *Individualized interventions help to promote self-care, foster motivation, and avoid incontinence.*

• Incorporate patient's suggestions for managing incontinent episodes into plan of care *to foster motivation.*

• Encourage patient to express feelings regarding incontinence *to provide emotional support and identify areas for further patient teaching.*

• Explain urge incontinence to patient and family members, especially preventive measures and potential underlying causes, *to foster compliance.*

• Note if patient expresses concern about effect of incontinence on sexuality. If appropriate, refer to a sex therapist *to promote sexual health.*

• Refer patient and family members to community resources such as support groups, as appropriate, *to help ensure continuity of care.*

Evaluations for expected outcomes

• Patient states if he is able to anticipate when episodes of incontinence are likely to occur.

• Patient states understanding of potential causes of urge incontinence and its treatment.

• Patient avoids complications of urge incontinence or complications are minimized.

• Patient discusses potential effects of urologic dysfunction on self and family members.

• Patient or family members demonstrate skill in managing incontinence.

• Patient and family members identify community resources to help them cope with alterations in urinary status.

Documentation

• Patient's urologic status
• Episodes of urge incontinence
• Nursing interventions and patient's response
• Instruction given to patient and family and their response
• Demonstrated ability to meet self-care needs
• Patient's expression of concern about potential changes in urologic status and its impact on body image and lifestyle
• Patient's statements indicating motivation to meet self-care needs
• Evaluations for expected outcomes

■ Injury, risk for

related to elder abuse

Definition

Accentuated risk for neglect or abuse of older adult by a family member

Assessment

• Age
• Sex
• Patient's health status, including presence of acute or chronic illness and changes or deterioration in mental or physical functioning
• Family status, including communication patterns and presence or absence of extended family
• Family members' willingness and ability to provide physical and emotional support to patient
• Evidence of physical abuse, including malnutrition, imprint of hand or fingers, marks from restraints, and

unexplained bruises, burns, welts, cuts, dislocations, or abrasions
• Evidence of emotional abuse, including observation or reports of insults, ridicule, or humiliation
• Evidence of financial abuse, including unexplained changes in bank accounts and transfer of funds to caregivers
• Evidence of neglect, including inappropriate clothing, unsanitary living conditions, inadequate food supplies, lack of medication, and absence of needed eyeglasses, hearing aids, cane, or walker

Risk factors
• Dependence on family members for daily care (patient)
• Deteriorating health, frailty, or impaired mobility (patient)
• Expressed frustration over responsibilities of caring for older family member (caregiver)
• Isolation from community, without relatives living nearby (caregiver)
• Limited education or inadequate financial resources (caregiver)
• Reported lack of social contacts outside family (patient)

Associated medical diagnoses (selected)
Alzheimer's disease, cerebrovascular accident, chronic obstructive pulmonary disease, coronary artery disease, dementia, depression, elder abuse, end-stage cardiac disease, hip fracture, hypertension, osteoarthritis, rheumatoid arthritis

Expected outcomes
• Patient will remain free from injury and will state that incidents of abuse no longer occur.
• Patient will express understanding of right to be free from abuse.
• Patient will report increased social contact outside family.

• Patient will establish "buddy system," whereby he and friend visit or telephone each other at regularly scheduled intervals.
• Patient will maintain control over mail, telephone, and other personal effects.
• Caregiver will state intention to contact respite care services, support groups, and other community resources.
• Caregiver will report increased ability to cope with responsibilities of caring for older family member.
• Patient and caregiver will report improved communication patterns.

Interventions and rationales
• Monitor patient closely at each visit for evidence of physical or mental abuse or neglect. Observe for bruises or abrasions, body odor, or dirty, unkempt appearance *to ensure his safety and well-being.* Question him privately about findings *to encourage trust and promote open communication.*
• Encourage patient to discuss incidents of abuse or threats of abuse. Be willing to listen and be careful to convey nonjudgmental attitude. *Older patients may be reluctant to discuss abuse or threats of abuse because of fear of retaliation, embarrassment, or reluctance to report family members to authorities. By communicating that you care and are willing to listen, you may help patient overcome these barriers.*
• Teach patient about his right to be free from abuse. Discuss responsibility of law enforcement agencies to investigate incidents of abuse. Provide list of social service agencies that can provide counseling *to empower patient to resist or prevent episodes of abuse.*
• Encourage patient to maintain use of personal telephone and open his own

mail *to promote sense of control and self-worth and maintain contact with people outside home.*

• Encourage patient to participate in community activities, such as church groups and senior volunteer organizations, *to establish social contacts and develop strong support network.*

• Suggest use of Meals On Wheels or community geriatric outreach for homebound patient *to prevent isolation and provide respite for family caregiver.*

• Encourage friends to visit patient at home. Suggest that patient and friend develop "buddy system," whereby each takes turns telephoning or visiting other at regular intervals *to provide social contact, respite for caregiver, and additional safeguard against abuse.*

• If appropriate, encourage patient and family members to periodically hold conferences. Help patient and family members identify productive topics for discussion, such as strategies for dealing with patient's self-care deficits or scheduling respite care, *to foster open communication, defuse tension, and develop solutions to practical problems of caring for older family member.*

• Inform caregiver about state and county services for elderly, respite services, adult day-care, support groups for children of aging parents, and other community resources *to enhance caregiver's ability to cope and thereby diminish likelihood of abuse.*

• Report actual or suspected elder abuse to local authorities and provide follow-up or emergency care, if needed. *Nearly every state has laws mandating that suspected elder abuse be reported to authorities.*

Evaluations for expected outcomes

• Patient doesn't exhibit injuries and states that incidents of abuse have stopped.

• Patient expresses understanding of right to be protected from abuse.

• Patient reports satisfaction with ability to maintain or increase social contacts outside family.

• Patient establishes "buddy system" with friend outside home.

• Patient maintains control over mail, telephone, and other personal effects.

• Caregiver regularly attends community support group and contacts appropriate social service agencies and other sources of support.

• Caregiver reports increased ability to cope with responsibilities of caring for older family member.

• Patient and caregiver report improved communication.

Documentation

• Evidence of emotional, physical, or financial neglect or abuse

• Patient's statements that indicate risk for abuse

• Caregiver's statements indicating feelings about caring for older family member

• Caregiver's statements indicating willingness to attend support groups or use community resources

• Patient's and caregiver's expressed understanding of teaching provided by nurse

• Patient's response to nursing interventions

• Evaluations for expected outcomes

■ Knowledge deficit

related to difficulty understanding disease process and its effect on self-care

Definition

Lack of knowledge regarding any aspect of health care, including disease process, medications, treatment plan, community resources, and coping strategies

Assessment

• Current knowledge level
• Interest and motivation to learn
• Preferred learning style
• Comprehension ability and reading level
• Other factors that may affect learning, such as cultural influences; religious practices and beliefs; sensory, cognitive, or physical impairment; support systems; economic status; and feelings of anger, depression, or hopelessness

Defining characteristics

• Inability to follow through with instruction
• Inappropriate or exaggerated behaviors (hysteria, hostility, agitation, apathy)
• Poor performance on test of knowledge
• Verbalization of problem

Associated medical diagnoses (selected)

Cerebrovascular accident, chronic bronchitis, chronic obstructive pulmonary disease, diabetes mellitus, digitalis toxicity, emphysema, heart failure

Expected outcomes

• Patient will express understanding of disease process, medication regimen, and treatment plan.
• Patient will make informed choices when addressing health care problems and self-care deficits.
• Patient will demonstrate ability to effectively implement chosen health care strategy.

Interventions and rationales

• Consider older patient's life experiences when developing teaching plan. *New information is easier to assimilate if it is built on existing knowledge.*
• Provide quiet, calm environment for learning *to enable patient to process information without distraction from background noise or stress.*
• Limit length of each teaching session *to avoid information overload.*
• Ask patient if he wants to learn new or additional information. If not, discuss why. *Open discussion helps to identify barriers to learning and determine if these barriers may be eliminated. Discussion also promotes acceptance of patient's right to choose his own level of participation.*
• Encourage patient to use memory aids, such as preset alarms on watch, calendar for noting scheduled appointments, and small notepad for recording questions or symptoms, *to help compensate for memory lapses.*
• Write instructions in large letters, using black ink or contrasting colors. *Older patients see black best and may have difficulty distinguishing pastels or monochromatic color schemes.*
• Modify teaching style to accommodate normal aging changes:
– Face patient when speaking.
– Use well-modulated voice.
– Allow ample time for teaching sessions.

Understanding normal age-related changes enhances teaching effectiveness.
• Set aside time during each session for answering questions and clarifying information. *Older patient may need affirmation that knowledge he possesses is current and correct. Discussion may also stimulate exchange of ideas and further learning.*
• Encourage patient to join support group, such as club for stroke survivors or support group for cancer patients, *to reinforce education and promote contact with others in same situation.*
• Involve caregiver in teaching sessions, when appropriate, *to reinforce information and ensure continuity of care at home.*

Evaluations for expected outcomes
• Patient expresses increased understanding of disease process, medication regimen, and treatment plan, describing at least three basic concepts relevant to disease process and its impact on activities of daily living.
• Patient states at least four strategies to improve self-care and expresses understanding of how chosen strategies will provide relief from disease process and improve his ability to perform activities of daily living.
• Patient demonstrates ongoing ability to implement chosen health care strategies.

Documentation
• Patient's verbal statements and behavior that indicate knowledge deficit
• Teaching provided and patient's or caregiver's response, including questions and comments made during teaching sessions
• Patient's description of chosen intervention strategies

• Patient's statements and behaviors that indicate implementation of strategies
• Evaluations for expected outcomes

■ Mobility, impaired bed
related to neuromuscular dysfunction

Definition
Limitation of ability to move about in bed

Assessment
• Age and sex
• Vital signs
• History of neuromuscular disorder or dysfunction
• Drug history
• Musculoskeletal status, including coordination, muscle size and strength, muscle tone, range of motion (ROM), and functional mobility as follows:
0 = completely independent
1 = requires use of equipment or device
2 = requires help, supervision, or teaching from another person
3 = requires help from another person and equipment or device
4 = dependent; doesn't participate in activity
• Neurologic status, including level of consciousness, motor ability, and sensory ability

Defining characteristics
• Altered or limited ability to move in bed
• Altered postural reflexes
• Fatigue
• Flaccidity
• Inability to coordinate movement
• Paraplegia

- Paresis
- Quadriplegia
- Spasticity
- Weakness

Associated medical diagnoses (selected)

Brain abscess, cerebral aneurysm, cerebrovascular accident, Guillain-Barré syndrome, head injury, multiple sclerosis, muscular dystrophy, myasthenia gravis, paralysis, paresis, Parkinson's disease, spinal cord injury or tumor

Expected outcomes

- Patient won't exhibit complications associated with impaired bed mobility, such as altered skin integrity, contractures, venous stasis, thrombus formation, depression, altered health maintenance, and falls.
- Patient will maintain or improve muscle strength and joint ROM.
- Patient will achieve highest level of bed mobility possible (independence, independence with device, verbalization of needs for assistance with bed mobility, requires assistance of one person, requires assistance of two people).
- Patient will maintain safety while in bed.
- Patient will demonstrate ability to use equipment or devices to assist with moving about in bed safely.
- Patient will adapt to alteration in ability to move about in bed.
- Patient will participate in social, physical, and occupational activities to the greatest extent possible.

Interventions and rationales

- Perform ROM exercises to affected joints, unless contraindicated, at least once per shift. Progress from passive to active ROM, as tolerated, *to prevent joint contractures and muscle atrophy.*

- Assist patient in maintaining anatomically correct and functional body positioning. Encourage repositioning every 2 hours while in bed. Establish turning schedule for immobile patients. *Proper positioning relieves pressure, thereby preventing skin breakdown, and helps prevent fluid accumulation in dependent extremities.*
- Identify patient's level of independence using functional mobility scale. Communicate your findings to staff *to provide continuity of care and preserve documented level of independence.*
- Monitor and record daily evidence of complications related to altered bed mobility (contractures, venous stasis, skin breakdown, thrombus formation, depression, altered health maintenance or self-care skills, falls). *Patients with neuromuscular dysfunction are at risk for complications.*
- Perform medical regimen to manage or prevent complications (for example, administer prophylactic heparin for venous stasis) *to promote patient's health and well-being.*
- Assess patient's skin every 2 hours *to maintain skin integrity.*
- Help patient move about in bed. Encourage progressive mobility up to the limits imposed by patient's condition *to maintain muscle tone, prevent complications associated with immobility, and promote self-care.*
- Refer patient to a physical therapist for development of a program to improve bed mobility *to assist with rehabilitation of musculoskeletal deficits.*
- Refer patient to an occupational therapist for development of a program to maximize self-care *to promote restoration of self-care skills.*
- Encourage patient to participate in physical and occupational therapy

sessions. Incorporate equipment, devices, and techniques used by therapists into your care. Request written instructions from patient's therapists to use as a reference *to help ensure continuity of care and reinforce learned skills.*

• If you're uncertain about your ability to move patient safely, request help from colleagues *to maintain safety.*

• Instruct patient and family members in techniques to improve bed mobility and ways to prevent complications *to help prepare patient and family members for discharge.*

• Demonstrate patient's bed mobility regimen and note date. Have patient and family members perform a return demonstration *to ensure continuity of care and use of proper technique.*

• Assist patient in identifying and contacting resources for social and spiritual support *to promote patient's reintegration into the community and help him maintain psychosocial health.*

Evaluations for expected outcomes

• Patient doesn't exhibit complications associated with impaired bed mobility, such as altered skin integrity, contractures, venous stasis, thrombus formation, depression, altered health maintenance, and falls.

• Patient maintains or improves muscle strength and joint ROM.

• Patient achieves highest level of bed mobility possible (independence, independence with device, verbalization of needs for assistance with bed mobility, requires assistance of one person, requires assistance of two people).

• Patient maintains safety while in bed.

• Patient demonstrates ability to use equipment or devices to assist with moving about in bed safely.

• Patient adapts to alteration in ability to move about in bed.

• Patient participates in social, physical, and occupational activities to the greatest extent possible.

Documentation

• Patient's bed mobility status
• Presence of complications
• Referrals for physical or occupational therapy
• Response to program to improve or restore bed mobility
• Patient's statements regarding the loss of bed mobility skills and his goals for improving bed mobility
• Teaching provided to patient and family members
• Patient's and family members' demonstrated skill in carrying out bed mobility program
• Evaluations for expected outcomes

■ Mobility, impaired wheelchair

related to neuromuscular disorder or dysfunction

Definition

Limitation in ability to move about in wheelchair

Assessment

• Age and sex
• Vital signs
• History of neuromuscular disorder or dysfunction
• Drug history
• Musculoskeletal status, including coordination, gait, muscle size and strength, muscle tone, range of motion (ROM), and functional mobility as follows:
0 = completely independent

1 = requires use of equipment or device

2 = requires help, supervision, or teaching from another person

3 = requires help from another person and equipment or device

4 = dependent; doesn't participate in activity

• Neurologic status, including level of consciousness, motor ability, and sensory ability

• Characteristics of the patient's wheelchair (for example, whether standard or motorized) and adequacy of wheelchair for meeting the patient's needs (right size, appropriate safety features, and easy for patient to operate)

• Endurance (length of time patient can operate wheelchair before becoming fatigued)

Defining characteristics

• Alteration in ability to use wheelchair to move about

• Alteration in postural reflexes

• Fatigue

• Flaccidity

• Inability to coordinate movement

• Paraplegia

• Paresis

• Quadriplegia

• Spasticity

• Weakness

Associated medical diagnoses (selected)

Brain abscess, cerebral aneurysm, cerebrovascular accident, Guillain-Barré syndrome, head injury, multiple sclerosis, muscular dystrophy, myasthenia gravis, paralysis, paresis, Parkinson's disease, spinal cord injury or tumor

Expected outcomes

• Patient won't exhibit complications associated with impaired wheelchair mobility, such as skin breakdown, contractures, venous stasis, thrombus formation, depression, alteration in health maintenance, and falls.

• Patient will maintain or improve muscle strength and joint ROM.

• Patient will achieve highest level of independence possible with regard to wheelchair use.

• Patient will express feelings regarding alteration in ability to use wheelchair.

• Patient will maintain safety when using wheelchair.

• Patient will adapt to alteration in ability.

• Patient will participate in social and occupational activities to the greatest extent possible.

• Patient will demonstrate understanding of techniques to improve wheelchair mobility.

Interventions and rationales

• Perform ROM exercises for affected joints, unless contraindicated, at least once per shift. Progress from passive to active ROM, as tolerated, *to prevent joint contractures and muscle atrophy.*

• Make sure patient maintains anatomically correct and functional body positioning while in wheelchair *to promote comfort.* Explain to patient where vulnerable pressure points are and teach him to shift and reposition his weight *to prevent skin breakdown.*

• Assess whether patient's wheelchair is adequate to meet his needs *to help maintain mobility and independence.* Consider the following:

– Is seat the right size? It should be wide and deep enough to support patient's thighs and allow him to sit comfortably. It should be low enough so that patient's feet touch floor but high enough to allow easy transfer from bed to chair. The chair's back should be tall enough to support patient's upper body.

– Is chair easy for patient to operate when weak? If patient has little or no arm strength, he may need a motorized wheelchair.

– Is chair safe? All wheelchairs have safety features, such as brakes that lock the wheels, but some safety features can be modified to meet patient's needs. For example, seat belts can be attached at the waist, hips, or chest.

• Identify patient's level of independence using functional mobility scale. Communicate findings to staff *to promote continuity of care and preserve documented level of independence.*

• Monitor and record daily evidence of complications related to alteration in wheelchair mobility (contractures, venous stasis, skin breakdown, thrombus formation, depression, and alteration in health maintenance or self-care skills). *Patients with neuromuscular dysfunction are at risk for complications.*

• Encourage patient to operate his wheelchair independently to the limits imposed by his condition *to maintain muscle tone, prevent complications of immobility, and promote independence in self-care and health maintenance skills.*

• Refer to physical therapist for development of program to enhance wheelchair mobility *to assist with rehabilitation of musculoskeletal deficits.*

• Encourage attendance at physical therapy sessions and reinforce prescribed activities on the unit by using equipment, devices, and techniques used in the therapy session. Request a written copy of patient's rehabilitation program to use as a reference *to maintain continuity of care and promote patient safety.*

• Assess patient's skin on return to bed and request wheelchair cushion, if necessary, *to maintain patient's skin integrity.*

• Demonstrate techniques to promote wheelchair mobility to patient and family members, and note date *to help prepare patient for discharge and maintain safety.* For example, teach patient and family members how to perform wheelchair push-ups. If patient can move his arms, have him grip arms of chair and push down hard with his hands and arms to try to raise his body off the seat. Have patient and family members perform a return demonstration *to ensure continuity of care and use of proper technique.*

• Assist in identifying resources for helping patient maintain the highest level of mobility, such as a community stroke program, sports associations for people with disabilities, or the National Multiple Sclerosis Society, *to promote the patient's reintegration into the community.*

Evaluations for expected outcomes

• Patient doesn't exhibit complications associated with impaired wheelchair mobility, such as skin breakdown, contractures, venous stasis, thrombus formation, depression, alteration in health maintenance, and falls.

• Patient maintains or improves muscle strength and joint ROM.

• Patient achieves highest level of independence possible with regard to wheelchair use.

• Patient expresses feelings regarding alteration in ability to use wheelchair.

• Patient maintains safety when using wheelchair.

• Patient adapts to alteration in ability.

• Patient participates in social and occupational activities to the greatest extent possible.
• Patient demonstrates understanding of techniques to improve wheelchair mobility.

Documentation
• Observations of changes in patient's mobility status and related complications
• Patient's expression of concern about loss of wheelchair mobility
• Patient's goals for future regarding mobility status
• Teaching provided to patient
• Patient's return demonstration of skills in carrying out wheelchair mobility program
• Patient's response to nursing interventions
• Evaluations for expected outcomes

■ Nutrition alteration: More than body requirements

related to a decline in basal metabolic rate and physical activity

Definition
Change in normal eating pattern or activity level that results in increased body weight

Assessment
• Activity level
• Health history, including evidence of impaired mobility, chronic illness, use of appetite-stimulating medications, lack of exercise, and family history of obesity
• Nutritional status, including height and weight, usual dietary pattern, stated food preferences, and weight fluctuations

• Psychosocial factors, including lifestyle, ethnic background, socioeconomic status, education level, mode of transportation, internal and external cues that trigger desire to eat, motivation to lose weight, and rate of food consumption
• Home environment, including presence of family members or significant other, responsibility for grocery shopping and meal preparation, food storage and preparation facilities, and access to transportation

Defining characteristics
• Body weight 10% or more over ideal weight
• Dysfunctional eating patterns, such as concentrating food intake at end of day, eating in response to internal cue other than hunger (such as boredom), eating in response to external cues (such as social situations), and pairing food with other activities
• Sedentary lifestyle
• Triceps skin-fold measurement greater than 15 mm in men and 25 mm in women

Associated medical diagnoses (selected)
Chronic obstructive pulmonary disease, depression, heart failure, hypertension, osteoarthritis

Expected outcomes
• Patient will express understanding of why obesity is a problem.
• Patient will develop realistic goals for weight reduction and will plan to achieve these goals.
• Patient will lose specified amount of weight per week.
• Patient will carry out exercise and activity plan.

Interventions and rationales
• Assess patient's perception of weight problem. Determine whether

patient understands that obesity affects lifestyle and creates health risks *to evaluate patient's motivation to lose weight and determine appropriate plan of action.*

• Encourage patient to keep food diary *to track dietary intake accurately.*

• Teach patient about changes in nutrient and vitamin needs that occur with aging *to promote well-informed food choices. Dietary requirements diminish with age; older patient's caloric requirements decrease by 10% to 25%.*

• If patient lacks motivation or resources for preparing balanced meals, provide information on appropriate community services, such as Meals On Wheels or federally sponsored nutrition programs, *to help patient obtain healthier meals.*

• Encourage patient to make gradual improvements in eating habits; for example, slowly introduce low-calorie, nutritious foods into diet. Keep in mind that older patient has developed current habits over many years. *Planning for gradual changes increases chances of success.*

• Set realistic goal for weight loss; weekly loss of ½ to 1 lb (0.2 to 0.45 kg) is adequate. *Realistic goals increase motivation and ensure success of weight-control program.*

• If appropriate, have registered dietitian discuss meal planning and food preparation with patient, taking into account physical, psychological, socioeconomic, and cultural factors, *to provide appropriate nutritional guidance.*

• Help patient develop modified exercise plan, such as regular walking, *to burn calories, increase endurance, and maintain musculoskeletal strength. Regular exercise enhances patient's motivation and self-concept.*

• Provide ongoing support and recognition of patient's progress *to reinforce changes in eating habits and help patient assess progress accurately.*

• Provide patient with information on social events and artistic, cultural, and educational programs *to stimulate patient to become more active.*

Evaluations for expected outcomes

• Patient expresses understanding of consequences of continued obesity.

• Patient actively participates in developing weight-reduction goals.

• Patient loses specified amount of weight per week.

• Patient carries out exercise and activity plan.

Documentation

• Patient's weight

• Patient's expression of feelings about obesity

• Observations of patient's eating patterns

• Weight-reduction plan

• Teaching provided and patient's response

• Evaluations for expected outcomes

■ Poisoning, risk for

related to drug toxicity or polypharmacy

Definition

Accentuated risk of ingestion of drugs or dangerous products in doses sufficient to cause poisoning

Assessment

• Age

• Sex

• Drug history, including prescription and over-the-counter medications

- Use of alcoholic beverages
- Health history, including evidence of hepatic or renal impairment
- Nutritional status, including weight changes, protein intake, and fluid status
- Psychosocial history, including activity level, knowledge level, financial status, mental status, and living arrangements
- Laboratory studies, including toxicology screening; serum digitalis, serum electrolyte, blood urea nitrogen, serum creatinine, and bilirubin levels; liver enzymes, such as aspartate aminotransferase, alanine aminotransferase, and alkaline phosphatase; and total serum protein and albumin to globulin ratio

Risk factors
- Cognitive or emotional difficulties, including forgetfulness or confusion
- Drugs stored near bedside
- History of drug abuse or alcoholism
- Impaired vision
- Inability to read medication labels
- Living alone
- Multiple health care providers, drug prescriptions, and pharmacies
- Poor bowel habits, including chronic use of enemas or laxative abuse
- Poor understanding of drug interactions
- Poor understanding of drug usage
- Poor understanding of precautions necessary for safe drug therapy

Associated medical diagnoses (selected)
Chronic obstructive pulmonary disease, digitalis toxicity, drug overdose or toxicity, end-stage renal disease, poisoning

Expected outcomes
- Patient will express understanding of medication regimen.

- Patient won't experience episodes of toxicity.
- Patient's medical condition will remain under control.
- Patient will take only prescribed medications in correct quantities at correct times.

Interventions and rationales
- Instruct patient or family member in drug regimen, including reasons for taking drugs, safety precautions, and how to monitor effectiveness of drugs, *to increase compliance.*
- Regularly review and document patient's medication regimen *to monitor medication use, assess whether certain medications should be discontinued, and monitor for drug interactions.*
- Instruct patient or family member to store drugs in secure area away from bedside *to prevent accidental ingestion. Many older patients keep medications at their bedside to decrease need to arise during night.*
- If color-coding medications, use only bright, contrasting colors. *Older patients can't distinguish pastel colors well.*
- Help patient or family member identify behaviors that contribute to risk of toxicity, such as obtaining prescriptions from various health care providers or using different pharmacies, *to raise awareness of potential hazards.*
- Encourage patient or family member to retain primary doctor who coordinates care. *Older patients with multiple health problems may receive care from various providers who are unaware of each other's treatment plans and medication regimens.*
- Provide instructions for use of medications, including quantity, frequency, and number of doses, *to enhance understanding of medication regimen*

and increase compliance. Make sure instructions are clearly written in black or blue ink. *Older patients can read black or blue ink more easily.*
• Be sure all medication labels are inscribed in large print and include dosage instructions *to avoid medication errors.*
• Help patient maintain accurate and effective system for following medication regimen, such as check-off calendar system or separate pill boxes labeled for each day of week, *to reduce errors.* Encourage patient to work with pharmacist when developing this system.
• Monitor patient's urine and serum toxicity levels when indicated *to reduce risk of toxicity. Age-related changes in body function may lead to decreased renal, liver, and GI clearance of drugs, increasing patient's risk of toxicity. Also, variety of drugs commonly used by older patient increases risk of toxicity from drug interactions.*
• Discuss with doctor possibility of using alternative drugs, such as long-acting preparations or drugs that require only one dose per day, *to simplify drug regimen and thereby decrease risk of toxicity.*

Evaluation for expected outcomes
• Patient expresses understanding of medication regimen.
• Patient doesn't experience episodes of toxicity.
• Patient's existing medical condition remains under control.
• Patient takes only prescribed drugs in correct quantities at correct times.

Documentation
• Evidence of patient's or family member's lack of understanding of or poor compliance with medication regimen

• Additional factors that increase patient's risk of drug toxicity
• Physical findings
• Instructions provided about safe drug practices
• Patient's or family member's response to instructions
• Patient's responses to nursing interventions
• Evaluations for expected outcomes

■ Powerlessness

related to perceived loss of control over life situation

Definition
Feeling of helplessness, hopelessness, and lack of control

Assessment
• Environmental factors, such as institutional setting
• Impact of therapeutic regimens on lifestyle, including use of cane or walker, changes in diet, and medication regimen
• Economic status, including retirement income, medical expenses such as ongoing home care or placement in nursing home, and Medicare or other insurance coverage
• Emotional status, including recent loss of spouse and history of dependence on others
• Physical impairments, including arthritic conditions, loss of limb use, diminished vision, and lengthy or chronic illness

Defining characteristics
• Apathy
• Depression over physical deterioration
• Failure to defend self-care practices

- Failure to monitor progress
- Failure to seek information about care
- Irritability because of dependence on others
- Passivity
- Expressed resentment, anger, and guilt
- Reluctance to express true feelings because of fear of alienating caregivers
- Reluctance to participate in decisions about health
- Uncertainty about fluctuating energy levels
- Expressed dissatisfaction over inability to perform previous tasks
- Expressed self-doubt
- Expressed lack of control over self-care, current situation, and outcome

Associated medical diagnoses (selected)
Cerebrovascular accident, chronic obstructive pulmonary disease, dementia, depression, heart failure, hip fracture, macular degeneration

Expected outcomes
- Patient will identify aspects of life still under his control.
- Patient will help develop schedule for self-care activities.
- Patient will participate in decisions about his care and lifestyle.
- Patient will express more realistic expectations and increased satisfaction with current situation.

Interventions and rationales
- Guide patient through life review. Encourage patient to reflect on past achievements *to foster sense of satisfaction and promote acceptance of current status.*
- Help patient establish realistic expectations and goals. *Having realistic expectations helps prevent failures,*

which might exacerbate feelings of powerlessness.
- Help patient identify aspects of his life that are still under his control. For example, offer patient chance to request changes to arrangement of furniture in room. Recognize patient's right to express feelings. *Empowering older patient in any way possible may prevent feelings of powerlessness from becoming overwhelming.*
- Encourage patient to make choices in scheduling daily routine, including personal hygiene, dressing and grooming, meals, and physical therapy. Emphasize that patient, not staff members, has authority to make scheduling decisions. *This helps patient reassert control.*
- Ask patient open-ended questions rather than questions that he can answer with "yes" or "no." *Open-ended questions encourage patient to assert his opinions and thereby regain feeling of control.*
- Encourage staff members to express interest in patient's progress and set aside time to listen attentively to patient *to acknowledge and reinforce efforts to regain control.*
- Encourage patient to take an active role in choosing among social and recreational activities *to enhance patient's lifestyle and further diminish feelings of powerlessness.*

Evaluation for expected outcomes
- Patient identifies aspects of life still under his control and describes actions he can take to improve or modify his routine.
- Patient displays an appropriate sense of responsibility in scheduling self-care activities.
- Patient takes part in decisions about his care and lifestyle.

• Patient expresses more realistic expectations and increased satisfaction with current situation.

Documentation
• Patient's verbal and behavioral expressions of powerlessness
• Patient's level of involvement in self-care activities
• Patient's level of participation in therapeutic and social milieu
• Patient's responses to nursing interventions
• Patient's statements indicating increased feelings of control
• Evaluations for expected outcomes

■ Role performance alteration

Definition
Disruption in ability to perform social, vocational, and family roles

Assessment
• Age
• Sex
• Patient's perception of social, vocational, and family roles
• Neurologic status, including level of consciousness, memory, mental status, orientation, and cognitive and perceptual functioning
• Physical disabilities or limitations
• Coping behaviors
• Developmental status, including evaluation of age-appropriate task resolution, such as accepting changes in mental and physical capacities, relinquishing past roles, creating new social relationships, substituting new activities and interests for those that can no longer be pursued, and revising goals, values, and self-concept to accommodate lifestyle changes

• Family status, including roles of family members, effect of illness on patient's family, and family members' understanding of patient's illness
• Family members' perceptions of patient's ability to perform social, vocational, and family roles

Defining characteristics
• Altered role perceptions
• Change in ability to perform social, vocational, and family roles
• Changes in mental or physical capacity that affect ability to perform social, vocational, and family roles
• Inadequate role competence
• Role strain

Associated medical diagnoses (selected)
This nursing diagnosis may be seen with any chronic medical condition or age-related change that may affect an older patient's role performance. Examples include end-stage disease (renal or cardiac), heart failure, hip fracture, macular degeneration, and Parkinson's disease.

Expected outcomes
• Patient will express feelings about limitations imposed by aging.
• Patient will discuss plans to reevaluate social, family, and vocational roles and adapt them to present physical and mental status.
• Family members will express willingness to take over responsibilities previously performed by patient.
• Patient will continue to perform usual social, family, and vocational roles to extent possible.
• Family members will express willingness to provide emotional support as patient adjusts to altered role performance.

Interventions and rationales

• Discuss with patient factors that make it difficult to fulfill his usual vocational role. For example, has patient recently been forced to retire? How does patient cope with free time? How does patient feel about no longer being family breadwinner? *Discussion helps patient gain insight and rationally define problems and potential solutions.*

• Help patient develop activity program and explore ways patient can contribute to society, such as participation in senior volunteer program, *to help restore patient's sense of purpose.*

• Discuss factors that make it difficult for patient to fulfill usual social roles. For example, have many of patient's close friends died? Is it difficult for patient to obtain transportation to social events? *This will help patient identify causes of diminished social interaction.*

• Investigate support groups, senior citizen centers, and other community resources *to help patient find new outlets for forming social relationships.*

• Discuss with family members ways they can help patient cope with altered role performance, such as visiting frequently, providing emotional support, and requesting patient's input into family decisions, *to help maintain patient's self-esteem.*

• Encourage patient to fulfill life roles within constraints imposed by aging *to maintain sense of purpose and preserve connection with others.*

• Encourage family members to express feelings about patient's altered role performance. Discuss alternative ways for family members to partially or fully assume roles once performed by patient *to enhance family coping.*

• Provide patient and family members with information about developmental tasks that patient must perform to master process of aging. These may include accepting changes in mental and physical capacities, relinquishing past roles, creating new social relationships, substituting new activities and interests for those he can no longer pursue, and revising goals, values, and self-concept to accommodate lifestyle changes. *Helping patient and family members understand that these tasks are normal part of aging process may enhance coping.*

Evaluations for expected outcomes

• Patient expresses feelings about limitations imposed by aging.

• Patient describes plans to adapt to role changes related to aging and chronic illness.

• Family members express willingness to take on responsibilities formerly held by patient.

• Patient continues to fulfill family, social, and vocational responsibilities to extent possible.

• Family members express willingness to provide emotional support for patient as he adjusts to altered role performance.

Documentation

• Patient's expression of feelings and concerns associated with altered role performance

• Nursing interventions to help patient understand and accept changes in role performance

• Patient's response to nursing interventions

• Statements by family members indicating their attitude toward patient's altered role performance

• Referrals to support services for patient and family members

• Evaluations for expected outcomes

■ Self-esteem, situational low

related to hospitalization and forced dependence on health care team

Definition
Negative self-image that develops in response to a loss or change in individual who previously had a positive self-image

Assessment
• Changes in physical appearance, including wrinkles, sagging skin, gray hair, aging spots, scoliosis, dowager's hump, and increased truncal fat
• Changes in social status, including recent retirement (forced or voluntary)
• Changes in sleep patterns, including trouble falling asleep, frequent awakenings, and restless sleep
• Family status, including recent loss of spouse or significant other
• Reason for current hospitalization
• Medical history, including chronic illnesses
• Mental status, including evidence of depression, hopelessness, discouragement, preoccupation with bodily functions, and unrealistic fear of developing serious disease

Defining characteristics
• Difficulty making decisions
• Evaluation of self as unable to handle life events
• Expression of negative feelings about self (such as helplessness or uselessness)
• Expressions of self-negating thoughts
• Expressed shame or guilt
• Negative self-appraisal in response to life events in a patient who previously exhibited positive self-evaluation

Associated medical diagnoses (selected)
Cataracts, hypertension, myocardial infarction, obesity

Expected outcomes
• Patient will participate in care.
• Patient will maintain eye contact and initiate conversations.
• Patient will maintain upright and open posture.
• Patient's body language and speech content will be congruent.
• Patient will talk about impact of changes caused by chronic illness or aging on lifestyle.
• Patient will express (verbally or through behavior) increased acceptance of changes caused by chronic illness or aging.
• Patient will express increased self-esteem.

Interventions and rationales
• Ask permission to enter patient's personal space, including areas around his bed, bedside tables, and closet. *As patient's self-esteem decreases, significance of personal space increases. Asking permission provides patient with sense of control and raises self-esteem.*
• Encourage patient to wear own pajamas or gowns and robes *to contribute to positive self-identity.*
• Arrange patient's personal items on bedside stand so that they are in easy reach *to maintain patient's independence.*
• Incorporate appropriate exercise activities into patient's daily care *to enhance strength, endurance, and coordination and improve self-esteem.*

• Encourage patient to reminisce *to focus patient's attention on past accomplishments.*
• If patient has limited mobility, install over-the-bed trapeze *to promote independence.*
• Incorporate tactile stimulation into daily activities through such techniques as back rubs, foot massages, and touching of hand or arm. *Frequent touching enhances patient's sense of self-worth.*
• Encourage patient to express feelings about chronic illness or aging and fears about loss of independence and ability to participate in work and leisure activities. *This allows patient to gain insight and to rationally define problems and possible solutions.*
• Provide information about appropriate support groups and encourage interacting with individuals who have successfully adapted to illness or limitations *to increase patient's coping skills.*

Evaluations for expected outcomes
• Patient carries out activities of daily living while in hospital.
• Patient maintains eye contact and initiates conversations.
• Patient is open and receptive to others.
• Patient's body language and speech are congruent.
• Patient states at least two ways that chronic illness or aging will affect his lifestyle.
• Patient discusses feelings about aging, chronic illness, loss of independence, and diminished ability to participate in work and leisure activities.
• At least once each day, patient makes statements reflecting greater self-esteem.

Documentation
• Patient's expressions that indicate lowered self-esteem
• Mental status assessment (baseline and ongoing)
• Interventions to improve patient's self-esteem
• Patient's response to nursing interventions
• Evaluations for expected outcomes

■ Sensory or perceptual alteration (auditory)

related to illness or the aging process

Definition
Changes in the sense of hearing

Assessment
• Mental status, including mood, affect, comprehension level, and recent stressors
• Occupational hazards
• Auditory status, including physical examination of ears (cerumen buildup, excessive hair in canal), previous ear trauma or surgery, and use of hearing aid
• Audiometric evaluation, including Rinne, Weber's, Schwabach's, and speech and noise tests
• Adaptive or maladaptive communication-related behaviors, such as lip reading, gestures, withdrawal, and isolation
• Medication history, including drugs that may cause hearing loss, such as aspirin, streptomycin, kanamycin, and neomycin

Defining characteristics
• Altered communication pattern
• Auditory distortions

• Change in behavior pattern
• Change in problem-solving abilities
• Change in usual response to auditory stimuli
• Disorientation
• Hallucinations
• Irritability
• Poor concentration
• Reported or measured change in auditory acuity
• Restlessness

Associated medical diagnoses (selected)
Acoustic tumors, deafness, diabetes mellitus, otosclerosis, presbycusis, recurrent otitis media, tinnitus, trauma, tumors of the nasopharynx, vascular lesions, viral infections

Expected outcomes
• Patient will express understanding of normal hearing changes that occur with age.
• Patient will express feelings about hearing changes and impact on lifestyle.
• Patient will demonstrate correct use of hearing aids.
• Patient will incorporate alternative communication techniques, such as lip reading, gestures, and written information, into daily activities.
• Patient will express interest in attending community support groups.
• Patient will take steps to enhance communication where possible, such as decreasing background noise and looking at speaker's mouth while listening.

Interventions and rationales
• Provide information about progressive hearing loss that occurs with age (presbycusis) *to enhance patient's understanding of hearing deficits.*
• Support and encourage patient's expression of feelings about hearing loss

to help overcome self-consciousness. Because of stigma attached to hearing loss, older patient may be reluctant to discuss this problem.
• Incorporate written (flash cards and word lists) and visual (sign language, gestures, and facial expressions) communication methods into daily care *to provide patient with alternative means of communication and to enhance his sense of control.*
• When speaking to patient, eliminate background noises, such as television, air conditioning, fans, chatter, and radios, *to help patient concentrate on what you're saying.*
• Speaking slowly and carefully, orient patient to topic of conversation *to reduce feelings of paranoia that may cause patient to withdraw from social interaction.*
• Speak to patient in moderate, low-pitched voice, maintaining even volume throughout each sentence, *to maximize patient's hearing. Speaking louder won't improve patient's hearing because presbycusis first causes loss in high-pitched sound recognition.*
• Face patient when speaking and enunciate words, especially consonant sounds, carefully, *to help patient read lips.*
• If patient has difficulty understanding sentence, rephrase it *to overcome possible barriers in language comprehension.*
• Encourage patient to participate in activities such as cards or checkers that don't require high level of verbal communication *to promote social activity.*
• Describe types of adaptive hearing devices and their care *to help patient make informed choices and maintain independence.*
• Provide information about support groups, such as nationally affiliated

hearing-impaired support group Self Help for Hard of Hearing People (SHHH), *to promote continuity of care through community support.*
• Make sure other staff members are aware of patient's hearing deficit, which may be related to patient's decreased ability to hear high frequencies. Explain that fatigue or environmental distractions may contribute to hearing deficits. *Teaching colleagues about presbycusis will help ensure high-quality care.*

Evaluations for expected outcomes
• Patient expresses understanding of hearing loss that occurs with aging.
• Patient expresses feelings about hearing deficit and discusses how to modify lifestyle to adapt to deficit.
• Patient demonstrates correct care and use of adaptive hearing devices.
• Patient uses alternative communication techniques to express needs or wants.
• Patient expresses interest in attending appropriate community support groups.
• Patient takes appropriate steps to enhance communication where possible.

Documentation
• Patient's statements that indicate feelings about hearing deficits
• Patient's behavioral response to hearing loss
• Nursing interventions to help patient cope with hearing deficits
• Patient teaching, including explanation of hearing loss, instructions on how to care for hearing aids, and instructions on alternative communication techniques
• Patient's responses to nursing interventions
• Evaluations for expected outcomes

■ Sensory or perceptual alteration (visual)
related to illness or the aging process

Definition
Change in the sense of sight

Assessment
• Age
• Vision status, including visual fields, corneal reflexes, extraocular movements, visual acuity, intraocular pressure, accommodation, night blindness, physical examination of eye including ophthalmoscopy, use of glasses, and previous eye trauma, infection, or surgery
• State of other senses
• Patient's lifestyle and physical environment
• Mental status, including behavior, mood, affect, and coping mechanisms
• Family history of visual problems

Defining characteristics
• Altered communication pattern
• Change in behavior pattern
• Change in problem-solving abilities
• Change in usual response to stimuli
• Disorientation
• Hallucinations
• Irritability
• Poor concentration
• Reported or measured change in visual acuity
• Restlessness
• Visual distortions

Associated medical diagnoses (selected)
Cataracts, detached retina, glaucoma, macular degeneration, presbyopia

Expected outcomes
• Patient will discuss impact of vision loss on lifestyle.
• Patient will regain vision to extent possible and begin to come to terms with potentially permanent vision loss.
• Patient will express feelings of safety, comfort, and security.
• Patient will show interest in external environment.
• Patient will use adaptive devices to compensate for vision loss.

Interventions and rationales
• Teach patient about normal age-related eye changes (presbyopia) *to increase patient's understanding of vision changes.*
• Encourage patient to undergo annual eye examinations *to monitor for progressive vision loss. Decreased vision can exacerbate acute confusion.*
• Install night-lights in patient's room and strategically arrange lighting *to avoid abrupt changes in light. Aging eyes take longer to accommodate to changes in lighting levels.*
• Provide adequate light for performing activities of daily living (ADLs). *Patient over age 60 needs twice as much illumination for close tasks as patient age 20.*
• Adjust lighting to reduce glare from shiny surfaces, such as magazine paper and walls. *Aging eyes are more sensitive to glare.*
• If color-coding medications, use only bright, contrasting colors. *Pastel colors, such as light blues and greens, look alike to aging eyes.*
• When teaching patient, use large black print, *which is easier to see and read.*
• Provide large-print objects, such as clocks, calendars, and telephone dials, *to promote sense of independence.*

• Confer with patient before moving furniture or other items in room *to help patient maintain independence in ADLs.*
• Place brightly colored strip on edge of bedside tray and table *to prevent objects from falling on bed or floor as result of depth perception problems.*
• Touch patient *to communicate that you're listening.*
• Provide patient with low-vision aids, such as large-print books and magnifying glasses, *to help increase patient's independence.*

Evaluations for expected outcomes
• Patient describes effects of vision loss on lifestyle.
• Patient regains vision to extent possible and begins to come to terms with potentially permanent vision loss.
• Patient expresses feelings of safety, comfort, and security.
• Patient expresses interest in external environment.
• Patient uses adaptive devices to compensate for vision loss.

Documentation
• Patient's expression of feelings about vision loss
• Patient's behavioral response to vision loss
• Use of adaptive equipment or devices
• Teaching provided to patient and patient's response
• Patient's response to nursing interventions
• Evaluations for expected outcomes

■ Sexuality pattern alteration (female patient)

related to illness, medical treatment, or age-related changes

Definition
State in which a person expresses concern about personal sexuality

Assessment
• Changes in female reproductive organs related to aging
• Hormone replacement therapy (postmenopause or postoophorectomy), including estrogen, progesterone, or both
• Relationship with spouse or significant other
• Psychosocial status, including self-perception, ability to cope with aging process, usual sexual activity pattern, and social interaction patterns
• Chronic illnesses
• Impaired mobility
• Perceived changes in sexual activity resulting from surgery or illness

Defining characteristics
• Reported difficulties, limitations, or changes in sexual behavior or activity

Associated medical diagnoses (selected)
Diabetes mellitus, hip fracture, hypothyroidism, menopause, multiple sclerosis, osteoporosis, Parkinson's disease, rheumatoid arthritis

Expected outcomes
• Patient will express feelings about sexuality and self-concept.
• Patient will discuss options for maintaining intimacy throughout her life span.
• Patient will express understanding of normal physiologic changes in reproductive organs that occur with aging.
• Patient will express understanding of options to relieve discomfort associated with menopause or hysterectomy.

Interventions and rationales
• Provide information about hysterectomy and menopause. *After menopause or hysterectomy, older women may need reassurance that sexual activity can still be enjoyable.*
• Teach patient about impact of normal physiologic changes caused by aging on sexuality. For example, vagina becomes smaller and less elastic, vaginal walls become thin and smooth, and external genitalia may become softer. Also, vaginal lubrication may take longer. Patient may also have abdominal pain or bladder irritability during intercourse. *Explaining how aging affects sexuality may help patient to accept these physiologic changes.*
• Encourage patient to express feelings about sexuality *to reassure patient that you're willing to discuss her concerns.*
• Discuss other options for intimacy, such as hugging, touching, and closeness, *to reaffirm patient's identity as sexual being.*
• Provide information about alternative techniques and adaptations that can assist sexual satisfaction *to encourage patient to explore and accept her sexuality.* Topics may include use of lubricants, Kegel exercises (for vaginal muscle tone), self-stimulation, and alternative sexual positions and activities.
• Discuss impact that chronic illness or adverse drug reactions can have on patient's sexuality *to explore ways of eliminating barriers to sexual enjoy-*

ment. Discuss with doctor possibility of providing alternative medications.

• Teach patient benefits and risks associated with hormone replacement therapy, including:
– reduced postmenopausal osteoporosis
– decreased risk of cardiovascular disease
– increased risk of endometrial cancer (with estrogen therapy alone)
– presence of monthly period with combined estrogen and progestin therapy
– increased risk of breast cancer with combined estrogen and progestin therapy
Education helps patient make most informed decision possible.

• Discuss psychosocial issues that may affect patient's sexuality, such as financial concerns about remarriage or family member's objections to her relationship with male companion, *to help patient focus on specific concerns and avoid misunderstandings.*

• If patient lives in long-term care facility or life-care community, encourage her to participate in social activities *to enhance opportunities for sexual expression.*

Evaluations for expected outcomes

• Patient discusses feelings related to sexuality and self-concept.

• Patient discusses options for maintaining intimacy throughout her life.

• Patient describes physiologic changes in reproductive organs that occur with aging.

• Patient describes options to relieve discomfort associated with menopause or hysterectomy, including risks and benefits of hormone replacement therapy.

Documentation

• Patient's expression of feelings about sexuality and aging

• Teaching provided and patient's response

• Patient's behavioral responses to care

• Patient's expression of improved ability to achieve sexual enjoyment and intimacy

• Evaluations for expected outcomes

■ Skin integrity impairment, risk for

related to the aging process and impaired mobility

Definition
Presence of risk factors for interruption in skin integrity

Assessment

• Age

• Physical examination, including inspection of lower limbs, testing for sensation in lower limbs, palpation of peripheral pulses, and presence of edema

• Integumentary status, including color, elasticity, hygiene, lesions, moisture, quantity and distribution of hair, sensation, temperature and blood pressure, texture, turgor, and condition of nails

• Psychosocial status, including coping patterns, lifestyle, presence of family members or significant other, mental status, self-concept, and body image

• Mobility status, including activity level, joint range of motion, contractures, muscle mass, and tone

• Mental status

• Evidence of incontinence

• Recent changes in medication regimen
• History of skin problems, including pressure ulcers, dermatitis, and trauma
• Ability to perform skin care regimen

Risk factors
• External factors, including pressure, friction and shearing, restraints, physical immobilization, humidity and moisture, chemical substances, radiation, excretions and secretions, hypothermia or hyperthermia, and age
• Internal factors, including effects of medications, skeletal prominences, immunologic responses, altered nutritional status (obesity or emaciation), sensation, pigmentation, metabolic state, circulation, and skin turgor

Associated medical diagnoses (selected)
Anemia, cerebrovascular accident, chronic renal failure, cirrhosis, diabetes mellitus, hip fracture, hyperparathyroidism, obesity, peripheral vascular disease, Raynaud's disease, thrombophlebitis

Expected outcomes
• Patient will maintain intact skin.
• Patient or caregiver will describe normal aging changes in skin and risk factors for disturbance in skin integrity.
• Patient or caregiver will implement strategies to prevent skin breakdown and will carry out skin care regimen.

Interventions and rationales
• Educate patient or caregiver about changes to skin caused by aging *to motivate patient or caregiver to implement skin care regimen. Physiologic changes associated with aging increase risk of skin breakdown. For example, older patients, especially those immobilized with chronic health problems, are at high risk for pressure ulcers. Physiologic changes also leave older patients vulnerable to problems associated with dry skin.*
• Help patient to obtain appropriate evaluation and treatment of underlying skin condition *to promote healing and minimize complications.*
• Help patient or caregiver implement pressure-relief movement and massage program *to prevent pressure ulcers.* Patient should change position at least every 2 hours. *Frequent turning and massage promotes adequate tissue perfusion and prevents necrosis.*
• Use preventive skin care devices as needed, such as foam mattress, alternating pressure mattress, sheepskin, pillows, or padding, *to avoid discomfort and skin breakdown. These measures don't replace need for turning.*
• Teach patient about need for good nutrition, including importance of meeting caloric requirements and benefits of adequate vitamin and protein intake. *Good nutrition helps to maintain adequate tissue nourishment, perfusion, and oxygenation.*
• Help patient or caregiver develop and implement daily routine of skin inspection and care. Discuss need to maintain good personal hygiene; use nonirritating (nonalkaline) soap; pat rather than rub skin dry; inspect skin regularly; avoid prolonged exposure to water, sun, cold, and wind; and recognize and report signs of skin breakdown (redness, blisters, and discoloration). *Daily program of skin inspection and maintenance will protect older patient's skin integrity.*
• Encourage patient or caregiver to seek immediate attention if skin injury or trauma occurs *to help prevent further injury and conditions that may require extensive treatment.*

• Monitor wounds or incisions for infection and follow prescribed treatment regimen *to prevent infection, which may delay healing.*

Evaluations for expected outcomes
• Patient's skin remains intact.
• Patient or caregiver describes skin changes that result from aging and lists risk factors for impaired skin integrity.
• Patient or caregiver implements daily program of skin inspection and care, including frequent turning and movement.

Documentation
• Observations of patient's skin
• Presence of risk factors for impaired skin integrity
• Patient teaching provided and patient's response
• Patient's response to nursing interventions
• Evaluations for expected outcomes

■ Social isolation

related to physiologic, environmental, or emotional barriers

Definition
Self-imposed or environmentally imposed lack of contact with others

Assessment
• Age
• Psychosocial status, including support systems, financial resources, coping and problem-solving ability, cultural background, and activities or hobbies
• Health status, including vision or hearing deficits, chronic illness, incontinence, and pain
• Self-care abilities, including knowledge and use of adaptive equipment and supplies, and technical and mechanical skills
• Living conditions, including home environment, site of activities and resources, and transportation
• Mental status, including behavior, mood, and affect
• Musculoskeletal status, including coordination, functional ability, gait, range of motion, presence of tremor or paralysis, and muscle tone, size, and strength

Defining characteristics
• Culturally unacceptable behavior
• Description of lifestyle as solitary or circumscribed by membership in subculture
• Evidence of physical or mental handicap or altered state of wellness
• Expressed feelings of being different from others
• Expressed feelings of rejection or aloneness
• Expressed frustration over inability to meet expectations of others
• Inappropriate interests or activities
• Insecurity in public
• Lack of family, friends, and social groups
• Lack of purpose in life
• Preoccupation with own thoughts
• Projection of hostility in voice and behavior
• Repetitive, meaningless actions
• Sad, dull affect
• Uncommunicative and withdrawn behavior, with poor eye contact

Associated medical diagnoses (selected)
Alzheimer's disease, cerebrovascular accident, depression, Parkinson's disease

Expected outcomes

• Patient will express feelings associated with social isolation.
• Patient will seek assistance or information from staff to overcome social isolation.
• Patient will make use of community resources.
• Patient will describe increased number of social contacts.
• Patient will express satisfaction with level of social contacts.

Interventions and rationales

• Assign primary nurse or case manager to patient *to provide consistency and promote trust.*
• Discuss with patient causes and contributing factors of social isolation. Find out what factors patient believes interfere most with his ability to develop relationships with others *to determine patient's wants and needs.*
• Determine if patient is willing to make changes in lifestyle or daily routine to increase contact with others. *Patient needs to have motivation for nursing interventions to succeed.*
• If appropriate, address physical limitations that interfere with patient's ability to form social relationships. For example, if patient has hearing deficit, make referral to audiologist for hearing aid; if patient has mobility impairment, make referral to physical therapist for exercise program or for recommendations for assistive devices. *Patient may need physical limitations addressed before he can overcome social isolation.*
• Assess influence of home environment on patient's social life. For example, is patient afraid to go outside because of high crime rate in neighborhood? If so; consider investigating options, such as retirement community or residential care facility, that

might offer better social opportunities. *Patient may not be aware of alternative living options.*
• Investigate activity groups, support groups, senior citizens centers, health education programs, and other community resources *to develop activity program for patient.*
• Investigate availability and cost of public transportation. Familiarize patient with route to planned activities. *Patient must overcome barriers to transportation to gain access to outside world.*
• Involve patient in planning activities that will enhance his social life and assist him in identifying resources *to individualize care planning and reduce feelings of dependency and helplessness.*

Evaluations for expected outcomes

• Patient expresses feelings associated with social isolation.
• Patient expresses desire to overcome social isolation and seeks help from staff to increase participation in social activities.
• Patient makes use of resources, such as social services, senior citizens centers, American Association of Retired Persons, and religious organizations.
• Patient indicates that social contacts have increased and feelings of social isolation have diminished.
• Patient expresses satisfaction with level of social contacts.

Documentation

• Factors that have caused or contributed to patient's social isolation
• Patient's statements indicating dissatisfaction with social situation
• Community resources identified for patient

• Planning done by patient, family member, primary nurse, and case manager
• Patient's use of community resources
• Evaluations for expected outcomes

■ Verbal communication impairment

related to physiologic or psychosocial changes

Definition

Decreased ability to appropriately speak, understand, or use words that is caused by organic and environmental factors

Assessment

• History of neurologic disease
• Speech characteristics, including pattern (rate of speech, phrase length, effort, fluency, prosody, repetition, and information content), vocabulary, level of comprehension, and presence of aphasia (Broca's, Wernicke's, transcortical, receptive, or global) or dysarthria
• Ability to use alternative forms of communication (eye blinks, gestures, pictures, nods, or written notes)
• Auditory status, including use of hearing aid, history of hearing deficits, and presence of cerumen
• Vision status, including use of eyeglasses, history of vision deficits, visual acuity (near and distant), and visual fields
• Neurologic status, including level of consciousness, orientation, cognition, memory (recent and remote), insight, judgment, cranial nerves (IX, X, XII), primitive reflexes (snout, suck, and palm-chin), and results of diagnostic studies (arteriogram, electroenceph-

alogram, and computed tomography and magnetic resonance imaging scans)
• Psychosocial status, including family, friends, other support systems, recent relocation, recent losses, and efforts to express sadness, frustration, anxiety, or other emotions associated with verbal communication impairment
• Medication status, including use of prescription and over-the-counter medications

Defining characteristics

• Disorientation
• Difficulty expressing thought verbally (aphasia, dysphasia, apraxia, dyslexia)
• Difficulty comprehending and maintaining usual communication pattern
• Difficulty forming words or sentences (aphonia, dyslalia, dysarthria)
• Difficulty using or inability to use facial expressions or body language
• Dyspnea
• Impaired articulation
• Inability or lack of desire to speak
• Inability to speak dominant language
• Inappropriate verbalizations
• Lack of eye contact or poor selective attention
• Stuttering or slurring
• Vision deficit (partial or total)

Associated medical diagnoses (selected)

Alzheimer's disease, amyotrophic lateral sclerosis, brain tumors, cerebrovascular accident, deafness, dementia, Huntington's disease

Expected outcomes

• Patient will improve communication skills to extent possible.
• Patient will attend sessions with speech therapist.

• Visitors and staff members will demonstrate appropriate respect when speaking with patient.
• Patient will communicate needs without excessive frustration.
• Patient will take steps to decrease isolation from friends and family members.
• Patient or family member will identify and contact appropriate support services.
• Patient will indicate through gestures, behavior, writing, or speaking that he is coming to terms with his impaired ability to communicate.

Interventions and rationales
• When initiating communication, face patient, maintain eye contact, speak slowly, and enunciate clearly *to make it easier for patient to receive and process your message.*
• Take steps to enhance communication while providing care:
– Communicate one idea at a time.
– Use "yes" and "no" questions.
– Avoid abstract thoughts and controversial topics.
– Use plain, everyday vocabulary.
– Allow longer response time.
– Guess at meaning of incorrect words.
– Reduce distractions.
– Eliminate unnecessary noise.
– Encourage patient to use gestures or other alternative means of communication.
Facilitating communication efforts will help decrease patient's frustration.
• If patient's communication problems are exacerbated by hearing deficits, use appropriate techniques to overcome hearing problems:
– Minimize glare in patient's room *to make it easier for patient to read your lips.*

– Use normal voice when speaking. *Shouting makes your voice frequency higher and doesn't assist hearing.*
– Check for proper use of adaptive hearing devices. If patient wears hearing aid, be sure battery is working and hearing aid is in place correctly *to enhance hearing ability.*
– Use paper and pencil if hearing is severely impaired *to provide alternative means of communication.*
• If patient doesn't follow your conversation, rephrase ideas using simpler wording *to overcome differences in language or culture that may block communication.*
• Don't rush patient when he is struggling to express his thoughts. Demonstrate tact and willingness to listen. Even if you can't understand patient, let him know you accept his efforts to communicate and you empathize with his frustration. *Patient with impaired verbal communication experiences isolation, despair, and frustration. Demonstrating compassion and fostering therapeutic relationship is most important step for improving communication.*
• Avoid conversing with patient when he's tired. *Patient's attention span may deteriorate when he's fatigued, thereby making efforts to communicate even more frustrating.*
• Encourage patient to engage in social activities, such as attending therapy sessions and eating with other patients at group tables, *to reduce feelings of isolation.*
• If appropriate, help patient reintegrate into family life; for example, arrange for patient to attend family gatherings. *Impaired speech may affect patient's role in family. Providing opportunity to reintegrate patient into family life may diminish loneliness and anxiety.*

• Encourage patient to reminisce. Use photographs, gestures, and visits from family members and friends to stimulate patient's desire to express himself. *Recalling meaningful experiences may motivate patient to try to communicate and may enhance feelings of self-worth.*
• Encourage family members and colleagues to use speech appropriate for adults when talking to patient and not to talk about him within his range of hearing *to convey respect.*
• Obtain referral to speech therapist. Educate family members and colleagues about methods prescribed by therapist to enhance communication *to ensure continuity of care.*
• Refer patient and family members to appropriate community resources, such as club for stroke survivors or support group for relatives of Alzheimer's patients, *to help them cope with communication impairment after discharge.*

Evaluation for expected outcomes
• Patient improves communication skills to extent possible.
• Patient attends sessions with speech therapist ___ times per week.
• Visitors and staff demonstrate appropriate respect when speaking with patient by using adult speech and not talking about him within his hearing range.
• Patient communicates needs, using gestures, behavior, writing, or speech, without excessive frustration.
• Patient takes steps to decrease isolation from friends and family members.
• Patient or family member identifies and contacts appropriate support services.
• Patient indicates that he is coming to terms with his impaired ability to communicate.

Documentation
• Observations of impaired speaking ability, use of communication aids, and expressions of frustration
• Interventions implemented to decrease barriers to effective communication
• Patient's efforts to communicate using gestures, behavior, writing, and speech
• Patient teaching and patient's response
• Referrals to speech therapist and other support services
• Evaluations for expected outcomes

■ Violence, risk for: Self-directed

related to recurrent losses or changes in physical or mental condition

Definition
Presence of risk factors for attempted suicide

Assessment
• Age
• Sex
• Race
• Religion
• Marital status (widowed, divorced, married, or single)
• Life situation, including isolation (living alone or in urban area) and recent retirement, unemployment, or move to new area
• Mental health history, including coping behaviors, statements of low self-esteem, family dynamics, and communication patterns
• Recent stressors, including divorce, death of spouse, and relocation

• Mental status, including orientation, level of consciousness, and thought processes
• Support systems

Risk factors
• Changes in mood or affect
• Changes in physical or mental status
• Confusion
• Direct or indirect statements of intent to commit suicide
• Evidence of getting affairs in order, such as changing or making will
• Evidence of giving away money or valuables
• Experience of multiple losses, such as loss of spouse, income, and friends
• Expressed feelings of hopelessness, helplessness, or depression
• History of attempted suicide
• Hoarding of medications
• Purchasing of gun or other weapon
• Suicidal ideation
• Frequent medical visits about somatic complaints

Associated medical diagnoses (selected)
This nursing diagnosis may be associated with any mental or physical illness that decompensates patient and in which prognosis is poor, such as dementia, depression, drug or alcohol addiction, metastatic disease, and traumatic injury.

Expected outcomes
• Patient won't harm himself and will remain in safe environment.
• Patient will discuss sadness, despair, and other feelings.
• Patient will discuss events that led up to current crisis.
• Patient will acknowledge suicidal thoughts.
• Patient will receive referral to mental health professional.

• Patient will express improved self-concept.
• Patient will report decreased desire to kill himself.
• Patient will discuss appropriate coping skills to avoid future suicidal episodes.

Interventions and rationales
• Be aware of key facts about suicide in older patients:
– Suicide among older adults is a serious problem. Those with highest risk of suicide are at least 85 years old, depressed, with high self-esteem and need to control life.
– Suicide rate for older adult men is seven times that for older women.
– Most suicides by older patients are planned and aren't just gestures or threats; even frail nursing home residents can find strength to carry out suicide if sufficiently determined. *Awareness of suicide risks may help prevent attempts.*
• Remove items from patient's surroundings that could be used in suicide attempt *to ensure patient's safety.*
• Set aside time for listening to patient *to communicate that you care.*
• Approach patient with understanding and concern *to alleviate angry or embarrassed feelings related to emotional breakdown or previous unsuccessful suicide attempt.*
• Communicate nonjudgmental attitude *to build trust and rapport.*
• Assess patient for signs and symptoms of depression, such as persistent depressed mood, diminished interest in daily activities, sleep disturbances, inappropriate guilt, loss of energy, poor concentration, changes in appetite, psychomotor retardation or agitation, and passive wish for death. *Elderly patients are at increased risk for depression. Depression increases*

in both frequency and intensity with advancing age. Factors that contribute to increase in depression include changes in neurotransmitter levels, multiple losses, diminished health, and decreased resources. Depression may also occur in early stages of dementia.

• Discuss problems that led patient to episode of depression. *Talking about specific events may help patient achieve catharsis and develop appropriate coping skills.* Events that may contribute to depression in older patients include recent major loss, experience of rejection by or isolation from family or friends, recent disability, loss of partner, loss of sexual function, and loss of social, family, or occupational role.

• Recognize patient's feelings of inadequacy and take steps to bolster self-esteem. Encourage patient to participate in life review, revisit places where significant past events took place, put together scrapbook, research family genealogy, or attend family, class, or church reunions. *These activities help patient experience emotions, which ultimately promotes improved self-esteem.*

• Avoid comparing patient with others *to reduce stereotyping and foster individuality.*

• Support patient but don't give false reassurances that everything will work out. Let him know that, although no easy answer exists, help is available and you'll help him find alternative solutions *to ease despair.*

• Supervise administration of prescribed medications. Be aware of drug actions and adverse effects and make sure that patient doesn't hoard medications *to ensure he won't harm himself, even inadvertently.*

• Decrease environmental stimuli when necessary and provide safe outlet for releasing emotions and anger. Review situations that cause stress for patient and help him develop plans for dealing with them. *These measures will help patient cope better with depression.*

• Assess for signs of suicidal thinking that warrant further investigation, such as sudden hoarding of medications, giving away possessions, sudden interest in guns, and despondent remarks, *to determine if patient is at risk for suicide.*

• Ask patient directly, "Have you thought about killing yourself?" If so, ask, "What do you plan to do?" *to assess for suicidal ideation.*

• If you suspect that patient is at risk for suicide, refer him to mental health professional for immediate evaluation *to ensure safety.*

• Educate patient or family member in use of prescribed antidepressants. Explain that geriatric doses differ from those for younger patients. *Knowledge of medications and careful monitoring help guard against adverse effects.*

• Help patient identify community resources *to obtain continued therapy and support after hospitalization.*

• Encourage family members to talk with one another and develop improved coping strategies *to foster enhanced family functioning.*

Evaluations for expected outcomes
• Patient doesn't harm himself and his environment is safe, with items that could be used in suicide attempt removed.

• Patient expresses feelings and thoughts in way that promotes healing process.

• Patient discusses events that led up to current crisis.
• Patient acknowledges suicidal thoughts.
• Patient receives referral to mental health professional.
• Patient states that he feels better about himself.
• Patient states that he experiences fewer suicidal thoughts.
• Patient expresses understanding of importance of increased social support and improved coping skills in avoiding future suicidal episodes.

Documentation

• Patient's exact description of suicidal thoughts and recent suicide attempt
• Observations of patient's behavior
• Interventions to prevent suicide
• Patient's responses to therapy
• Evaluations for expected outcomes

PART SIX

PSYCHIATRIC AND MENTAL HEALTH

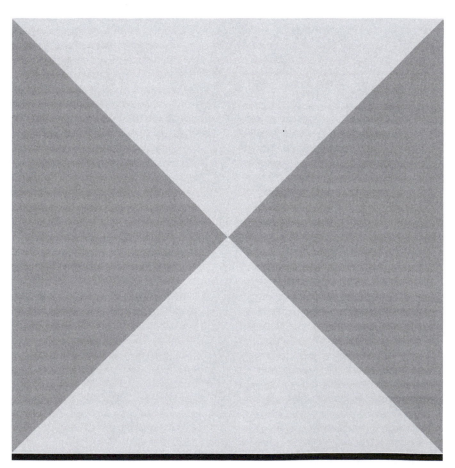

INTRODUCTION

Whether or not you work in mental health nursing, you need to develop skills in dealing with patients who have psychiatric disorders or psychological health problems. As a practitioner, you have a responsibility to respond to the psychological as well as the physical needs of your patients. This section includes plans of care for patients with such diverse needs as anxiety, coping, fear, and posttraumatic stress syndrome. The establishment and maintenance of a therapeutic relationship is an essential skill in providing mental health care. The nurse should also maintain a nonjudgmental attitude and be open to the prospect of recovery throughout care.

As increased attention is being paid to substance abuse, domestic violence, sexual abuse, and related problems, you'll be called on to provide comprehensive care for these patients in outpatient settings, hospitals, and nontraditional health care settings. Recent improvements in drug therapy now allow mental health patients to live in community settings with supervision of their medication regimen.

As more patients cope with the effects of chronic disease, nurses are called on to provide support and instruction for families and friends. Likewise, as more patients are cared for across the managed care spectrum, attention to the mental health aspect of care is crucial in meeting patient outcomes. The plans of care in this section will aid you in providing care in the areas of psychological and social health.

Altered family processes
related to dysfunctional behavior

Definition
A change in family relationship or functioning

Assessment
• Family status, including marital status, developmental stage of family, family roles, family rules, communication patterns, family goals, and socioeconomic status
• Family health history, including history of mental illness, stress-related illnesses, history of substance abuse, and sexual abuse of spouse or children
• Parental status, including ages of dependent children and knowledge of normal child behavior
• Psychological status, including self-image and self-esteem, functional ability, independence level, and problem-solving and decision-making skills

Defining characteristics
• Changes in:
– availability for emotional support
– communication patterns
– expressions of conflict within family
– expressions of conflict with or isolation from community resources
– mutual support
– participation in problem solving
– patterns and rituals
– somatic complaints
– stress-reduction behaviors

Associated medical diagnoses (selected)
Anxiety disorders; attention-deficit disorder; conduct disorder; delirium, dementia, and amnestic and other cognitive disorders; dissociative disorder; factitious disorder; personality disorders; schizophrenia; sexual disorders; somatoform disorder; substance abuse–related disorders

Expected outcomes
• Family members will not experience verbal, physical, emotional, or sexual abuse.
• Family members will communicate clearly, honestly, consistently, and directly.
• Family members will establish clearly defined roles and equitable responsibilities.
• Family members will express understanding of rules and expectations.
• Family members will report that methods of solving problems and resolving conflicts have improved.
• Family members will report a decrease in the number and intensity of family crises.
• Family members will seek ongoing treatment.

Interventions and rationales
• Meet with family members *to establish levels of authority and responsibility in the family.*
• In family meeting, arrange seating so adults present unified front *to reinforce their function as a decision-making unit.*
• Hold adults accountable for their alcohol or substance abuse and have them sign a "Use Contract" *to decrease denial, increase trust, and promote change.*
• Assist family to set limits on abusive behaviors and have them sign "Abuse Contracts" *to foster feelings of safety and trust.*
• Teach family to communicate clearly and honestly *to increase their ability to express thoughts and feelings in a positive way.*
• Encourage family members to evaluate communication patterns periodi-

cally *to reinforce benefits of effective communication skills.*
• Refer to outside agencies, if needed, *to ensure continuing support.*

Evaluation for expected outcomes
• Family members don't experience any type of abuse.
• Family members report that family communication is clear, honest, and respectful.
• Family members describe clearly defined roles and responsibilities.
• Family members demonstrate understanding of roles and responsibilities.
• Family members identify problems and work together to solve them.
• Family members report fewer family crises.
• Family members recognize the need for professional assistance.

Documentation
• Problems and conflicts described by family members
• Behavioral contracts signed by family members
• Changes in roles and responsibilities and information about how these changes were negotiated
• Evidence of changes in family communication patterns
• Family responses to nursing interventions
• Evaluations for expected outcomes

■ Altered family processes: Alcoholism

Definition
Ineffective family functioning related to alcohol abuse in one or more members, often leading to conflict, denial of problems, resistance to change, ineffective problem solving, and a series of self-perpetuating crises

Assessment
• Family status, including alcoholic family member's ability to function in occupational and family roles, ability of other family members to function in their roles, family conflicts, financial status, and rituals during holidays and family celebrations
• Coping patterns, including type and number of changes family has recently experienced, usual response to stress, ability to adapt to change, and use of support systems
• Family health history, including medication use, mental illness, stress-related illnesses, history of alcohol or drug abuse, and evidence of emotional, physical, or sexual abuse of spouse or children
• Parental status, including age, marital status, number and ages of dependent children, and knowledge of normal child behavior
• Drinking pattern, including continuous or binge drinking, periods of abstinence and relapse, use of other substances, symptoms of withdrawal, and past drinking patterns and treatment
• Psychological status, including self-image and self-esteem, functional ability, independence level, and problem-solving and decision-making skills
• Spiritual status, including affiliation with a religious group and religious practices

Defining characteristics
• Changes in:
– availability for affective responsiveness and intimacy
– mutual support
– participation in decision making
– communication patterns
– power alliances
– satisfaction with family and in expressions of conflict within the family
– somatic complaints

Associated medical diagnoses (selected)
Antisocial personality disorder, anxiety disorder, cirrhosis, depression, drug or alcohol addiction, esophageal varices, fetal alcohol syndrome

Expected outcomes
• Family members will acknowledge there is a problem with alcoholism within the family.
• Alcoholic family member will sign a contract stating that he agrees to abstain from alcohol.
• Family members will sign contracts stating that they won't engage in abusive behavior.
• Family members will communicate their needs using "I" statements.
• Parents will take steps to reassert appropriate boundaries with children and resume parental responsibilities.
• Family members will discuss problems in an open, safe environment.
• Family members will acknowledge their strengths and their progress in resolving problems.
• Number and intensity of family crises will diminish.
• Family members will state their plans to continue to seek counseling and attend appropriate support group meetings.

Interventions and rationales
• Encourage family members to acknowledge that alcoholism is a problem within family *to break through family denial*. Encourage individual family members to take responsibility for their problems. *Problems can't be addressed until family members take responsibility for them.*
• Inform alcoholic family member that he'll have to address his alcoholism before progress can be made in rebuilding family relations. Tell him that abstinence with the help of a support group such as Alcoholics Anonymous (AA) is the only proven effective treatment for alcoholism *to establish abstinence as basis for treatment.*
• Ask alcoholic family member to sign a contract stating he'll abstain from alcohol *to help him take responsibility for his behavior.*
• Help family members evaluate consequences of abusive and violent behavior. Inform them that any suspected abuse will be reported. Ask family members to sign contracts stating they won't abuse each other *to help ensure safety of family members.*
• Teach family members to communicate their needs assertively. Encourage family members to use "I" statements to express feelings — for example, "I'm mad because you didn't show up for the school play like you promised." — *to help family members get in touch with and talk about feelings.*
• Discuss with parents their ideas and beliefs regarding parental authority. Ask if they feel they have abdicated authority. Work with parents to develop steps to reassert parental authority *to reestablish appropriate boundaries and relieve children of need to assume parental roles.*
• Provide opportunity for family members to discuss conflicts in an open, safe atmosphere *to decrease anxiety and help family members develop confidence in their ability to resolve problems.*
• Assist family members in identifying their strengths and their progress in addressing problems *to build self-esteem.*
• Encourage family members to continue to seek counseling *to enhance interpersonal skills and strengthen the family unit.*
• Encourage family members to participate in Al-Anon, or Alateen *to foster recovery.*

Evaluations for expected outcomes
• Family members acknowledge that alcoholism is a problem in the family.
• Alcoholic family member signs a contract stating that he agrees to abstain from alcohol.
• Family members sign contracts stating that they won't engage in abusive behavior.
• Family members communicate their needs using "I" statements.
• Parents take steps to reassert appropriate boundaries with children and to resume parental responsibilities.
• Family members discuss problems in an open, safe environment.
• Family members acknowledge their strengths and the progress they have made in resolving problems.
• Number and intensity of family crises diminish.
• Family members state their plans to continue to seek counseling and attend appropriate support groups.

Documentation
• Family's reactions to and experience with alcoholism
• Interventions to assist family and family's responses to them
• Referrals to community agencies
• Evaluations for expected outcomes

■ Anxiety

related to environmental conflict (phobia)

Definition
Feeling of threat or danger to self arising from an unidentifiable source

Assessment
• History of panic symptoms (choking feeling in throat, hyperventilation, light-headedness, dizziness, and other physical signs and symptoms of anxiety)
• Psychological status, including patient's explanation of problem, onset, duration, precipitating events, past coping, present coping (note use of repression and denial and escape-avoidance behaviors), insight (note patient's understanding of irrationality of fears), motivation to change, anxiety level (+1, +2, +3, +4), secondary gains (what kind and from whom), current stressors, results of mental status examination (note expression of anxiety in terms of personal fears, concentration, judgment, affect, and impulse control as well as all other aspects of mental status), and personal abilities, talents, and strengths
• Sociologic status, including support systems, hobbies, interests, work history, family makeup, family roles (evidence of harmony or disharmony), family coping mechanisms, evidence of reinforcement of problem by family, and lifestyle (how this reinforces irrational fears)
• Medication history (response, effectiveness, and adverse effects)

Defining characteristics
• Diarrhea
• Dry mouth
• Fidgeting
• Focus on self
• Heart pounding
• Increased blood pressure
• Increased respirations
• Increased wariness
• Shakiness
• Tendency to become rattled
• Worrying

Associated medical diagnoses (selected)
Anorexia nervosa, anxiety disorder, phobic disorder, schizophrenia

Expected outcomes

• Patient will experience reduced anxiety by identifying precipitating situations.
• Patient will connect life events to occurrence of anxiety.
• Patient will identify current stressors.
• Patient will set limits and compromises on behavior when ready.
• Patient will develop effective coping behaviors.
• Patient will maintain autonomy and independence without handicapping fears or use of phobic behavior.

Interventions and rationales

• Identify your feelings toward patient *to keep them from interfering with treatment.*
• Accept patient as is. *Forcing patient to change before he's ready causes panic.*
• Explore factors that precipitate phobic reactions and anxiety. *This is important for understanding patient's dynamics.*
• Reassure patient he is safe. *Patient may perceive that he is at risk.*
• Support patient with desensitization techniques *to help him overcome problem.*
• Give patient chance to ventilate feelings. *This reduces patient's tendency to suppress or repress; bottled-up feelings continue to affect behavior even though patient may be unaware of them.*
• Teach relaxation techniques (breathing exercises, progressive muscle relaxation, guided imagery, meditation) *to counteract fight-or-flight response.*
• Help patient set limits and compromises on behavior when ready and allow patient to be afraid. *Fear is a feeling, neither right nor wrong.*
• Give patient facts about fear and anxiety and their consequences *to reduce anxiety and encourage patient to help in managing problem.*
• Encourage patient not to run away when afraid *to help patient learn that fear can be faced and managed.*
• Help patient develop own techniques for dealing with fears *to establish alternatives to escape or avoidance behaviors.*

Evaluations for expected outcomes

• Patient identifies precipitating situations and demonstrates fewer physical symptoms of anxiety, improved concentration, and reduced preoccupation with fears.
• Patient discusses possible relationship between anxiety and past and present experiences.
• Patient lists stressors.
• Patient limits phobic behavior when ready.
• Patient participates in desensitization therapy and learns to better manage stress, health, and responsibilities.
• Patient makes decisions, shows greater independence, and decreases behaviors that limit spontaneous activity.

Documentation

• Observation of subjective and objective data
• Interventions to reduce anxiety and increase coping
• Patient's response to interventions
• Evaluations for expected outcomes

■ Caregiver role strain

related to unpredictability of the care situation

Definition

A caregiver's felt or exhibited difficulty in performing a family caregiver role

Assessment
- Caregiver's age, sex, level of education, occupation, and marital status
- Caregiver's physical and mental status, including chronic health problems, self-care abilities and limitations, and level of cognitive function
- Patient's physical and mental status, including history of psychiatric illness, self-care limitations, and level of cognitive functioning
- Support systems, including financial resources, family members and friends, community services, health-related services such as geriatric or psychiatric day care, and church affiliation
- Cultural, ethnic, and religious background of family
- Family roles, coping patterns, family alliances, goals, and values

Defining characteristics
- Apprehension about patient's care when caregiver is ill or deceased
- Apprehension about patient's health and caregiver's ability to provide care in future
- Apprehension about possible institutionalization of patient
- Preoccupation with care routine

Associated medical diagnoses (selected)
Alzheimer's disease, anxiety disorder, depressive disorder, psychoactive substance use, somatic disorder

Expected outcomes
- Family members will discuss how patient's illness has altered established roles and responsibilities within the family.
- Family members will assign responsibilities to prevent too much from falling on one individual's shoulders.
- Family members will establish limits on the patient's behavior and will work together to uphold them.
- Family members will refrain from using destructive coping mechanisms, such as substance abuse and physical or mental abuse of care recipient.
- Family members will make use of outside support systems, such as community resources, religious organizations, and day hospitals.
- Family members will recognize need for professional assistance.

Interventions and rationales
- Encourage discussion among family members about role changes and added responsibilities that have occurred as a result of patient's health status *to establish open and honest communication among family members.*
- Encourage discussion of family's past experience with crises, comparing them with present situation *to help family see they have survived difficulties together and encourage them to seek viable solutions.*
- Assist family members to clarify needs, set individual goals, and develop plans to meet them. *This will instill in each person a sense of empowerment and control over his life.*
- Encourage family members to retain involvement with social and religious networks *to avoid feelings of isolation and abandonment.*
- Refer family to appropriate professional services *to ensure their needs are being met.*

Evaluations for expected outcomes
- Family members adjust to changes in roles and responsibilities.
- Family members share responsibilities of caregiving equitably.
- Patient behaves within limits set by caregiver.
- Family members don't exhibit signs of stress.

• Family members use community resources as necessary.
• Family members attend support groups or seek other forms of professional assistance.

Documentation
• Family members' beliefs and attitudes about patient's illness
• Role adjustment and flexibility of family members
• Coping patterns
• Patient's behavior
• Goals articulated by family members
• Use of support systems
• Referrals for professional help
• Patient's and family members' responses to nursing interventions
• Evaluations for expected outcomes

■ Coping, ineffective individual

related to personal vulnerability

Definition
Inability to use adaptive behaviors in response to difficult life situations

Assessment
• Patient's perception of present health problem or crisis
• Coping behaviors
• Usual problem-solving techniques used to cope with life problems
• Physical or emotional impairment
• Occupation
• Diversional activities
• Financial resources
• Support systems, including family members, friends, and clergy
• Reactions of family members to patient's crisis

Defining characteristics
• Change in communication patterns

• Decreased use of social support
• Destructive behavior toward self or others
• Difficulty asking for help
• Fatigue
• High illness rate
• Inability to meet basic needs and role expectations
• Lack of goal-directed behavior, such as inability to attend, difficulty organizing information, poor concentration, and poor problem-solving abilities
• Maladaptive coping behaviors
• Risk-taking behaviors
• Sleep disturbance
• Statements indicating inability to cope
• Substance abuse

Associated medical diagnoses (selected)
This nursing diagnosis may occur whenever an individual uses maladaptive strategies to cope with life's tasks. Associated diagnoses include affective disorders, antisocial personality disorder, bipolar disorder (depressive and manic phases), borderline personality disorder, dependent personality disorder, depression, drug or alcohol addiction, drug overdose, hypochondriasis, narcissistic personality disorder, obsessive-compulsive disorder, panic disorder, passive-aggressive personality disorder, phobic disorder, and schizophrenia.

Expected outcomes
• Patient will express understanding of the relationship between emotional state and behavior.
• Patient will become actively involved in planning own care.
• Patient will reduce use of manipulative behavior to gratify needs.
• Patient will accept responsibility for behavior.

• Patient will identify effective and ineffective coping techniques.
• Patient will use available support systems, such as family, friends, and psychotherapist, to develop and maintain effective coping skills.

Interventions and rationales

• If possible, assign primary nurse to patient *to provide continuity of care and promote development of a therapeutic relationship.*
• Spend consistent, uninterrupted time with patient. Encourage open expression of feelings. *An open environment will help patient ventilate intense emotion. Through discussion, you can help patient understand the personal meaning attached to recent events and foster a realistic assessment of his situation.*
• As patient becomes able to express feelings more openly, discuss relationship between feelings and behavior. *To change, patient must understand this relationship.*
• Discourage dependent behavior by assisting patient only when necessary. Provide positive reinforcement for independent behavior *to enhance self-esteem, encourage repetition of desired behavior, and promote effective coping.*
• Encourage patient to make decisions about care *to reduce feelings of helplessness and enhance patient's sense of mastery over current situation.*
• Set limits on manipulative behavior. Provide patient with clear expectations for behavior and describe consequences if limits are violated. *If patient can't curb inappropriate behavior, consistent limit-setting imposes external controls.*
• Recognize that manipulative behaviors reduce patient's sense of insecurity by increasing feelings of power. *Understanding patient's motivation*

may help you deal better with manipulative behavior.
• Help patient recognize and accept responsibility for actions. Discourage patient from unfairly placing blame on others. *Developing a sense of responsibility is necessary before change can occur.*
• Help patient recognize and feel good about positive personal qualities and accomplishments. *As self-esteem increases, patient will feel less need to manipulate others.*
• Help patient analyze current situation and evaluate effectiveness of coping strategies *to foster an objective outlook.*
• Praise patient for identifying and using effective coping techniques *to reinforce appropriate behavior.*
• Suggest alternatives to ineffective behaviors identified by patient. Encourage patient to determine what new behaviors can be effectively incorporated into lifestyle. *Fostering patient participation in care promotes feelings of independence.*
• Encourage patient to use support systems, such as psychotherapist, family, and friends, *to maintain effective coping skills.*

Evaluations for expected outcomes

• Patient describes emotions triggered by illness or personal crisis and usual coping behaviors.
• Patient works with primary nurses to plan care.
• Patient describes two instances in which needs were met through direct communication.
• Patient describes one difficult interpersonal situation that was solved by identifying the problem, choosing alternative ways to communicate, and taking action.
• Patient identifies two effective and two ineffective coping behaviors.

• Patient enlists support and assistance from family and friends.

Documentation
• Patient's perception of present situation
• Emotions expressed by patient
• Observations of patient's behaviors
• Interventions performed to help patient develop coping skills
• Patient's responses to nursing interventions
• Evaluations for expected outcomes

■ Hopelessness
related to child's mood disturbance

Definition
A subjective feeling in which a child sees limited or no alternatives or personal choices available and is unable to mobilize energy on own behalf

Assessment
• Family status, including family composition, level of education of family members, parents' occupation, child's grade level, ability of family to meet child's physical and emotional needs, coping patterns, and evidence of abuse
• Psychological status, including changes in appetite, energy level, motivation, and personal hygiene
• Sleep pattern
• Social status, including quality of relationships, degree of trust in others, level of self-esteem, and ability to function in social or academic roles

Defining characteristics
• Decreased affect
• Decreased appetite
• Decreased or increased sleep
• Decreased verbalization

• Lack of initiative
• Passivity

Associated medical diagnoses (selected)
Adjustment disorders, anxiety disorders, conduct disorder, posttraumatic stress syndrome, reactive attachment disorder of infancy or early childhood, separation anxiety disorder

Expected outcomes
• Child won't harm himself while in hospital.
• Child will complete activities of daily living (ADLs) with assistance.
• Child will identify feelings and seek help when they are overwhelming.
• Child will identify ways to deal with stress at home and school.
• Child will begin making positive statements about himself and others.

Interventions and rationales
• Provide safe environment *to maintain child's safety.*
• Spend time each shift with child. Allow child to play in lieu of talking. *Playing is a form of communication for children.*
• Encourage child to perform self-care activities to extent possible and praise smallest efforts *to enhance self-esteem and reduce feelings of hopelessness.*
• Help child make contact with other children *to reduce feelings of hopelessness.*
• Have family members bring toys, pictures, and other personal belongings *to reduce child's stress.*
• Teach child, parents, and teachers about interventions that increase self-esteem *so that child continues to receive support after discharge.*

Evaluations for expected outcomes
• Child remains safe and unharmed.
• Child completes ADLs.

• Child asks for help when unable to cope with feelings.
• Child demonstrates positive methods of dealing with stress.
• Child attempts to make positive statements about himself and others.

Documentation
• Observations of child's behavior
• Child's participation in self-care activities
• Child's expressions during play therapy
• Nursing interventions that stabilize mood and maintain safety
• Child's response to nursing interventions
• Evaluations for expected outcomes

■ Injury, risk for

related to elder abuse

Definition
A state in which an individual is at risk of injury as a result of environmental conditions interacting with the individual's adaptive and defensive resources

Assessment
• Age
• Health history, including accidents, falls, exposure to environmental hazards, marks from restraints, and unexplained bruising
• Evidence of neglect, including inappropriate clothing, unsanitary living conditions, inadequate food supplies, lack of medication, and absence of needed eyeglasses, hearing aid, cane, or walker
• Family status, including caregiver relationship to patient; time and resources available for caregiving; willingness and ability to meet the patient's physical, social, and psychological needs; feelings of frustration; and history of abuse of any family member

Risk factors
• Affective orientation
• Design, structure, and arrangement of community, building, and equipment
• Developmental age
• Mode of transportation
• People or provider (nosocomial agents and staffing patterns)
• Pollutants, drugs, alcohol, caffeine, nicotine, and preservatives

Associated medical diagnoses (selected)
Alzheimer's disease, bipolar disorder, dementia, fractures, malnutrition, osteoarthritis, rheumatoid arthritis, schizophrenia

Expected outcomes
• Patient will remain free from injury.
• Patient will state that no incidents of abuse occur.
• Patient will maintain control of mail, telephone, and other personal effects.
• Caregiver will state intention to contact respite care services and support groups.
• Patient and caregiver will report improved communication patterns.

Interventions and rationales
• Monitor patient closely for signs of physical or mental abuse or neglect (bruises, abrasions, body odor, and unkept appearance) *to ensure patient's safety and well-being.*
• Encourage patient to discuss abuse or threats of abuse. Be willing to listen and be careful to convey a nonjudgmental attitude. *Patient may be hesitant to talk openly for fear of retaliation.*

• Report actual or suspected abuse to local authorities. *Every state has an agency that investigates and makes decisions about how a patient can best be protected from further abuse.*
• Encourage patient to answer his own telephone and open his own mail. *This gives patient a sense of control and self-worth.*
• Inform patient and caregiver about state and county services for elderly people, respite services, adult day care, and support groups for children of aging parents *to enhance caregiver's ability to cope.*

Evaluations for expected outcomes
• Patient shows no physical or mental signs of abuse.
• Patient reaffirms there has been no abuse.
• Patient is able to manage his own mail and telephone messages.
• Caregiver contacts community agencies that offer assistance.
• Patient and family demonstrate improved communication.

Documentation
• Evidence of abuse
• Comments by patient that indicate abuse
• Reports made to state agencies
• Changes in caregiver-patient relationship
• Outside agencies contacted by caregiver
• Changes occurring as a result of using outside resources
• Evaluations for expected outcomes

■ Knowledge deficit
related to informed consent

Definition
Absence or deficiency of cognitive information related to a specific topic

Assessment
• Age
• Developmental stage
• Educational level
• Ethnic group
• Religion
• Beliefs, values, and attitudes about health and illness
• Family status, including marital status, family roles, and family communication patterns
• Mental status, including level of consciousness, thought and speech, mood and affect, orientation, memory, capacity to read and write, and judgment
• Legal status, including patient's authority to give consent, presence of a legal guardian, and nature of treatment

Defining characteristics
• Inability to understand prescribed treatment
• Inappropriate or exaggerated behavior

Associated medical diagnoses (selected)
Developmental disability, mental illness

Expected outcomes
• Patient will describe the treatment and name the person who will perform it.
• Patient will express an awareness of his right to refuse treatment.

Interventions and rationales

- Ask patient to describe his understanding of procedure to be performed *to determine how much patient can assimilate.*
- Answer questions in terms patient can understand. If patient can't understand, refer to doctor *to ensure patient's right to informed consent is protected.*
- If patient is unable to understand, make sure patient's legal guardian understands procedure and reason for doing it. *Nurse can be held liable if informed consent isn't obtained.*
- If treatment is ongoing, continue to educate patient about his care and legal rights *to ensure continuity of care.*

Evaluations for expected outcomes

- Patient can explain treatment accurately.
- Patient states understanding of legitimate right to refuse treatment.

Documentation

- Patient's or guardian's understanding of treatment
- Actions taken to ensure informed consent
- Signed consent (or refusal to sign)
- Evaluations for expected outcomes

■ Personal identity disturbance

related to lowered self-esteem

Definition

Uncertainty about components of self regarding choices of vocation, intimacy, and lifestyle

Assessment

- Choices of vocation, sexual orientation, religious orientation, and friendships
- Ability to defend choices regarding long-range goals, recognize alternatives, and appreciate consequences
- Comfort level with decisions made about long-range goals
- Degree of anxiety or depression about long-range goals
- Loss of interest or social isolation from usual activities or friends
- Level of irritability about long-range goals
- Sleep difficulties
- Changes in eating habits
- Family status, including method of dealing with general conflicts, level of patient's communication with parents, handling of negotiations regarding restriction of freedom, degree of patient's separation from family, tolerance of patient's expressed opinions, reaction of parents to patient's long-range goals, and age-appropriateness of dating, curfew regulation, and money responsibilities
- Family and cultural standards related to separation issues

Defining characteristics

- Inadequate sense of self
- Relationship problems
- Social, emotional, or psychological immaturity

Associated medical diagnoses (selected)

Acquired immunodeficiency syndrome, anorexia nervosa, antisocial personality disorder, borderline personality disorder, brain abscess, bulimia nervosa, chronic pain, dependent personality disorder, hemophilia, incest, multiple personality disorder, narcissistic personality disorder, obsessive-compulsive disorder, passive-aggressive personality disorder, phobic disorder, urinary diversion

Expected outcomes
• Patient will establish trusting relationship with caregiver.
• Patient's issues will be discussed.
• Family's issues will be discussed.
• Patient will establish a firm, positive sense of self and personal identity.
• Patient will choose long-range goals using problem-solving techniques and will be comfortable with choices.
• Family will accept patient's choices of long-range goals.

Interventions and rationales
• Assess patient alone, without family, *to gather baseline data and begin therapeutic relationship.*
• Explain your role as patient advocate; negotiate rules of interaction, including confidentiality and depth and breadth of discussion *to establish your role as resource for patient rather than as family's agent.*
• Explore personal identity issues distressing to patient *to isolate issues into smaller, more solvable units.*
• Help patient identify values, beliefs, hopes, dreams, skills, and interests. *Patient's deficits may lie in lack of self-exploration, problem-solving methods used, or separation issues with parents.*
• Integrate personal identity issues into decisions and choices *to help patient develop skill in problem-solving methods.*
• Help patient identify likely consequences of each choice. *Discussion and explanation aid problem-solving skills.*
• Promote choices with most likelihood of success. *Specific instructions can help patient gain problem-solving ability and maturity.*

• Encourage family conferences to explore potential reactions to patient's choices, and promote support for patient's independent decision-making. *Meetings can help patient and family members identify problems and find better ways to interact. Meetings also allow patient and family members to ventilate true feelings in safe environment.*
• Encourage peer support groups to explore and share personal identity experiences. *Adolescents and young adults often accept support from peers more readily than from older adults.*
• Promote outpatient counseling and family meetings as appropriate to reinforce progress. *Establishing outpatient support systems can reduce regression.*
• Listen to patient's personal values and beliefs, but remain nonjudgmental, even if his values and beliefs differ from your own. *Remaining nonjudgmental but attentive shows your support.*

Evaluations for expected outcomes
• Patient openly discusses concerns with caregiver.
• Patient describes personal identity struggles.
• Family members discuss their reactions to patient's personal identity choices.
• Patient describes values, beliefs, skills, and interests in positive way.
• Patient identifies choices and possible alternatives, postulates consequences, and makes decisions about long-range goals.
• Family members accept patient's choices of long-range goals.

Documentation
• Assessment of patient's initial issues and problem-solving ability, includ-

ing family's reactions, as well as assessment of level of separation achieved by patient
• Patient's level of emotional distress and changes in sleep and eating, initially and as hospitalization continues
• Patient's progress in problem solving and making choices
• Patient-family interactions and content of family meetings
• Patient's interaction in peer-group meetings
• Outpatient resources identified and suggested to patient and family members
• Evaluations for expected outcomes

■ Posttrauma syndrome

related to assault

Definition
Sustained painful response to an unexpected life event

Assessment
• History and circumstances of assault
• Patient's perception of event
• Physical injuries sustained, including cardiopulmonary, genitourinary, integumentary, and musculoskeletal
• Neurologic status
• Emotional reactions, including grief reaction and changes in self-concept and sleep pattern
• Cognitive reactions, including concentration, memory, and orientation
• Behavioral reactions, including coping patterns and social interactions
• Available support systems

Defining characteristics
• Avoidance, alienation, and altered moods
• Denial, grief, fear, and depression
• Detachment

• Exaggerated startle response and flashbacks
• Guilt
• Hypervigilance
• Intrusive dreams, nightmares, or thoughts and difficulty concentrating
• Irritability
• Panic attacks
• Repression
• Shame

Associated medical diagnoses (selected)
This nursing diagnosis may occur in any patient injured as a result of physical assault, such as battered wives, physically abused children and elderly persons, victims of gunshot wounds or stabbing, prisoners of war, and hostages. Examples of associated diagnoses include incest, posttraumatic stress syndrome, rape, sexual assault, and spouse abuse.

Expected outcomes
• Patient will recover from physical injuries to extent possible.
• Patient will state feelings related to alleged assault and will express feelings of guilt.
• Patient will express feelings of physical safety.
• Patient will use effective coping mechanisms to reduce fear.
• Patient will mobilize support systems and professional resources as necessary.
• Patient will reestablish and maintain adaptive interpersonal relationships.

Interventions and rationales
• Follow medical regimen to manage physical injuries. *This reduces anxiety as patient perceives body's ability to recover from injury.*
• Provide patient with psychological support:

– Visit frequently *to decrease patient's fear of being left alone and to encourage trusting relationship.*
– Be available to listen *to express empathy with patient's feelings.*
– Accept patient's feelings and behaviors *to reassure patient that they're appropriate and valid.*
– Reassure patient of safety and take appropriate measures to ensure it. *Patient's feelings of safety are compromised by fear of repeated assaults.*
• Avoid care-related activities and environmental stimuli (loud noises, bright lights, abrupt entrances to room, painful procedures or treatments) that may intensify symptoms. *Patient's traumatic experience may be intensified by misinterpreting procedures or environmental factors as repeated assaults.*
• Monitor mental status, reorienting patient to surroundings and interpreting reality as often as necessary, *to alleviate psychic numbing, a characteristic symptom of assault.*
• Instruct patient in at least one fear-reducing behavior, such as seeking support from others when frightened, *to help patient gain sense of mastery over current situation.*
• Support family members:
– Provide time for them to express feelings.
– Help them understand phases of crisis and patient's reactions to them. *These measures help reduce anxiety.*
• Offer referrals to community or professional resources, including clergy, mental health professional, social services, and support groups, *to help patient regain sense of universality, decrease isolation, share fears, and deal constructively with feelings.*
• Recognize that patient's culture may affect his response to assault; remain supportive and nonjudgmental *to show*

patient you support and accept his response.*

Evaluations for expected outcomes
• Patient recovers from injuries to extent possible and resumes normal or near-normal activities of daily living.
• Patient expresses feelings of anger, blame, fear, and guilt. Patient spends less time recriminating himself.
• Patient reports feeling safe.
• Patient demonstrates at least one fear-reducing behavior during times of panic (specify).
• Patient uses available support groups or mental health crisis center.
• Patient interacts socially with others.

Documentation
• Patient's perception of event
• Observations of patient's verbal and nonverbal behaviors
• Observations of patient's interaction with others
• Patient's responses to nursing interventions
• Referrals to other support systems
• Evaluations for expected outcomes

■ Posttrauma syndrome

related to incest

Definition
A sustained maladaptive response to a traumatic, overwhelming event

Assessment
• Age
• Sex
• Education level
• Customs and rituals, especially pertaining to sexuality
• Family roles, rules, and subsystems

• Evidence of physical, sexual, or emotional abuse within family
• Ability of family members to protect children and correctly judge situations as being safe or unsafe
• Family history of alcoholism, substance abuse, or incarceration of family members

Defining characteristics
• Detachment
• Difficulty in concentrating
• Expressed feelings of denial or shame
• Fear
• Flashbacks
• Irritability
• Panic attacks
• Repression

Associated medical diagnoses (selected)
Anxiety disorders, behavioral disorders, depressive disorders, eating disorders, parent-child relational problem, physical abuse of child, posttraumatic stress syndrome, sexual abuse of child

Expected outcomes
• Child won't harm himself or others.
• Child will agree to maintain personal safety.
• Child will begin expressing feelings in words.
• Child will describe steps to take to maintain safety.
• Child will express awareness of placement after discharge (home, foster care, group home, day treatment program).

Interventions and rationales
• Inform members of treatment team and appropriate community agencies that child may be victim of incest. *You have a responsibility to ensure child's safety after discharge.*

• Observe child for changes in mood or behavior and for statements of intention to harm himself. *Children who have recently disclosed sexual abuse have high rate of suicide.*
• Ask child to agree to verbal and written safety contracts stating he won't harm himself *to provide child with a tangible reminder of how to cope with crises.*
• If child wants to talk about the traumatic event, actively listen *to reassure him that what he tells you is important.*
• Praise child for participating in one-on-one therapy sessions *to enhance his participation and sense of self-worth.*
• Help child identify adults who can be trusted, such as school counselor, clergy person, or school nurse, *to help prevent further episodes of incest.*
• Make appropriate referrals to mental health professionals and social service agencies *to ensure child's safety in community.*

Evaluations for expected outcomes
• Child doesn't harm himself or others.
• Child enters into a contract to refrain from injuring himself or others.
• Child finds positive ways of expressing feelings.
• Child follows steps defined in his plan to maintain safety.
• Child cooperates in looking at a positive living environment after discharge.

Documentation
• Written or verbal safety contract
• Exact quotes of child if any disclosures are made regarding incest
• Child's behavior with peers, staff, and family during visits
• Responses to nursing interventions
• Evaluations for expected outcomes

■ Powerlessness

related to physical, sexual, or emotional abuse by partner

Definition

Perception that one's own action won't significantly affect an outcome

Assessment

• Age
• Sex
• Level of education
• Occupation
• Ethnic group
• Family status, including marital status; developmental stage; socioeconomic status; support systems; history of physical, sexual, or emotional support; and family health history
• Beliefs, values, and attitudes about health and illness
• History of substance abuse
• Description of physical, sexual, or emotional abuse

Defining characteristics

• Expressed feelings of anger, guilt, apathy, or depression
• Inability to seek information regarding care
• Passivity
• Reluctance to express true feelings
• Verbal expressions of having no control over outcome
• Verbal expressions of having no control over present situation

Associated medical diagnoses (selected)

Anxiety disorder, cognitive disorder, dementia, dependent personality disorder, head trauma, mood disorder, posttraumatic stress syndrome

Expected outcomes

• Patient will identify feelings of powerlessness.
• Patient will identify risks to personal safety.
• Patient will make decisions related to care.
• Patient will identify life situations over which she has no control.
• Patient will develop a plan to take control of her life.

Interventions and rationales

• Evaluate patient's potential for harm. *Ensuring patient's safety is your primary responsibility.*
• Discuss patient's abusive relationship with her. Help her to identify feelings of powerlessness and the circumstances that lead to such situations *to help her recognize things that threaten her loss of control.*
• Contact social services *to ensure patient receives legal and financial support as needed.*
• Assist patient to take responsibility for making decisions about self-care by setting care goals and making an activity schedule *to increase her feelings of control over her life.*
• Help patient recognize situations in which she exhibited determination and control over her life *to reinforce past successes and develop a foundation for establishing future goals.*
• Refer patient to a women's shelter *to ensure continued safety after discharge.*

Evaluations for expected outcomes

• Patient discusses feelings of powerlessness.
• Patient describes circumstances in which safety is threatened.
• Patient makes choices in relation to care.
• Patient understands situations in her life over which she has no control.
• Patient develops a plan that will help her take control of her life.

Documentation
• Observations of patient's behavior
• Visits and phone calls from abusive spouse
• Patient's plan for her future
• Patient's responses to nursing interventions
• Referrals to specialized professionals and support groups
• Evaluations for expected outcomes

■ Rape-trauma syndrome

Definition
Physical and emotional trauma that occurs as a result of sexual assault

Assessment
• History and circumstances of traumatic event
• Physical injuries sustained, including genitourinary, integumentary, musculoskeletal, and neurologic
• Emotional reactions, including grief reaction, changes in self-concept, and spiritual distress
• Support systems available to patient, including clergy, family members, and friends
• Problem-solving techniques usually employed by patient

Defining characteristics
• Aggression, anger, and depression
• Agitation
• Changes in relationships
• Embarrassment or shame
• Fear or paranoia
• Guilt and self-blame
• Loss of self-esteem
• Nightmares, sleep disturbances, and phobias
• Sexual dysfunction
• Shock

Associated medical diagnoses (selected)
Incest, rape, sexual assault, spouse abuse

Expected outcomes
• Patient will recover from physical injuries.
• Patient will express feelings and fears.
• Patient will use support systems.

Interventions and rationales
• Follow medical regimen to manage physical injuries caused by traumatic event. *This is first step in meeting patient's hierarchy of needs and depends on extent of patient's other injuries and intensity of psychological response.*
• Follow facility's protocol regarding legal responsibilities. Be aware of potential legal issues of rape and of role nurses may play as witnesses in legal proceedings. *These steps will help protect patient's legal rights.*
• Provide emotional support:
– Be available to listen. Active listening allows empathetic response to patient's feelings while being aware of own thoughts and behaviors.
– Accept patient's feelings to let patient know her feelings are valid and acceptable.
– Approach patient in a warm, caring manner *to cultivate her trust and cooperation.*
– Provide privacy during physical examination and interviewing process. *To protect patient's rights, no information should be released without prior consent.*
– Assure patient of safety and take all necessary measures to ensure it. *This reduces patient's fears of repeated assault.*
• Support patient's family members in their reactions to the traumatic event:

– Provide time for them to express their feelings and concerns.
– Help them understand patient's reactions.
Giving them time to talk and providing accurate information helps them support their loved one.
• Offer referral to other support persons or groups, such as clergy, crisis center, mental health professionals, rape counselors, and Women Organized Against Rape. *This will help patient express feelings and develop coping skills.*

Evaluations for expected outcomes
• Patient recovers from physical injuries.
• Patient expresses feelings common to rape victims, such as anger, blame, humiliation, and fear of disease or pregnancy.
• Patient contacts local mental health, rape-counseling, or crisis center.

Documentation
• Patient's expressions of feelings about herself and traumatic event
• Physical findings and treatment
• Observations of family's interaction with patient
• Referrals to support persons
• Patient's response to nursing interventions
• Evaluations for expected outcomes

■ Rape-trauma syndrome: Compound reaction

Definition
Trauma syndrome that develops after rape or attempted rape in which patient undergoes an acute phase of disorganization and a long-term reorganization; patient experiences drastic changes in behavior, psychological
equilibrium, and ability to function as a consequence of rape

Assessment
• History and circumstances of traumatic event
• Physical symptoms reported by patient
• Physical injuries sustained, including genitourinary, integumentary, musculoskeletal, and neurologic
• Emotional reactions
• Behavioral and cognitive changes, such as expansive mood and affect, agitation, extreme alertness, and narrowed attention span
• Symptoms associated with posttrauma response, including hypervigilance and reexperience of assault
• Available support systems
• Past experience with physical or psychological trauma, including coping strategies and problem-solving skills
• Occupation, educational background, and lifestyle

Defining characteristics
• Changes in lifestyle (change in residence or recurring nightmares)
• Emotional reaction (anger, embarrassment, and fear)
• Multiple physical symptoms (GI irritability, muscle tension, and sleep pattern disturbance)
• Reactivated symptoms of previous physical or psychiatric conditions
• Reliance on alcohol or drugs

Associated medical diagnoses (selected)
Incest, rape, sexual assault, spouse abuse

Expected outcomes
• Patient will recover from physical injuries to fullest extent possible.
• Patient will express feelings about the rape.

- Patient will report feeling safe.
- Patient will contact appropriate support persons or groups.
- Patient will report desire to reestablish and maintain interpersonal relationships.

Interventions and rationales
- Follow medical regimen to manage physical injuries. *This is first step in meeting patient's needs.*
- Document and report rape or attempted rape to appropriate authorities *to help protect patient's legal rights.*
- When interviewing patient, use open-ended questions and listen intently *to encourage patient to talk about trauma and express her feelings, both verbally and through behavior.*
- Show patient that you accept her feelings, but set limits on aggressive behavior. *Demonstrating acceptance reassures patient that her response to trauma is valid. Setting limits provides patient with necessary structure.*
- Take appropriate measures to reassure patient of her safety:
– Approach patient carefully with open hands.
– Stay with patient.
– Have female staff conduct patient interview and physical examination. *Safety measures help to decrease patient's anxiety and reduce fears of another assault.*
- Direct patient to perform purposeful activities, such as taking medications and following instructions of health care personnel, *to help reduce patient's anxiety and restore her sense of control.*
- Educate patient about the variety of responses to trauma. *Patient with a compound reaction may feel that extreme emotional turmoil she experiences after rape is abnormal. Learning that others have undergone the same experience may help reassure her and decrease her isolation.*

- Provide patient's family members with opportunities to express their reactions to the trauma and patient's response. Educate family members about compound reaction to rape *to help them support patient.*
- Refer patient to appropriate support persons, such as clergy, mental health professional, or rape counselor. Encourage patient to participate in support groups or therapy groups offered by rape counseling center. *Patient may need long-term care to cope with psychological consequences of rape.*
- Provide ongoing support as patient struggles to regain psychological equilibrium. Encourage her efforts to renew involvement in usual activities. *To achieve long-term personality reorganization, patient will require time, consistent support, and ongoing counseling.*

Evaluations for expected outcomes
- Patient recovers from physical injuries and resumes normal or near-normal activities of daily living.
- Patient expresses feelings associated with the rape.
- Patient reports feeling safe.
- After discharge, patient participates in ongoing counseling sessions or support group.
- Patient reports increased ability to cope with psychological consequences of rape and increased social interactions and activities.

Documentation
- Patient's expressions of feelings related to trauma
- Observations of patient's behavior and interactions with others
- Nursing interventions
- Patient's response to interventions
- Referrals accepted by patient
- Evaluations for expected outcomes

■ Rape-trauma syndrome: Silent reaction

Definition
Trauma syndrome that develops after rape, attempted rape, or sexual assault, in which patient undergoes an acute phase of disorganization and a long-term reorganization; patient doesn't tell anyone about the rape nor does she deal with her feelings about it

Assessment
• Symptoms associated with posttrauma response
• Evidence of emotional distress, including shock, fear, anger, and guilt
• Behavioral and cognitive changes, such as lack of affect, agitation, decreased alertness, and narrowed attention span
• Evidence of physical injuries
• Available support systems
• Past experience with physical or psychological trauma, including coping strategies and problem-solving skills
• Laboratory studies, including tests for pregnancy and sexually transmitted diseases

Defining characteristics
• Abrupt changes in relationships with men
• Increased anxiety during interview (blocking of associations, long periods of silence, and minor stuttering)
• Increase in nightmares
• No expression that rape, attempted rape, or sexual assault occurred
• Pronounced changes in sexual behavior
• Sudden onset of phobic reactions

Associated medical diagnoses (selected)
Incest, rape, sexual assault, spouse abuse

Expected outcomes
• Patient will disclose that rape, attempted rape, or sexual assault occurred.
• Patient will recover from physical injuries to fullest extent possible.
• Patient will make contact with appropriate sources of support.
• Patient will express willingness to address psychosocial problems associated with traumatic experience.

Interventions and rationales
• Establish an atmosphere of trust *to help patient overcome silence about the rape or sexual assault.*
• Confront patient directly but gently with the question of whether she is a victim of rape or sexual assault. For example, you might say, "You seem very upset and you've told me about increased nightmares and a sudden loss of interest in sexual relations. These are common characteristics of victims of sexual assault. If you've been sexually assaulted, you can tell me. I'll help you." *Patient with silent reaction needs patience and encouragement to overcome anxiety about disclosing rape or sexual assault.*
• Clear up misconceptions patient may have about nature of rape or sexual assault. *If, for example, intercourse didn't take place or attacker was a boyfriend, spouse, or family member, patient may not believe that sexual assault occurred. Tell patient that sexual assault can take different forms and that all can be equally traumatic.*
• If patient remains unwilling to disclose the rape or sexual assault, tell her that you'll continue to be available to help. Encourage her to contact you if she feels the need *to provide a resource for future help and to maintain communication.*

• If patient discloses the rape or sexual assault, be careful to respond in a caring, nonjudgmental manner *to cultivate trust and cooperation.* Follow medical regimen to manage physical injuries (if rape or sexual assault was recent) and follow facility protocol for documenting rape or sexual assault and reporting it to authorities *to ensure patient's physical well-being and protect her legal rights.* Use open-ended questions and listen intently *to encourage patient to talk about the trauma.* If patient is withdrawn, be understanding and supportive when gathering information *to allow patient to proceed at her own pace.*

• Emphasize to patient that attack wasn't her fault. *Patient with silent reaction may feel intense guilt and shame over assault.*

• Educate patient about variety of emotional responses to trauma. Rapetrauma syndrome is a variant of posttraumatic stress syndrome. Responses such as suicidal ideation, disorientation, confusion, extreme detachment, nightmares, flashbacks, guilt, and depression are common. *Patient may believe that emotional turmoil she experiences after rape or sexual assault is abnormal. Pointing out that others have undergone the same experience may lessen patient's isolation, help her talk about her symptoms, and motivate her to seek follow-up care.*

• Offer referral to appropriate support persons or groups, such as clergy, mental health professionals, or rape counselor. Contact a local rape crisis center for information about support groups or therapy groups. Note that, if only a single assault has occurred, short-term counseling may be sufficient. However, if patient is a survivor of several assaults or repeated incest, she may need long-term psychotherapy. *Appropriate referrals help ensure that patient gets needed care.*

Evaluations for expected outcomes

• Patient discloses that rape, attempted rape, or sexual assault occurred.
• Patient recovers from physical injuries and resumes normal or near-normal activities of daily living.
• Patient contacts rape counselor and agrees to participate in therapy group.
• Patient acknowledges that rape or sexual assault wasn't her fault and that she needs to deal with psychological consequences of trauma.

Documentation

• Evidence that patient has been raped or sexually assaulted, including patient's behavior and physical evidence
• Efforts made to help patient discuss rape or sexual assault and patient's response
• Nursing interventions
• Patient's response to interventions
• Referrals accepted by patient
• Evaluations for expected outcomes

■ Self-mutilation, risk for

related to emotional illness

Definition

State in which an individual is at risk for performing a deliberate act of self-harm that is intended to produce immediate tissue damage

Assessment

• Age
• Sex
• Developmental history
• Current stress level and coping behaviors
• Mental status, including judgment, thought content, and mood

• Family history, including abusive behavior
• Previous episodes of self-mutilation or suicide attempts
• Substance abuse history
• Social history, including sexual activity and aggression within peer group

Risk factors
• Borderline personality disorder (especially in females ages 16 to 25)
• Command hallucinations
• Dysfunctional family
• Feelings of depression, rejection, self-hatred, guilt, or depersonalization
• History of physical or sexual abuse, emotional abuse or deprivation, or emotional disturbance
• History of self-injury
• Inability to cope with increased physical or emotional tension
• Labile affect
• Mental retardation and autism
• Psychotic state (typically young adult males)
• Separation anxiety

Associated medical diagnoses (selected)
Autism, borderline personality disorder, developmental disability, factitious disorder with physical symptoms, malingering, multiple personality disorder, sexual masochism

Expected outcomes
• Patient won't harm himself while in facility.
• Patient will express increased sense of security.
• Patient will report being able to cope better with disorganization, aggressive impulses, anxiety, and hallucinations.
• Patient will experience fewer or no dissociative states.
• Patient will participate in therapeutic milieu.

• Patient will report suicidal thoughts to staff members.

Interventions and rationales
• Limit number of staff members interacting with patient *to provide continuity of care and increase patient's sense of security.*
• Have staff members make frequent, short contacts with patient *to reassure patient without stifling independence.*
• Remove all dangerous objects from patient's environment *to promote safety.*
• Make short-term verbal contracts with patient in which patient states he won't harm himself *to make patient aware he's ultimately responsible for his own safety and that he's capable of guaranteeing it.*
• Administer psychotropic medications as ordered *to reduce tension, impulsive behavior, hallucinations, and panic.*
• If patient enters dissociative state or hallucinates, move him to quiet room with reduced stimuli. If he needs restraints, remain with him and provide reassurance *to calm him and orient him to reality.*
• As ordered, place patient under observation *to provide protection and increase patient's sense of security.* If hospitalized, patient can be "zoned" or asked to remain in areas within sight of staff members.
• If patient is participating in therapeutic milieu, discuss patient's risk of self-harm with community members *to provide enhanced protection and psychological support.*
• If patient harms himself, care for injuries in a calm, nonjudgmental manner. Encourage patient to talk about feelings that prompted self-mutilation. *Discussion may help patient connect self-destructive behavior to feelings that preceded it and allow*

exploration of alternative ways of dealing with negative thoughts and feelings.
• If self-destructive acts persist, consider developing behavior modification program, in which patient is rewarded with benefits (personal attention, material items) for demonstrating self-control *to reinforce self-control.*
• Ask patient directly whether he's thinking of suicide and, if so, what plan he has. *A self-destructive patient may become suicidal and may require additional precautions.*
• Hold frequent treatment team meetings *to ensure consistent care that is appropriate to patient's current behavior.*

Evaluations for expected outcomes
• Patient keeps terms of verbal contract that he won't harm himself.
• Patient expresses increased sense of security.
• Patient describes coping skills that help him deal better with disorganization, aggressive impulses, anxiety, and hallucinations.
• Patient experiences fewer or no dissociative states.
• Patient participates in therapeutic milieu.
• Patient tells staff member about suicidal thoughts.

Documentation
• Nursing interventions performed and patient's response to them
• Verbal contracts between patient and nurse
• Patient's responses to medication and behavior modification program
• Revisions to treatment plan
• Drawing of self-inflicted injuries
• Evidence of suicidal ideation
• Evaluations for expected outcomes

■ Sexual dysfunction
related to decreased libido caused by depression

Definition
Presence of physiologic or emotional factors that alter one's usual pattern of sexual function

Assessment
• Comprehensive sexual history, including attitude toward sex, sexual preference, sexual responsiveness of partner, previous sexual response patterns, and sexual desire, enjoyment, and performance
• Psychological factors, including self-esteem, body image, guilt, symptoms of depression, and suicidal ideation
• Support systems, including family, friends, and clergy
• Attitude of spouse or significant other
• Sociocultural factors, including educational level, socioeconomic status, ethnic group, and religious beliefs and practices
• Physiologic factors, including medication history (response, effectiveness, and adverse reactions), current medication regimen (including tricyclic antidepressants or monoamine oxidase [MAO] inhibitors), and substance abuse history (type and effect on mental status)
• Coping and problem-solving ability and ability to concentrate

Defining characteristics
• Actual or perceived limitation imposed by disease or therapy
• Change in relationship with spouse or significant other
• Change of interest in himself and others
• Conflicts involving values

• Inability or change in ability to achieve sexual satisfaction
• Need for confirmation of desirability
• Verbal expression of problem

Associated medical diagnoses (selected)
Bipolar disorder (depressive phase), cyclothymia, dysthymia, hyperpituitarism, hypoactive sexual desire disorder, major depression (single episode or recurrent), major depressive episode (melancholic type), sexual aversion disorder

Expected outcomes
• Patient will acknowledge depressive episode and problem in sexual function.
• Patient will voice feelings about decreases in sexual desire.
• Patient will identify ways to enhance pleasure and improve interpersonal communication with partner.
• Patient will regain sexual desire with recovery from depression.
• Patient will accept referral for sex therapy if necessary.

Interventions and rationales
• Initiate trusting therapeutic relationship with patient. Make purpose, nature, and parameters of this relationship clear *to help patient feel secure and develop trust.*
• Educate patient and family members about nature of depression, its treatment, and its effect on sexual desire. *Understanding link between depression and sexual desire may diminish feelings of guilt and worthlessness and help raise self-esteem.*
• Allow patient to express feelings openly in nonthreatening, nonjudgmental atmosphere *to foster communication and help patient cope with unresolved issues.* Offer feedback *to validate patient's feelings and promote self-esteem.*

• Include patient and partner in planning care and interventions *to enhance feeling of control for both partners.*
• Reinforce compliance with treatment plan for depression. *Even though tricyclic antidepressants and MAO inhibitors may diminish sexual desire, patient needs to comply to resolve depression.*
• Discuss with patient and partner alternative expressions of affection to enhance their relationship during treatment *to help couple preserve intimacy during temporary loss of libido.*
• Refer patient for sex counseling or therapy if low sexual desire persists after resolution of depression. *Sexual desire should return to its usual level after successful treatment for depression. If it doesn't, patient should receive professional therapy.*

Evaluations for expected outcomes
• Patient describes depressive episode, treatment plan, and effects on sexual desire.
• Patient expresses concerns to staff and family members.
• Patient identifies at least three activities to enhance pleasure and communication with partner.
• Patient reports return of sexual fantasies and desire for sexual activity.
• Patient communicates willingness to follow through with referral for sex therapy.

Documentation
• Patient's perceptions and concerns
• Observation of patient's behavior, depressive symptoms, and suicidal risk
• Interventions to assist patient and family members
• Patient's and partner's responses to nursing interventions
• Evaluations for expected outcomes

■ Sexual dysfunction

related to hypersexuality

Definition
Presence of physiologic or emotional factors that alter one's usual pattern of sexual function

Assessment
• History of behaviors indicating excessive elation, such as hypersexuality, intrusiveness, grandiose thoughts, looseness of association, flight of ideas, extreme levels of energy, lack of sleep, lack of proper nutrition, poor judgment, elevated mood, expansiveness, pressured and rapid speech, and strained interpersonal relationships
• History of psychiatric illness, including personality disorders exemplified by lack of impulse control
• Sexual history, including attitude toward sex, previous sexual patterns, sexual preference, sexual response of partners, and appropriateness of sexual behavior
• Sociocultural factors, including educational level, socioeconomic status, and ethnic group
• Patient's perception of sexual behaviors and practices
• Partner's perception of patient's sexual behaviors
• Coping and problem-solving abilities
• Health history, including medication history (response, effectiveness, and adverse reactions), use of psychosis-inducing drugs (such as phencyclidine and amphetamines), use of disinhibiting drugs (such as alcohol, amphetamines, and cocaine), and other substance abuse (type and effect on mental status)

Defining characteristics
• Disturbances in interpersonal relationships caused by inappropriate sexual behavior
• Excessive motor activity
• Excessive sexual activity
• Frustration and anger if sexual behavior is thwarted
• General lack of impulse control
• Impulsive acting out of sexual urges
• Inability to conform sexual behavior to social norms
• Inability to control outcome of sexual encounters
• Inappropriate and provocative verbalizations that are sexual in content
• Intrusiveness with peers, including excessive physical closeness and inappropriate touching
• Periods of excessive elation or cycles of elation and depression
• Poor perception of reality caused by psychosis or organic mental disorders
• Sexual encounters that appear self-destructive; inability to maintain lasting relationships because of sexual behavior

Associated medical diagnoses (selected)
Affective disorders, bipolar disorder (manic phase), drug-induced psychotic states, exhibitionism, fetishism, frottage, organic mental disorder, pedophilia, personality disorders, schizophrenia, sexual masochism, sexual sadism, transvestism, voyeurism

Expected outcomes
• Patient will meet sexual needs in socially appropriate manner.
• Patient will reduce or eliminate sexual behaviors that may harm himself or others.
• Patient will learn how to recognize indicators of impending episodes of hypersexuality and how to prevent such episodes from occurring.

• Patient will state plan to participate in recommended therapy.

Interventions and rationales
• Help patient recognize potentially harmful sexual behavior. Set limits on high-risk sexual behavior. *Indiscriminate, impulsive sexual behavior can lead to unwanted pregnancy, sexually transmitted diseases, and physical and emotional trauma.*
• Encourage patient to express sexual urges in socially acceptable ways (including masturbation in private setting) *to help patient discover positive methods of relieving sexual tension.*
• Discuss with patient hypersexual behaviors and feelings associated with hypersexuality *to promote insight into behavior.*
• Refer patient to medical and psychiatric specialist or sex therapist if needed. *Indiscriminate and impulsive hypersexuality usually indicates physical or psychiatric illness that requires further evaluation and treatment by an appropriate professional.*

Evaluations for expected outcomes
• Patient states desire to express sexual drive in socially acceptable manner.
• Patient reports sexual relationships that aren't harmful to himself or others.
• Patient develops increased understanding of hypersexual urges and the ability to cope with intense sexual desire.
• Patient expresses willingness to participate in psychiatric care or sex therapy if needed.

Documentation
• Patient's perception of sexual behaviors and level of sexual activities
• Patient's statements about sexual behaviors

• Observations of patient's behavior, including inappropriate sexual expression
• Interventions to help patient set limits on hypersexuality
• Patient's response to nursing interventions
• Evaluations for expected outcomes

■ Social isolation
related to dysfunctional interpersonal relations

Definition
Aloneness experienced by an individual and perceived as a negative or threatened state imposed by others

Assessment
• Age
• Sex
• Level of education
• Ethnic group
• Family status, including marital status, family roles, ability of family to meet patient's physical and emotional needs, and communication style
• Coping patterns
• Evidence of physical, sexual, or emotional abuse
• Mental status, including motor activity, thought and speech, mood and affect, perceptions, orientation, memory, general information, attention span, abstraction, and judgment

Defining characteristics
• Absence of supportive significant other
• Behavior unacceptable to the dominant cultural group
• Expressed feelings of aloneness imposed by others
• Expressed feelings of difference from others

- No eye contact
- Projection of hostility in voice
- Sad, dull affect
- Uncommunicative behavior
- Withdrawal

Associated medical diagnoses (selected)

Anxiety disorder, dementia, mental retardation, mood disorder, personality disorders (antisocial, avoidant, borderline, paranoid, schizoid), schizophrenia

Expected outcomes

- Patient will articulate feelings of isolation.
- Patient will agree to spend time daily talking to others.
- Patient will express comfort in talking to others.
- Patient will plan to continue social interactions with family and friends after discharge.

Interventions and rationales

- Spend time with patient each shift *to establish a trusting relationship.*
- Encourage patient to articulate his feelings. Listen nonjudgmentally *to let patient know his ideas are valued.*
- Demonstrate eye contact, appropriate physical boundaries, and other socially appropriate behavior *to provide a model for patient.*
- Encourage patient to begin relating to others through participation in unit activities *to help practice newly acquired social skills.*
- Encourage patient to increase his level of social contact gradually *to avoid becoming overwhelmed.*
- Help patient locate community resources and support groups *to decrease isolation and provide support.*

Evaluations for expected outcomes

- Patient discusses his difficulty interacting with others.

- Patient is observed communicating with others.
- Patient appears to communicate with increasing ease.
- Patient has developed a personal plan for continued ease in communicating with others.

Documentation

- Patient's comments about his interpersonal problems
- Patient's expression of loneliness
- Patient's participation in group activities
- Resources provided to patient for ongoing care
- Evaluations for expected outcomes

■ Social isolation

related to inadequate personal resources

Definition

Self-imposed or environmentally imposed lack of contact with support systems

Assessment

- Reason for hospitalization (physiologic or psychiatric)
- Support systems, including clergy, family members, and friends
- Diversional interests
- Attitudes of family members toward patient in this situation
- Financial resources
- Occupation
- Level of education and intelligence
- Coping and problem-solving ability
- Self-esteem

Defining characteristics

- Description of lifestyle as solitary or circumscribed by membership in subculture

• Evidence of physical or mental handicap or altered state of wellness
• Expressed feelings of being different from others
• Expressed feelings of rejection or aloneness
• Expressed frustration over inability to meet expectations of others
• Inappropriate or immature interests or activities
• Insecurity in public
• Lack of family, friends, and social groups
• Lack of purpose in life
• Uncommunicative and withdrawn behavior, with poor eye contact

Associated medical diagnoses (selected)
This diagnosis occurs among elderly patients, homeless people, patients with current or past history of psychiatric disorders, and patients who have no family or friends to support them. Examples of associated medical diagnoses include alcoholism, antisocial personality disorder, borderline personality disorder, obsessive-compulsive disorder, and phobic disorder.

Expected outcomes
• Patient will interact positively with caregivers.
• Patient will express feelings about lack of supportive relationships.
• Patient will express desire to be involved with others.
• Patient will express desire to improve himself and current condition — for example, by obtaining further education or learning how to better manage finances.
• Patient will use available resources (social services, home health care, psychology services, self-improvement classes) to establish realistic plan for future.
• Patient will state plan to participate in social activity.

Interventions and rationales
• Assign same caregivers to patient *to promote trusting relationships with staff members. Consistent care promotes patient's ability to communicate openly.*
• Assign primary nurse to coordinate patient's care. *This reduces potential for fragmented nursing interventions.*
• Plan 15-minute period each shift to sit with patient. If patient doesn't wish to talk, remain silent. *Active listening communicates concern, allows time to collect thoughts, and encourages patient to initiate interaction.*
• Involve patient in planning care and have him participate in self-care continuously *to provide structure, reduce feelings of helplessness, and foster independent action.*
• Discuss patient's living accommodations and lifestyle outside facility to *help you understand patient and facilitate discharge planning.*
• Refer patient to social services for follow-up, if necessary, *to ensure comprehensive approach to care.*
• Help patient identify social outlets (peer group, associations, group activity) *to draw patient's attention to specific data and promote goal-directed interaction.*

Evaluations for expected outcomes
• Patient seeks information from and expresses feelings to caregivers.
• Patient acknowledges concern about absence of supportive relationships.
• Patient expresses desire to develop meaningful relationships.
• Patient states at least two methods of achieving personal growth and improving current situation.
• Patient identifies and contacts social service agencies.
• Patient states plan to participate in social activities.

Documentation
• Patient's perceptions of current situation
• Patient's expressions of plans for future
• Observations of patient's behavior
• Planning done by patient with nurse, doctor, social worker, and others
• Patient's response to nursing interventions
• Evaluations for expected outcomes

■ Sorrow, chronic

related to change in physical, social, or psychological status

Definition
A cyclical, recurring, and potentially progressive pattern of pervasive sadness that is experienced in response to continual loss throughout the trajectory of an illness or disability

Assessment
• Age and sex
• History of recent loss
• Patient's usual pattern of coping with loss, including cultural, intellectual, and emotional responses
• Expressed feelings of loss of control over current situation
• Behavioral manifestations of grieving, including their intensity
• Somatic problems associated with grieving, including changes in appetite, sleep patterns, activity level, and libido
• Lifestyle changes related to illness (mobility restrictions, risk of complications, and medication regimen)
• Psychosocial status, including religious beliefs and practices, personal philosophy, educational background, and effect of altered health status on social life
• Physical and social environment
• Sources of support, including family members, friends, and clergy

Defining characteristics
• Expressed feelings that vary in intensity, are periodic, may progress and intensify over time, and may interfere with patient's ability to reach highest level of personal and social well-being
• Expressions of one or more of the following: anger, being misunderstood, confusion, depression, disappointment, emptiness, fear, frustration, guilt or self-blame, helplessness, hopelessness, loneliness, low self-esteem, recurring loss, and being overwhelmed
• Expressions of periodic, recurrent feeling of sadness

Associated medical diagnoses (selected)
Cancer, cerebrovascular accident, head injury, spinal cord injury

Expected outcomes
• Patient will identify losses associated with changes in health status.
• Patient will express feelings about changes in health status.
• Patient will seek assistance in dealing with emotions related to loss.
• Patient will begin to develop healthful coping mechanisms, such as open expression of grief.
• Patient will seek out support from family, friends, clergy, or others when necessary.
• Patient will begin to plan for discharge and for future.
• Patient will express realistic expectations with regard to health status.

Interventions and rationales
• Spend at least 15 minutes each shift with patient to focus on expression of feelings. Encourage patient to express thoughts and feelings openly. *Dys-*

functional grieving may result from inability to freely express feelings.
• Communicate to the patient that feelings of anger are acceptable, but place limits on destructive behavior. *Inability to identify anger as normal response to loss may cause patient to express aggression inappropriately.*
• Help patient focus realistically on changes in health status because of loss *to help patient plan for future.*
• Encourage patient to reach out to people who can offer support, such as family, friends, and clergy, *to increase emotional strength.*
• Encourage patient and family members to reminisce. *Engaging in life review promotes a peaceful atmosphere and helps in understanding meaning of loss in relation to health and life.*
• Inform patient and family members about additional sources of support within facility or community *to facilitate adaptive responses to loss and encourage community integration.*
• Encourage patient to take an active part in setting goals for health care *to facilitate independence and enhance self-esteem.*
• Help patient and family set realistic goals for discharge and future *to help patient to place loss in perspective and move on to new opportunities and relationships.*
• Encourage patient to be as independent as possible in self-care activities *to enhance self-esteem and promote optimal functioning.*
• Refer patient to psychologist, psychiatrist, or social worker as appropriate. *Restoring emotional health may require assistance from a mental health professional.*

Evaluations for expected outcomes
• Patient identifies losses associated with changes in health status.

• Patient expresses feelings about changes in health status.
• Patient seeks assistance in dealing with emotions related to loss.
• Patient begins to develop healthful coping mechanisms, such as open expression of grief.
• Patient seeks out support from family, friends, clergy, or others when necessary.
• Patient begins to plan for discharge and for future.
• Patient expresses realistic expectations with regard to health status.

Documentation
• Patient's statements regarding loss
• Patient's behavioral response to loss, including interactions with family members and staff
• Nursing interventions to help patient overcome chronic sorrow
• Patient's response to nursing interventions
• Patient's statements indicating understanding that grief is normal
• Patient's statements regarding goals for discharge and future
• Referrals to a mental health professional
• Evaluations for expected outcomes

■ Spiritual well-being, potential for enhanced

Definition
Process of developing the inner self by interconnecting physical, psychological, and spiritual strengths

Assessment
• Spiritual status, including personal religious habits, religious or church affiliation, embarrassment at practicing religious rituals, and opposition to

beliefs by family, peers, and health care providers
• Health history, including medical conditions that change body image, chronic or terminal illness, and debilitating disease
• Psychological status, including reactions to illness and disability; change in appetite, energy level, motivation, personal hygiene, self-image, sleep, and sex drive; alcohol or drug abuse; moodiness; recent divorce, job loss, or losses through separation or death; personality traits; and relationships with peers
• Self-care status, including neurologic, musculoskeletal, sensory, or psychological impairment and ability to carry out activities and adapt
• Family status, including marital status and communication patterns
• Nutritional status, including malabsorption or nutritional deficiencies, obesity, anorexia, bulimia, weight loss or gain, nausea, vomiting, fainting, constipation, diarrhea, pallor, irritability, cravings, food hoarding, alteration in such personal habits as exercise, drug and alcohol use, and use of laxatives
• Sleep pattern status, including hours of sleep, energy level before and after sleep, difficulty falling asleep, nocturnal awakening, early morning awakening, hypersomnia, insomnia, and sleep pattern reversal

Defining characteristics
• Harmonious interconnectedness (harmony and connection with self, others, higher power, and environment)
• Inner strengths, such as inner core, transcendence, self-consciousness, and sense of awareness
• Sense of unfolding mystery

Associated medical diagnoses (selected)
This nursing diagnosis may apply to any individual who desires a higher level of spirituality.

Expected outcomes
• Patient will discuss spiritual conflicts.
• Patient will have opportunity to meet with chosen religious figure.
• Patient will receive support in his efforts to pursue enhanced spiritual well-being.
• Patient will pursue religious or spiritual practices to extent he feels comfortable.
• Patient will openly discuss effects of illness on his beliefs and other spiritual issues.
• Patient will describe plan to continue to enhance spiritual well-being.
• Patient will receive referrals for continued support.

Interventions and rationales
• Monitor for potential signs of spiritual distress that might harm patient's well-being (altered self-care, sleep pattern disturbance, and change in exercise and eating habits) *to plan appropriate interventions.*
• Assess significance of spirituality in patient's life and ability to cope with illness. Note whether patient participates in religious rituals, observes religious practices (prayer, meditation, and dietary restrictions), or wishes to discuss spiritual beliefs. Keep an open view of what constitutes spirituality. *Before you can intervene in spiritual matters, you must determine the significance of spirituality for patient.*
• Ask patient whether his illness has affected his spiritual outlook and tell him you're willing to help him address spiritual issues if he wishes *to reduce isolation and help bring issues*

related to spiritual distress out into open.

• Ask patient whether he wishes to discuss spiritual concerns with religious figure *to allow access to expert spiritual care resources.*

• Encourage patient to pursue spiritual questions. Reassure him that spiritual concerns are valid and that by strengthening his spirituality, he can enhance his overall well-being *to demonstrate acceptance.*

• Provide patient with resources for coping with spiritual distress (referrals to religious or spiritual organizations and books on prayer and meditation) *to enhance his opportunity to attend to spiritual needs.* Make sure he receives materials appropriate to religious affiliation and spiritual beliefs *to demonstrate respect for his beliefs and values.* If you lack knowledge about patient's beliefs and practices, consult religious figure *to best meet patient's needs.*

• Help patient arrange travel to place selected for prayer, reflection, or contemplation. Use such resources as church-affiliated vans or volunteer escorts *to enhance patient's contact with outside sources of support.*

• Demonstrate to patient that you're willing to discuss issues related to spirituality, such as patient's view of God, how illness has affected his religious beliefs, and how hospital stays affect his spiritual practices, *to bring spiritual issues into open.* Keep an open mind when listening. Keep conversation focused on patient's spiritual values and role they play in recovering from illness and coping with changes in body image *to ensure that interaction between you and patient remains therapeutic.*

• Discuss with patient importance of maintaining healthy diet, getting regular exercise and sleep, and maintain-

ing healthy interaction with family and friends. *A patient in spiritual distress may neglect his day-to-day well-being.*

• Praise patient for taking time to attend to his spiritual needs and encourage him to continue to develop his spirituality once he leaves facility *to provide continued encouragement.*

• Provide patient with referrals to appropriate religious groups, spiritually centered organizations, and social service organizations. Consider such resources as parish nurses, home-visiting services, and computer networks *to help provide continued opportunity for spiritual development and to ensure continuity of care.*

Evaluations for expected outcomes

• Patient discusses spiritual conflicts.

• Patient has opportunity to meet with chosen religious figure.

• Patient recognizes and expresses support he has received in his efforts to pursue enhanced spiritual well-being.

• Patient pursues religious or spiritual practices to extent he feels comfortable.

• Patient discusses effects of illness on his beliefs and other spiritual issues openly.

• Patient describes plan to continue to enhance spiritual well-being.

• Patient identifies religious resources offered outside facility or agency.

Documentation

• Statements about spiritual conflicts

• Visits with religious representative

• Engagement in religious or spiritual practices

• Religious resources suggested outside facility or agency

• Statements about ability to cope with changes in body image as a result of illness, to maintain spiritual

values in the face of long-term or chronic illness, and to pursue spiritual practices during hospital stays
• Eating patterns, exercise schedules, and sleep patterns
• Stated plans to continue to enhance spiritual well-being
• Evaluations for expected outcomes

■ Verbal communication impairment

related to psychological barriers

Definition

Decreased ability to speak, understand, or use words appropriately

Assessment

• Neurologic status, including history of neurologic disorders, mental status (orientation, level of consciousness, mood or behavior, knowledge and intelligence, vocabulary, and memory), and speech (pattern, language, level of comprehension and expression, and ability to use other forms of communication, such as gestures, pictures, and drawings)
• Psychological status, including history of mental or psychiatric disorders, history of alcohol or psychoactive drug use, stressors, phobias, and coping strategies

Defining characteristics

• Disorientation
• Difficulty comprehending and maintaining usual communication pattern
• Difficulty expressing thought verbally (aphasia, dysphasia, apraxia, dyslexia)
• Difficulty using or inability to use facial expressions or body language
• Dyspnea
• Inability or lack of desire to speak

• Inappropriate verbalizations
• Stuttering or slurring
• Visual deficit (partial or total)

Associated medical diagnoses (selected)

Bipolar disorder (manic phase), dementia, Huntington's disease, intoxication

Expected outcomes

• Patient will communicate needs and desires to staff, family, or friends.
• Staff members will meet patient's needs.
• Patient will incur no injury or harm.
• Patient's communication ability will return to baseline level.
• Patient will explain relationship of causative factors such as alcohol to inability to communicate effectively.
• Patient will begin to make plans to use self-help groups and other resources to improve psychological status.

Interventions and rationales

• Observe patient closely *to anticipate needs* (for example, restlessness may indicate need to urinate).
• Minimize environmental stimuli and maintain a quiet, nonthreatening environment *to reduce anxiety.*
• Introduce yourself and explain procedures in simple terms. Encourage consistent use of same terms for common objects. *Treating patient as normal may enhance responsiveness.*
• Encourage communication attempts and allow patient time to say or write words in response *to decrease frustration.*
• Assess patient's communication status daily and record. Match communication needs to interventions: For disorientation, use reality orientation techniques; for manic state, reduce environmental stimuli and talk softly and calmly; for alcohol withdrawal

syndrome, reassure patient, don't reinforce presence of hallucinations, and provide quiet environment; for stuttering, use rhythm or song. *Each patient needs communication status interventions tailored to his situation.*
• Determine patient's past interests and habits from family members and discuss them with patient *to stimulate nonthreatening two-way conversation.*
• Maintain safe environment by using side rails, soft restraints, and other safety measures according to established policies *to protect patient.*
• Refer patient to psychiatric liaison nurse, social services, community agencies, and self-help groups such as Alcoholics Anonymous. *Resolution of communication problems may require long-term follow-up.*

Evaluations for expected outcomes
• Patient consistently communicates needs to staff, family, or friends.
• Staff members meet patient's basic needs.
• Patient doesn't show signs of neglect (weight loss, dehydration, and constipation) or evidence of falls (bruises, contusions, and cuts).
• Patient demonstrates return to baseline communication level by stating name, place, and time.
• Patient describes relationship between causative factors and impaired communication.
• Patient expresses intent to attend self-help groups and identifies resources appropriate to resolving underlying psychological problem.

Documentation
• Patient's concern with level of communication
• Observations of patient's needs, communication attempts, orientation, and safety measures

• Interventions carried out to promote communication
• Contributing factors to poor communication and plans to improve psychological status
• Patient's response to nursing interventions
• Evaluations for expected outcomes

■ Violence, risk for: Directed at others

related to excitement or antisocial behavior

Definition
Presence of risk factors for violence directed at others

Assessment
• Age
• Sex
• Recent stressors and coping strategies
• Patient history, including health history, substance abuse history (type and effects on mental status), and previous episodes of violence (circumstances, behavior, and arrests)
• Reactions of family members to episodes of violence
• Mental status examination (with emphasis on insight and judgment)
• Physical findings, including neurologic examination
• Laboratory studies, including electroencephalogram, toxicology screening, and blood chemistry

Risk factors
• Cognitive impairment
• History of violence, verbal threats, childhood abuse, or substance abuse
• Psychotic symptoms

Associated medical diagnoses (selected)
Affective disorder, antisocial personality disorder, bipolar disorder (manic phase), impulse control disorder, intermittent explosive disorder, spouse abuse, substance abuse

Expected outcomes
• Patient will maintain control over anger.
• Patient will successfully rechannel hostility into socially acceptable behaviors.
• Patient will discuss angry feelings and will verbalize ways to tolerate frustration appropriately.
• Patient will express need for long-term treatment by appropriate professional.

Interventions and rationales
• Maintain low level of stimuli in patient's environment *to avoid increasing agitation and provoking violent behavior.*
• Remove all objects from environment that patient could use to injure others *to provide for patient's safety and protect potential victims of violence.*
• Instruct staff members to maintain and convey calm attitude toward patient. *Anxiety is contagious and can be transferred to patient. Calm attitude reinforces feeling of safety.*
• Explain in firm, calm voice that you'll help patient remain in control. *Communicating willingness to help patient maintain self-control encourages patient to take control of behavior.*
• Set limits on patient's behavior *to reinforce expectation that patient will act in responsible, controlled manner.*
• Express understanding of patient's feelings and encourage open discussion *to provide support, reassurance,*

and positive reinforcement for desirable behaviors.
• Administer prescribed medications to help patient control aggressive behavior and remain calm. Monitor for effectiveness. *When used appropriately, medications commonly remove need for physical restraint.*
• Explain medication program to patient *to promote compliance* and make sure he takes medications as prescribed *to help keep him calm.*
• According to facility policy, restrain or seclude patient, as necessary, *to prevent serious injury to himself or others.* Use seclusion or restraint only after less restrictive measures have failed. Both measures require a doctor's order as well as accurate documentation.
• Establish daily routine of strenuous exercise and encourage patient to adhere to it. *Exercise provides alternative way to handle frustration.*
• Encourage patient to gradually begin discussing hostile feelings *to help him develop more appropriate ways of dealing with hostility.*
• Refer patient for appropriate long-term treatment — for example, to drug or alcohol rehabilitation center, psychiatrist, or psychologist. *Patient may require help from specialized professionals or agencies.*

Evaluations for expected outcomes
• Patient behaves in nonaggressive manner.
• Patient participates in strenuous physical exercise on daily basis.
• Patient states what precipitates anger and describes consequences of failing to control it.
• Patient expresses need for ongoing treatment.

Documentation
• Patient behaviors that indicate escalating agitation
• Other observations about patient's verbal and nonverbal behavior
• Factors that precipitate acts of violence
• Nursing interventions performed to reduce or prevent violent behavior
• Nursing interventions performed to ensure safety of other patients and staff members
• Patient's behavior in response to nursing interventions
• Referrals to specialized professionals and agencies
• Evaluations for expected outcomes

■ Violence, risk for: Self-directed

related to suicide attempt

Definition
Presence of risk factors for self-directed violence

Assessment
• Age
• Sex
• Medical history
• Patient's life situation
• Recent stressors and coping behaviors
• Available support systems
• History of suicide attempts, including aggressiveness of suicide attempts, lethality of suicide attempts, and prior suicide attempts
• History of substance abuse (type and effects on mental status)
• Reaction of family members
• Safety hazards
• Mental status, including abstract thinking, affect, content of thought, general information, insight, judgment, mood, orientation, recent and remote memory, and thought processes

Risk factors
• Age: 15 to 19 or over 45
• Conflicting interpersonal relationships
• Evidence of giving away personal items
• History of suicide attempts
• Suicidal ideation, plan, and available resources

Associated medical diagnoses (selected)
This diagnosis can be associated with any illness resulting in long-term disability or incapacity (terminal diseases, degenerative diseases, traumatic injury) as well as with bipolar disorder (depressive phase), borderline personality disorder, depression, schizophrenia, self-destructive or suicidal behavior, and sexual assault.

Expected outcomes
• Patient's environment will be free from potential suicide weapons.
• Patient will recover from suicidal episode.
• Patient will discuss feelings that precipitated suicide attempt.
• Patient will consult mental health professional.
• Patient will describe available resources for crisis prevention and management.
• Patient will voice improvement in self-worth.

Interventions and rationales
• Ask patient directly, "Have you thought about killing yourself?" If so, ask, "What do you plan to do?" *Suicide risk increases if patient has definite plan.*
• Initiate appropriate safety protocols by removing from patient's environment anything that could be used to

inflict further self-injury (razor blades, belts, glass objects, and pills) *to help ensure patient's safety.*
• Make short-term contract with patient that he won't harm himself during specific period. Continue negotiating until no evidence of suicidal ideation exists. *Contract gets subject of suicide out in open, places some responsibility for safety on patient, and conveys acceptance of patient as worthwhile person.*
• Supervise administration of prescribed medications. *Medications may be appropriate alternative to verbal interventions.* Be aware of drug actions and adverse effects. Make sure that patient doesn't hoard medications.
• Provide supervision (one-on-one observation when possible) for patient based on facility policy *to ensure compliance with legal requirements to protect patient and to reassure patient of staff concern.*
• Use warm, caring, nonjudgmental manner *to show unconditional positive regard.*
• Listen carefully to patient and don't challenge him *to communicate caring and support.*
• Demonstrate understanding, but don't reinforce denial of current situation *because denial can mask roots of suicidal feelings.*
• Make appropriate referrals to mental health professionals *to help patient work through suicidal feelings and develop healthier alternatives.*
• Help patient set goal for obtaining long-term psychiatric care. *Ambivalence about psychiatric care or refusal to consult with therapist marks suicidal patient's lack of insight and use of denial.*
• Provide patient with telephone numbers and other information about crisis centers, hot lines, and counselors.

Alternatives may ease anxiety about perceived threat of long-term psychotherapy.

Evaluations for expected outcomes
• Patient won't harm himself in hospital.
• In aftermath of initial suicide attempt, patient makes commitment not to act on suicidal thoughts.
• Patient states reasons for suicide attempt.
• Patient contacts mental health professional.
• Patient identifies crisis prevention resources, such as hot line phone number, local crisis center, and name of therapist.
• Patient expresses positive feelings about himself.

Documentation
• Patient's comments about suicide attempt and current feelings about it
• Observations of patient's behavior
• Interventions to reduce or prevent self-destructive behavior
• Patient's observable responses to interventions
• Evaluations for expected outcomes

PART SEVEN

COMMUNITY-BASED HEALTH

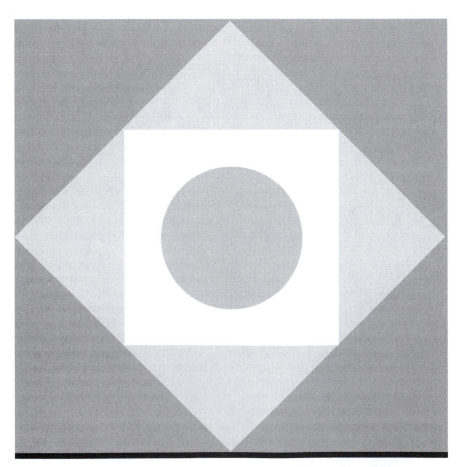

INTRODUCTION

Today, more and more nurses must provide care in nontraditional settings, including patients' homes, hospices, subacute care facilities, geriatric care centers, ambulatory care centers, schools, homeless shelters, prisons, day-care centers (child and geriatric), community nursing centers, centers for the disabled, and other community-based facilities. This section on community-based health will help you meet your care-planning needs in nontraditional clinical placements.

One of the most important recent changes in health care delivery is the reduction in hospital care and the subsequent shift toward home care. Nurses provide home care for patients with complex chronic illnesses, acute conditions, and postoperative care needs. In this section, you'll find plans written specifically to help you administer home care safely and effectively, including plans that focus on home infusion therapy and home ventilation therapy.

In all nontraditional settings, a key nursing role is fostering patient and family participation. Both patient and family must be knowledgeable about care and motivated to take responsibility for their health. This section provides plans of care that will help you manage the therapeutic relationship when working in the community. Several scenarios are depicted: helping an overburdened caregiver cope with a family member who has Alzheimer's disease, helping a patient understand the intricacies of managed care, helping a hospice patient adjust to the course of terminal illness, and more.

In the community setting, teaching patients effectively may demand a creative approach. In addition to educating patients about their health condition, your role may include helping patients access health information. What is more, patients may need help sorting through the vast amount of information available to them. Several plans of care directly address the opportunities and challenges of teaching patients in the community, including a plan about health care resources on the Internet.

Through teaching efforts, you may have the opportunity not only to improve the lives of individual patients but also to enhance the well-being of an entire community. Therefore, this section also includes plans of care that address community-wide health issues, such as high levels of teenage pregnancy, drug and alcohol abuse, and timely immunizations for children. These plans can help you meet your documentation needs when working in community-based health — and they can also give you a taste of the expanding horizons of contemporary nursing.

■ Caregiver role strain, risk for

related to caring for family member with Alzheimer's disease

Definition

Feeling of difficulty and frustration in caring for a family member with Alzheimer's disease

Assessment

• Caregiver's age, sex, and general health
• Cultural status, including level of education, occupation, nationality, area of residence (rural, suburban, or urban), beliefs and attitudes about Alzheimer's disease, and race, ethnicity, and religion
• Family status, including caregiver's relationship to patient, roles, rules, communication skills, family subsystems, support network, ability of family members to meet caregiver's and patient's physical and emotional needs, social and economic factors, coping patterns, and evidence of abuse
• Caregiver's psychological status, including quality of relationship with patient, sense of self-worth, hobbies, recreational activities, and recent life changes
• Patient's self-care status, including functional ability and ability to perform activities of daily living
• Caregiver's spiritual status, including religious affiliation, religious practices, and attitudes about life, death, suffering, and faith

Risk factors

• Codependency (between caregiver and patient)
• Competing role commitments (caregiver)
• Developmental delay or disability (caregiver or patient)
• Deviant, bizarre behavior (patient)
• Discharge of family member with significant home care needs
• Drug or alcohol addiction (caregiver or patient)
• Female gender (caregiver)
• History of poor relationship (between caregiver and patient)
• Impaired health (caregiver)
• Inadequate housing, transportation, community services, or equipment for providing care
• Isolation (caregiver)
• Lack of developmental readiness for caregiver role
• Lack of experience (caregiver)
• Lack of respite or recreation (caregiver)
• Numerous, complex caregiving tasks (caregiver)
• Poor coping ability (caregiver)
• Preexisting dysfunctional family coping patterns
• Preexisting role as spouse (caregiver)
• Presence of abuse or violence
• Presence of other stressors, such as significant personal loss, natural disaster, economic hardship, and major life events
• Probability of long duration of caregiving
• Psychological or cognitive problems (patient)
• Unpredictable course or severity of illness or instability of health (patient)

Associated medical diagnoses (selected)

Alzheimer's disease, Creutzfeldt-Jakob disease, Huntington's disease, multi-infarct dementia, Pick's disease

Expected outcomes

• Caregiver will realistically describe current obligations and challenges that lie ahead.

• Caregiver will distinguish obligations she must fulfill from those that she can control or limit.

• In conjunction with nurse, caregiver will develop plan of care for patient and demonstrate ability to follow plan of care.

• Caregiver will exhibit positive sense of self-worth.

• Caregiver will describe emotional response to caring for patient.

• Caregiver will express less role strain.

• Caregiver will describe help available from informal and formal support systems in community and will take steps to obtain help.

Interventions and rationales

• Assess caregiver's stress level. Several tools allow such assessment, including one in the book *Alzheimer's: A Caregiver's Guide and Source Book* by Howard Gruetzner. *Pinpointing specific areas of stress will enable nurse to assist caregiver more precisely in developing "stress relief" plan.*

• Describe five stages of Alzheimer's disease to caregiver (early and late confusional states and early, middle, and late dementia). Discuss characteristics of each stage and ways to respond to behavioral problems of each stage. *Understanding progressive nature of disease will help caregiver to cope.*

• Help caregiver develop realistic plan of care that considers patient's abilities and limitations. Plan will require modification as patient decompensates. *Plan provides consistency for both caregiver and patient.*

• Instruct caregiver to encourage patient to participate in social and self-care activities, such as bathing, dressing, dining out with friends, and playing cards, to greatest extent possible. *Allowing patient to become dependent too soon increases caregiver's stress.*

• Facilitate family meeting to help primary caregiver seek assistance from other family members. *Caregiver may feel guilty about asking for help. Nurse's presence may lend support and decrease caregiver's feelings of guilt and embarrassment.*

• Support caregiver and family members as they adjust to degenerative nature of disease. Be aware that over time stress associated with caring for patient increases. *Providing ongoing support will help family members avoid physical and emotional problems associated with stress.*

• Identify community resources that may offer caregiver relief from constant supervision of patient. Examples of resources include home health aides, respite care, and adult day care. *Caregivers can use outside resources to provide care for patient while caregiver tends to own needs.*

• Help caregiver contact informal sources of support, such as church groups, extended family, and community volunteers, *for support and relief.*

• If patient is taking drug therapy for Alzheimer's disease, ensure that caregiver understands dosages, adverse effects, and signs and symptoms to report to doctor. *Patients receiving drug therapy for Alzheimer's disease require careful monitoring.*

• Encourage caregiver to accept help from care manager, *who can coordinate patient's care.*

• Encourage caregiver to attend Alzheimer's support group *for oppor-*

tunity to interact with people who share similar experiences.
• Refer caregiver to Alzheimer's Association *so caregiver can be aware of current advances in treatment.*

Evaluations for expected outcomes
• Caregiver develops realistic assessment of situation.
• Caregiver distinguishes obligations she must fulfill from those she can control or limit.
• Caregiver develops plan of care for patient and demonstrates ability to follow that plan.
• Caregiver exhibits positive sense of self-worth.
• Caregiver describes emotional response to caring for patient.
• Caregiver expresses less role strain.
• Caregiver describes and accepts help from informal and formal support systems and resources.

Documentation
• Caregiver's comments related to:
– fatigue
– family members' reactions to caregiver's experience
– feelings about patient's behavior
– financial concerns
– contact with friends or feelings of isolation
– attendance at support group meetings
– feelings of self-worth
• Contacts nurse made in community on behalf of caregiver
• Evaluations for expected outcomes

■ Coping, ineffective community

related to increased levels of teen pregnancy

Definition
Difficulty experienced by a community in confronting social, health, or economic problems

Assessment
• Community demographics, including age and sex distribution, education and income levels, and ethnic, racial, and religious groups
• Family status, including family composition (percentage of single-parent families in community), responsibilities assumed by teenagers in caring for siblings, and ability of families to meet their physical, social, emotional, and economic needs
• Community health status, including prevalence of health problems in community, attitudes toward sex and sexuality, availability of health care services, community members' use of health care services, and beliefs, values, and attitudes about health and illness
• Prevalence of teen pregnancies, attitudes toward teen mothers and their infants, and incidence of sexually transmitted diseases, low-birth-weight neonates, and congenital abnormalities
• Education system, including availability of sex education in schools, availability of programs to help pregnant teens complete their education, and willingness of parents to allow children to participate
• Teenagers' knowledge about sex and sexuality

• Political system, including government officials' support for or opposition to sex education
• Attitude of religious groups toward sex and sexuality and religious groups' influence on educators
• Transportation availability to clinics and other social services and recreation opportunities for adolescents
• Welfare and health care system and reliance of teen mothers on welfare for support

Defining characteristics
• Deficits in participation
• Excessive conflicts
• Expressed powerlessness and vulnerability
• Failure of community to meet its own expectations
• High illness rate
• Increased social problems (abuse, divorce, and unemployment)
• Perception of stressors as excessive

Associated medical diagnoses (selected)
Mother: drug and alcohol abuse, sexually transmitted diseases
Child: developmental delays, failure to thrive, fetal alcohol syndrome, hepatitis, human immunodeficiency virus infection, lack of immunizations, malnutrition, neglect, withdrawal

Expected outcomes
• Community members will express awareness of seriousness of high adolescent pregnancy rate in their community.
• Community members will express need for plan to reduce prevalence of teen pregnancies.
• Community members will develop and implement plans to reduce teen pregnancy.
• Community members will evaluate success of plan in meeting goals and objectives and will continue to revise it as necessary.
• Community members will report reduction in rate of teen pregnancy.

Interventions and rationales
• Assess teenagers' knowledge about sex and sexuality *to determine their educational needs.*
• Work with schools to develop pregnancy prevention programs *to provide adolescents with information about risks, problems, and complications of early pregnancy.*
• Work closely with individual pregnant adolescents *to assess their needs and provide care.*
• Implement outreach and health promotion program *to raise community members' awareness of need to approach teen pregnancy as community problem.* Consider these steps:
– Work with teachers, school psychologists, counselors, school nurses, students, and parent-teacher association to determine extent of teen pregnancy problem among adolescent population.
– Encourage local youth groups, churches, and social service organizations to feature guest speakers on pregnancy prevention at their meetings.
– Contact representatives of local corporations to ask for funding for educational programs.
– Help community members (school nurses, counselors, and teachers) recognize adolescent girls who need counseling about such issues as peer pressure to be sexually active and long-term consequences of pregnancy. Remind community members of importance of listening attentively and remaining nonjudgmental. *Adults who take nonjudgmental approach will have more success in effectively communicating advice to adolescents.*

– Provide education on birth-control measures (including abstinence from sex) and have this information available at school. *Access to information at school provides adolescents with safe environment in which to seek help.*

• Establish clubs for adolescent girls in community. During club meetings, members should have opportunity to discuss difficult questions openly, such as why girls consider babies as status symbols and how to respond to peer pressure to be sexually active. *Such clubs foster self-esteem, and improved self-esteem is the most effective way to reduce teen pregnancies.*

• Encourage adolescents to participate in peer-support networks that allow them to discuss social and dating pressure and other issues related to teen pregnancy *to give adolescents chance to express their feelings openly and obtain support from peers.*

• Encourage community members to establish school-based clinics that allow teens access to reproductive-system models, pregnancy tests, and nonprescription birth-control measures *to support teenagers who make the decision to protect themselves from unwanted pregnancies.*

• Develop referral list for teenagers that includes such resources as hospitals with human sexuality courses, charities that provide prenatal care and childbirth services, women's clinics, and Planned Parenthood *to compensate for restricted access to information in adolescent's home or school.*

• Encourage community members to implement information campaign to educate adolescents, parents, and community members about problems associated with teen pregnancy. *To effectively reduce pregnancy rates,*

education program must involve entire community.

• Work with community members to evaluate effectiveness of teen pregnancy prevention program and assist with modifying program as needed *to ensure program's effectiveness and promote use of program as model for preventive health.*

• Collect statistical data from schools to analyze teen pregnancy rates *to help evaluate effectiveness of the prevention program.*

Evaluations for expected outcomes

• Community members express awareness of seriousness of teen pregnancy problem.

• Community members express need for plan to reduce teen pregnancy.

• Community members develop and implement plan to reduce incidence of teen pregnancies, including outreach and health promotion and school-based sex education and self-esteem programs.

• Community members evaluate success of plan and revise it as needed.

• Community members report reduction in rate of teen pregnancy.

Documentation

• Community perception of problem
• Statistics that support existence of problem
• Community resources that already exist to alleviate problem
• Future plans to deal with problem
• Evaluations for expected outcomes

■ Coping, potential for enhanced community

related to immunization

Definition
Potential for a community to improve its ability to meet the social, economic, or health-related needs of its residents

Assessment
• Community demographics, including age and sex distribution, ethnic groups, racial groups, religious groups, and education and income levels
• Community health status, including availability of health care services, use of health care services, prevalence of childhood illnesses in the community, epidemiologic statistics, and beliefs, values, and attitudes about health and illness
• Education system, including educational level of adult population and state law or school system's requirements for immunization before school attendance
• Religious institutions and their support for or objections to immunization
• Social services, including availability of clinics and other social services, access to health care, welfare system, and parents' dependence on welfare for support

Defining characteristics
• Active planning to handle predicted stressors
• Active problem solving when faced with issues
• Agreement that community carries responsibility for stress management
• Deficits in one or more effective coping characteristics

• Existing relaxation and recreation programs
• Positive communication among community members and between members and larger community organizations
• Sufficient resources for managing stressors

Associated medical diagnoses (selected)
Diphtheria, hepatitis B, mumps, pertussis, polio, rubella, rubeola, tetanus, varicella

Expected outcomes
• Community members will express understanding of problems associated with failure to immunize population and will recognize need for plan to reduce number of children and adults who aren't immunized.
• Community members will establish plan to increase rate of immunizations and ensure adequate protection from communicable diseases.
• Community members will work to reduce spread of communicable diseases and increase rate of immunization within community.
• Community members will evaluate established plans for ensuring that all children become immunized and will make changes to plans as necessary.

Interventions and rationales
• Work with community members to pinpoint potential problems associated with inadequate immunization of population *to ensure adequate protection against communicable disease.* Consider taking these steps:
– Identify new members of community, such as immigrants and refugees, *to help reach parents who need information about immunization.*
– Identify parents who don't follow through with required series of immu-

nizations *to protect children from incomplete immunization.*
• Encourage community members to implement program to disseminate information about problems associated with inadequate immunization *to educate residents and promote community's established immunization program.*
• Provide extensive education about communicable disease and importance of immunizations *to empower community residents and help decrease risk of communicable disease.*
• Encourage health departments, clinics, and practitioners' offices to provide information on recommended childhood immunization schedule to public *to foster education about immunization.*
• Contact parents of children who aren't immunized in person or by handwritten note. Make it clear that your purpose in promoting immunization is to protect their child from illness *to build parents' trust in immunization programs.*
• Provide immunization information in parents' first language *to overcome lack of understanding caused by language barriers.*
• Develop list of referrals for parents of children who aren't immunized. Include information on low-cost health insurance, city health centers, and well-baby clinics *to encourage compliance.*
• Coordinate with local nursing schools, health department nurses, and other interested nursing groups to provide necessary number of professionals to deliver adequate immunizations *to reduce risk of communicable disease.*
• Conduct follow-up survey on immunization rates *to measure effectiveness of educational efforts.*

• Collect statistical data from community sources, such as health department and schools, *to continue to identify children who haven't been immunized.*

Evaluations for expected outcomes
• Community members understand risks of failing to immunize population and recognize need for plan.
• Community members put forth plan to meet community's immunization needs that contains definite actions yet allows for modifications.
• Community members implement plan to reduce spread of communicable disease and increase rate of immunization.
• Community members evaluate plan and make changes as needed to help solve problems and further goal of meeting community's immunization needs.

Documentation
• Evidence of need for immunization program
• Statistical data documenting problem
• Written plan to resolve problem
• Efforts made to disseminate written information to community
• Evaluations for expected outcomes

■ Fear

related to physical, emotional, or sexual abuse

Definition
Feeling of physical or emotional disturbance related to an episode of physical, emotional, or sexual abuse

Assessment
• Patient's age and sex

• Developmental status, including cognitive, psychosexual, and psychosocial stages; cognitive and motor capabilities; and communication and socialization skills
• Temperature, pulse rate, blood pressure, respiratory rate, and skin color and temperature
• Health history, especially past or present bruises, burns, fractures, dislocations, and other injuries
• Changes in behavior, eating or sleeping habits, and ability to concentrate
• Parental status, including parents' age and maturity level, marital status, stability of parental relationship, educational levels, financial needs and resources, employment status, developmental state of family, parent's knowledge of normal growth and development, relationship with child, understanding of child's fear, past responses to crises, and coping mechanisms

Defining characteristics
• Aggression
• Bedwetting
• Decreased self-assurance
• Expressed feelings of alarm, apprehension, dread, horror, panic, and terror
• Identification of and concentration on object of fear
• Immediate response to object of fear
• Impulsive behavior
• Increased alertness
• Increased heart rate
• Increased tension, worrying, and wariness
• Jitteriness
• Physical arousal
• Wide-eyed appearance
• Withdrawal

Associated medical diagnoses (selected)
This nursing diagnosis can occur in any child, regardless of setting.

Expected outcomes
• Child will identify sources of fear.
• Child will exhibit marked decrease in physiologic and behavioral manifestations of fear and will report feeling safe and comfortable.
• Child will experience no further injury or abuse.
• Child will attend school regularly, participate actively in activities, and develop positive relationships with peers, teachers, and school nurse.
• If removed from home, child will grieve loss of parents.
• Parents will acknowledge abuse and will do everything possible to protect child.
• Parents will seek individual and group support.
• Parents will receive counseling for problems that might lead to abuse, such as dysfunction in family and lack of food, shelter, or medical care.

Interventions and rationales
• Observe child for signs of possible abuse and elicit as much information from child about injuries as possible. *Discrepancies between physical evidence and reported history may be important signs of possible child abuse.* Report case to social service agency as soon as possible.
• Spend as much time as possible establishing rapport with child. Communicate at child's eye level. Speak in soft, reassuring voice. *Establishing rapport encourages child to express feelings and provides comfort.*
• Help child identify sources of fear *to enable child to put emotions into perspective.*
• During discussion with child, be careful not to condemn parents in any

way for their actions. *Listening non-judgmentally helps to maintain therapeutic relationship.*

• Refrain from asking child too many questions. *Excessive questioning may upset child and make it more difficult for professionals who will investigate incident formally.*

• Emphasize to child that he has done nothing wrong *to prevent feelings of guilt that may interfere with child's ability to communicate about problem.*

• Reassure child that no one is permitted to hurt him. Tell him he has a right to refuse to let anyone touch him in a way that makes him uncomfortable. *Accurate information dispels misconceptions that exacerbate child's fear.*

• Report suspected abuse to appropriate social service agency as soon as problem is discovered. *In many states, failure to report abuse constitutes a crime.*

• Evaluate whether to tell parents that you're reporting suspected abuse. *Child might be in danger if parents know they're being reported. Protecting child is first priority.*

• Be available to child if he wishes to talk about interactions with outside social service agencies or ways in which his life has changed. *Having someone he trusts will enhance child's ability to cope.*

Evaluations for expected outcomes
• Child discusses sources of fear.
• Child exhibits marked decrease in physiologic and behavioral manifestations of fear and reports feeling safe and comfortable.
• Child experiences no further injury or abuse.
• Child attends school regularly, participates in school activities and sup-

port groups, and reports improved relationships with peers and adults.
• If removed from home, child grieves loss of parents.
• Parents acknowledge abuse and do everything possible to protect child.
• Parents seek individual and group support.
• Parents receive counseling for problems that might lead to abuse.

Documentation
• Child's verbal and behavioral expressions of fear
• Physical manifestations of fear
• Communication with parents
• Details of report to social service agency
• Child's and parents' responses to nursing interventions
• Evaluations for expected outcomes

■ Grieving, anticipatory
related to the need for hospice care

Definition
Grief response in anticipation of perceived personal loss

Assessment
• Patient's status, including present condition, estimated life expectancy, and recent treatments and interventions
• Pain control and management, including patient's wishes and the family's expectations
• Patient's and family's status, including events leading to decision to use hospice services, family's cultural and religious beliefs, family members' understanding of hospice care, and family support, including family dy-

namics, family's special needs, and family member in charge
• Concepts of death, dying, and loss, including willingness of patient and family to discuss terminal illness, willingness to make plans, anger expressed by family members, communication patterns among family members and with health care professionals, awareness of processes and events leading up to death, understanding of what occurs at moment of death, and ethical, financial, and social decisions faced by family members
• Advance directives, including presence of living will
• Involvement with community resources such as church or support group

Defining characteristics
• Altered activity level
• Altered communication pattern
• Altered libido
• Bargaining with higher power
• Changes in eating habits
• Changes in sleep or dream patterns
• Denial of impending death
• Difficulty taking on new or different roles
• Expressed anger
• Expressed distress at impending death
• Expressed guilt
• Resolution of grief before death
• Sorrow

Associated medical diagnoses (selected)
This diagnosis is associated with patients requiring hospice care. Hospice care services may be appropriate for any terminally ill patient (life expectancy of 6 months or less).

Expected outcomes
• Patient will report no pain, show no sign of infection, and be as comfortable as possible.

• Patient will express his needs.
• Patient will grieve his loss of life.
• Patient will communicate with family and other members of support network.
• Patient will receive care from family or friends.
• Patient will remain as independent as possible for as long as possible.
• Patient will talk openly about illness and impending death.
• Patient will receive support through stages of dying.
• Patient will die with dignity.

Interventions and rationales
• On each hospice visit, conduct thorough physical assessment, monitor patient's vital signs, and note signs of complications or impending death. *Assessment provides information needed to modify plan of care.*
• Assess patient's and family members' psychosocial status *to determine need for continued support.*
• Answer all questions honestly *to support patient's and family members' right to know.*
• Help patient understand grieving process and accept feelings he experiences as normal. Discuss and help patient progress through psychological stages of anticipated death: shock and denial, anger, bargaining, depression, and acceptance. *Knowing these stages will help you and family members anticipate patient's needs. Remember that not all patients go through each stage.*
• Guide patient in reviewing his life. Encourage him to write or tape his life history as lasting gift to family members *to help patient give events from his past meaningful interpretation.*
• Encourage patient to make simple decisions related to care *to give*

patient sense of functional ability and control.

• Express acceptance of patient's response to his anticipated death, whatever that response: crying, sadness, anger, fear, or denial. *Each patient responds to dying in his own way. Helping patient to express feelings freely enhances coping.*

• Teach patient and family members about pain control, comfort measures, diet, medications, hydration, palliative care, skin care, and how to respond to complications or serious change in patient's condition. *Knowledge of how to meet basic needs of terminally ill enhances patient's and family members' feeling of control.*

• Perform skilled care related to indwelling urinary catheters, I.V. therapy, medications, supplemental oxygen, and other treatments prescribed by doctor *to fulfill professional nursing responsibilities.*

• Evaluate needs of patient and caregiver for additional resources that hospice can provide. *Commonly, family may be able to use social, financial, religious, or volunteer services.* Be aware that they may hesitate to ask about such services.

• Support patient's spiritual coping behaviors. For example, arrange for patient to have at bedside objects that provide spiritual comfort, such as bible, prayer shawl, pictures, statues, rosary beads, or other items. *Even nonobservant individuals commonly turn to religion when confronted by death.*

• Recommend that family call the American Cancer Society at 1-800-ACS-2345 and request publication *Caring for the Patient with Cancer at Home. This guide for patients and families is a good quick reference for caring for terminally ill patients. The*

information is also appropriate for patients with terminal illnesses other than cancer.

• If grief counseling is available, refer family members to this service. Also, provide support to family members after patient's death *to prevent feelings of being abandoned by the hospice staff.*

Evaluations for expected outcomes
• Patient reports no pain, shows no signs of infection, and indicates state of relative comfort.
• Patient expresses his needs.
• Patient grieves his loss of life.
• Patient communicates with family members and other members of support network.
• Patient receives care from family or friends.
• Patient remains as independent as possible for as long as possible.
• Patient talks openly about impending death and accepts death peacefully.
• Patient receives support through stages of dying.
• Patient dies with dignity.

Documentation
• Assessment of patient's physical and emotional status
• Patient's and family members' adaptation to situation
• Interventions to meet patient's needs
• Patient's response to nursing interventions
• Referrals to community agencies
• Evaluations for expected outcomes

■ Growth and development alteration

related to environmental and stimulation deficiencies

Definition
State in which child demonstrates deviations in norms for age-group

Assessment
- Psychosocial status, including age, sex, developmental stage, special education status, school attendance record, classroom difficulties or course failures, suspensions or expulsions, physical and mental health (diagnosed medical conditions, *DSM-IV* diagnoses, and medication use), child welfare (including guardianship), alcohol and drug abuse, and history of delinquency
- Family status, including parents' marital status; family configuration; level of education; employment, socioeconomic status, and public assistance eligibility; familial history of mental illness, substance abuse, criminal activity, or family violence; and types of agencies, placements, and services family members have contacted
- Cultural influences, including nationality, ethnicity, religious affiliation, and health beliefs and practices
- Parenting skills, including time spent daily with child by each parent, quality of parent-child interactions, disciplinary history and style of parenting, physical interaction with child, and support from other care providers
- Social skills and peer interactions, including amount, type, and frequency of interaction with peers and adults; ability to be understood by peers and adults; ability to maintain satisfactory relationships with peers and adults; and ability to maintain self-control, understand directions, and demonstrate appropriate behaviors and feelings
- Developmental assessment, including motor skills (gross and fine) and language acquisition and use (expressive and receptive ability)

Defining characteristics
- Altered physical growth
- Delay or difficulty in performing motor, social, or expressive skills typical of age-group
- Flat affect
- Inability to perform self-care activities or maintain self-control at age-appropriate level
- Listlessness and decreased responses

Associated medical diagnoses (selected)
Accidents, autism, cerebral palsy, child abuse and neglect, cystic fibrosis, Down syndrome, failure to thrive, fragile X syndrome, learning disabilities, poisonings

Expected outcomes
- Teachers, staff members, administrators, and parents will identify children who exhibit altered growth and development and will target these children for intervention.
- Teachers, staff, and administrators will identify children who may be at risk for abuse or neglect and will contact child protective services as necessary.
- Children will demonstrate improved motor skills, language acquisition and use, and personal social adaptive skills.
- Parents will report feeling more comfortable about their parenting skills.

• Parents will learn basic skills and how to initiate activities that help stimulate children.
• Children will participate in group activities and will show developmental progress.

Interventions and rationales
• Conduct team meetings to identify students with special needs *to initiate needed interventions for children in community.*
• Help teachers, staff members, and administrators identify students who may be at risk for child abuse or neglect. Contact child protective services as necessary *to initiate investigation and help ensure child's safety.*
• Educate teachers about each student's condition and about adaptations that may be needed in classroom *to promote independence and participation in activity for students with special needs.*
• Encourage parents, teachers, and staff members to identify socially skilled children and to encourage these children to participate in group activities with peers who exhibit altered growth and development *to promote interaction for developmentally delayed students.*
• Discuss with parents and teachers value of appropriate toys for promoting group activity, including cars, games, and gross motor equipment, as well as puppets, dolls, costumes, and other items that encourage emotional and creative expression. *Introducing toys may encourage children to play together. Limited number of materials available promotes sharing and positive peer interaction.*
• Work with parents and teachers to initiate activities among children that encourage interaction in small groups. *Groups of two to three children are most conducive for peer interaction.*

• Conduct special activities for children with altered growth and development, or encourage parents and teachers to conduct such activities. Appropriate activities might include reading to children, showing educational movies and television shows, and taking students on field trips *to provide stimulating experiences.*
• Work with school counselor and other school staff members to develop parenting skills class and make this class available to community members *to improve parents' self-esteem, help them to create more stimulating home environment, and foster realistic expectations about their children's behavior.*
• Work with parents and teachers to maintain structured program for children throughout school year *to ensure consistent intervention.*
• Continue to work with parents by following up with telephone calls or home visits, conducting conferences, and providing referrals *to monitor child's development and progress at home and to allow parents to express their needs and concerns about health of their child and family.*

Evaluations for expected outcomes
• Children who exhibit signs of altered growth and development receive appropriate interventions, such as participation in group activities (including small groups) and appropriate stimulation with books, toys, and activities.
• Children at risk for abuse or neglect receive help from child protective services as needed.
• Children demonstrate improved skills and language.
• Parents report feeling more comfortable about their parenting skills.

• Parents provide more stimulating activities and experiences for children.
• Children participate in group activities and show ongoing developmental progress.

Documentation
• Student visits to school nurse, including reason for visit, assessment findings, interventions performed, whether parent was contacted, and whether child was picked up at school or returned to class
• Information revealed during team meetings with school nurse, staff members, faculty, administrators, and parents, such as child's behavior, developmental progress, test results, planned course of action, and outside agency referrals
• Instances of suspected child abuse or neglect and date they were reported
• Evaluations for expected outcomes

■ Health maintenance alteration

related to lack of familiarity with neighborhood resources

Definition
Inability of community members to meet their needs due to a lack of awareness of community resources, such as social agencies, businesses, and service organizations

Assessment
• Community demographics, including age and sex distribution, ethnic and racial groups, education, and income levels
• Prevalence of health problems in community, availability of health care services, and use of health care services
• Psychosocial status of community members, including cognitive abilities, access to transportation, physical disabilities, communication problems, environmental factors, financial resources, support systems, and beliefs and practices regarding health

Defining characteristics
• History of lack of health-seeking behaviors
• Impaired personal support systems
• Inability to take responsibility for meeting basic health needs
• Interest in improving health behaviors
• Lack of adaptive behaviors to environmental changes
• Lack of knowledge regarding basic health practices
• Lack of necessary equipment or financial and other resources

Associated medical diagnoses (selected)
Alzheimer's disease, arthritis, cancer, cardiovascular disease, chronic or acute alteration in physical or mental health, multiple sclerosis, Parkinson's disease, pulmonary disease, stroke

Expected outcomes
• Community members will express desire to learn about available resources.
• Community members will identify local resources and how to access them.
• Community members will contact community agencies.
• Community organizations will develop resource information guides for their members and will promote increased access to needed resources.

Interventions and rationales

• Assess factors that hinder community members learning about neighborhood resources *to identify areas where education may bring about change.*

• Assist members in learning about community and resources available to them, such as American Heart Association, Agency on Aging, Cancer Society, Meals On Wheels, and Alzheimer's support group, *to help empower community members.*

• Plan specific programs to familiarize members of community organizations with neighborhood resources, such as having agency spokesperson attend senior citizen lunch meetings to distribute program materials, *to enhance acceptance and reach more people.*

• Help community members identify specific neighborhood resources they need. For example, senior citizen group may need nutrition support services, whereas young families may need information about immunizations and child safety. *Targeting resources that meet specific health needs increases chances that they'll be used.*

• Assist community organizations — such as neighborhood civic associations, church-sponsored groups, or social clubs — develop a manual describing health care resources available to group members *to provide ongoing resource and help community members become self-sufficient.*

• Ask members of community organizations to evaluate community resources. Discuss ways in which organizations may become politically active in requesting needed services. *Once members are aware of resources, evaluation may help point out need for changes.*

Evaluation for expected outcomes

• Community members express lack of familiarity with neighborhood resources and desire to learn about them.

• Community members seek out and obtain information about neighborhood resources.

• Community members contact appropriate neighborhood resources.

• Community organizations develop resource information guides for their members and promote increased access to needed resources.

Documentation

• Perception of problem as expressed by community members

• Responses of community members to presentations by agency spokespeople

• Evaluation of neighborhood resources

• Evaluations for expected outcomes.

Health-seeking behaviors

related to locating health-related information on the Internet

Definition

State in which a patient in stable health actively seeks ways to alter personal health habits or the environment to move toward optimal health

Assessment

• Current health status

• Risk factors, including age, sex, health history, family health history, and smoking history

• Psychosocial status, including lifestyle, motivation to learn about health, and recognition of potential for growth and autonomy

• Cognitive status, including level of consciousness, educational level, abstract thinking ability, and reasoning and problem-solving abilities
• Mobility status, including muscle strength and mass and use of assistive devices
• Internet access, including availability of computer, modem, and software to support Internet research

Defining characteristics
• Desire for increased control of health status
• Desire to seek higher level of wellness
• Expressed concern about effect of environmental conditions on health status
• Lack of knowledge about ways to promote health
• Unfamiliarity with sources for obtaining health-related information

Associated medical diagnoses (selected)
This diagnosis may coincide with any medical diagnosis, depending on the patient and his health care needs. It may be especially useful for newly diagnosed patients, homebound patients, patients with obscure conditions, and patients who seek information on controversial treatment options.

Expected outcomes
• Patient will state desire for additional health care information.
• Patient will identify health-related resources available on Internet.
• Patient will voice understanding of how to evaluate Internet health resources.
• Patient will share relevant information obtained from Internet with health care provider.

Interventions and rationales
• Inform patient that he can obtain information on health-related topics on Internet *to make patient aware of valuable resource for health information and help patient take active role in health care decisions.*
• Explain to patient that Internet is a large interconnected network of computers. No single entity owns it, and no person or organization controls it. The World Wide Web is a multimedia-based portion of Internet, which offers color, graphics, sound, video, and dynamic navigation systems. *Clear explanation will help patient understand depth and scope of Internet and World Wide Web.*
• Provide patient with basic information on how to use Internet. For example, discuss common Internet terms, such as:
– Universal resource locator (URL). Each Web site has its own unique address, or URL, a series of words and symbols that help identify the site. When seeking a particular Web site, patient must enter URL exactly as indicated.
– Home page. When visiting Web site, patient may first arrive at opening page, called home page.
– Hypertext links. Usually underlined and displayed in different color on Web document, hypertext links connect user to other web documents. Hypertext links may be called hyperlinks or simply links.
– Search engine. Type of Web site that lists different categories and allows user to search for information on chosen topics using key words. Popular search engines include AltaVista, Yahoo, Lycos, and Excite. One search engine dedicated to health-related topics is Health AtoZ (http://www. healthatoz.com). *The Internet world is filled with jargon.*

Helping patient understand this terminology will reduce anxiety about using Internet.

• Provide patient with information about getting on Internet. Explain that, in addition to a computer, patient will need a modem, browser, and Internet connection.

– Patient can obtain Internet connection through Internet Service Provider (ISP) or commercial on-line service, such as America Online (AOL), Compuserve, or Prodigy.

– Browsers such as Super Mosaic, Netscape Navigator, or Microsoft Internet Explorer are software applications that allow user to navigate and view Web. *Providing fundamental information will make exploring Web less intimidating.*

• Encourage patient to locate established Internet sites for health information. For more information on specific sites, recommend that patient read reference books, such as Dr. Tom Linden's *Guide to Online Medicine,* published by McGraw-Hill Book Co. *Reference publications will help patient gain general knowledge about Web and specific sites and help him find information he wants.*

• Help patient find general health information on Internet. Recommended sites include:

– Centers for Disease Control and Prevention (http://www.cdc.gov)

– Health and Medicine in the News, which provides information on medical advances reported in media (http://www.biomed.lib.umn.edu)

– Healthfinder, which provides consumer health and human services information (http://www.healthfinder.gov)

– Medical Matrix, which provides general medical information (http://www.medmatrix.org)

– National Institutes of Health (NIH) Information Center, which provides links to NIH Consumer Health Information, a list of on-line consumer health resources (http://www.nih.gov/health)

– Nursing World, sponsored by American Nurses Association, provides general nursing information (http://www.nursingworld.org)

– United States Department of Health and Human Services (http://www.os.dhhs.gov)

– The Virtual Hospital (http://vh.radiology.uiowa.edu). *Internet has huge volume of information available. Pointing patient to specific sites will make experience of using Web more efficient and productive.*

• Help patient locate Internet sites appropriate for his specific needs. Examples of useful sites are listed below:

– AIDS information from HIVNET Information Server (http://www.hivnet.org)

– Cancer information from CancerNet (http://www.cancernet.nci.nih.gov)

– OncoLink (http://www.oncolink.upenn.edu)

– National Cancer Institute (http://www.nci.nih.gov)

– Disability-related information from University of Washington (gopher://hawking.u.washington.edu)

– Information from Alcoholics Anonymous (http://www.alcoholics-anonymous.org)

– Information on diabetes mellitus (http://www.diabetes.com)

– Information on issues related to death and dying (http://www.katsden.com/webster/index.html)

– Information on multiple sclerosis (http://www.infosci.org)

– Information on spinal cord injury from Cure Paralysis Now (http://www.cureparalysis.org)

– Medication information from Pharmaceutical Information Network (http://pharminfo.com). *These Internet sites may provide relevant information and support for patients and families.*

• Help patient to evaluate health information obtained from Internet *to achieve maximum benefit from Internet and minimize potential harm.* Emphasize that information found on Internet can't always be relied on. Information may be reported inaccurately, findings may not be based on valid research methods, or information may be out of date. Patient may want to find original source of information, verify accuracy, or verify credentials of organization sponsoring site.

• If patient gains new insight on his own condition or treatment, encourage him to share this information with his primary health care practitioner *to foster sense of responsibility for obtaining health care.* Suggest patient provide practitioner with summary of his findings in advance of his appointment to allow practitioner time to evaluate information *to promote responsiveness to suggestions.*

Evaluations for expected outcomes

• Patient reports that he's able to locate sites on Internet with health care information.
• Patient identifies Internet sites for information on specific health-related topics.
• Patient evaluates information obtained from Internet for reliability and accuracy.
• Patient shares relevant information with health care practitioner.

Documentation

• Patient's expression of desire to find more information about health-related issues
• Instructions provided and patient's understanding of instructions
• Internet sites contacted and information obtained
• Evaluations for expected outcomes

■ Infection, risk for

related to home infusion therapy

Definition

Presence of risk factors associated with home infusion therapy that increase the possibility of bacterial, viral, or fungal infection

Assessment

• Patient's health status, including age, weight, reason for home infusion therapy, vital signs, nutritional status, and motor skills
• Health history, including drug allergies, substance abuse, chronic metabolic or systemic disease, and recent or present respiratory, urinary, or oral infection
• Current medical treatments, including radiation therapy, chemotherapy, antibiotic or antifungal therapy, steroid treatment, and anticoagulant, thrombolytic, or immunosuppressive therapy
• Mental status, including level of consciousness, orientation, judgment, and affect
• Caregiver's physical and mental status, including chronic health problems, self-care abilities, mobility limitations, and level of cognitive function
• Home environment, including structural barriers, availability of soap and water for hand washing, clean prepa-

ration area, access to telephone, and need for special equipment
• Financial status, including insurance coverage and understanding of co-payments and out-of-pocket expenses

Risk factors
• Absence or incompetence of care-giver in home
• Impaired cognitive or motor skills of patient or caregiver
• Implanted vascular access device
• Inadequate insurance coverage or financial resources
• Therapy that continues for more than 1 week
• Unsanitary household conditions

Associated medical diagnoses (selected)
Abscesses; acquired immunodefi-ciency syndrome (AIDS); amyotroph-ic lateral sclerosis; bacteremia; can-cer; Crohn's disease; cystic fibrosis; end-stage cardiac, renal, or pul-monary disease; osteomyelitis; pre-mature labor; thrombophlebitis

Expected outcomes
• Patient or caregiver will demon-strate ability to administer drugs and fluids as prescribed.
• Patient or caregiver will demon-strate ability to prevent infection from home infusion therapy.
• Patient or caregiver will monitor site and general condition of patient for complications (redness or tenderness at insertion site, swelling, burning, cool skin, decreased flow rate, blood backup in line, pain along vein, gen-eral discomfort, fever, chills, malaise, and respiratory distress) and will report complications immediately.
• Patient or caregiver will exhibit capability and comfort in carrying out all necessary procedures.

Interventions and rationales
• During initial visit, approach care in systematic and organized fashion. Have available written materials, checklists, supplies, equipment, and other items. Conduct teaching ses-sions in quiet place where you, patient, and caregiver will be undis-turbed. *Organized approach may re-duce anxiety and help patient and caregiver to perceive responsibility as series of well-defined tasks.*
• Use verbal and written instructions, demonstrate each step, and have patient and caregiver perform return demonstrations. *Some patients and caregivers may have difficulty learn-ing new skills and require repeated reinforcement.*
• Ensure that patient and caregiver understand purpose of treatment, and enlist their participation throughout course of therapy. *Understanding treatment and its goals helps home care patient assume greater role in administering, monitoring, and main-taining therapy.*
• Provide emotional support and encouragement *to decrease patient's and caregiver's anxiety regarding home infusion therapy.*
• Provide all necessary supplies, including solution, sterile I.V. tubing, pole and infusion pump, intake and output record, and dressings. Explain how to get additional supplies and help patient and caregiver to make these arrangements *to promote inde-pendence.*
• Stress need to use aseptic technique *to reduce risk of infection at access site.*
• Emphasize importance of following safety precautions when disposing of used supplies *to protect caregivers and patient from injury.*
• Tell patient to protect catheter from coming into contact with granular or

lint-producing surfaces. *Airborne particles and surface contaminants could cause localized infection.*
• Teach patient to change site dressing as ordered (usually every 2 to 3 days) or whenever it becomes wet, soiled, or nonocclusive *to reduce risk of infection.*
• Teach patient and family members drug names, treatment protocols, administration procedures, potential adverse affects and drug toxicity, and signs indicating need to call doctor or nurse immediately *to reinforce need to be precise in drug administration.*
• Teach patient and caregiver how to manage complications related to improper catheter placement and fluid administration. These may include redness, tenderness, swelling, heat, or fluid leakage at site; streaking or pain along vein; decreased flow rate or blood backflow in tubing; and fever, chills, malaise, or shortness of breath. *Detecting complications as early as possible may prevent more serious consequences.*

Evaluations for expected outcomes
• Patient receives drugs and fluids as prescribed.
• Patient remains free from infection associated with home infusion therapy.
• Patient or caregiver detects and immediately reports complications associated with home infusion therapy.
• Patient or caregiver exhibits capability and comfort in carrying out all necessary procedures.

Documentation
• Explanation and demonstration of each procedure and return demonstration by patient (documented on comprehensive teaching checklist)
• Times of care measures, especially dressing, tubing, and solution changes

• Observations of patient's condition, complications, and subsequent treatments
• Evidence of patient's and caregiver's learning
• Evaluations for expected outcomes

■ Infection, risk for

related to increased incidence of tuberculosis

Definition
Presence of risk factors that threaten physical well-being, such as homelessness, crowded and unsanitary living conditions, human immunodeficiency virus (HIV) infection, and other conditions

Assessment
• Age, sex, and national origin
• Health history, including illnesses, treatment, drug therapy, recent hospitalization, history of substance abuse, and time of last chest X-ray
• Current health beliefs and practices
• History of exposure to tuberculosis (TB)
• Living conditions, including number of occupants, sanitation, and ventilation
• Occupation and work history
• Sexual activity pattern
• Support systems, including family members and their willingness to provide support, friends, and community organizations
• Education level
• Nutritional status, including height, weight, daily food consumption, and sources of food
• Financial resources

Risk factors
- Crowded living conditions
- History of TB
- HIV infection
- Homelessness
- Incarceration
- Multiple sex partners
- Recent emigration from Africa, Asia, Mexico, or South America
- Recent exposure to TB
- Treatment with immunosuppressants or corticosteroids
- Unsanitary living conditions
- Weak immune system or disease that affects immune system, especially acquired immunodeficiency syndrome (AIDS)

Associated medical diagnoses (selected)
Conditions that increase the risk of active TB after infection (AIDS, bronchogenic carcinoma, chronic renal failure, diabetes mellitus, Hodgkin's disease, leukemia, lymphoma, silicosis), HIV infection, TB

Expected outcomes
- Infection won't be transmitted to other people with whom patient has contact.
- Patient's contacts will receive appropriate screening, monitoring, and education.
- Patient and contacts will comply with anti-infective regimen.
- Patient and contacts will learn about and demonstrate safety precautions, such as washing hands, covering nose and mouth when coughing, and properly disposing of used tissues.
- Patient will demonstrate normal respiratory pattern and absence of dyspnea, cough, and pain.
- Patient will remain free from infection and complications of TB.
- Patient will keep appointments for follow-up care.

Interventions and rationales
- Assess for history of exposure to TB or physical evidence of exposure. *Nurses in community settings contribute significantly to detection of patients with TB. Nurses working in heavily populated cities, especially with large numbers of disenfranchised individuals or immigrants, see a higher incidence of exposure and active disease. Also, nurses who work with patients with AIDS need to be alert for cases of active TB.*
- Perform purified protein derivative (PPD) test and read in 48 hours *to provide initial screening test.*
- If the PPD site shows positive reaction (measured by induration), refer patient to doctor *for further evaluation, chest X-ray, and drug prescriptions, if indicated.*
- Emphasize need to take drugs exactly as prescribed. *Skipping doses and other self-administration errors prolong length of treatment.*
- Teach patient about potential adverse effects of medications *to encourage patient to recognize and report adverse effects promptly.*
- Warn patients who are taking rifampin that it will turn their body secretions red-orange. Soft contact lenses worn by patient may become permanently discolored. *Preparation will help reduce patient's anxiety about adverse effects.*
- Teach patient and contacts about signs and symptoms of disease that require medical treatment: increased cough, hemoptysis, unexpected weight loss, fever, and night sweats. *Early detection and treatment helps to control spread of disease.*
- Teach patient and contacts specific precautions:
– Wash hands in hot, soapy water.
– Cough and sneeze into tissues and dispose of them properly.

– Wash eating utensils separately in hot, soapy water. *Such measures reduce spread of TB.*

• Stress importance of high-protein, well-balanced diet. When recommending specific foods, take into account patient's socioeconomic status. *Patient may require assistance in obtaining foods beneficial to his health.*

• Emphasize importance of scheduling and keeping follow-up appointments *to promote compliance with treatment. Sputum is cultured monthly during therapy, until cultures are negative, and then every 3 months for duration of therapy.*

• Refer patient to support group or other community resources, as appropriate, *to foster independence and use of available resources.*

Evaluations for expected outcomes

• Patient doesn't pass infection to others.

• Contacts receive appropriate screening, monitoring, and education.

• Patient and contacts comply with medication regimen.

• Patient and contacts practice safety measures, such as hand washing and proper disposal of tissues.

• Patient is free from cough, hemoptysis, dyspnea, and pain.

• Patient has negative cultures and remains afebrile.

• Patient keeps appointments for follow-up care.

Documentation

• Observations of patient's general condition

• Detailed assessment of patient's respiratory status

• Observations about patient's living environment that either support or interfere with recovery

• Referrals to support groups or other community agencies

• Evaluations for expected outcomes

■ Knowledge deficit

related to the Americans with Disabilities Act (ADA)

Definition

Inadequate understanding of information or inability to perform skills needed to practice health-related behaviors

Assessment

• Psychosocial status, including age, learning ability (affective, cognitive, and psychomotor domains), decision-making ability, developmental stage, financial resources, health beliefs and attitudes, interest in learning, knowledge and skill regarding current health problem, obstacles to learning, support systems, and usual coping pattern

• Neurologic status, including level of consciousness, memory, mental status, and orientation

• Musculoskeletal status, including coordination, gait, muscle size and strength, muscle tone, range of motion, and functional mobility as follows:

0 = completely independent

1 = requires use of equipment or device

2 = requires help, supervision, or teaching from another person

3 = requires help from another person and equipment or device

4 = dependent; doesn't participate in activity

Defining characteristics
• Difficulty gaining access to public places
• Expressed concern about possible discrimination because of disability
• Lack of familiarity with information about rights of disabled
• Requests for information about rights of individuals with disabilities

Associated medical diagnoses (selected)
This diagnosis may be associated with any medical diagnosis that results in disability, such as amputation, blindness, head injury, hearing impairment, multiple sclerosis, muscular dystrophy, polio, rheumatoid arthritis, and spinal cord injury.

Expected outcomes
• Patient will express need for information about rights of individuals with disabilities.
• Patient will state understanding of rights as disabled person under ADA.
• Patient will state intention to seek adaptations to work environment or other accommodations as consequence of learning about ADA.

Interventions and rationales
• Establish environment of mutual trust and respect *to enhance learning.*
• Listen to patient's concerns about coping with disability in society. *As a community health nurse, you should be concerned not only with patient's physiologic well-being but also with his ability to function to his maximum potential in community.*
• Discuss with patient whether he feels fully informed about his rights under law. Ask whether he is aware of laws that protect rights of disabled. *Open, direct discussion will establish need for information.*
• Inform patient about ADA *to enhance his understanding of legal*

rights. Tell him Congress passed this law in 1990. Explain that many important rights of disabled people, defined as anyone "with a physical or mental impairment that substantially limits one or more major life activities, are set out in the law"
• Teach patient about his rights under ADA. Explain that ADA:
– provides for equal employment opportunities for people with disabilities. Explain that law doesn't mandate for quotas, affirmative action, preferential treatment, or guarantee of job.
– states that employers must make work-related accommodation for qualified person with disability.
– prohibits discrimination against qualified person with disability by department or agency of any state or local government.
– requires that programs and services of all state and local governments be readily accessible to and usable by individuals with disabilities.
– provides for access to public accommodations and services; for example, widening or enlarging doors, removing architectural and communication barriers, or providing alternative arrangements if accommodation isn't possible. This provision affects hotels, theaters, shopping centers, professional offices, pharmacies, banks, schools, health centers, and other establishments.
– provides for access to telecommunications for people with hearing and speech impairments. *Discussion of specific provisions of law may help patient to reevaluate past experiences and alert him to possibility of taking appropriate action to assert his rights.*
• If patient requests more information, refer him to resources available from library or Internet *to help him increase his knowledge about issues related to*

disability. For example, tell him to read *Complying with the Americans with Disabilities Act: A Guidebook for Management and People with Disabilities* by Don Fersh and Peter W. Thomas, Esq., published by Quorum Books, or to contact *Americans with Disabilities Act Document Center* Web site (http://janweb.icdi. wvu.edu/kinder).

Evaluations for expected outcomes
• Patient expresses desire to obtain information about ADA.
• Patient demonstrates initiative in searching for information about ADA and develops realistic understanding of rights under ADA.
• Patient identifies specific changes he'll seek in response to information about ADA, such as accommodation to disabilities by employer.

Documentation
• Patient's statements of desire for information related to disability
• Patient's stated goals of learning more about rights of disabled under law
• Methods used to teach patient
• Patient's statements indicating enhanced understanding of ADA
• Evaluations for expected outcomes

■ Knowledge deficit
related to lack of familiarity with managed care

Definition
Inadequate understanding of procedures that must be followed when obtaining health care through a managed care plan

Assessment
• Psychosocial status, including age, developmental stage, learning ability, decision-making ability, health beliefs and attitudes, interest in learning, knowledge and skills regarding current health problem, obstacles to learning, financial resources, support systems, and usual coping pattern
• Neurologic status, including level of consciousness, memory, mental status, and orientation

Defining characteristics
• Expressed lack of understanding of managed care system
• Lack of familiarity with available resources for information
• Requests for information about procedures for obtaining care

Associated medical diagnoses (selected)
This nursing diagnosis can occur with any medical diagnosis. It's prevalent among the elderly and patients who are new to managed care.

Expected outcomes
• Patient will keep insurance card, written material about plan requirements, and name and phone numbers of primary care doctor and managed care plan readily available.
• Patient will express understanding of how to use managed care plan, discuss benefits of managed care, and describe role of primary care doctor.
• Patient will demonstrate understanding of co-payments, deductibles, and other financial issues and will explain how to get additional information when needed.
• Patient will schedule preventive screening appointments to which he's entitled.

Interventions and rationales

• Allow patient time to identify his frustrations about managed care. *Managed care concepts are complex and difficult to understand. Providing patient with opportunity to express his current understanding of managed care may allow you to identify misperceptions. Patient may view managed care as mechanism for denying patient's choice of doctors, hospitals, and other health care options.*

• Provide simple explanation of managed care and its benefits. Point out advantages and disadvantages of managed care to health consumer. Explain difference between HMO and PPO in simple terms:

– HMO stands for Health Maintenance Organization. There are four different HMO models. A staff-model HMO employs doctors who care for enrollees. In network, group practice, and IPA (individual practice association) models, the HMO contracts directly with doctors, either individually or in groups, to provide care to their enrollees.

– PPO stands for Preferred Provider Organization. This is a slightly more flexible type of plan. It's less restrictive than an HMO but has many built-in safeguards. In this case, the managed care organization contracts with a group of selected or preferred providers for its members. These doctors then agree to accept whatever reimbursement the PPO determines is fair. *Understanding structure of managed care may help patients who are accustomed to fee-for-service plans adjust to new system.*

• Review highlights of patient's plan. Explain importance of keeping insurance card and phone numbers for plan handy at all times. *Better understanding of how to use plan will enhance patient's opportunity to obtain needed health care.*

• Explore patient's understanding of role of primary care doctor. Stress importance of always going through primary care doctor to meet health care needs. *Understanding role of primary care doctor is key to using managed care plan successfully.*

• Determine what screening examinations are covered under the plan and how often they are allowed. Screening examinations may include routine physical examinations, mammograms, prostate-specific antigen screening, eye examinations, and other procedures. *Accessing these benefits may allow for diagnosis of major illnesses at earlier stage.*

• Have patient incorporate learned material into plan that defines how to use managed care plan for specific medical problems, how and when to obtain referrals, and whom to contact for billing problems. *Developing plan allows patient to use new information and receive feedback.*

• Urge patient to ask questions *to clarify need for further information and allow you to evaluate patient's understanding.*

Evaluations for expected outcomes

• Patient carries his insurance card and keeps essential phone numbers readily available for himself or caregivers.

• Patient expresses understanding of how to use managed care plan, discusses benefits of plan, and describes role of primary care doctor.

• Patient demonstrates understanding of co-payments, deductibles, and other financial issues, and explains how to get additional information when needed.

• Patient schedules preventive screening appointments to which he is entitled.

Documentation
• Information provided to patient
• Patient's response to teaching
• Appointments made by patient as result of teaching
• Evaluations for expected outcomes

■ Management of therapeutic regimen, ineffective community

related to drug and alcohol abuse among teenagers

Definition
An unsatisfactory pattern of integrating programs for preventing and treating health problems in the community

Assessment
• Community demographics, including age and sex distribution, ethnic groups, and education and income levels
• Prevalence of health problems in community, availability of health care services, and community use of health care services
• Drug and alcohol use among teenagers, including reports of episodes of blackouts, injuries, accidents, and mental health problems; reports from teachers about changes in student behaviors and attitudes and failing grades; increased incidence of school absenteeism, dropouts, and encounters with police and legal system; and reports from school psychologist and counselors
• Problems that may be associated with drug and alcohol abuse in teenagers, such as school violence, automobile accidents, homicides, suicides, domestic violence, burglaries, and increased teenage pregnancy, sex-

ually transmitted diseases, low-birth-weight neonates, and congenital abnormalities

Defining characteristics
• Deficient community activities for secondary and tertiary prevention
• Higher-than-normal drug and alcohol abuse rate among teenagers
• Insufficient advocates for teenagers
• Insufficient number or unavailable health care resources for teenage drug and alcohol abuse
• Insufficient people and programs to be accountable for care of teenage drug and alcohol abusers
• Unexpected acceleration of teenage drug and alcohol abuse rate

Associated medical diagnoses (selected)
Adolescent antisocial behavior, alcoholism, mood disorders, oppositional defiant disorder, parent-child relational problem, substance-related disorders (intoxication, withdrawal, dependence, psychoses)

Expected outcomes
• Community members will express need for and develop plan to reduce prevalence of drug and alcohol abuse.
• Community members will demonstrate commitment to maintaining drug education and outreach programs for local teenagers.
• Teenagers will report understanding of negative effects of drug and alcohol abuse on their health, families, and community.

Interventions and rationales
• Implement outreach and health promotion program *to raise community members' awareness of need to approach drug and alcohol abuse as community problem.* Consider these steps:

– Work with teachers, school psychologists, counselors, students, and parent-teacher association *to educate parents and teenagers about risk factors and signs and symptoms of drug abuse.*

– Place drug education posters in schools and local teenage hangouts.

– Encourage local youth groups, churches, and social service organizations *to feature guest speakers on teen drug and alcohol abuse at their meetings.*

– Contact representatives of local corporations *to develop partnerships and sources of funding for educational and recreational programs.*

• Encourage community members to establish drug and alcohol counseling program *to provide early identification of teenagers at high risk for drug and alcohol abuse.* Educate people who will be working with teenagers about importance of remaining non-judgmental and open-minded and of maintaining confidentiality *to foster trust.*

• Counsel teenagers to participate in outreach and health promotion programs *to allow for early identification, intervention, treatment, and anticipatory guidance.*

• Establish school-based drug and alcohol education program *to teach about risks of drug and alcohol abuse.* Drug and alcohol education program should include teaching about self-esteem issues, assertiveness skills, stress management, coping with peer pressure, and factual information about drugs and alcohol. Participation in recreational activities should also be part of program. *To be effective, drug and alcohol education program should use holistic approach that supports teenagers' emotional needs and encourages them to make informed choices.*

• Develop learning packet for community residents *to increase community's understanding of drug and alcohol abuse.* With this knowledge, parents and others can act as advocates for teenagers.

• Conduct follow-up survey on drug and alcohol use *to measure effectiveness of screening, education, and treatment programs.*

Evaluations for expected outcomes

• Community members express need for and develop plan to reduce incidence (new cases) and prevalence (current number of people with problem) of drug and alcohol abuse.

• Community members establish outreach and health promotion programs and school-based drug and alcohol abuse programs.

• Teenagers report increased understanding of negative effects of drug and alcohol use on their health, families, and community.

Documentation

• Description of outreach and health promotion programs developed in community
• Evidence of participation
• Results of follow-up survey on drug and alcohol abuse
• Evaluations for expected outcomes

■ Nutrition alteration: Less than body requirements

related to lack of resources or knowledge

Definition

Change in normal eating pattern that results in changed body weight

Assessment
- Age, sex, height, and weight
- Nutritional history, hereditary influences, usual daily intake, meal preparation habits, and use of alcohol or drugs
- Cultural influences, including education level, occupation, nationality or ethnic group; beliefs, values, and attitudes about health and illness; and health practices and customs

For child:
- Parents' educational level and knowledge of child development
- Home environment and financial resources
- Child's capabilities, including communication skills, motor skills, cognitive abilities, and socialization skills

Defining characteristics
- Abdominal pain or cramping, with or without pathology
- Altered taste sensation
- Aversion to or lack of interest in eating
- Body weight 20% or more under ideal weight
- Diarrhea and steatorrhea
- Evidence of lack of food
- Excessive hair loss
- Fragile capillaries
- Hyperactive bowel sounds
- Inadequate food intake (less than recommended daily allowances)
- Lack of information or misinformation about nutrition
- Loss of body weight despite adequate food intake
- Pale conjunctivae and mucous membranes
- Perceived inability to ingest food
- Poor muscle tone
- Satiety immediately upon eating
- Sore, inflamed buccal cavity
- Weakness of muscles required for chewing or swallowing

Associated medical diagnoses (selected)
Alcohol abuse, calcium imbalance, chloride imbalance, failure to thrive, kwashiorkor, malnutrition, marasmus, phosphorus imbalance, psychiatric disorders, sodium deficiency, substance abuse, vitamin deficiency

Expected outcomes
- Patient will describe reasons for not obtaining adequate nutrition.
- Patient will state food preferences.
- Patient will consume adequate calories daily.
- Patient will gain specified amount of weight weekly.
- Patient will eat independently without constant encouragement.
- Patient will use community resources to improve nutritional status, as needed.

Interventions and rationales
For adult:
- Identify patients who don't have resources to eat properly or who neglect nutritional needs. *Nurses working in community settings frequently encounter patients whose nutritional needs aren't met. Nursing responsibilities include identifying these individuals and intervening on their behalf.*
- Encourage patient to discuss reasons for not eating *to assess cause of problem and develop plan of care.*
- Determine patient's food preferences and attempt to obtain preferred foods. Offer foods that appeal to the senses *to enhance patient's appetite.*
- Suggest patient eat high-protein, high-calorie foods *to prevent body protein breakdown and provide caloric energy.*
- If patient is entitled to food stamps, help him to obtain them and teach him how to use them *to buy foods that provide well-balanced meals.*

• Depending on patient's resources, help locate soup kitchens for homeless, senior centers that serve meals for nominal fee, Meals On Wheels, or similar programs *to promote access to appropriate community resources.*
For child:
• Assess child for evidence of balanced nutrition patterns. Stress to parents importance of good nutrition *to reinforce to child and parents value of good nutrition to growth and development.*
• Encourage child to take advantage of school breakfast program *to begin school day with adequate nutrients.*
• Determine child's food preferences *to use as basis for teaching child and parents.*
• Teach child and parents about required daily nutrients. Stress need for parents to supervise child's meals. *Parental support helps child develop good eating habits.*
• If you work in school, confer with teachers to develop stimulating lessons on nutrition. *Working together, teachers and school nurses can reinforce lessons about nutrition.*
• Document cases of undernourished children and noncompliant parents. If necessary, refer family to appropriate social service agency. *Cases in which parents can't or won't cooperate on child's behalf may require further intervention.*

Evaluations for expected outcomes
• Patient describes reasons for not obtaining adequate nutrition.
• Patient states food preferences.
• Patient consumes adequate calories daily.
• Patient gains specified amount of weight weekly.
• Patient eats independently without constant encouragement.

• Patient uses community resources as needed.

Documentation
• Patient's weight
• Daily intake
• Teaching provided
• Referrals
• Patient's response to nursing interventions
• Evaluations for expected outcomes

■ Poisoning, risk for

related to ingestion of lead

Definition
Risk of accidental exposure to or ingestion of dangerous products (or some folk remedies) in doses sufficient to cause lead poisoning

Assessment
• Age and sex
• Results of test for blood lead concentration
• Sources of lead in child's environment, such as living in or frequently visiting older building, living in area with heavy traffic, or living near lead smelter
• Occupations and hobbies of family members that include use of lead
• Cultural use of folk remedies that contain lead
• History of pica, such as biting nails or sucking on pencils or other items
• Nutritional deficiencies, such as inadequate amounts of protein, iron, calcium, and zinc
• Mental status, including ability to concentrate and mental acuity
• History of developmental delays
• Behavior such as irritability, restlessness, and hyperactivity

Risk factors
- History of lead poisoning among siblings or peers
- Home located near lead-related industries
- Household members who have lead-related occupations or hobbies
- Old or deteriorated home or remodeled home in restored urban area
- Pica
- Poor nutrition
- Poverty
- Use of certain folk remedies

Associated medical diagnoses (selected)
Lead poisoning

Expected outcomes
- Laboratory tests will indicate blood lead concentration of less than 9 mcg/dl.
- Patient will have no signs or symptoms of elevated blood lead levels.
- Environmental factors for lead poisoning in home will be eliminated as much as possible.
- Parents and teachers will demonstrate understanding of safety guidelines and will promote them at home and in school.
- Children will practice safety measures to prevent lead poisoning.

Interventions and rationales
- Assess patient for anemia, distractibility, hearing impairment, hyperactivity, impulsivity, and mild intellectual deficit *to detect low-dose lead poisoning. Blindness, coma, seizures, mental retardation, or paralysis may indicate high-dose poisoning.*
- If there is any indication that a child needs blood level tested, request order to have test performed. *Early intervention reduces levels and prevents more serious complications. When children are registered for preschool, kindergarten, or first grade, their blood should be tested for elevated lead levels. All children under age 6, or as state regulations dictate, should be tested for elevated blood lead levels.*
- In cases of elevated blood levels, communicate with child's primary doctor to determine what actions must be taken. *Nursing responsibilities include following up when child's health may be jeopardized.*
- Set up educational programs for children, parents, and teachers about dangers of lead poisoning. Tailor sessions to appropriate educational level. *Education is first defense against lead poisoning.* Make sure parent understand these critical concepts:
  –Before eating, carefully wash hands with hot soapy water. Dirt and dust on hands may contain lead that may be ingested while eating.
  – Teach children to keep hands, toys, and all other objects out of mouth because they contain dirt. Wash pacifiers and other items meant to be put into mouth (especially if item falls on floor or other dirty surface).
  – Provide children with healthy, balanced diet to ensure that they receive adequate amounts of iron, protein, calcium, and zinc. Make sure to provide fresh fruits, vegetables, whole grains, and meat. Eating regularly is important because lead is absorbed more quickly on empty stomach.
  – Allow water to run for 2 minutes before using for drinking, cooking, or making formula to decrease amount of lead in water. This is especially important in areas where lead content of water is high.
  – Don't store food in open cans, and be cautious about using cookware and ceramic dishes that may contain lead or may have been fired incorrectly. These can be insidious sources of lead.

• Assess whether child or family members use folk remedies. *Various cultures use folk remedies that contain lead. For example, Mexican azacron or greta and Asian paylooah are used as remedies for diarrhea and vomiting.* Suggest alternative remedies.
• Teach parents to be alert for stomachaches, irritability, and headaches. *These may be early signs of higher-than-normal lead levels.*

Evaluations for expected outcomes
• Screening results show normal blood lead levels.
• Patient doesn't have signs and symptoms of elevated blood lead levels.
• Environmental factors for lead poisoning in home are eliminated.
• Parents and teachers promote safety guidelines at home and in school.
• Children practice safety measures to prevent lead poisoning.

Documentation
• Blood lead levels
• Physical and behavioral manifestations of elevated blood lead levels
• Referrals to doctor for treatment and follow-up visits
• Teaching provided
• Response to nursing interventions
• Evaluations for expected outcomes

■ Spiritual well-being, potential for enhanced
related to parish nursing

Definition
Process of developing the inner self by enhancing physical, psychological, and spiritual strengths

Assessment
• Spiritual status, including personal religious habits; religious or church affiliation; perceptions of life, faith, death, and suffering; support network; embarrassment at practicing religious rituals; opposition to beliefs by family, peers, or health care providers; and conflicts with belief system
• Health history, including medical conditions that change body image, chronic or terminal illness, and debilitating disease
• Psychological status, including reactions to illness and disability, job loss, loss through separation or death, relationships with peers, and change in appetite, energy level, motivation, personal hygiene, self-image, and sleep habits
• Self-care status, including neurologic, musculoskeletal, sensory, or psychological impairment and ability to carry out activities and adapt
• Family status, including marital status, communication skills and methods of conflict resolution, cultural factors that affect health practices, socioeconomic factors, family goals, family health history, ability of family to meet physical, social, and emotional needs

Defining characteristics
• Harmonious interconnectedness (harmony and connection with self, others, higher power, and environment)
• Inner strengths, such as inner core, transcendence, self-consciousness, and sense of awareness
• Sense of unfolding mystery

Associated medical diagnoses (selected)
This diagnosis can be associated with any illness, condition, or circumstance in which the parish nurse can

help the patient or family to find spiritual support in the community

Expected outcomes
• Patient will discuss spiritual concerns.
• Patient will meet with appropriate religious figure.
• Patient will openly discuss effect of illness on beliefs and other spiritual issues.
• Patient will receive referrals for continued support.
• Patient will receive support in effort to pursue enhanced spiritual well-being.

Interventions and rationales
• Assess patient's desire for spiritual intervention as part of his care *to promote physical, emotional, and spiritual health.*
• Listen attentively to patient's concerns *to ascertain impact of spirituality in patient's life.*
• Ask patient if health concerns or other circumstances have affected his spiritual outlook and tell him you're willing to help him address spiritual issues if he wishes to do so. *This reduces patient's feeling of isolation and allows for open discussion of spiritual distress.*
• Discuss ways in which patient believes community can provide support. *Learning how patient defines his expectations will help you assess feasibility of meeting expectations.*
• Help patient determine mechanism for soliciting support from community, such as placing request for assistance in parish bulletin or requesting visit from member of clergy. *Patient may know type of support he needs but may not know how to go about getting it.*
• Demonstrate to patient that you're willing to discuss issues related to spirituality or to pray with patient if he wishes. Keep an open mind. Keep conversation focused on patient's spiritual values *to maintain therapeutic value of interaction between patient and nurse.*
• Provide information about other community resources that might benefit patient and family members *to help provide continuity of care.*

Evaluations for expected outcomes
• Patient discusses spiritual concerns.
• Patient receives opportunity to meet with clergy member.
• Patient recognizes and verbalizes support given to his efforts to pursue enhanced spiritual well-being.
• Patient openly discusses effects of illness on beliefs and other spiritual issues.
• Patient receives referrals for continued support.

Documentation
• Spiritual needs as defined by patient and nurse
• Interventions initiated by nurse
• Referrals to outside agencies
• Patient's statements about spiritual well-being
• Evaluations for expected outcomes

■ Ventilation, spontaneous: Inability to sustain

related to home ventilation therapy

Definition
Inability to breathe adequately without artificial support

Assessment
• Age and sex
• Health history, including previous respiratory problems, neurologic or

neuromuscular disease, and recent hospitalization
• Respiratory status, including rate and depth of respiration, chest excursion and symmetry, presence of cyanosis, use of accessory muscles for respiration, effectiveness of cough, suctioning demands, and sputum characteristics
• Neuromuscular strength and endurance
• Mental and emotional status, including cognitive state and ability to follow directions
• Functional status, including ability to perform activities of daily living (ADLs)
• Family status, including usual coping patterns, family roles, communication patterns, financial resources, effect of patient's illness on family, and beliefs and attitudes about health, illness, death, and other issues
• Home environment, including electrical safety, availability of hot water, house layout, lighting, and fire hazards
• Knowledge of safety precautions

Defining characteristics
• Apprehension
• Decreased arterial oxygen saturation
• Decreased cooperation
• Decreased partial pressure of oxygen
• Decreased tidal volume
• Dyspnea
• Increased metabolic rate
• Increased partial pressure of arterial carbon dioxide
• Increased restlessness
• Increased use of accessory muscles of respiration
• Tachycardia

Associated medical diagnoses (selected)
Amyotrophic lateral sclerosis, chronic obstructive pulmonary disease, Guillain-Barré syndrome, multiple sclerosis, Parkinson's disease, spinal cord injury

Expected outcomes
• Patient will exhibit clear breath sounds.
• Patient will not exhibit signs of respiratory distress or infection.
• Patient will incorporate mechanical ventilation into ADLs and family life.
• Patient will demonstrate adequate use of communication aids.
• Patient will remain free from complications.
• Caregiver will demonstrate ease in using equipment and procedures to keep patient comfortable and free from infection.
• Caregiver will implement and maintain safety measures for using oxygen in home.

Interventions and rationales
• Ascertain what patient and family members already know about home ventilation therapy *to determine what patient needs to learn. Building on current knowledge enhances learning.*
• Teach patient and family members set up, use, and care of all parts of equipment *to promote independence and decrease anxiety.*
• Explain meanings of ventilator alarms and what to do if alarms sound *to help reduce anxiety and minimize complications.*
• Explain how to get help in case of emergency *to decrease potential for injury.*
• Emphasize importance of patient's involvement in family activities, even though he's on mechanical ventilation, *to increase patient's sense of well-being.*
• Emphasize to family members that patient needs to be attended at all times *to ensure ongoing care.*

• Demonstrate to family members how to clean and disinfect equipment *to ensure that patient doesn't develop infection.*
• Teach home oxygen safety *to avoid fire or injury to patient and family members.*
• Inform patient and family members about signs and symptoms of complications, such as atelectasis, fluid overload, respiratory infection, and tension pneumothorax. Encourage immediate reporting of complications *to ensure early intervention for respiratory distress.*

Evaluations for expected outcomes
• Patient has clear breath sounds.
• Patient doesn't exhibit respiratory distress or infection.
• Patient incorporates mechanical ventilation into daily life.
• Patient demonstrates use of communication aids.
• Patient remains free from complications.
• Caregiver demonstrates ease in using equipment and procedures to keep patient comfortable and free from infection.
• Caregiver implements and maintains safety measures for using oxygen in home.

Documentation
• Assessment results, such as vital signs and breath sounds
• Checks of ventilator settings, alarms, and backup equipment
• Arterial blood gas results
• Patient's response to respiratory treatment
• Patient's response to nursing interventions
• Patient teaching and patient's and family member's responses to teaching
• Evaluations for expected outcomes

APPENDICES

SELECTED NURSING DIAGNOSES BY MEDICAL DIAGNOSIS

Abnormal rupture of membranes
- Fluid volume deficit *related to postpartum hemorrhage*
- Hyperthermia *related to infection*
- Infection, risk for *related to labor and delivery*

Abortion
- Grieving, dysfunctional *related to actual object loss*
- Self-esteem disturbance
- Tissue perfusion alteration (specify) *related to hypovolemia*

Abruptio placentae
- Anxiety *related to situational crisis*
- Grieving, dysfunctional *related to actual object loss*
- Pain *related to physiologic response to labor*
- Tissue perfusion alteration *related to decreased cellular exchange*

Acoustic neuroma
- Breathing pattern, ineffective *related to decreased energy or fatigue*
- Fluid volume deficit, risk for *related to presence of risk factors that may cause fluid and electrolyte imbalance*
- Nutrition alteration: Less than body requirements *related to inability to ingest foods*
- Pain *related to physical, biological, or chemical agents*
- Sensory or perceptual alteration (auditory) *related to altered sensory reception, transmission, or integration*
- Skin integrity impairment *related to external (environmental) factors*
- Tissue perfusion alteration (cerebral) *related to decreased cellular exchange*

Acquired immunodeficiency syndrome
- Altered protection *related to myelosuppression and immunosuppression*
- Caregiver role strain *related to discharge of a family member with significant home care needs*
- Caregiver role strain, risk for *related to developmental state*
- Confusion, chronic
- Coping, defensive *related to perceived threat to positive self-regard*
- Coping, ineffective community *related to increased incidence of teen pregnancy*
- Death anxiety *related to terminal illness*
- Denial *related to fear or anxiety*
- Grieving, anticipatory *related to perceived potential loss of significant object (such as person, job, possessions)*
- Grieving, anticipatory *related to chronic or terminal illness*
- Hopelessness *related to failing or deteriorating physiologic condition*
- Infection, risk for *related to external factors*
- Infection, risk for *related to increased incidence of tuberculosis*
- Infection, risk for *related to neonate's immature immune system*
- Loneliness, risk for
- Management of therapeutic regimen, ineffective: Individual *related to health beliefs*
- Management of therapeutic regimen, ineffective: Family *related to family conflict, complex therapy, economic difficulties, or difficulty coping with the health care system*
- Memory impairment *related to neurologic disturbance*
- Parental role conflict *related to home care of a child with special needs*
- Personal identity disturbance *related to lowered self-esteem*
- Powerlessness *related to chronic illness*
- Sexuality pattern alteration *related to illness or medical treatment*
- Social isolation *related to altered state of wellness*

Acute pancreatitis
- Knowledge deficit *related to lack of exposure*
- Nausea *related to irritation to the GI system*

663

Acute renal failure

- Cardiac output, decreased *related to reduced stroke volume as a result of mechanical or structural problems*
- Death anxiety *related to terminal illness*
- Family process alteration *related to situational crisis*
- Fear *related to unfamiliarity*
- Fluid volume deficit *related to active loss*
- Fluid volume excess *related to compromised regulatory mechanisms*
- Infection, risk for *related to external factors*
- Mobility impairment, physical *related to pain or discomfort*
- Self-care deficit *related to musculoskeletal impairment*
- Sexual dysfunction *related to altered body structure or function*
- Skin integrity impairment *related to internal (somatic) factors*
- Sleep pattern disturbance *related to internal factors*
- Thought process alteration *related to physiologic causes*
- Tissue perfusion alteration (renal) *related to decreased cellular exchange*

Acute respiratory failure

- Activity intolerance *related to imbalance between oxygen supply and demand*
- Aspiration, risk for *related to absence of protective mechanisms*
- Cardiac output, decreased *related to reduced stroke volume as a result of mechanical or structural problems*
- Death anxiety *related to terminal illness*
- Fear *related to unfamiliarity*
- Gas exchange impairment *related to altered oxygen supply*
- Infection, risk for *related to external factors*
- Powerlessness *related to health care environment*
- Sensory or perceptual alteration *related to sensory overload*
- Sleep pattern disturbance *related to external factors*
- Spiritual distress *related to situational crisis*
- Suffocation, risk for *related to external factors*
- Thought process alteration *related to physiologic causes*

- Tissue perfusion alteration (cardiopulmonary) *related to decreased cellular exchange*
- Verbal communication impairment *related to decreased circulation to brain*
- Verbal communication impairment *related to developmental factors*
- Verbal communication impairment *related to physical barriers*

Adrenal insufficiency

- Body image disturbance
- Body temperature alteration, risk for *related to decreased sensitivity of thermoreceptors*
- Coping, ineffective family: Compromised *related to caring for dependent, aging family member*
- Hypothermia *related to exposure to cold or cold environment*
- Infection, risk for *related to external factors*
- Pain *related to physical, biological, or chemical agents*
- Self-esteem, chronic low
- Sexual dysfunction *related to altered body structure or function*
- Sleep pattern disturbance *related to internal factors*

Adrenocortical insufficiency

- Growth, altered, risk for

Adult respiratory distress syndrome

- Airway clearance, ineffective *related to presence of tracheobronchial obstruction or secretions*
- Breathing pattern, ineffective *related to decreased energy or fatigue*
- Coping, ineffective individual *related to situational crisis*
- Fluid volume deficit *related to active loss*
- Gas exchange impairment *related to altered oxygen supply*
- Infection, risk for *related to external factors*
- Nutrition alteration: Less than body requirements *related to inability to ingest foods*
- Self-care deficit *related to musculoskeletal impairment*
- Skin integrity impairment *related to external (environmental) factors*
- Tissue perfusion alteration (cardiopulmonary) *related to decreased cellular exchange*

• Ventilation, spontaneous: Inability to sustain
• Ventilatory weaning response, dysfunctional *related to diminished ventilator support*
• Verbal communication impairment *related to physical barriers*

Affective disorders
• Anxiety *related to obsessive-compulsive behavior*
• Coping, ineffective individual *related to personal vulnerability*
• Hopelessness *related to chronic illness*
• Loneliness, risk for
• Role performance alteration *related to ineffective coping*
• Sensory or perceptual alteration (specify) *related to hallucinations*
• Sexual dysfunction *related to hypersexuality*
• Thought process alteration *related to psychological causes*
• Violence, risk for: Directed at others *related to excitement or antisocial behavior*

Alcohol addiction and abuse
• Altered family processes: Alcoholism
• Confusion, acute
• Coping, defensive *related to perceived threat to positive self-regard*
• Coping, ineffective individual *related to personal vulnerability*
• Denial *related to fear or anxiety*
• Incontinence, functional *related to sensory or mobility deficits*
• Knowledge deficit *related to lack of exposure*
• Management of therapeutic regimen, ineffective community *related to drug and alcohol abuse among teenagers*
• Management of therapeutic regimen, ineffective family *related to family conflict, complex therapy, economic difficulties, or difficulty coping with the health care system*
• Mobility impairment, physical *related to perceptual or cognitive impairment*
• Nutrition alteration: Less than body requirements *related to lack of resources or knowledge*
• Poisoning, risk for *related to substance abuse*
• Powerlessness *related to illness-related regimen*
• Self-care deficit *related to perceptual or cognitive impairment*

• Sexual dysfunction *related to impotence*
• Sleep pattern disturbance *related to internal factors*
• Social isolation *related to inadequate personal resources*
• Spiritual well-being, potential for enhanced
• Violence, risk for: Self-directed *related to recurrent losses or changes in physical or mental condition*

Alzheimer's disease
• Adult failure to thrive *related to illness, disability, or environmental deprivation*
• Anxiety *related to situational crisis*
• Caregiver role strain *related to discharge of a family member with significant home care needs*
• Caregiver role strain *related to unpredictability of the care situation*
• Caregiver role strain, risk for
• Confusion, chronic
• Coping, ineffective family: Compromised *related to caring for dependent, aging family member*
• Coping, ineffective family: Compromised *related to inadequate or incorrect information held by primary caregiver*
• Coping, ineffective individual *related to inability to solve problems or adapt to demands of daily living*
• Environmental interpretation syndrome, impaired
• Family process alteration *related to situational crisis*
• Grieving, anticipatory *related to perceived potential loss of significant object (such as person, job, possessions)*
• Health maintenance alteration *related to lack of familiarity with neighborhood resources*
• Health maintenance alteration *related to perceptual or cognitive impairment*
• Home maintenance management impairment *related to impaired cognitive or emotional functioning*
• Hopelessness *related to chronic illness*
• Incontinence, bowel *related to perceptual or cognitive impairment*
• Incontinence, functional *related to cognitive deficits*
• Incontinence, stress
• Injury, risk for *related to elder abuse*
• Injury, risk for *related to lack of awareness of environmental hazards*

- Knowledge deficit *related to cognitive impairment*
- Memory impairment *related to neurologic disturbance*
- Nutrition alteration: Less than body requirements *related to inability to ingest foods*
- Poisoning, risk for *related to external factors*
- Poisoning, risk for *related to internal factors (biological, psychological, developmental)*
- Relocation stress syndrome *related to inadequate preparation for admission, transfer, or discharge*
- Role performance alteration *related to ineffective coping*
- Self-care deficit *related to perceptual or cognitive impairment*
- Self-esteem, chronic low
- Sensory or perceptual alteration *related to sensory deprivation*
- Sexuality pattern alteration *related to illness or medical treatment*
- Social isolation *related to physiologic, environmental, or emotional barriers*
- Thought process alteration *related to loss of memory*
- Trauma, risk for *related to external factors (environmental, physical, chemical agents)*
- Verbal communication impairment *related to physiologic or psychosocial changes*

Amniotic fluid embolism
- Injury, risk for *related to internal and external neonatal risk factors*

Amputation
- Adjustment impairment *related to disability*
- Body image disturbance *related to alterations in health or invasive medical procedures*
- Decisional conflict *related to health care options*
- Energy field disturbance
- Grieving, anticipatory *related to perceived potential loss of significant object (such as person, job, possessions)*
- Injury, risk for *related to sensory or motor deficits*
- Knowledge deficit *related to the Americans with Disabilities Act*
- Pain *related to physical, biological, or chemical agents*
- Pain *related to psychological factors*

- Pain, chronic *related to physical disability*
- Self-esteem disturbance
- Surgical recovery, delayed

Amyotrophic lateral sclerosis
- Airway clearance, ineffective *related to presence of tracheobronchial obstruction or secretions*
- Aspiration, risk for *related to absence of protective mechanisms*
- Breathing pattern, ineffective *related to decreased energy or fatigue*
- Caregiver role strain *related to discharge of a family member with significant home care needs*
- Caregiver role strain, risk for *related to developmental state*
- Coping, ineffective family: Compromised *related to inadequate or incorrect information held by primary caregiver*
- Coping, ineffective individual *related to situational crisis*
- Death anxiety *related to terminal illness*
- Grieving, anticipatory *related to perceived potential loss of significant object (such as person, job, possessions)*
- Health maintenance alteration *related to lack of motor skills*
- Hopelessness *related to failing or deteriorating physiologic condition*
- Incontinence, bowel *related to neuromuscular involvement*
- Infection, risk for *related to home infusion therapy*
- Mobility impairment, physical *related to perceptual or cognitive impairment*
- Self-care deficit *related to musculoskeletal impairment*
- Self-esteem, chronic low
- Sexuality pattern alteration *related to illness or medical treatment*
- Skin integrity impairment *related to external (environmental) factors*
- Social isolation *related to altered state of wellness*
- Ventilation, spontaneous: Inability to sustain
- Ventilatory weaning response, dysfunctional *related to diminished ventilator support*
- Verbal communication impairment *related to physiologic or psychosocial changes*

Anaphylactic shock
- Cardiac output, decreased *related to reduced stroke volume as a result of mechanical or structural problems*
- Tissue perfusion alteration (cardiopulmonary) *related to decreased cellular exchange*
- Tissue perfusion alteration (renal) *related to decreased cellular exchange*

Anemias
- Activity intolerance *related to imbalance between oxygen supply and demand*
- Adult failure to thrive *related to illness, disability, or environmental deprivation*
- Altered protection *related to myelosuppression and immunosuppression*
- Breathing pattern, ineffective *related to inability to maintain adequate rate and depth of respirations*
- Cardiac output, decreased *related to reduced myocardial perfusion*
- Cardiac output, decreased *related to reduced stroke volume as a result of mechanical or structural problems*
- Fatigue
- Gas exchange impairment *related to altered oxygen supply*
- Infection, risk for *related to external factors*
- Skin integrity impairment *related to external (environmental) factors*
- Tissue perfusion alteration (cardiopulmonary) *related to decreased cellular exchange*

Angina pectoris
- Anxiety *related to situational crisis*
- Cardiac output, decreased *related to reduced stroke volume as a result of mechanical or structural problems*
- Denial *related to fear or anxiety*
- Environmental interpretation syndrome, impaired
- Pain *related to physical, biological, or chemical agents*
- Role performance alteration *related to ineffective coping*
- Sexuality pattern alteration *related to illness or medical treatment*

Anorexia nervosa
- Anxiety *related to environmental conflict (phobia)*
- Anxiety *related to situational crisis*
- Body image disturbance

- Constipation *related to inadequate intake of fluid and bulk*
- Constipation, risk of
- Denial *related to fear or anxiety*
- Family process alteration *related to situational crisis*
- Fluid volume deficit *related to active loss*
- Hyperthermia *related to dehydration*
- Nutrition alteration: Less than body requirements *related to psychological factors*
- Personal identity disturbance *related to lowered self-esteem*
- Sleep pattern disturbance *related to internal factors*
- Social isolation *related to altered state of wellness*

Antisocial personality disorder
- Altered family processes: Alcoholism
- Coping, ineffective individual *related to personal vulnerability*
- Home maintenance management impairment *related to impaired cognitive or emotional functioning*
- Personal identity disturbance *related to lowered self-esteem*
- Role performance alteration *related to ineffective coping*
- Self-esteem, chronic low
- Self-mutilation, risk for *related to emotional illness*
- Sensory or perceptual alteration *related to hallucinations*
- Sexual dysfunction *related to hypersexuality*
- Social isolation *related to inadequate personal resources*
- Violence, risk for: Directed at others *related to excitement or antisocial behavior*

Anxiety disorder
- Altered family processes *related to dysfunctional behavior*
- Anxiety *related to environmental conflict (phobia)*
- Anxiety *related to situational crisis*
- Caregiver role strain *related to unpredictability of the care situation*
- Constipation *related to diet, fluid intake, activity level, and personal bowel habits*
- Coping, defensive *related to perceived threat to positive self-regard*
- Denial *related to fear or anxiety*
- Diarrhea *related to stress and anxiety*

- Home maintenance management impairment *related to impaired cognitive or emotional functioning*
- Hopelessness *related to child's mood disturbance*
- Loneliness, risk for
- Nutrition alteration: More than body requirements *related to excessive intake*
- Nutrition alteration, risk for: More than body requirements *related to excessive intake*
- Posttrauma syndrome *related to incest*
- Posttrauma syndrome, risk for
- Powerlessness *related to physical, sexual, or emotional abuse by partner*
- Self-esteem, chronic low
- Sensory or perceptual alteration *related to sensory overload*
- Social isolation *related to dysfunctional interpersonal relations*
- Thought process alteration *related to psychological causes*

Aortic aneurysm

- Fluid volume excess *related to compromised regulatory mechanisms*
- Gas exchange impairment *related to altered oxygen supply*
- Pain *related to physical, biological, or chemical agents*
- Tissue perfusion alteration (cardiopulmonary) *related to decreased cellular exchange*
- Tissue perfusion alteration (peripheral) *related to reduced arterial blood flow*
- Tissue perfusion alteration (renal) *related to decreased cellular exchange*

Aortic insufficiency

- Activity intolerance *related to imbalance between oxygen supply and demand*
- Cardiac output, decreased *related to reduced stroke volume as a result of mechanical or structural problems*
- Knowledge deficit *related to lack of exposure*
- Tissue perfusion alteration (cardiopulmonary) *related to decreased cellular exchange*

Aortic stenosis

- Activity intolerance *related to imbalance between oxygen supply and demand*
- Cardiac output, decreased *related to reduced stroke volume as a result of mechanical or structural problems*

- Knowledge deficit *related to lack of exposure*
- Tissue perfusion alteration (cardiopulmonary) *related to decreased cellular exchange*

Appendicitis

- Infection, risk for *related to surgical incision*
- Nutrition alteration: Less than body requirements *related to inability to ingest foods*
- Pain *related to physical, biological, or chemical agents*

Arterial insufficiency

- Tissue integrity impairment *related to peripheral vascular changes*

Arterial occlusion

- Pain *related to physical, biological, or chemical agents*
- Sensory or perceptual alteration (tactile)
- Skin integrity impairment *related to internal (somatic) factors*
- Tissue perfusion alteration (peripheral) *related to reduced arterial blood flow*

Asphyxia

- Aspiration, risk for *related to absence of protective mechanisms*
- Breathing pattern, ineffective *related to decreased energy or fatigue*
- Growth and development alteration *related to effects of physical disability*
- Hypothermia *related to exposure to cold or cold environment*
- Suffocation, risk for *related to external factors*

Asthma

- Activity intolerance *related to imbalance between oxygen supply and demand*
- Airway clearance, ineffective *related to presence of tracheobronchial obstruction or secretions*
- Airway clearance, ineffective *related to decreased energy or fatigue*
- Anxiety *related to situational crisis*
- Breathing pattern, ineffective *related to decreased energy or fatigue*
- Breathing pattern, ineffective *related to inability to maintain adequate rate and depth of respirations*
- Coping, family: Potential for growth *related to self-actualization needs*

- Coping, ineffective individual *related to situational crisis*
- Gas exchange impairment *related to altered oxygen supply*
- Infection, risk for *related to external factors*
- Latex allergy response
- Latex allergy response, risk for
- Management of therapeutic regimen, ineffective: Individual *related to health beliefs*
- Oral mucous membrane alteration *related to dehydration*
- Self-care deficit *related to musculoskeletal impairment*

Atelectasis
- Airway clearance, ineffective *related to presence of tracheobronchial obstruction or secretions*
- Anxiety *related to situational crisis*
- Breathing pattern, ineffective *related to decreased energy or fatigue*
- Gas exchange impairment *related to altered oxygen supply*
- Mobility impairment, physical *related to pain or discomfort*
- Self-care deficit *related to musculoskeletal impairment*

Attention deficit hyperactivity disorder
- Altered family processes *related to dysfunctional behavior*
- Development, altered, risk for

Autism
- Development, altered, risk for
- Growth and development alteration *related to environmental and stimulation deficiencies*
- Self-mutilation, risk for *related to emotional illness*

Bell's palsy
- Body image disturbance
- Neglect, unilateral *related to neurologic illness or trauma*
- Self-esteem, chronic low
- Sensory or perceptual alteration (gustatory)
- Sexuality pattern alteration *related to illness or medical treatment*
- Social isolation *related to altered state of wellness*
- Swallowing impairment *related to neuromuscular impairment*

- Verbal communication impairment *related to physical barriers*

Benign prostatic hypertrophy
- Sexual dysfunction *related to altered body structure or function*
- Sexuality pattern alteration *related to illness or medical treatment*
- Urinary elimination alteration *related to obstruction*
- Urinary retention *related to obstruction, sensory or neuromuscular impairment*

Bipolar disorder: Depressive phase
- Constipation *related to inadequate intake of fluid and bulk*
- Coping, ineffective individual *related to personal vulnerability*
- Denial *related to fear or anxiety*
- Health maintenance alteration *related to perceptual or cognitive impairment*
- Hopelessness *related to chronic illness*
- Injury, risk for *related to elder abuse*
- Nutrition alteration: Less than body requirements *related to psychological factors*
- Self-care deficit *related to perceptual or cognitive impairment*
- Self-esteem, chronic low
- Sensory or perceptual alteration *related to sensory deprivation*
- Sexual dysfunction *related to decreased libido caused by depression*
- Sleep pattern disturbance *related to internal factors*
- Social isolation *related to altered state of wellness*
- Thought process alteration *related to psychological causes*
- Violence, risk for: Self-directed *related to suicide attempt*

Bipolar disorder: Manic phase
- Coping, ineffective individual *related to personal vulnerability*
- Denial *related to fear or anxiety*
- Home maintenance management impairment *related to impaired cognitive or emotional functioning*
- Injury, risk for *related to elder abuse*
- Mobility impairment, physical *related to perceptual or cognitive impairment*
- Self-care deficit *related to perceptual or cognitive impairment*
- Self-esteem, chronic low
- Sensory or perceptual alteration *related to sensory overload*

• Sexual dysfunction *related to hypersexuality*
• Sleep pattern disturbance *related to internal factors*
• Thought process alteration *related to psychological causes*
• Verbal communication impairment *related to psychological barriers*
• Violence, risk for: Directed at others *related to excitement or antisocial behavior*

Bladder cancer
• Fear *related to unfamiliarity*
• Incontinence, urge *related to decreased bladder capacity*
• Pain *related to physical, biological, or chemical agents*
• Tissue integrity impairment *related to radiation*
• Urinary elimination alteration *related to obstruction*

Blindness
• Body image disturbance
• Diversional activity deficit *related to lack of environmental stimulation*
• Fear *related to unfamiliarity*
• Injury, risk for *related to lack of awareness of environmental hazards*
• Knowledge deficit *related to the Americans with Disabilities Act*
• Loneliness, risk for
• Mobility impairment, physical *related to perceptual or cognitive impairment*
• Parent-infant attachment, altered, risk for
• Powerlessness *related to chronic illness*
• Role performance alteration *related to ineffective coping*
• Sensory or perceptual alteration (visual) *related to altered sensory reception, transmission, or integration*

Bone marrow transplantation
• Activity intolerance *related to imbalance between oxygen supply and demand*
• Altered protection *related to myelosuppression and immunosuppression*
• Body image disturbance
• Cardiac output, decreased *related to reduced stroke volume as a result of mechanical or structural problems*
• Diarrhea *related to malabsorption, inflammation, or irritation of bowel*
• Diversional activity deficit *related to prolonged illness and separation from friends and family*

• Fluid volume excess *related to excess fluid intake or retention, or excess sodium intake or retention*
• Infection, risk for *related to external factors*
• Nutrition alteration: Less than body requirements *related to inability to digest or absorb nutrients because of biological factors*
• Oral mucous membrane alteration *related to pathologic condition*
• Skin integrity impairment *related to external (environmental) factors*

Bone sarcomas
• Activity intolerance *related to immobility*
• Mobility impairment, physical *related to pain or discomfort*
• Pain *related to physical, biological, or chemical agents*
• Tissue integrity impairment *related to radiation*

Borderline personality disorder
• Coping, ineffective individual *related to personal vulnerability*
• Fear *related to separation from support system*
• Personal identity disturbance *related to lowered self-esteem*
• Self-esteem, chronic low
• Self-mutilation, risk for *related to emotional illness*
• Social isolation *related to inadequate personal resources*
• Violence, risk for: Self-directed *related to suicide attempt*

Bowel fistula
• Fluid volume deficit, risk for *related to excessive loss*

Bowel resection
• Infection, risk for *related to surgical incision*
• Surgical recovery, delayed

Brain abscess
• Aspiration, risk for *related to absence of protective mechanisms*
• Body image disturbance
• Incontinence, urinary urge, risk for
• Injury, risk for *related to lack of awareness of environmental hazards*
• Intracranial adaptive capacity, decreased

• Mobility impairment, physical *related to neuromuscular impairment*
• Pain *related to physical, biological, or chemical agents*
• Personal identity disturbance *related to lowered self-esteem*
• Sexuality pattern alteration *related to illness or medical treatment*
• Skin integrity impairment *related to external (environmental) factors*
• Tissue perfusion alteration (cerebral) *related to decreased cellular exchange*

Brain tumors
• Constipation, colonic
• Coping, ineffective individual *related to situational crisis*
• Environmental interpretation syndrome, impaired
• Fear *related to unfamiliarity*
• Grieving, anticipatory *related to perceived potential loss of life*
• Incontinence, bowel *related to perceptual or cognitive impairment*
• Incontinence, total *related to neuropathy, trauma, or disease affecting spinal nerves*
• Injury, risk for *related to sensory or motor deficits*
• Intracranial adaptive capacity, decreased
• Sensory or perceptual alteration
• Thermoregulation, ineffective *related to child's illness or trauma*
• Thought process alteration *related to physiologic causes*
• Tissue integrity impairment *related to radiation*
• Urinary elimination alteration *related to sensory or neuromuscular impairment*
• Verbal communication impairment *related to physiologic or psychosocial changes*

Breast cancer
• Body image disturbance
• Coping, ineffective individual *related to situational crisis*
• Decisional conflict *related to health care options*
• Fear *related to unfamiliarity*
• Grieving, anticipatory *related to perceived potential loss of significant object (such as person, job, possessions)*
• Grieving, dysfunctional *related to actual object loss*
• Pain *related to physical, biological, or chemical agents*

• Skin integrity impairment *related to external (environmental) factors*

Breast engorgement
• Breast-feeding, ineffective *related to limited maternal experience*
• Infection, risk for *related to external factors*
• Pain *related to physical, biological, or chemical agents*
• Skin integrity impairment *related to external (environmental) factors*

Bronchiectasis
• Airway clearance, ineffective *related to presence of tracheobronchial obstruction or secretions*
• Breathing pattern, ineffective *related to decreased energy or fatigue*
• Coping, ineffective family: Compromised *related to prolonged disease*
• Gas exchange impairment *related to altered oxygen supply*
• Infection, risk for *related to external factors*
• Nutrition alteration: Less than body requirements *related to inability to ingest foods*

Bulimia nervosa
• Anxiety *related to situational crisis*
• Body image disturbance
• Body image disturbance *related to an eating disorder*
• Constipation *related to inadequate intake of fluid and bulk*
• Constipation, risk of
• Denial *related to fear or anxiety*
• Family process alteration *related to situational crisis*
• Fluid volume deficit *related to active loss*
• Hyperthermia *related to dehydration*
• Nutrition alteration: Less than body requirements *related to psychological factors*
• Personal identity disturbance *related to lowered self-esteem*
• Sleep pattern disturbance *related to internal factors*
• Social isolation *related to altered state of wellness*

Burns
• Body image disturbance
• Body temperature alteration, risk for *related to dehydration*

• Breathing pattern, ineffective *related to inability to maintain adequate rate and depth of respirations*
• Constipation *related to inadequate intake of fluid and bulk*
• Coping, ineffective family: Disabling *related to long-term illness*
• Diversional activity deficit *related to prolonged illness and separation from friends and family*
• Fluid volume deficit *related to active loss*
• Fluid volume deficit, risk for *related to excessive loss*
• Grieving, anticipatory *related to perceived potential loss of significant object (such as person, job, possessions)*
• Hyperthermia *related to infection*
• Hypothermia *related to exposure to cold or cold environment*
• Infection, risk for *related to external factors*
• Injury, risk for *related to lack of awareness of environmental hazards*
• Mobility impairment, physical *related to pain or discomfort*
• Nutrition alteration: Less than body requirements *related to inability to digest or absorb nutrients because of biological factors*
• Pain *related to physical, biological, or chemical agents*
• Parenting alteration, risk for *related to lack of knowledge or ineffective role model*
• Powerlessness *related to illness-related regimen*
• Skin integrity impairment *related to external (environmental) factors*
• Tissue perfusion alteration (renal) *related to decreased cellular exchange*
• Ventilation, spontaneous: Inability to sustain
• Ventilatory weaning response, dysfunctional *related to diminished ventilator support*

Bursitis
• Activity intolerance *related to immobility*
• Mobility impairment, physical *related to pain or discomfort*
• Role performance alteration *related to ineffective coping*

Calcium imbalance
• Nutrition alteration: Less than body requirements *related to lack of resources or knowledge*

Cancer
• Adult failure to thrive *related to illness, disability, or environmental deprivation*
• Coping, ineffective family: Disabling *related to long-term illness*
• Death anxiety *related to terminal illness*
• Energy field disturbance
• Grieving, anticipatory *related to chronic or terminal illness*
• Health maintenance alteration *related to lack of familiarity with neighborhood resources*
• Infection, risk for *related to home infusion therapy*
• Sorrow, chronic *related to change in physical, social, or psychological status*
• Spiritual distress, risk for

Cardiac arrhythmias
• Cardiac output, decreased *related to reduced myocardial perfusion*
• Cardiac output, decreased *related to reduced stroke volume as a result of electrophysiologic problems*
• Coping, ineffective individual *related to situational crisis*
• Fear *related to unfamiliarity*
• Fluid volume excess *related to compromised regulatory mechanisms*
• Sexuality pattern alteration *related to illness or medical treatment*
• Tissue perfusion alteration (cardiopulmonary) *related to decreased cellular exchange*

Cardiac disease: End-stage
• Activity intolerance *related to imbalance between oxygen supply and demand*
• Adult failure to thrive *related to illness, disability, or environmental deprivation*
• Cardiac output, decreased *related to reduced stroke volume as a result of mechanical or structural problems*
• Caregiver role strain, risk for
• Caregiver role strain *related to discharge of a family member with significant home care needs*
• Coping, defensive *related to perceived threat to positive self-regard*
• Coping, ineffective individual *related to inability to solve problems or adapt to demands of daily living*
• Decisional conflict *related to health care options*
• Fluid volume excess *related to compromised regulatory mechanisms*

- Grieving, anticipatory *related to perceived potential loss of life*
- Hopelessness *related to failing or deteriorating physiologic condition*
- Infection, risk for *related to home infusion therapy*
- Injury, risk for *related to elder abuse*
- Role performance alteration
- Self-esteem, situational low

Cardiogenic shock

- Cardiac output, decreased *related to reduced stroke volume as a result of mechanical or structural problems*
- Fluid volume excess *related to compromised regulatory mechanisms*
- Gas exchange impairment *related to altered oxygen supply*
- Tissue perfusion alteration *related to decreased cellular exchange*

Carpal tunnel syndrome

- Mobility impairment, physical *related to pain or discomfort*
- Pain *related to physical, biological, or chemical agents*
- Peripheral neurovascular dysfunction, risk for
- Tissue perfusion alteration (peripheral) *related to reduced arterial blood flow*

Cataracts

- Body image disturbance *related to negative self-image*
- Coping, ineffective individual *related to inability to solve problems or adapt to demands of daily living*
- Health maintenance alteration *related to perceptual or cognitive impairment*
- Injury, risk for *related to lack of awareness of environmental hazards*
- Mobility impairment, physical *related to perceptual or cognitive impairment*
- Sensory or perceptual alteration (visual) *related to illness or the aging process*

Cellulitis

- Anxiety *related to situational crisis*
- Knowledge deficit *related to lack of exposure*
- Mobility impairment, physical *related to pain or discomfort*
- Pain *related to physical, biological, or chemical agents*
- Skin integrity impairment *related to internal (somatic) factors*

Cerebral aneurysm

- Airway clearance, ineffective *related to presence of tracheobronchial obstruction or secretions*
- Breathing pattern, ineffective *related to pain*
- Injury, risk for *related to sensory or motor deficits*
- Intracranial adaptive capacity, decreased
- Mobility impairment, physical *related to neuromuscular impairment*
- Skin integrity impairment *related to external (environmental) factors*
- Tissue perfusion alteration *related to decreased cellular exchange*

Cerebral edema

- Thermoregulation, ineffective *related to child's illness or trauma*

Cerebral palsy

- Caregiver role strain, risk for *related to developmental state*
- Growth and development alteration *related to environmental and stimulation deficiencies*
- Growth and development alteration *related to perinatal insult or injury*
- Incontinence, total *related to neuropathy, trauma, or disease affecting spinal nerves*
- Mobility impairment, physical *related to neuromuscular impairment*
- Self-care deficit *related to musculoskeletal impairment*

Cerebrovascular accident

- Activity intolerance, risk for *related to immobility*
- Airway clearance, ineffective *related to presence of tracheobronchial obstruction or secretions*
- Aspiration, risk for *related to absence of protective mechanisms*
- Body image disturbance
- Breathing pattern, ineffective *related to decreased energy or fatigue*
- Caregiver role strain *related to discharge of a family member with significant home care needs*
- Caregiver role strain, risk for
- Confusion, acute
- Confusion, chronic
- Constipation *related to diet, fluid intake, activity level, and personal bowel habits*

- Coping, ineffective family: Compromised *related to caring for dependent, aging family member*
- Death anxiety *related to terminal illness*
- Disuse syndrome, risk for
- Environmental interpretation syndrome, impaired
- Family process alteration *related to situational crisis*
- Fatigue
- Gas exchange impairment *related to altered oxygen-carrying capacity of the blood*
- Health maintenance alteration *related to lack of familiarity with neighborhood resources*
- Health maintenance alteration *related to lack of motor skills*
- Home maintenance management impairment *related to impaired cognitive, emotional, or psychomotor functioning*
- Hopelessness *related to failing or deteriorating physiologic condition*
- Incontinence, bowel *related to neuromuscular involvement*
- Incontinence, functional *related to sensory or mobility deficits*
- Incontinence, stress
- Incontinence, total *related to neurologic dysfunction*
- Injury, risk for *related to elder abuse*
- Injury, risk for *related to sensory or motor deficits*
- Intracranial adaptive capacity, decreased
- Knowledge deficit *related to cognitive impairment*
- Memory impairment *related to neurologic disturbance*
- Mobility impairment, physical *related to neuromuscular impairment*
- Neglect, unilateral *related to neurologic illness or trauma*
- Nutrition alteration: Less than body requirements *related to inability to ingest foods*
- Nutrition alteration: More than body requirements *related to excessive intake*
- Poisoning, risk for *related to external factors*
- Powerlessness *related to perceived loss of control over life situation*
- Self-care deficit *related to musculoskeletal impairment*
- Self-esteem, situational low
- Sensory or perceptual alteration (tactile)
- Sexuality pattern alteration *related to illness or medical treatment*

- Skin integrity impairment, risk for *related to the aging process and impaired mobility*
- Sleep deprivation
- Social interaction impairment *related to altered thought processes*
- Social isolation *related to physiologic, environmental, or emotional barriers*
- Sorrow, chronic *related to change in physical, social, or psychological status*
- Swallowing impairment *related to neuromuscular impairment*
- Thermoregulation, ineffective *related to trauma or illness*
- Tissue perfusion alteration (cerebral) *related to decreased cellular exchange*
- Urinary elimination alteration *related to sensory or neuromuscular impairment*
- Verbal communication impairment *related to physiologic or psychosocial changes*
- Walking, impaired *related to neuromuscular dysfunction*

Cervical cancer
- Body image disturbance
- Fatigue
- Fear *related to unfamiliarity*
- Pain *related to physical, biological, or chemical agents*
- Skin integrity impairment *related to external (environmental) factors*

Chemotherapy
- Altered protection *related to myelosuppression and immunosuppression*
- Constipation *related to inadequate intake of fluid and bulk*
- Diarrhea *related to malabsorption, inflammation, or irritation of bowel*
- Diversional activity deficit *related to prolonged illness and separation from friends and family*
- Fluid volume deficit *related to active loss*
- Gas exchange impairment *related to altered oxygen-carrying capacity of the blood*
- Infection, risk for *related to external factors*
- Mobility impairment, physical *related to pain or discomfort*
- Nausea *related to irritation of the GI system*
- Nutrition alteration: Less than body requirements *related to inability to ingest foods*
- Oral mucous membrane alteration *related to pathologic condition*

• Sensory or perceptual alteration (auditory) *related to altered sensory reception, transmission, or integration*
• Sexual dysfunction *related to altered body structure or function*
• Skin integrity impairment, risk for
• Tissue perfusion alteration *related to decreased cellular exchange*

Chest trauma
• Airway clearance, ineffective *related to decreased energy or fatigue*
• Aspiration, risk for *related to absence of protective mechanisms*
• Breathing pattern, ineffective *related to pain*
• Ventilation, spontaneous: Inability to sustain
• Ventilatory weaning response, dysfunctional *related to diminished ventilator support*

Child abuse
• Growth and development alteration *related to environmental and stimulation deficiencies*
• Parent-infant attachment, altered, risk for
• Parenting alteration *related to lack of knowledge*
• Parenting alteration, risk for *related to lack of knowledge or ineffective role model*

Childbirth
• Family process alteration *related to inclusion of new member*
• Knowledge deficit *related to neonatal care*

Chlamydia
• Infection, risk for *related to external factors*
• Infection, risk for *related to neonate's immature immune system*
• Sexuality pattern alteration *related to illness or medical treatment*

Chloride imbalance
• Nutrition alteration: Less than body requirements *related to lack of resources or knowledge*

Cholecystitis
• Fluid volume deficit *related to active loss*
• Infection, risk for *related to external factors*
• Nutrition alteration: Less than body requirements *related to inability to digest or absorb nutrients because of biological factors*

• Pain *related to physical, biological, or chemical agents*
• Pain *related to physiologic changes of pregnancy*

Chronic bronchitis
• Activity intolerance *related to imbalance between oxygen supply and demand*
• Airway clearance, ineffective *related to decreased energy or fatigue*
• Airway clearance, ineffective *related to presence of tracheobronchial obstruction or secretions*
• Breathing pattern, ineffective *related to decreased energy or fatigue*
• Fatigue
• Fear *related to unfamiliarity*
• Gas exchange impairment *related to carbon dioxide retention or excess mucus production*
• Hopelessness *related to chronic illness*
• Infection, risk for *related to external factors*
• Knowledge deficit *related to difficulty understanding disease process and its effect on self-care*
• Knowledge deficit *related to lack of motivation*
• Ventilation, spontaneous: Inability to sustain

Chronic fatigue syndrome
• Fatigue
• Hopelessness *related to chronic illness*
• Management of therapeutic regimen, ineffective: Individual *related to health beliefs*
• Pain *related to physical, biological, or chemical agents*
• Sleep pattern disturbance *related to internal factors*

Chronic obstructive pulmonary disease
• Activity intolerance *related to imbalance between oxygen supply and demand*
• Adult failure to thrive *related to illness, disability, or environmental deprivation*
• Airway clearance, ineffective *related to presence of tracheobronchial obstruction or secretions*
• Breathing pattern, ineffective *related to decreased energy or fatigue*
• Caregiver role strain *related to discharge of a family member with significant home care needs*
• Coping, defensive *related to perceived threat to positive self-regard*

- Coping, ineffective family: Compromised *related to prolonged disease*
- Denial *related to fear or anxiety*
- Fatigue
- Fear *related to unfamiliarity*
- Fluid volume deficit *related to active loss*
- Gas exchange impairment *related to altered oxygen supply*
- Health maintenance alteration *related to perceptual or cognitive impairment*
- Home maintenance management impairment *related to impaired cognitive, emotional, or psychomotor functioning*
- Hopelessness *related to chronic illness*
- Infection, risk for *related to external factors*
- Injury, risk for *related to elder abuse*
- Knowledge deficit *related to difficulty understanding disease process and its effect on self-care*
- Nutrition alteration: Less than body requirements *related to inability to digest or absorb nutrients because of biological factors*
- Nutrition alteration: More than body requirements *related to a decline in basal metabolic rate and physical activity*
- Oral mucous membrane alteration *related to dehydration*
- Powerlessness *related to perceived loss of control over life situation*
- Sleep pattern disturbance *related to internal factors*
- Suffocation, risk for *related to external factors*
- Tissue perfusion alteration (cardiopulmonary) *related to decreased cellular exchange*
- Ventilation, spontaneous: Inability to sustain
- Ventilatory weaning response, dysfunctional *related to diminished ventilator support*
- Verbal communication impairment *related to physical barriers*

Chronic pain
- Adjustment impairment *related to disability*
- Coping, defensive *related to perceived threat to positive self-regard*
- Hopelessness *related to chronic illness*
- Pain, chronic *related to physical disability*
- Personal identity disturbance *related to lowered self-esteem*
- Self-esteem, chronic low

Chronic renal failure
- Body image disturbance
- Coping, ineffective family: Compromised *related to prolonged disease*
- Death anxiety *related to terminal illness*
- Denial *related to fear or anxiety*
- Family process alteration *related to situational crisis*
- Fluid volume excess *related to compromised regulatory mechanisms*
- Infection, risk for *related to external factors*
- Knowledge deficit *related to lack of exposure*
- Powerlessness *related to chronic illness*
- Sexual dysfunction *related to altered body structure or function*
- Skin integrity impairment, risk for
- Tissue perfusion alteration (renal) *related to decreased cellular exchange*

Cirrhosis
- Altered family processes: Alcoholism
- Breathing pattern, ineffective *related to decreased energy or fatigue*
- Coping, ineffective family: Compromised *related to prolonged disease*
- Fluid volume deficit *related to active loss*
- Incontinence, stress
- Injury, risk for *related to external factors*
- Nutrition alteration: Less than body requirements *related to inability to digest or absorb nutrients because of biological factors*
- Skin integrity impairment, risk for *related to the aging process and impaired mobility*
- Thought process alteration *related to physiologic causes*

Cleft lip or palate
- Aspiration, risk for *related to ineffective swallow reflex*
- Breast-feeding, ineffective *related to limited maternal experience*
- Coping, ineffective family: Compromised *related to neonatal health problems*
- Infant feeding pattern, ineffective *related to neurologic impairment or developmental delay*
- Nutrition alteration: Less than body requirements *related to ineffective suck reflex*
- Verbal communication impairment *related to physical barriers*

Colic
- Infant behavior, disorganized *related to pain, prematurity, oral problems, motor*

problems, feeding intolerance, environmental overstimulation, or lack of stimulation

Colitis
- Adjustment impairment *related to disability*
- Body image disturbance
- Body temperature alteration, risk for *related to dehydration*
- Diarrhea *related to stress and anxiety*
- Diarrhea *related to primary bowel pathology*
- Fluid volume deficit *related to active loss*
- Nutrition alteration: Less than body requirements *related to inability to absorb nutrients or insufficient intake*
- Pain *related to physical, biological, or chemical agents*
- Tissue perfusion alteration (GI) *related to decreased cellular exchange*

Colon and rectal cancer
- Constipation *related to GI obstruction*
- Diarrhea *related to malabsorption, inflammation, or irritation of bowel*
- Fluid volume deficit *related to active loss*
- Pain *related to physical, biological, or chemical agents*

Colostomy
- Body image disturbance
- Fluid volume deficit *related to active loss*
- Nutrition alteration: Less than body requirements *related to inability to digest or absorb nutrients because of biological factors*
- Self-esteem disturbance
- Sexuality pattern alteration *related to illness or medical treatment*
- Skin integrity impairment *related to external (environmental) factors*
- Tissue perfusion alteration (GI) *related to decreased cellular exchange*

Conduct disorder
- Altered family processes *related to dysfunctional behavior*
- Hopelessness *related to child's mood disturbance*
- Self-esteem disturbance *related to problematic relationship with parents*

Congenital anomalies
- Coping, ineffective family: Disabling *related to long-term illness*

- Incontinence, total *related to neuropathy, trauma, or disease affecting spinal nerves*

Congenital heart disease
- Activity intolerance *related to imbalance between oxygen supply and demand*
- Breathing pattern, ineffective *related to inability to maintain adequate rate and depth of respirations*
- Cardiac output, decreased *related to reduced stroke volume as a result of mechanical or structural problems*
- Family process alteration *related to situational crisis*
- Growth, altered, risk for
- Infection, risk for *related to external factors*
- Injury, risk for *related to internal and external neonatal risk factors*

Coronary artery disease
- Activity intolerance *related to imbalance between oxygen supply and demand*
- Anxiety *related to situational crisis*
- Cardiac output, decreased *related to reduced stroke volume as a result of mechanical or structural problems*
- Gas exchange impairment *related to altered oxygen-carrying capacity of the blood*
- Health-seeking behaviors *related to absence of aerobic exercise as a risk factor for coronary artery disease*
- Health-seeking behaviors *related to elevated serum cholesterol level as a risk factor for coronary artery disease*
- Health-seeking behaviors *related to smoking as a risk factor for coronary artery disease*
- Health-seeking behaviors *related to stress as a risk factor for coronary artery disease*
- Home maintenance management impairment *related to inadequate support system*
- Injury, risk for *related to elder abuse*
- Knowledge deficit *related to lack of exposure*
- Nutrition alteration: More than body requirements *related to excessive intake*
- Pain *related to physical, biological, or chemical agents*
- Role performance alteration *related to ineffective coping*
- Sexuality pattern alteration *related to illness or medical treatment*
- Tissue perfusion alteration (cardiopulmonary) *related to decreased cellular exchange*

Cor pulmonale

- Activity intolerance *related to imbalance between oxygen supply and demand*
- Airway clearance, ineffective *related to presence of tracheobronchial obstruction or secretions*
- Breathing pattern, ineffective *related to decreased energy or fatigue*
- Cardiac output, decreased *related to reduced stroke volume as a result of mechanical or structural problems*
- Coping, ineffective individual *related to situational crisis*
- Fatigue
- Fluid volume excess *related to excess fluid intake or retention, or excess sodium intake or retention*
- Gas exchange impairment *related to altered oxygen supply*
- Grieving, anticipatory *related to perceived potential loss of life*
- Hopelessness *related to chronic illness*
- Infection, risk for *related to external factors*

Craniotomy

- Airway clearance, ineffective *related to presence of tracheobronchial obstruction or secretions*
- Body image disturbance
- Breathing pattern, ineffective *related to decreased energy or fatigue*
- Infection, risk for *related to surgical incision*
- Intracranial adaptive capacity, decreased
- Mobility impairment, physical *related to neuromuscular impairment*
- Pain *related to physical, biological, or chemical agents*
- Self-care deficit *related to musculoskeletal impairment*
- Sensory or perceptual alteration *related to sensory overload*
- Skin integrity impairment *related to external (environmental) factors*
- Sleep pattern disturbance *related to external factors*
- Surgical recovery, delayed
- Tissue perfusion alteration (cerebral) *related to decreased cellular exchange*

Crohn's disease

- Anxiety *related to situational crisis*
- Coping, ineffective family: Compromised *related to prolonged disease*
- Diarrhea *related to malabsorption, inflammation, or irritation of bowel*
- Diarrhea *related to primary bowel pathology*
- Fear *related to unfamiliarity*
- Fluid volume deficit *related to excessive loss of fluids and electrolytes*
- Fluid volume imbalance, risk for *related to excessive loss, intake, or retention*
- Infection, risk for *related to home infusion therapy*
- Nausea *related to irritation to the GI system*
- Nutrition alteration: Less than body requirements *related to inability to absorb nutrients or insufficient intake*
- Pain *related to physical, biological, or chemical agents*
- Skin integrity impairment *related to external (environmental) factors*

Cushing's syndrome

- Activity intolerance *related to imbalance between oxygen supply and demand*
- Body image disturbance
- Body temperature alteration, risk for *related to decreased sensitivity of thermoreceptors*
- Coping, ineffective individual *related to situational crisis*
- Fluid volume excess *related to compromised regulatory mechanisms*
- Grieving, dysfunctional *related to actual object loss*
- Hopelessness *related to chronic illness*
- Nutrition alteration: More than body requirements *related to excessive intake*
- Skin integrity impairment *related to internal (somatic) factors*
- Thought process alteration *related to loss of memory*

Cystic fibrosis

- Activity intolerance *related to imbalance between oxygen supply and demand*
- Airway clearance, ineffective *related to presence of tracheobronchial obstruction or secretions*
- Body temperature alteration, risk for *related to dehydration*
- Breathing pattern, ineffective *related to inability to maintain adequate rate and depth of respirations*
- Coping, family: Potential for growth *related to self-actualization needs*
- Coping, ineffective family: Compromised *related to inadequate or incorrect information held by primary caregiver*

• Diversional activity deficit *related to prolonged illness and separation from friends and family*
• Fluid volume deficit *related to excessive loss of fluids and electrolytes*
• Fluid volume deficit, risk for *related to excessive loss*
• Fluid volume imbalance, risk for *related to excessive loss, intake, or retention*
• Gas exchange impairment *related to altered oxygen-carrying capacity of the blood*
• Growth, altered, risk for
• Infection, risk for *related to home infusion therapy*
• Nutrition alteration: Less than body requirements *related to inability to absorb nutrients or insufficient intake*
• Parental role conflict *related to home care of a child with special needs*
• Parental role conflict *related to child's hospitalization*

Cystitis
• Incontinence, urge *related to decreased bladder capacity*
• Incontinence, urinary urge, risk for
• Noncompliance *related to patient's value system*
• Pain *related to physical, biological, or chemical agents*
• Sleep pattern disturbance *related to internal factors*
• Urinary elimination alteration *related to obstruction*

Deafness
• Coping, defensive *related to perceived threat to positive self-regard*
• Coping, ineffective individual *related to inability to solve problems or adapt to demands of daily living*
• Fear *related to unfamiliarity*
• Injury, risk for *related to sensory or motor deficits*
• Parent-infant attachment, altered, risk for
• Role performance alteration *related to ineffective coping*
• Self-esteem disturbance
• Sensory or perceptual alteration (auditory) *related to illness or the aging process*
• Verbal communication impairment *related to physiologic or psychosocial changes*

Delusional disorder
• Home maintenance management impairment *related to impaired cognitive or emotional functioning*
• Thought process alteration *related to psychological causes*

Dementia
• Activity intolerance *related to functional changes accompanying the aging process*
• Altered family processes *related to dysfunctional behavior*
• Caregiver role strain *related to discharge of a family member with significant home care needs*
• Confusion, acute
• Confusion, chronic
• Environmental interpretation syndrome, impaired
• Family process alteration *related to situational crisis*
• Incontinence, functional *related to sensory or mobility deficits*
• Injury, risk for *related to elder abuse*
• Injury, risk for *related to lack of awareness of environmental hazards*
• Memory impairment
• Powerlessness *related to perceived loss of control over life situation*
• Social isolation *related to dysfunctional interpersonal relations*
• Thought process alteration *related to psychological causes*
• Verbal communication impairment *related to physiologic or psychosocial changes*
• Violence, risk for: Self-directed *related to recurrent losses or changes in physical or mental condition*

Depression
• Adult failure to thrive *related to illness, disability, or environmental deprivation*
• Body image disturbance *related to an eating disorder*
• Caregiver role strain *related to unpredictability of the care situation*
• Constipation *related to diet, fluid intake, activity level, and personal bowel habits*
• Constipation, risk of
• Coping, ineffective individual *related to situational crisis*
• Denial *related to fear or anxiety*
• Diversional activity deficit *related to lack of environmental stimulation*
• Fatigue

• Home maintenance management impairment *related to impaired cognitive or emotional functioning*
• Hopelessness *related to chronic illness*
• Incontinence, functional *related to cognitive deficits*
• Injury, risk for *related to elder abuse*
• Injury, risk for *related to lack of awareness of environmental hazards*
• Loneliness, risk for
• Nutrition alteration: Less than body requirements *related to psychological factors*
• Nutrition alteration: More than body requirements *related to a decline in basal metabolic rate and physical activity*
• Nutrition alteration: More than body requirements *related to excessive intake*
• Nutrition alteration, risk for: More than body requirements *related to excessive intake*
• Poisoning, risk for *related to substance abuse*
• Posttrauma syndrome *related to incest*
• Posttrauma syndrome, risk for
• Powerlessness *related to perceived loss of control over life situation*
• Self-esteem, chronic low
• Sexual dysfunction *related to decreased libido caused by depression*
• Sleep pattern disturbance *related to internal factors*
• Social isolation *related to physiologic, environmental, or emotional barriers*
• Violence, risk for: Self-directed *related to recurrent losses or changes in physical or mental condition*

Detached retina

• Anxiety *related to situational crisis*
• Injury, risk for *related to sensory or motor deficits*
• Pain *related to physical, biological, or chemical agents*
• Sensory or perceptual alteration (visual) *related to altered sensory reception, transmission, or integration*
• Sensory or perceptual alteration (visual) *related to illness or the aging process*

Developmental disorder

• Coping, ineffective family: Disabling *related to long-term illness*
• Injury, risk for *related to developmental factors*
• Parental role conflict *related to home care of a child with special needs*

• Parent-infant attachment, altered, risk for
• Self-mutilation, risk for *related to emotional illness*

Diabetes insipidus

• Body temperature alteration, risk for *related to decreased sensitivity of thermoreceptors*
• Fluid volume deficit *related to excessive loss of fluids and electrolytes*
• Fluid volume deficit, risk for *related to excessive loss*
• Oral mucous membrane alteration *related to dehydration*

Diabetes mellitus

• Adjustment impairment *related to disability*
• Body image disturbance
• Body temperature alteration, risk for *related to decreased sensitivity of thermoreceptors*
• Cardiac output, decreased *related to reduced stroke volume as a result of mechanical or structural problems*
• Constipation *related to diet, fluid intake, activity level, and personal bowel habits*
• Coping, ineffective family: Compromised *related to prolonged disease*
• Coping, ineffective individual *related to situational crisis*
• Fluid volume deficit, risk for *related to excessive loss*
• Fluid volume deficit, risk for *related to excessive loss through physiologic routes*
• Grieving, anticipatory *related to chronic or terminal illness*
• Health maintenance alteration *related to type 1 diabetes mellitus*
• Hopelessness *related to chronic illness*
• Hyperthermia *related to dehydration*
• Incontinence, total *related to neurologic dysfunction*
• Infection, risk for *related to external factors*
• Injury, risk for *related to lack of awareness of environmental hazards*
• Knowledge deficit *related to difficulty understanding disease process and its effect on self-care*
• Management of therapeutic regimen, ineffective: Individual *related to health beliefs*
• Noncompliance *related to patient's value system*
• Nutrition alteration: More than body requirements *related to excessive intake*

• Nutrition alteration, risk for: More than body requirements *related to excessive intake*
• Oral mucous membrane alteration *related to dehydration*
• Powerlessness *related to chronic illness*
• Role performance alteration *related to ineffective coping*
• Self-esteem, chronic low
• Sensory or perceptual alteration *related to illness or the aging process*
• Sexuality pattern alteration *related to illness or medical treatment*
• Skin integrity impairment *related to internal (somatic) factors*
• Skin integrity impairment, risk for
• Social isolation *related to altered state of wellness*
• Tissue perfusion alteration (peripheral) *related to reduced arterial blood flow*
• Tissue perfusion alteration (renal) *related to decreased cellular exchange*
• Urinary elimination alteration *related to sensory or neuromuscular impairment*

Diabetic ketoacidosis
• Body temperature alteration, risk for *related to decreased sensitivity of thermoreceptors*
• Fluid volume deficit *related to active loss*
• Thought process alteration *related to physiologic causes*

Diarrhea
• Body image disturbance *related to an eating disorder*
• Diarrhea *related to malabsorption, inflammation, or irritation of bowel*
• Diarrhea *related to stress and anxiety*
• Fluid volume deficit *related to excessive loss of fluids and electrolytes*
• Fluid volume deficit, risk for *related to excessive loss*
• Fluid volume imbalance, risk for *related to excessive loss, intake, or retention*

Digitalis toxicity
• Cardiac output, decreased *related to reduced stroke volume as a result of electrophysiologic problems*
• Knowledge deficit *related to difficulty understanding disease process and its effect on self-care*
• Poisoning, risk for *related to drug toxicity or polypharmacy*

Disseminated intravascular coagulation
• Cardiac output, decreased *related to reduced stroke volume as a result of mechanical or structural problems*
• Fear *related to unfamiliarity*
• Fluid volume deficit *related to active loss*
• Gas exchange impairment *related to altered oxygen supply*

Dissociative disorder
• Altered family processes *related to dysfunctional behavior*
• Home maintenance management impairment *related to impaired cognitive or emotional functioning*
• Thought process alteration *related to loss of memory*

Diverticulitis
• Constipation *related to diet, fluid intake, activity level, and personal bowel habits*
• Constipation *related to GI obstruction*
• Diarrhea *related to malabsorption, inflammation, or irritation of bowel*
• Fluid volume deficit *related to active loss*
• Fluid volume deficit *related to excessive loss of fluids and electrolytes*
• Nutrition alteration: Less than body requirements *related to inability to digest or absorb nutrients because of biological factors*
• Pain *related to physical, biological, or chemical agents*

Down syndrome
• Aspiration, risk for *related to ineffective swallow reflex*
• Coping, ineffective family: Compromised *related to prolonged disease*
• Development, altered, risk for
• Family process alteration *related to situational crisis*
• Growth and development alteration *related to physical disability or environmental deprivation*
• Infection, risk for *related to external factors*
• Injury, risk for *related to lack of awareness of environmental hazards*
• Knowledge deficit *related to cognitive impairment*
• Parental role conflict *related to home care of a child with special needs*
• Self-care deficit *related to perceptual or cognitive impairment*
• Self-esteem, situational low

Drug addiction

- Adult failure to thrive *related to illness, disability, or environmental deprivation*
- Altered family processes: Alcoholism
- Confusion, acute
- Coping, defensive *related to perceived threat to positive self-regard*
- Coping, ineffective individual *related to personal vulnerability*
- Coping, ineffective individual *related to situational crisis*
- Decisional conflict *related to substance abuse*
- Denial *related to fear or anxiety*
- Health maintenance alteration *related to perceptual or cognitive impairment*
- Management of therapeutic regimen, ineffective: Community *related to drug and alcohol abuse among teenagers*
- Management of therapeutic regimen, ineffective: Family *related to family conflict, complex therapy, economic difficulties, or difficulty coping with the health care system*
- Poisoning, risk for *related to substance abuse*
- Sexual dysfunction *related to impotence*
- Sleep pattern disturbance *related to internal factors*
- Violence, risk for: Self-directed *related to recurrent losses or changes in physical or mental condition*

Drug overdose

- Coping, ineffective individual *related to personal vulnerability*
- Coping, ineffective individual *related to situational crisis*
- Gas exchange impairment *related to altered oxygen supply*
- Hyperthermia *related to dehydration*
- Hypothermia *related to exposure to cold or cold environment*
- Incontinence, functional *related to cognitive deficits*
- Incontinence, functional *related to sensory or mobility deficits*
- Poisoning, risk for *related to drug toxicity or polypharmacy*
- Suffocation, risk for *related to external factors*
- Thermoregulation, ineffective *related to trauma or illness*
- Thought process alteration *related to physiologic causes*
- Trauma, risk for *related to external factors (environmental, physical, chemical agents)*

Drug toxicity

- Gas exchange impairment *related to altered oxygen supply*
- Hyperthermia *related to dehydration*
- Hypothermia *related to exposure to cold or cold environment*
- Incontinence, functional *related to sensory or mobility deficits*
- Poisoning, risk for *related to drug toxicity or polypharmacy*

Duodenal ulcer

- Anxiety *related to situational crisis*
- Nutrition alteration: Less than body requirements *related to inability to digest or absorb nutrients because of biological factors*
- Pain *related to physical, biological, or chemical agents*
- Tissue perfusion alteration (GI) *related to decreased cellular exchange*

Eating disorders (anorexia nervosa and bulimia nervosa)

- Body image disturbance
- Body image disturbance *related to an eating disorder*
- Decisional conflict *related to sexual activity*
- Loneliness, risk for
- Nutrition alteration: Less than body requirements *related to inability to absorb nutrients or insufficient intake*
- Posttrauma syndrome *related to incest*

Ectopic pregnancy

- Fluid volume deficit *related to active loss*
- Pain *related to physical, biological, or chemical agents*
- Tissue perfusion alteration (cardiopulmonary) *related to decreased cellular exchange*

Emphysema

- Activity intolerance *related to imbalance between oxygen supply and demand*
- Airway clearance, ineffective *related to decreased energy or fatigue*
- Airway clearance, ineffective *related to presence of tracheobronchial obstruction or secretions*
- Breathing pattern, ineffective *related to decreased energy or fatigue*
- Fatigue
- Fear *related to unfamiliarity*

• Gas exchange impairment *related to carbon dioxide retention or excess mucus production*
• Hopelessness *related to chronic illness*
• Infection, risk for *related to external factors*
• Knowledge deficit *related to difficulty understanding disease process and its effect on self-care*
• Knowledge deficit *related to lack of motivation*
• Noncompliance *related to patient's value system*
• Nutrition alteration: Less than body requirements *related to inability to digest or absorb nutrients because of biological factors*
• Ventilation, spontaneous: Inability to sustain

Empyema
• Breathing pattern, ineffective *related to pain*
• Fluid volume deficit *related to active loss*
• Gas exchange impairment *related to altered oxygen supply*
• Infection, risk for *related to external factors*

Encephalitis
• Activity intolerance *related to immobility*
• Anxiety *related to situational crisis*
• Constipation *related to inadequate intake of fluid and bulk*
• Coping, ineffective individual *related to situational crisis*
• Fluid volume deficit *related to active loss*
• Growth and development alteration *related to physical disability or environmental deprivation*
• Hyperthermia *related to infection*
• Infection, risk for *related to external factors*
• Mobility impairment, physical *related to pain or discomfort*
• Pain *related to physical, biological, or chemical agents*
• Thermoregulation, ineffective *related to trauma or illness*
• Thought process alteration *related to physiologic causes*

Endocarditis
• Activity intolerance *related to imbalance between oxygen supply and demand*
• Anxiety *related to situational crisis*
• Cardiac output, decreased *related to reduced stroke volume as a result of mechanical or structural problems*

• Fluid volume excess *related to compromised regulatory mechanisms*
• Knowledge deficit *related to lack of exposure*
• Nutrition alteration: Less than body requirements *related to inability to ingest foods*

Endometrial cancer
• Fear *related to unfamiliarity*
• Grieving, anticipatory *related to perceived potential loss of significant object (such as person, job, possessions)*
• Pain *related to physical, biological, or chemical agents*
• Tissue integrity impairment *related to radiation*

Endometriosis
• Anxiety *related to situational crisis*
• Fluid volume deficit *related to active loss*
• Infection, risk for *related to external factors*
• Knowledge deficit *related to lack of exposure*
• Sexual dysfunction *related to altered body structure or function*

Esophageal cancer
• Aspiration, risk for *related to absence of protective mechanisms*
• Fatigue
• Fear *related to unfamiliarity*
• Fluid volume deficit, risk for *related to excessive loss*
• Infection, risk for *related to external factors*
• Nutrition alteration: Less than body requirements *related to inability to ingest foods*
• Pain *related to physical, biological, or chemical agents*

Esophageal fistula
• Aspiration, risk for *related to infant's immature cough or gag reflex*
• Fluid volume deficit, risk for *related to excessive loss*
• Nutrition alteration: Less than body requirements *related to ineffective suck reflex*

Esophageal varices
• Altered family processes: Alcoholism
• Fluid volume deficit *related to active loss*
• Fluid volume deficit, risk for *related to excessive loss*
• Nutrition alteration: Less than body requirements *related to inability to digest or*

absorb nutrients because of biological factors
• Skin integrity impairment, risk for

Failure to thrive
• Coping, ineffective community *related to increased levels of teen pregnancy*
• Fluid volume deficit *related to excessive loss of fluids and electrolytes*
• Fluid volume deficit, risk for *related to presence of risk factors for fluid and electrolyte imbalance*
• Growth and development alteration *related to environmental and stimulation deficiencies*
• Growth and development alteration *related to physical disability or environmental deprivation*
• Infant behavior, disorganized *related to pain, prematurity, oral problems, motor problems, feeding intolerance, environmental overstimulation, or lack of stimulation*
• Infant behavior, disorganized, risk for *related to pain, prematurity, oral problems, motor problems, feeding intolerance, environmental overstimulation, or lack of stimulation*
• Nutrition alteration: Less than body requirements *related to inability to absorb nutrients or insufficient intake*
• Nutrition alteration: Less than body requirements *related to lack of resources or knowledge*
• Parenting alteration *related to lack of knowledge*
• Parenting alteration, risk for *related to lack of knowledge or ineffective role model*

Fetal alcohol syndrome
• Altered family processes: Alcoholism
• Coping, ineffective community *related to increased levels of teen pregnancy*
• Coping, ineffective family: Compromised *related to neonatal health problems*
• Growth, altered, risk for
• Growth and development alteration *related to physical disability or environmental deprivation*

Food poisoning
• Breathing pattern, ineffective *related to decreased energy or fatigue*
• Diarrhea *related to malabsorption, inflammation, or irritation of bowel*
• Hyperthermia *related to infection*

• Mobility impairment, physical *related to pain or discomfort*
• Nausea *related to irritation to the GI system*
• Sensory or perceptual alteration (visual) *related to altered sensory reception, transmission, or integration*
• Verbal communication impairment *related to decreased circulation to brain*

Fractures
• Activity intolerance *related to immobility*
• Breathing pattern, ineffective *related to pain*
• Constipation, risk of
• Coping, ineffective family: Compromised *related to caring for dependent, aging family member*
• Coping, ineffective family: Compromised *related to prolonged disease*
• Denial *related to fear or anxiety*
• Disuse syndrome, risk for
• Diversional activity deficit *related to lack of environmental stimulation*
• Fluid volume deficit *related to active loss*
• Hopelessness *related to prolonged activity restriction, creating isolation*
• Injury, risk for *related to sensory or motor deficits*
• Mobility impairment, physical *related to pain or discomfort*
• Pain *related to physical, biological, or chemical agents*
• Parenting alteration *related to lack of knowledge*
• Peripheral neurovascular dysfunction, risk for
• Role performance alteration *related to ineffective coping*
• Self-care deficit *related to musculoskeletal impairment*
• Sensory or perceptual alteration
• Skin integrity impairment *related to external (environmental) factors*
• Trauma, risk for *related to external factors (environmental, physical, chemical agents)*
• Trauma, risk for *related to feelings of personal invulnerability*

Gallbladder disease
• Pain *related to physiologic changes of pregnancy*

Gastric cancer

- Nutrition alteration: Less than body requirements *related to inability to ingest foods*
- Tissue perfusion alteration (GI) *related to decreased cellular exchange*

Gastric ulcer

- Anxiety *related to situational crisis*
- Nutrition alteration: Less than body requirements *related to inability to digest or absorb nutrients because of biological factors*
- Nutrition alteration: Less than body requirements *related to inability to absorb nutrients or insufficient intake*
- Pain *related to physical, biological, or chemical agents*
- Tissue perfusion alteration (GI) *related to decreased cellular exchange*

Gastroenteritis

- Body temperature alteration, risk for *related to dehydration*
- Diarrhea *related to primary bowel pathology*
- Fluid volume deficit *related to excessive loss of fluids and electrolytes*
- Fluid volume deficit, risk for *related to excessive loss*
- Fluid volume deficit, risk for *related to presence of risk factors for fluid and electrolyte imbalance*

Genital herpes

- Coping, ineffective community *related to increased levels of teen pregnancy*
- Infection, risk for *related to external factors*
- Loneliness, risk for
- Powerlessness *related to chronic illness*
- Sexuality pattern alteration *related to illness or medical treatment*
- Social isolation *related to altered state of wellness*

Gestational diabetes

- Infection, risk for *related to altered primary defenses during the postpartum period*

Glaucoma

- Anxiety *related to situational crisis*
- Grieving, anticipatory *related to perceived potential loss of significant object (such as person, job, possessions)*
- Injury, risk for *related to sensory or motor deficits*

- Knowledge deficit *related to lack of exposure*
- Pain *related to physical, biological, or chemical agents*
- Sensory or perceptual alteration (visual) *related to altered sensory reception, transmission, or integration*
- Sensory or perceptual alteration (visual) *related to illness or the aging process*

Glomerulonephritis

- Coping, ineffective family: Compromised *related to prolonged disease*
- Fluid volume excess *related to compromised regulatory mechanisms*
- Infection, risk for *related to external factors*
- Nutrition alteration: Less than body requirements *related to inability to digest or absorb nutrients because of biological factors*
- Tissue perfusion alteration (renal) *related to decreased cellular exchange*

Gonorrhea

- Coping, ineffective community *related to increased levels of teen pregnancy*
- Infection, risk for *related to external factors*
- Infection, risk for *related to neonate's immature immune system*
- Sexuality pattern alteration *related to illness or medical treatment*

Gout

- Activity intolerance *related to immobility*
- Body image disturbance
- Knowledge deficit *related to lack of exposure*
- Mobility impairment, physical *related to pain or discomfort*
- Nutrition alteration: More than body requirements *related to excessive intake*
- Pain *related to physical, biological, or chemical agents*
- Self-care deficit *related to musculoskeletal impairment*

Guillain-Barré syndrome

- Activity intolerance *related to immobility*
- Airway clearance, ineffective *related to decreased energy or fatigue*
- Airway clearance, ineffective *related to presence of tracheobronchial obstruction or secretions*
- Anxiety *related to situational crisis*
- Breathing pattern, ineffective *related to decreased energy or fatigue*

• Coping, ineffective individual *related to situational crisis*
• Fatigue
• Gas exchange impairment *related to altered oxygen supply*
• Incontinence, bowel *related to neuromuscular involvement*
• Incontinence, urinary urge, risk for
• Mobility impairment, physical *related to neuromuscular impairment*
• Pain *related to physical, biological, or chemical agents*
• Self-care deficit *related to musculoskeletal impairment*
• Ventilation, spontaneous: Inability to sustain
• Ventilation, spontaneous: Inability to sustain *related to home ventilation therapy*

Headaches
• Pain, chronic *related to physical mobility*

Head injury
• Activity intolerance *related to immobility*
• Activity intolerance, risk for *related to immobility*
• Aspiration, risk for *related to absence of protective mechanisms*
• Body image disturbance
• Body temperature alteration, risk for *related to dehydration*
• Confusion, acute
• Confusion, chronic
• Constipation, risk of
• Development, altered, risk for
• Disuse syndrome, risk for
• Environmental interpretation syndrome, impaired
• Fear *related to unfamiliarity*
• Fluid volume imbalance, risk for *related to excessive loss, intake, or retention*
• Gas exchange impairment *related to altered oxygen supply*
• Growth and development alteration *related to physical disability or environmental deprivation*
• Incontinence, bowel *related to neuromuscular involvement*
• Incontinence, bowel *related to perceptual or cognitive impairment*
• Incontinence, total *related to neurologic dysfunction*
• Incontinence, urinary urge, risk for
• Injury, risk for *related to sensory or motor deficits*
• Intracranial adaptive capacity, decreased

• Knowledge deficit *related to the Americans with Disabilities Act*
• Knowledge deficit *related to lack of exposure*
• Memory impairment *related to neurologic disturbance*
• Mobility impairment, physical *related to neuromuscular impairment*
• Neglect, unilateral *related to neurologic illness or trauma*
• Nutrition alteration: Less than body requirements *related to inability to ingest foods*
• Parenting alteration *related to lack of knowledge*
• Parenting alteration, risk for *related to lack of knowledge or ineffective role model*
• Posttrauma syndrome *related to accidental injury*
• Powerlessness *related to physical, sexual, or emotional abuse by partner*
• Self-care deficit *related to musculoskeletal impairment*
• Sensory or perceptual alteration
• Sleep deprivation
• Social interaction impairment *related to altered thought processes*
• Sorrow, chronic *related to change in physical, social, or psychological status*
• Swallowing impairment *related to neuromuscular impairment*
• Thermoregulation, ineffective *related to trauma or illness*
• Thought process alteration *related to physiologic causes*
• Tissue perfusion alteration *related to decreased cellular exchange*
• Trauma, risk for *related to external factors (environmental, physical, chemical agents)*
• Trauma, risk for *related to feelings of personal invulnerability*
• Verbal communication impairment *related to decreased circulation to brain*
• Verbal communication impairment *related to developmental factors*

Head or neck cancer
• Airway clearance, ineffective *related to presence of tracheobronchial obstruction or secretions*
• Body image disturbance
• Oral mucous membrane alteration *related to pathologic condition*
• Pain *related to physical, biological, or chemical agents*

- Sensory or perceptual alteration (gustatory)
- Tissue integrity impairment *related to radiation*
- Verbal communication impairment *related to physical barriers*

Heart failure

- Activity intolerance *related to imbalance between oxygen supply and demand*
- Activity intolerance, risk for *related to immobility*
- Airway clearance, ineffective *related to decreased energy or fatigue*
- Breathing pattern, ineffective *related to inability to maintain adequate rate and depth of respirations*
- Cardiac output, decreased *related to reduced myocardial perfusion*
- Cardiac output, decreased *related to reduced stroke volume as a result of electrophysiologic problems*
- Cardiac output, decreased *related to reduced stroke volume as a result of mechanical or structural problems*
- Caregiver role strain *related to discharge of a family member with significant home care needs*
- Caregiver role strain, risk for
- Death anxiety *related to terminal illness*
- Fatigue
- Fluid volume excess *related to compromised regulatory mechanisms*
- Fluid volume excess *related to excess fluid intake or retention or excess sodium intake or retention*
- Fluid volume imbalance, risk for *related to excessive loss, intake, or retention*
- Gas exchange impairment *related to altered oxygen supply*
- Home maintenance management impairment *related to impaired cognitive or emotional functioning*
- Hopelessness *related to chronic illness*
- Injury, risk for *related to sensory or motor deficits*
- Knowledge deficit *related to difficulty understanding disease process and its effect on self-care*
- Knowledge deficit *related to lack of exposure*
- Nutrition alteration: More than body requirements *related to a decline in basal metabolic rate and physical activity*
- Pain *related to physical, biological, or chemical agents*

- Powerlessness *related to illness-related regimen*
- Role performance alteration
- Tissue perfusion alteration *related to decreased cellular exchange*

Hemodialysis

- Body image disturbance
- Family process alteration *related to situational crisis*
- Fluid volume deficit *related to active loss*
- Fluid volume excess *related to compromised regulatory mechanisms*
- Infection, risk for *related to external factors*
- Knowledge deficit *related to lack of exposure*
- Thought process alteration *related to physiologic causes*

Hemophilia

- Altered protection *related to myelosuppression and immunosuppression*
- Body temperature alteration, risk for, *related to dehydration*
- Coping, family: Potential for growth *related to self-actualization needs*
- Gas exchange impairment *related to altered oxygen-carrying capacity of the blood*
- Injury, risk for *related to lack of awareness of environmental hazards*
- Pain *related to physical, biological, or chemical agents*
- Parental role conflict *related to home care of a child with special needs*
- Personal identity disturbance *related to lowered self-esteem*
- Self-esteem, chronic low
- Trauma, risk for *related to external factors (environmental, physical, chemical agents)*

Hemorrhage

- Aspiration, risk for *related to absence of protective mechanisms*
- Fluid volume deficit *related to active loss*
- Fluid volume deficit *related to postpartum hemorrhage*
- Oral mucous membrane alteration *related to dehydration*
- Thermoregulation, ineffective *related to trauma or illness*
- Tissue perfusion alteration (renal) *related to decreased cellular exchange*

Hemorrhoids

- Constipation *related to personal habits*

• Knowledge deficit *related to lack of exposure*
• Pain *related to physical, biological, or chemical agents*
• Pain *related to physiologic changes of pregnancy*

Hemothorax
• Breathing pattern, ineffective *related to pain*
• Fear *related to unfamiliarity*
• Fluid volume deficit *related to active loss*
• Gas exchange impairment *related to altered oxygen supply*
• Pain *related to physical, biological, or chemical agents*
• Tissue perfusion alteration *related to hypovolemia*
• Ventilation, spontaneous: Inability to sustain

Hepatic coma
• Fluid volume deficit *related to active loss*
• Infection, risk for *related to external factors*
• Injury, risk for *related to sensory or motor deficits*
• Nutrition alteration: Less than body requirements *related to inability to digest or absorb nutrients because of biological factors*
• Sensory or perceptual alteration *related to sensory overload*
• Skin integrity impairment *related to external (environmental) factors*
• Thought process alteration *related to physiologic causes*

Hepatitis
• Coping, ineffective community *related to increased levels of teen pregnancy*
• Coping, potential for enhanced community *related to immunization*
• Nausea *related to irritation to the GI system*

Hip fracture
• Activity intolerance, risk for *related to immobility*
• Coping, ineffective family: Compromised *related to caring for dependent, aging family member*
• Denial *related to fear or anxiety about aging*
• Injury, risk for *related to elder abuse*
• Powerlessness *related to perceived loss of control over life situation*

• Role performance alteration
• Sexuality pattern alteration (female patient) *related to illness, medical treatment, or age-related changes*
• Skin integrity impairment, risk for *related to the aging process and impaired mobility*

Hodgkin's disease
• Altered protection *related to myelosuppression and immunosuppression*
• Breathing pattern, ineffective *related to decreased energy or fatigue*
• Grieving, anticipatory *related to perceived potential loss of life*
• Infection, risk for *related to external factors*
• Infection, risk for *related to increased incidence of tuberculosis*
• Mobility impairment, physical *related to pain or discomfort*
• Nutrition alteration: Less than body requirements *related to inability to ingest foods*
• Skin integrity impairment *related to external (environmental) factors*
• Tissue integrity impairment *related to radiation*

Human immunodeficiency virus
• Caregiver role strain, risk for *related to caring for a family member with Alzheimer's disease*
• Environmental interpretation syndrome, impaired
• Infection, risk for *related to increased incidence of tuberculosis*

Huntington's disease
• Caregiver role strain *related to discharge of a family member with significant home care needs*
• Coping, ineffective family: Compromised *related to inadequate or incorrect information held by primary caregiver*
• Health maintenance alteration *related to perceptual or cognitive impairment*
• Incontinence, bowel *related to perceptual or cognitive impairment*
• Injury, risk for *related to lack of awareness of environmental hazards*
• Knowledge deficit *related to cognitive impairment*
• Mobility impairment, physical *related to neuromuscular impairment*
• Self-care deficit *related to perceptual or cognitive impairment*

• Verbal communication impairment *related to physiologic or psychosocial changes*
• Verbal communication impairment *related to psychological barriers*

Hydatidiform mole
• Fluid volume deficit *related to active loss*
• Grieving, anticipatory *related to perceived potential loss of life*
• Pain *related to physiologic changes of pregnancy*
• Pain *related to physiologic response to labor*

Hydrocephalus
• Anxiety *related to situational crisis*
• Body image disturbance
• Coping, ineffective family: Compromised *related to prolonged disease*
• Family process alteration *related to situational crisis*
• Growth and development alteration *related to effects of physical disability*
• Infection, risk for *related to external factors*
• Nutrition alteration: Less than body requirements *related to inability to ingest foods*
• Pain *related to physical, biological, or chemical agents*
• Skin integrity impairment, risk for

Hyperbilirubinemia
• Breast-feeding, interrupted *related to a contraindicating condition*
• Injury, risk for *related to internal and external neonatal risk factors*

Hyperemesis gravidarum
• Fluid volume deficit *related to active loss*
• Nutrition alteration: Less than body requirements *related to inability to digest or absorb nutrients because of biological factors*
• Nutrition alteration: Less than body requirements *related to ineffective suck reflex*
• Pain *related to physiologic changes of pregnancy*

Hyperosmolar hyperglycemic nonketotic syndrome
• Fluid volume deficit *related to active loss*
• Infection, risk for *related to external factors*
• Skin integrity impairment *related to internal (somatic) factors*
• Thought process alteration *related to physiologic causes*

• Tissue perfusion alteration *related to hypovolemia*

Hyperparathyroidism
• Anxiety *related to situational crisis*
• Body temperature alteration, risk for *related to decreased sensitivity of thermoreceptors*
• Breathing pattern, ineffective *related to decreased energy or fatigue*
• Coping, ineffective individual *related to situational crisis*
• Hopelessness *related to failing or deteriorating physiologic condition*
• Nutrition alteration: Less than body requirements *related to inability to ingest foods*
• Pain *related to physical, biological, or chemical agents*
• Skin integrity impairment, risk for *related to the aging process and impaired mobility*

Hyperpituitarism
• Body image disturbance
• Coping, ineffective individual *related to situational crisis*
• Pain *related to physical, biological, or chemical agents*
• Sexual dysfunction *related to decreased libido caused by depression*

Hypertension
• Cardiac output, decreased *related to reduced stroke volume as a result of mechanical or structural problems*
• Denial *related to fear or anxiety about aging*
• Environmental interpretation syndrome, impaired
• Fluid volume excess *related to compromised regulatory mechanisms*
• Health-seeking behaviors *related to hypertension as a risk factor for coronary artery disease*
• Knowledge deficit *related to lack of exposure*
• Knowledge deficit *related to lack of motivation*
• Management of therapeutic regimen, ineffective: Individual *related to health beliefs*
• Noncompliance *related to patient's value system*
• Nutrition alteration: More than body requirements *related to a decline in basal metabolic rate and physical activity*

• Nutrition alteration: More than body requirements *related to excessive intake*
• Powerlessness *related to illness-related regimen*
• Self-esteem, situational low *related to hospitalization and forced dependence on health care team*
• Sexuality pattern alteration *related to illness or medical treatment*

Hyperthermia
• Hyperthermia *related to dehydration*
• Hyperthermia *related to infection*
• Knowledge deficit *related to lack of exposure*
• Oral mucous membrane alteration *related to dehydration*
• Thermoregulation, ineffective *related to trauma or illness*

Hyperthyroidism
• Activity intolerance *related to imbalance between oxygen supply and demand*
• Body image disturbance
• Body temperature alteration, risk for *related to decreased sensitivity of thermoreceptors*
• Cardiac output, decreased *related to reduced stroke volume as a result of electrophysiologic problems*
• Sleep pattern disturbance *related to internal factors, such as illness, psychological stress, drug therapy, biorhythm disturbance*
• Thought process alteration *related to psychological causes*

Hypochondriasis
• Coping, ineffective individual *related to personal vulnerability*
• Health maintenance alteration *related to perceptual or cognitive impairment*
• Thought process alteration *related to psychological causes*

Hypoparathyroidism
• Anxiety *related to situational crisis*
• Cardiac output, decreased *related to reduced stroke volume as a result of electrophysiologic problems*
• Coping, ineffective family: Compromised *related to prolonged disease*
• Coping, ineffective individual *related to situational crisis*
• Nutrition alteration: Less than body requirements *related to inability to digest or*

absorb nutrients because of biological factors
• Trauma, risk for *related to internal factors*

Hypopituitarism
• Growth, altered, risk for

Hypothermia
• Hypothermia *related to exposure to cold or cold environment*
• Knowledge deficit *related to lack of exposure*
• Thermoregulation, ineffective *related to trauma or illness*

Hypothyroidism
• Activity intolerance *related to imbalance between oxygen supply and demand*
• Body image disturbance
• Body temperature alteration, risk for *related to decreased sensitivity of thermoreceptors*
• Cardiac output, decreased *related to reduced stroke volume as a result of electrophysiologic problems*
• Constipation *related to diet, fluid intake, activity level, and personal bowel habits*
• Coping, ineffective family: Compromised *related to prolonged disease*
• Coping, ineffective individual *related to situational crisis*
• Development, altered, risk for
• Growth, altered, risk for
• Incontinence, functional *related to cognitive deficits*
• Sexuality pattern alteration (female patient) *related to illness, medical treatment, or age-related changes*
• Thought process alteration *related to physiologic causes*

Ileostomy
• Body image disturbance
• Fluid volume deficit *related to active loss*
• Infection, risk for *related to external factors*
• Nutrition alteration: Less than body requirements *related to inability to digest or absorb nutrients because of biological factors*
• Self-esteem disturbance
• Sexuality pattern alteration *related to illness or medical treatment*
• Skin integrity impairment *related to external (environmental) factors*
• Tissue perfusion alteration (GI) *related to decreased cellular exchange*

Impotence
- Body image disturbance
- Self-esteem, situational low
- Sexual dysfunction *related to impotence*
- Urinary retention *related to obstruction, sensory or neuromuscular impairment*

Incest
- Coping, ineffective individual *related to situational crisis*
- Family process alteration *related to situational crisis*
- Personal identity disturbance *related to lowered self-esteem*
- Posttrauma syndrome *related to assault*
- Rape-trauma syndrome: Compound reaction
- Rape-trauma syndrome: Silent reaction

Infant respiratory distress syndrome
- Airway clearance, ineffective *related to presence of tracheobronchial obstruction or secretions*
- Breathing pattern, ineffective *related to decreased energy or fatigue*
- Gas exchange impairment *related to altered oxygen supply*
- Infection, risk for *related to neonate's immature immune system*
- Thermoregulation, ineffective *related to immaturity*

Infertility
- Coping, ineffective individual *related to situational crisis*
- Grieving, dysfunctional *related to actual object loss*
- Knowledge deficit *related to lack of exposure*
- Self-esteem, situational low
- Self-esteem disturbance

Inhalation injuries
- Injury, risk for *related to lack of awareness of environmental hazards*
- Suffocation, risk for *related to external factors*
- Thermoregulation, ineffective *related to trauma or illness*

Interstitial pulmonary fibrosis
- Activity intolerance *related to imbalance between oxygen supply and demand*
- Breathing pattern, ineffective *related to decreased energy or fatigue*

- Gas exchange impairment *related to altered oxygen supply*

Intestinal obstruction
- Aspiration, risk for *related to absence of protective mechanisms*
- Constipation *related to GI obstruction*
- Fluid volume deficit, risk for *related to excessive loss*
- Fluid volume imbalance, risk for *related to excessive loss, intake, or retention*
- Nutrition alteration: Less than body requirements *related to inability to ingest foods*
- Nutrition alteration: Less than body requirements *related to inability to absorb nutrients or insufficient intake*
- Pain *related to physical, biological, or chemical agents*
- Tissue perfusion alteration (GI) *related to decreased cellular exchange*
- Urinary retention *related to obstruction, sensory or neuromuscular impairment*

Intoxication
- Aspiration, risk for *related to absence of protective mechanisms*
- Hypothermia *related to exposure to cold or cold environment*
- Management of therapeutic regimen, ineffective community *related to drug and alcohol abuse among teenagers*
- Sensory or perceptual alteration *related to hallucinations*
- Sensory or perceptual alteration *related to altered sensory reception, transmission, or integration*
- Thought process alteration *related to psychological causes*
- Verbal communication impairment *related to psychological barriers*

Joint replacement
- Coping, ineffective family: Compromised *related to caring for dependent, aging family member*
- Infection, risk for *related to surgical incision*
- Injury, risk for *related to lack of awareness of environmental hazards*
- Mobility impairment, physical *related to pain or discomfort*
- Pain *related to physical, biological, or chemical agents*
- Sensory or perceptual alteration (kinesthetic)

• Tissue perfusion alteration *related to decreased cellular exchange*

Juvenile rheumatoid arthritis
• Grieving, anticipatory *related to perceived potential loss of significant object or person*
• Grieving, anticipatory *related to chronic or terminal illness*
• Health maintenance alteration *related to lack of familiarity with neighborhood resources*
• Mobility impairment, physical *related to pain or discomfort*
• Sensory or perceptual alteration (tactile)

Kidney transplantation
• Altered protection *related to myelosuppression and immunosuppression*
• Body image disturbance
• Family process alteration *related to situational crisis*
• Fluid volume deficit *related to active loss*
• Infection, risk for *related to surgical incision*
• Knowledge deficit *related to lack of exposure*
• Surgical recovery, delayed

Labor and delivery
• Anxiety *related to situational crisis*
• Breast-feeding, effective
• Coping, ineffective individual *related to labor and delivery*
• Incontinence, total *related to neurologic dysfunction*
• Injury, risk for *related to induction or augmentation of labor*
• Knowledge deficit *related to lack of information about birth process*
• Knowledge deficit *related to postpartum self-care*
• Pain *related to physiologic changes of pregnancy*
• Pain *related to physiologic response to labor*
• Self-esteem disturbance *related to behavior during labor and delivery*
• Skin integrity impairment *related to episiotomy or abdominal incision*
• Urinary elimination alteration *related to sensory impairment during labor*

Laryngeal cancer
• Grieving, anticipatory *related to perceived potential loss of significant object (such as person, job, possessions)*

Leukemia
• Altered protection *related to myelosuppression and immunosuppression*
• Body temperature alteration, risk for *related to decreased sensitivity of thermoreceptors*
• Gas exchange impairment *related to altered oxygen-carrying capacity of the blood*
• Grieving, anticipatory *related to perceived potential loss of life*
• Grieving, anticipatory *related to chronic or terminal illness*
• Hopelessness *related to failing or deteriorating physiologic condition*
• Infection, risk for *related to external factors*
• Infection, risk for *related to increased incidence of tuberculosis*
• Nutrition alteration: Less than body requirements *related to inability to ingest foods*
• Oral mucous membrane alteration *related to pathologic condition*
• Pain *related to physical, biological, or chemical agents*
• Tissue integrity impairment *related to physical, chemical, or electrical hazards during surgery*
• Tissue integrity impairment *related to radiation*
• Tissue perfusion alteration (cardiopulmonary) *related to decreased cellular exchange*
• Tissue perfusion alteration (renal) *related to decreased cellular exchange*

Liver transplantation
• Altered protection *related to myelosuppression and immunosuppression*
• Coping, ineffective family: Compromised *related to prolonged disease*
• Coping, ineffective individual *related to situational crisis*
• Fear *related to unfamiliarity*
• Infection, risk for *related to surgical incision*
• Surgical recovery, delayed
• Tissue perfusion alteration (cardiopulmonary) *related to decreased cellular exchange*
• Tissue perfusion alteration (GI) *related to decreased cellular exchange*
• Tissue perfusion alteration (renal) *related to decreased cellular exchange*

Lung abscess
- Airway clearance, ineffective *related to presence of tracheobronchial obstruction or secretions*
- Anxiety *related to situational crisis*
- Body temperature alteration, risk for *related to decreased sensitivity of thermoreceptors*
- Breathing pattern, ineffective *related to pain*
- Coping, ineffective individual *related to situational crisis*
- Gas exchange impairment *related to altered oxygen supply*
- Pain *related to physical, biological, or chemical agents*
- Tissue perfusion alteration (cardiopulmonary) *related to decreased cellular exchange*

Lung cancer
- Activity intolerance *related to imbalance between oxygen supply and demand*
- Airway clearance, ineffective *related to decreased energy or fatigue*
- Breathing pattern, ineffective *related to decreased energy or fatigue*
- Fear *related to unfamiliarity*
- Gas exchange impairment *related to altered oxygen-carrying capacity of the blood*
- Nutrition alteration: Less than body requirements *related to inability to ingest foods*
- Powerlessness *related to chronic illness*
- Tissue integrity impairment *related to radiation*
- Verbal communication impairment *related to physical barriers*

Lupus erythematosus
- Adjustment impairment *related to disability*
- Cardiac output, decreased *related to reduced stroke volume as a result of mechanical or structural problems*
- Hopelessness *related to chronic illness*
- Infection, risk for *related to external factors*
- Mobility impairment, physical *related to pain or discomfort*
- Mobility impairment, physical *related to perceptual or cognitive impairment*
- Nutrition alteration: Less than body requirements *related to inability to digest or absorb nutrients because of biological factors*

- Tissue perfusion alteration *related to decreased cellular exchange*

Lyme disease
- Activity intolerance *related to imbalance between oxygen supply and demand*
- Fatigue
- Hyperthermia *related to infection*
- Pain *related to physical, biological, or chemical agents*
- Skin integrity impairment *related to external (environmental) factors*

Lymphomas
- Altered protection *related to myelosuppression and immunosuppression*
- Hopelessness *related to failing or deteriorating physiologic condition*
- Infection, risk for *related to external factors*
- Tissue integrity impairment *related to radiation*

Macular degeneration
- Activity intolerance *related to functional changes accompanying the aging process*
- Caregiver role strain, risk for *related to developmental state*
- Denial *related to fear or anxiety about aging*
- Powerlessness *related to perceived loss of control over life situation*
- Role performance alteration
- Sensory or perceptual alteration (visual) *related to altered sensory reception, transmission, or integration*
- Sensory or perceptual alteration (visual) *related to illness or the aging process*

Malnutrition
- Coping, ineffective community *related to increased levels of teen pregnancy*
- Injury, risk for *related to elder abuse*
- Nutrition alteration: Less than body requirements *related to lack of resources or knowledge*

Maternal psychological stress
- Anxiety *related to hospitalization and birth process*
- Anxiety *related to situational crisis*
- Breast-feeding, ineffective *related to dissatisfaction with breast-feeding process*
- Breast-feeding, ineffective *related to limited maternal experience*
- Breast-feeding, interrupted *related to a contraindicating condition*

• Powerlessness *related to illness-related regimen*

Meconium aspiration syndrome
• Breathing pattern, ineffective *related to adjustment to extrauterine existence*
• Injury, risk for *related to internal and external neonatal risk factors*

Melanoma
• Body image disturbance
• Coping, defensive *related to perceived threat to positive self-regard*
• Decisional conflict *related to health care options*
• Fatigue
• Oral mucous membrane alteration *related to pathologic condition*
• Powerlessness *related to illness-related regimen*
• Spiritual distress *related to situational crisis*

Ménière's disease
• Mobility impairment, physical *related to perceptual or cognitive impairment*
• Nausea *related to irritation to the GI system*
• Sensory or perceptual alteration (auditory) *related to altered sensory reception, transmission, or integration*
• Trauma, risk for *related to internal factors*

Meningitis
• Airway clearance, ineffective *related to decreased energy or fatigue*
• Breathing pattern, ineffective *related to decreased energy or fatigue*
• Fear *related to unfamiliarity*
• Fluid volume deficit *related to active loss*
• Fluid volume excess *related to compromised regulatory mechanisms*
• Fluid volume imbalance, risk for *related to excessive loss, intake, or retention*
• Hyperthermia *related to infection*
• Incontinence, bowel *related to perceptual or cognitive impairment*
• Infection, risk for *related to external factors*
• Pain *related to physical, biological, or chemical agents*
• Sensory or perceptual alteration (auditory) *related to altered sensory reception, transmission, or integration*
• Sensory or perceptual alteration (visual) *related to altered sensory reception, transmission, or integration*

Menopause
• Self-esteem disturbance
• Sexual dysfunction *related to altered body structure or function*
• Sexuality pattern alteration (female patient) *related to illness, medical treatment, or age-related changes*

Metabolic acidosis
• Breathing pattern, ineffective *related to decreased energy or fatigue*
• Injury, risk for *related to sensory or motor deficits*
• Knowledge deficit *related to cognitive impairment*
• Oral mucous membrane alteration *related to dehydration*
• Thought process alteration *related to physiologic causes*

Metabolic alkalosis
• Breathing pattern, ineffective *related to decreased energy or fatigue*
• Breathing pattern, ineffective *related to inability to maintain adequate rate and depth of respirations*
• Fluid volume deficit *related to active loss*
• Injury, risk for *related to sensory or motor deficits*
• Oral mucous membrane alteration *related to dehydration*
• Thought process alteration *related to physiologic causes*

Mitral insufficiency
• Activity intolerance *related to imbalance between oxygen supply and demand*
• Cardiac output, decreased *related to reduced stroke volume as a result of mechanical or structural problems*
• Fatigue
• Knowledge deficit *related to lack of exposure*
• Tissue perfusion alteration (cardiopulmonary) *related to decreased cellular exchange*

Mitral stenosis
• Activity intolerance *related to imbalance between oxygen supply and demand*
• Cardiac output, decreased *related to reduced stroke volume as a result of mechanical or structural problems*
• Fatigue
• Knowledge deficit *related to lack of exposure*

• Tissue perfusion alteration (cardiopulmonary) *related to decreased cellular exchange*

Mitral valve prolapse
• Breathing pattern, ineffective *related to decreased energy or fatigue*
• Cardiac output, decreased *related to reduced stroke volume as a result of mechanical or structural problems*
• Fatigue
• Tissue perfusion alteration (cardiopulmonary) *related to decreased cellular exchange*

Mood disorders
• Management of therapeutic regimen, ineffective community *related to drug and alcohol abuse among teenagers*
• Powerlessness *related to physical, sexual, or emotional abuse by partner*
• Social isolation *related to dysfunctional interpersonal relations*

Multiple births
• Anxiety *related to hospitalization and birth process*
• Coping, ineffective individual *related to labor and delivery*
• Incontinence, stress *related to weak pelvic musculature*
• Injury, risk for *related to labor*
• Knowledge deficit *related to lack of information about birth process*
• Parenting alteration *related to inadequate attachment to high-risk neonate*

Multiple myeloma
• Activity intolerance *related to imbalance between oxygen supply and demand*
• Fatigue
• Fluid volume excess *related to compromised regulatory mechanisms*
• Grieving, anticipatory *related to perceived potential loss of life*
• Infection, risk for *related to external factors*
• Nutrition alteration: Less than body requirements *related to inability to ingest foods*
• Pain *related to physical, biological, or chemical agents*
• Tissue perfusion alteration (cerebral) *related to decreased cellular exchange*

Multiple sclerosis
• Activity intolerance, risk for *related to immobility*
• Adjustment impairment *related to disability*
• Airway clearance, ineffective *related to decreased energy or fatigue*
• Caregiver role strain *related to discharge of a family member with significant home care needs*
• Caregiver role strain, risk for *related to developmental state*
• Coping, family: Potential for growth *related to self-actualization needs*
• Death anxiety *related to terminal illness*
• Fatigue
• Grieving, anticipatory *related to perceived potential loss of life*
• Health maintenance alteration *related to lack of familiarity with neighborhood resources*
• Health maintenance alteration *related to lack of motor skills*
• Incontinence, bowel *related to neuromuscular involvement*
• Incontinence, total *related to neurologic dysfunction*
• Incontinence, urinary urge, risk for
• Infection, risk for *related to external factors*
• Knowledge deficit *related to the Americans with Disabilities Act*
• Management of therapeutic regimen, ineffective: Individual *related to health beliefs*
• Memory impairment *related to neurologic disturbance*
• Mobility impairment, physical *related to neuromuscular impairment*
• Nutrition alteration: Less than body requirements *related to inability to digest or absorb nutrients because of biological factors*
• Pain *related to physical, biological, or chemical agents*
• Self-care deficit *related to musculoskeletal impairment*
• Self-esteem, chronic low
• Sensory or perceptual alteration
• Sexuality pattern alteration *related to illness or medical treatment*
• Spiritual distress, risk for
• Urinary elimination pattern alteration *related to sensory or neuromuscular impairment*
• Ventilation, spontaneous: Inability to sustain

Multisystem trauma

- Anxiety *related to situational crisis*
- Fluid volume deficit *related to active loss*
- Infection, risk for *related to external factors*
- Powerlessness *related to the health care environment*
- Self-care deficit *related to musculoskeletal impairment*
- Suffocation, risk for *related to internal factors*
- Tissue perfusion alteration *related to decreased cellular exchange*
- Trauma, risk for *related to internal factors*
- Ventilatory weaning response, dysfunctional *related to diminished ventilator support*

Muscular dystrophy

- Adjustment impairment *related to disability*
- Caregiver role strain *related to discharge of a family member with significant home care needs*
- Caregiver role strain, risk for
- Coping, family: Potential for growth *related to self-actualization needs*
- Health maintenance alteration *related to lack of motor skills*
- Hopelessness *related to failing or deteriorating physiologic condition*
- Incontinence, urinary urge, risk for
- Knowledge deficit *related to the Americans with Disabilities Act*
- Mobility impairment, physical *related to neuromuscular impairment*
- Self-care deficit *related to musculoskeletal impairment*
- Sensory or perceptual alteration (kinesthetic)

Myasthenia gravis

- Airway clearance, ineffective *related to presence of tracheobronchial obstruction or secretions*
- Fatigue
- Gas exchange impairment *related to altered oxygen-carrying capacity of the blood*
- Incontinence, bowel *related to neuromuscular involvement*
- Incontinence, urinary urge, risk for
- Mobility impairment, physical *related to neuromuscular impairment*
- Self-care deficit *related to musculoskeletal impairment*
- Self-esteem, chronic low

- Ventilatory weaning response, dysfunctional *related to diminished ventilator support*
- Verbal communication impairment *related to physical barriers*

Myocardial infarction

- Activity intolerance *related to imbalance between oxygen supply and demand*
- Adjustment impairment *related to disability*
- Anxiety *related to situational crisis*
- Cardiac output, decreased *related to reduced myocardial perfusion*
- Cardiac output, decreased *related to reduced stroke volume as a result of electrophysiologic problems*
- Cardiac output, decreased *related to reduced stroke volume as a result of mechanical or structural problems*
- Coping, ineffective family: Compromised *related to inadequate or incorrect information held by primary caregiver*
- Coping, ineffective individual *related to situational crisis*
- Death anxiety *related to terminal illness*
- Denial *related to fear or anxiety*
- Pain *related to physical, biological, or chemical agents*
- Role performance alteration *related to ineffective coping*
- Self-esteem, situational low *related to hospitalization and forced dependence on health care team*
- Sexual dysfunction *related to altered body structure or function*
- Sexuality pattern alteration *related to illness or medical treatment*
- Sleep pattern disturbance *related to internal factors*
- Spiritual distress *related to situational crisis*
- Spiritual distress, risk for
- Tissue perfusion alteration *related to decreased cellular exchange*

Narcissistic personality disorder

- Coping, ineffective individual *related to personal vulnerability*
- Fear *related to unfamiliarity*
- Personal identity disturbance *related to lowered self-esteem*

Neonatal asphyxia

- Aspiration, risk for *related to neonate's immature cough or gag reflex*

• Breathing pattern, ineffective *related to adjustment to extrauterine existence*
• Coping, ineffective family: Compromised *related to neonatal health problems*
• Growth and development alteration *related to perinatal insult or injury*
• Hypothermia *related to cold, stress, or sepsis*
• Injury, risk for *related to internal and external neonatal risk factors*

Neonatal hyperbilirubinemia
• Breast-feeding, interrupted *related to a contraindicating condition*

Neurologic impairment (neonatal)
• Coping, ineffective family: Compromised *related to neonatal health problems*
• Infant feeding pattern, ineffective *related to neurologic impairment or developmental delay*

Neuromuscular trauma
• Aspiration, risk for *related to absence of protective mechanisms*
• Constipation, risk of
• Disuse syndrome, risk for
• Disuse syndrome, risk for *related to prolonged inactivity*
• Incontinence, total *related to neurologic dysfunction*
• Posttrauma syndrome *related to accidental injury*
• Skin integrity impairment *related to external (environmental) factors*

Nutritional deficiencies
• Infection, risk for *related to external factors*
• Nutrition alteration: Less than body requirements *related to inability to ingest foods*
• Parenting alteration, risk for *related to lack of knowledge or ineffective role model*
• Skin integrity impairment *related to internal (somatic) factors*
• Thought process alteration *related to physiologic causes*

Obesity
• Constipation, risk of
• Incontinence, stress
• Incontinence, stress *related to weak pelvic musculature*
• Nutrition alteration: More than body requirements *related to excessive intake*

• Self-esteem, situational low *related to hospitalization and forced dependence on health care team*
• Skin integrity impairment, risk for *related to the aging process and impaired mobility*

Obsessive-compulsive disorder
• Anxiety *related to obsessive-compulsive behavior*
• Coping, ineffective individual *related to personal vulnerability*
• Decisional conflict *related to sexual activity*
• Denial *related to fear or anxiety*
• Home maintenance management impairment *related to impaired cognitive or emotional functioning*
• Personal identity disturbance *related to lowered self-esteem*
• Sleep pattern disturbance *related to internal factors*
• Social isolation *related to inadequate personal resources*

Organic brain syndrome
• Adult failure to thrive *related to illness, disability, or environmental deprivation*
• Fluid volume deficit, risk for *related to excessive loss*

Osteoarthritis
• Activity intolerance *related to functional changes accompanying the aging process*
• Activity intolerance *related to immobility*
• Body image disturbance
• Body image disturbance *related to negative self-image*
• Coping, ineffective family: Compromised *related to caring for dependent, aging family member*
• Health maintenance alteration *related to lack of familiarity with neighborhood resources*
• Home maintenance management impairment *related to impaired cognitive, emotional, or psychomotor functioning*
• Injury, risk for *related to elder abuse*
• Knowledge deficit *related to lack of exposure*
• Mobility impairment, physical *related to pain or discomfort*
• Nutrition alteration: More than body requirements *related to a decline in basal metabolic rate and physical activity*
• Pain *related to physical, biological, or chemical agents*

• Self-care deficit *related to musculoskeletal impairment*

Osteomyelitis
• Body image disturbance
• Coping, ineffective individual *related to situational crisis*
• Infection, risk for *related to home infusion therapy*
• Injury, risk for *related to lack of awareness of environmental hazards*
• Mobility impairment, physical *related to pain or discomfort*
• Pain *related to physical, biological, or chemical agents*
• Skin integrity impairment *related to external (environmental) factors*
• Tissue perfusion alteration *related to hypovolemia*

Osteoporosis
• Body image disturbance
• Body image disturbance *related to negative self-image*
• Denial *related to fear or anxiety about aging*
• Injury, risk for *related to lack of awareness of environmental hazards*
• Powerlessness *related to illness-related regimen*
• Sexuality pattern alteration *related to illness or medical treatment*
• Social isolation *related to altered state of wellness*
• Sexuality pattern alteration (female patient) *related to illness, medical treatment, or age-related changes*
• Trauma, risk for *related to external factors (environmental, physical, chemical agents)*

Ovarian cancer
• Constipation *related to GI obstruction*
• Fear *related to unfamiliarity*
• Grieving, anticipatory *related to perceived potential loss of significant object (such as person, job, possessions)*
• Nutrition alteration: Less than body requirements *related to inability to ingest foods*
• Spiritual distress *related to situational crisis*
• Tissue integrity impairment *related to radiation*
• Urinary elimination alteration *related to obstruction*

Panic disorder
• Anxiety *related to situational crisis*
• Coping, ineffective individual *related to personal vulnerability*
• Fear *related to unfamiliarity*
• Knowledge deficit *related to lack of exposure*
• Posttrauma syndrome, risk for
• Powerlessness *related to chronic illness*
• Self-esteem, chronic low
• Sleep pattern disturbance *related to external factors, such as environmental changes*

Paralysis
• Adjustment impairment *related to disability*
• Caregiver role strain *related to discharge of a family member with significant home care needs*
• Caregiver role strain, risk for *related to developmental state*
• Coping, ineffective family: Compromised *related to inadequate or incorrect information held by primary caregiver*
• Coping, ineffective individual *related to inability to solve problems or adapt to demands of daily living*
• Grieving, dysfunctional *related to actual object loss*
• Health maintenance alteration *related to lack of motor skills*
• Hopelessness *related to chronic illness*
• Incontinence, bowel *related to neuromuscular involvement*
• Incontinence, reflex *related to sensory or neuromuscular impairment*
• Mobility impairment, physical *related to neuromuscular impairment*
• Powerlessness *related to health care environment*
• Powerlessness *related to illness-related regimen*
• Role performance alteration *related to ineffective coping*
• Sexuality pattern alteration *related to illness or medical treatment*
• Skin integrity impairment *related to external (environmental) factors*
• Skin integrity impairment, risk for

Parkinson's disease
• Activity intolerance *related to functional changes accompanying the aging process*
• Activity intolerance *related to immobility*
• Aspiration, risk for *related to absence of protective mechanisms*
• Body image disturbance

- Breathing pattern, ineffective *related to decreased energy or fatigue*
- Caregiver role strain, risk for *related to developmental state*
- Coping, ineffective family: Compromised *related to caring for dependent, aging family member*
- Coping, ineffective family: Compromised *related to prolonged disease*
- Coping, ineffective individual *related to inability to solve problems or adapt to demands of daily living*
- Coping, ineffective individual *related to situational crisis*
- Death anxiety *related to terminal illness*
- Health maintenance alteration *related to lack of familiarity with neighborhood resources*
- Home maintenance management impairment *related to impaired cognitive, emotional, or psychomotor functioning*
- Hopelessness *related to chronic illness*
- Incontinence, bowel *related to neuromuscular involvement*
- Incontinence, urinary urge, risk for
- Injury, risk for *related to external factors*
- Knowledge deficit *related to lack of exposure*
- Loneliness, risk for
- Management of therapeutic regimen, ineffective: Individual *related to health beliefs*
- Mobility impairment, physical *related to neuromuscular impairment*
- Nutrition alteration: Less than body requirements *related to inability to ingest foods*
- Powerlessness *related to chronic illness*
- Role performance alteration
- Self-care deficit *related to musculoskeletal impairment*
- Self-esteem, chronic low
- Sensory or perceptual alteration (tactile)
- Sexuality pattern alteration *related to illness or medical treatment*
- Social isolation *related to altered state of wellness*
- Social isolation *related to physiologic, environmental, or emotional barriers*

Passive-aggressive personality disorder
- Anxiety *related to situational crisis*
- Coping, ineffective individual *related to personal vulnerability*
- Personal identity disturbance *related to lowered self-esteem*

Pelvic inflammatory disease
- Fluid volume deficit *related to active loss*
- Pain *related to physical, biological, or chemical agents*
- Sexual dysfunction *related to altered body structure or function*

Pericarditis
- Anxiety *related to situational crisis*
- Cardiac output, decreased *related to reduced stroke volume as a result of mechanical or structural problems*
- Pain *related to physical, biological, or chemical agents*
- Tissue perfusion alteration (cardiopulmonary) *related to decreased cellular exchange*

Perinatal trauma
- Growth and development alteration *related to perinatal insult or injury*
- Hypothermia *related to cold, stress, or sepsis*
- Injury, risk for *related to internal and external neonatal risk factors*

Peripheral vascular disease
- Activity intolerance *related to imbalance between oxygen supply and demand*
- Diversional activity deficit *related to long-term hospitalization or frequent, lengthy treatments*
- Infection, risk for *related to external factors*
- Mobility impairment, physical *related to pain or discomfort*
- Pain *related to physical, biological, or chemical agents*
- Peripheral neurovascular dysfunction, risk for
- Skin integrity impairment *related to internal (somatic) factors*
- Skin integrity impairment, risk for
- Skin integrity impairment, risk for *related to the aging process and impaired mobility*
- Tissue integrity impairment *related to peripheral vascular changes*

Peritoneal dialysis
- Body image disturbance
- Family process alteration *related to situational crisis*
- Fluid volume deficit *related to active loss*
- Fluid volume excess *related to excess fluid intake or retention or excess sodium intake or retention*
- Infection, risk for *related to external factors*

• Knowledge deficit *related to lack of exposure*
• Nutrition alteration: Less than body requirements *related to inability to digest or absorb nutrients because of biological factors*

Peritonitis
• Anxiety *related to situational crisis*
• Cardiac output, decreased *related to reduced stroke volume as a result of mechanical or structural problems*
• Fluid volume deficit *related to active loss*
• Infection, risk for *related to labor and delivery*
• Nausea *related to irritation to the GI system*
• Pain *related to physical, biological, or chemical agents*

Personality disorders
• Altered family processes *related to dysfunctional behavior*
• Decisional conflict *related to sexual activity*
• Loneliness, risk for
• Sexual dysfunction *related to hypersexuality*
• Social isolation *related to dysfunctional interpersonal relations*
• Violence, risk for: Self-directed *related to suicide attempt*

Phobic disorder
• Anxiety *related to environmental conflict (phobia)*
• Coping, ineffective individual *related to personal vulnerability*
• Fear *related to unfamiliarity*
• Personal identity disturbance *related to lowered self-esteem*
• Social isolation *related to inadequate personal resources*

Placenta previa
• Anxiety *related to situational crisis*
• Denial *related to fear or anxiety*
• Fear *related to unfamiliarity*

Pleural effusion
• Breathing pattern, ineffective *related to pain*
• Hyperthermia *related to dehydration*
• Infection, risk for *related to external factors*

• Ventilatory weaning response, dysfunctional *related to diminished ventilator support*

Pleurisy
• Breathing pattern, ineffective *related to pain*
• Fatigue
• Gas exchange impairment *related to altered oxygen supply*
• Pain *related to physical, biological, or chemical agents*
• Pain *related to physiologic changes of pregnancy*

Pneumonia
• Airway clearance, ineffective *related to decreased energy or fatigue*
• Airway clearance, ineffective *related to presence of tracheobronchial obstruction or secretions*
• Aspiration, risk for *related to absence of protective mechanisms*
• Breathing pattern, ineffective *related to decreased energy or fatigue*
• Fluid volume deficit *related to active loss*
• Gas exchange impairment *related to altered oxygen supply*
• Infection, risk for *related to altered primary defenses during the postpartum period*
• Mobility impairment, physical *related to pain or discomfort*
• Nutrition alteration: Less than body requirements *related to inability to ingest foods*
• Self-care deficit *related to musculoskeletal impairment*
• Tissue perfusion alteration (cardiopulmonary) *related to decreased cellular exchange*
• Ventilation, spontaneous: Inability to sustain
• Verbal communication impairment *related to physical barriers*

Pneumothorax
• Breathing pattern, ineffective *related to pain*
• Fear *related to unfamiliarity*
• Gas exchange impairment *related to altered oxygen supply*
• Pain *related to physical, biological, or chemical agents*
• Tissue perfusion alteration (cardiopulmonary) *related to decreased cellular exchange*

- Ventilation, spontaneous: Inability to sustain

Poisoning
- Aspiration, risk for *related to absence of protective mechanisms*
- Aspiration, risk for *related to ineffective swallow reflex*
- Growth and development alteration *related to environmental and stimulation deficiencies*
- Injury, risk for *related to lack of awareness of environmental hazards*
- Poisoning, risk for *related to drug toxicity or polypharmacy*
- Sensory or perceptual alteration (olfactory)
- Sensory or perceptual alteration (tactile)
- Tissue perfusion alteration (renal) *related to decreased cellular exchange*

Polycystic kidney disease
- Family process alteration *related to situational crisis*
- Infection, risk for *related to external factors*
- Knowledge deficit *related to lack of motivation*
- Pain *related to physical, biological, or chemical agents*
- Tissue perfusion alteration (renal) *related to decreased cellular exchange*

Polycythemia vera
- Gas exchange impairment *related to altered oxygen-carrying capacity of the blood*
- Pain *related to physical, biological, or chemical agents*
- Sensory or perceptual alteration (visual) *related to altered sensory reception, transmission, or integration*
- Skin integrity impairment *related to internal (somatic) factors*

Postpartum hemorrhage
- Anxiety *related to situational crisis*
- Fluid volume deficit *related to postpartum hemorrhage*
- Tissue perfusion alteration (cardiopulmonary) *related to decreased cellular exchange*
- Tissue perfusion alteration (cerebral) *related to decreased cellular exchange*

Posttraumatic stress disorder
- Hopelessness *related to child's mood disturbance*
- Loneliness, risk for

- Posttrauma syndrome *related to accidental injury*
- Posttrauma syndrome *related to assault*
- Posttrauma syndrome *related to incest*
- Posttrauma syndrome, risk for
- Powerlessness *related to physical, sexual, or emotional abuse by partner*
- Self-esteem disturbance *related to problematic relationship with parents*
- Sensory or perceptual alteration *related to sensory overload*
- Thought process alteration *related to psychological causes*

Pregnancy
- Anxiety *related to hospitalization and birth process*
- Constipation, risk of
- Coping, ineffective individual *related to labor and delivery*
- Family process alteration *related to impending birth*
- Knowledge deficit *related to lack of information about birth process*
- Knowledge deficit *related to postpartum self-care*
- Knowledge deficit *related to self-care activities during pregnancy*
- Tissue integrity impairment *related to peripheral vascular changes*
- Tissue perfusion alteration (peripheral) *related to reduced venous blood flow*

Pregnancy-induced hypertension
- Activity intolerance *related to imbalance between oxygen supply and demand*
- Fear *related to unfamiliarity*
- Fluid volume deficit *related to altered intake during labor*
- Fluid volume excess *related to compromised regulatory mechanisms*
- Knowledge deficit *related to lack of exposure*
- Pain *related to physiologic changes of pregnancy*
- Pain *related to physiologic response to labor*
- Sensory or perceptual alteration (visual) *related to altered sensory reception, transmission, or integration*
- Tissue perfusion alteration (cerebral) *related to decreased cellular exchange*
- Urinary elimination alteration *related to sensory impairment during labor*

Premature labor

- Anxiety *related to hospitalization and birth process*
- Breast-feeding, effective
- Coping, ineffective individual *related to situational crisis*
- Infection, risk for *related to home infusion therapy*
- Infection, risk for *related to labor and delivery*
- Knowledge deficit *related to lack of information about birth process*
- Knowledge deficit *related to premature labor*
- Parenting alteration *related to inadequate attachment to high-risk neonate*
- Self-esteem disturbance *related to behavior during labor and delivery*

Premature rupture of membranes

- Fluid volume deficit *related to altered intake during labor*
- Fluid volume deficit *related to postpartum hemorrhage*
- Infection, risk for *related to altered primary defenses during the postpartum period*

Prematurity

- Aspiration, risk for *related to neonate's immature cough or gag reflex*
- Breast-feeding, ineffective *related to dissatisfaction with breast-feeding process*
- Breast-feeding, interrupted *related to a contraindicating condition*
- Breast-feeding, ineffective *related to limited maternal experience*
- Breathing pattern, ineffective *related to adjustment to extrauterine existence*
- Breathing pattern, ineffective, *related to inability to maintain adequate rate and depth of respirations*
- Coping, ineffective family: Compromised *related to neonatal health problems*
- Development, altered, risk for
- Growth and development alteration *related to perinatal insult or injury*
- Hypothermia *related to cold, stress, or sepsis*
- Infant behavior, disorganized *related to pain, prematurity, oral problems, motor problems, feeding intolerance, environmental overstimulation, or lack of stimulation*
- Infant behavior, risk for disorganization *related to pain, prematurity, oral problems, motor problems, feeding intolerance, envi-ronmental overstimulation, or lack of stimulation*
- Infant feeding pattern, ineffective *related to neurologic impairment or developmental delay*
- Nutrition alteration: Less than body requirements *related to ineffective suck reflex*
- Parental role conflict *related to child's hospitalization*
- Parent-infant attachment, altered, risk for
- Thermoregulation, ineffective *related to immaturity*
- Verbal communication impairment *related to developmental factors*

Pressure ulcers

- Altered protection *related to myelosuppression and immunosuppression*
- Fluid volume deficit, risk for *related to excessive loss*
- Infection, risk for *related to external factors*
- Mobility impairment, physical *related to pain or discomfort*
- Nutrition alteration: Less than body requirements *related to inability to digest or absorb nutrients because of biological factors*
- Skin integrity impairment *related to external (environmental) factors*
- Tissue integrity impairment *related to peripheral vascular changes*

Prolapsed intervertebral disk

- Incontinence, reflex *related to sensory or neuromuscular involvement*
- Mobility impairment, physical *related to neuromuscular impairment*
- Pain *related to physical, biological, or chemical agents*
- Urinary elimination alteration *related to sensory or neuromuscular impairment*

Prostate cancer

- Pain *related to physical, biological, or chemical agents*
- Sexual dysfunction *related to impotence*
- Sorrow *related to change in physical status*
- Tissue integrity impairment *related to radiation*
- Urinary elimination alteration *related to obstruction*

Prostatectomy

- Body image disturbance
- Infection, risk for *related to external factors*

- Skin integrity impairment *related to internal (somatic) factors*
- Urinary elimination alteration *related to obstruction*

Pseudomembranous colitis
- Diarrhea *related to malabsorption, inflammation, or irritation of bowel*
- Fluid volume deficit *related to active loss*
- Skin integrity impairment *related to external (environmental) factors*
- Tissue perfusion alteration (cardiopulmonary) *related to decreased cellular exchange*
- Tissue perfusion alteration (GI) *related to decreased cellular exchange*
- Tissue perfusion alteration (renal) *related to decreased cellular exchange*

Psoriasis
- Body image disturbance
- Body image disturbance *related to negative self-image*
- Body temperature alteration, risk for *related to dehydration*
- Powerlessness *related to chronic illness*
- Skin integrity impairment *related to internal (somatic) factors*
- Social isolation *related to altered state of wellness*

Pulmonary edema
- Activity intolerance *related to imbalance between oxygen supply and demand*
- Airway clearance, ineffective *related to presence of tracheobronchial obstruction or secretions*
- Breathing pattern, ineffective *related to decreased energy or fatigue*
- Cardiac output, decreased *related to reduced stroke volume as a result of mechanical or structural problems*
- Fear *related to unfamiliarity*
- Fluid volume excess *related to compromised regulatory mechanisms*
- Gas exchange impairment *related to altered oxygen supply*
- Self-care deficit *related to musculoskeletal impairment*
- Tissue perfusion alteration (cardiopulmonary) *related to decreased cellular exchange*
- Ventilatory weaning response, dysfunctional *related to diminished ventilator support*

- Verbal communication impairment *related to physical barriers*

Pulmonary embolus
- Activity intolerance *related to imbalance between oxygen supply and demand*
- Breathing pattern, ineffective *related to pain*
- Cardiac output, decreased *related to reduced stroke volume as a result of mechanical or structural problems*
- Fluid volume deficit *related to active loss*
- Gas exchange impairment *related to altered oxygen supply*
- Pain *related to physical, biological, or chemical agents*
- Pain *related to physiologic changes of pregnancy*
- Tissue perfusion alteration (cardiopulmonary) *related to decreased cellular exchange*
- Tissue perfusion alteration (venous) *related to reduced peripheral blood flow*
- Verbal communication impairment *related to physical barriers*

Pulmonary fibrosis
- Breathing pattern, ineffective *related to decreased energy or fatigue*
- Gas exchange impairment *related to altered oxygen supply*

Pyelonephritis
- Fluid volume excess *related to compromised regulatory mechanisms*
- Infection, risk for *related to external factors*
- Infection, risk for *related to labor and delivery*
- Mobility impairment, physical *related to pain or discomfort*
- Pain *related to physical, biological, or chemical agents*

Pyloric stenosis
- Aspiration, risk for *related to neonate's immature cough or gag reflex*
- Body temperature alteration, risk for *related to dehydration*
- Nutrition alteration: Less than body requirements *related to inability to absorb nutrients or insufficient intake*

Radiation therapy
- Diarrhea *related to malabsorption, inflammation, or irritation of bowel*
- Fluid volume deficit *related to active loss*

• Mobility impairment, physical *related to pain or discomfort*
• Nausea *related to irritation to the GI system*
• Nutrition alteration: Less than body requirements *related to inability to ingest foods*
• Oral mucous membrane alteration *related to pathologic condition*
• Pain *related to physical, biological, or chemical agents*
• Sexual dysfunction *related to altered body structure or function*
• Tissue integrity impairment *related to radiation*

Rape
• Posttrauma syndrome *related to assault*
• Rape-trauma syndrome
• Rape-trauma syndrome: Compound reaction
• Rape-trauma syndrome: Silent reaction
• Self-esteem disturbance
• Social isolation *related to behavior that fails to conform to social norms*

Raynaud's disease
• Sensory or perceptual alteration (tactile)
• Skin integrity impairment, risk for
• Skin integrity impairment, risk for *related to the aging process and impaired mobility*
• Tissue integrity impairment *related to peripheral vascular changes*
• Tissue perfusion alteration (peripheral) *related to reduced arterial blood flow*

Renal calculi
• Denial *related to fear or anxiety*
• Denial *related to fear or anxiety about aging*
• Infection, risk for *related to external factors*
• Pain *related to physical, biological, or chemical agents*
• Urinary elimination alteration *related to obstruction*

Renal cancer
• Fluid volume deficit *related to active loss*
• Pain *related to physical, biological, or chemical agents*

Renal disease: End-stage
• Caregiver role strain *related to discharge of a family member with significant home care needs*

• Caregiver role strain, risk for *related to developmental state*
• Coping, defensive *related to perceived threat to positive self-regard*
• Coping, ineffective individual *related to inability to solve problems or adapt to demands of daily living*
• Coping, ineffective individual *related to situational crisis*
• Decisional conflict *related to health care options*
• Denial *related to fear or anxiety*
• Disuse syndrome, risk for
• Fluid volume excess *related to excess fluid intake or retention or excess sodium intake or retention*
• Grieving, anticipatory *related to perceived potential loss of life*
• Hopelessness *related to failing or deteriorating physiologic condition*
• Infection, risk for *related to home infusion therapy*
• Poisoning, risk for *related to drug toxicity or polypharmacy*
• Role performance alteration
• Self-esteem, chronic low
• Sexuality pattern alteration *related to illness or medical treatment*
• Spiritual distress *related to situational crisis*
• Spiritual distress, risk for

Reye's syndrome
• Growth and development alteration *related to physical disability or environmental deprivation*
• Intracranial adaptive capacity, decreased
• Mobility impairment, physical *related to neuromuscular impairment*
• Thermoregulation, ineffective *related to trauma or illness*

Rheumatic fever
• Anxiety *related to situational crisis*
• Breathing pattern, ineffective *related to inability to maintain adequate rate and depth of respirations*
• Cardiac output, decreased *related to reduced stroke volume as a result of mechanical or structural problems*
• Fatigue
• Gas exchange impairment *related to altered oxygen supply*
• Hyperthermia *related to infection*
• Infection, risk for *related to external factors*

- Knowledge deficit *related to lack of exposure*
- Mobility impairment, physical *related to pain or discomfort*
- Pain *related to physical, biological, or chemical agents*

Rheumatoid arthritis
- Activity intolerance *related to immobility*
- Altered protection *related to myelosuppression and immunosuppression*
- Body image disturbance
- Coping, ineffective individual *related to inability to solve problems or adapt to demands of daily living*
- Denial *related to fear or anxiety*
- Denial *related to fear or anxiety about aging*
- Disuse syndrome, risk for
- Health maintenance alteration *related to lack of familiarity with neighborhood resources*
- Injury, risk for *related to elder abuse*
- Knowledge deficit *related to the Americans with Disabilities Act*
- Knowledge deficit *related to lack of exposure*
- Management of therapeutic regimen, ineffective: Individual *related to health beliefs*
- Mobility impairment, physical *related to pain or discomfort*
- Pain *related to physical, biological, or chemical agents*
- Self-care deficit *related to musculoskeletal impairment*
- Sexual dysfunction *related to altered body structure or function*
- Sleep pattern disturbance *related to internal factors*

Salmonella
- Constipation *related to GI obstruction*
- Diarrhea *related to malabsorption, inflammation, or irritation of bowel*
- Diarrhea *related to primary bowel pathology*
- Fluid volume deficit, risk for *related to excessive loss*
- Hyperthermia *related to infection*
- Infection, risk for *related to external factors*
- Urinary elimination alteration *related to sensory or neuromuscular impairment*

Sarcoidosis
- Activity intolerance *related to imbalance between oxygen supply and demand*

- Body image disturbance
- Breathing pattern, ineffective *related to decreased energy or fatigue*
- Cardiac output, decreased *related to reduced stroke volume as a result of electrophysiologic problems*
- Gas exchange impairment *related to altered oxygen-carrying capacity of the blood*
- Pain *related to physical, biological, or chemical agents*

Scarlet fever
- Hyperthermia *related to infection*
- Infection, risk for *related to external factors*
- Oral mucous membrane impairment *related to pathologic condition*
- Pain *related to physical, biological, or chemical agents*

Schizophrenia
- Altered family processes *related to dysfunctional behavior*
- Anxiety *related to environmental conflict (phobia)*
- Anxiety *related to obsessive-compulsive behavior*
- Caregiver role strain *related to discharge of a family member with significant home care needs*
- Caregiver role strain, risk for *related to developmental state*
- Coping, ineffective individual *related to personal vulnerability*
- Health maintenance alteration *related to perceptual or cognitive impairment*
- Home maintenance management impairment *related to impaired cognitive or emotional functioning*
- Hopelessness *related to chronic illness*
- Injury, risk for *related to elder abuse*
- Incontinence, functional *related to cognitive deficits*
- Poisoning, risk for *related to internal factors (biological, psychological, developmental)*
- Role performance alteration *related to ineffective coping*
- Self-care deficit *related to perceptual or cognitive impairment*
- Sensory or perceptual alteration *related to hallucinations*
- Sleep pattern disturbance *related to internal factors*
- Sexual dysfunction *related to hypersexuality*

- Social interaction impairment *related to altered thought processes*
- Social isolation *related to dysfunctional interpersonal relations*
- Thought process alteration *related to psychological causes*
- Violence, risk for: Self-directed *related to suicide attempt*

Seizure disorders
- Airway clearance, ineffective *related to presence of tracheobronchial obstruction or secretions*
- Anxiety *related to situational crisis*
- Breathing pattern, ineffective *related to decreased energy or fatigue*
- Coping, ineffective individual *related to situational crisis*
- Development, altered, risk for
- Environmental interpretation syndrome, impaired
- Growth and development alteration *related to physical disability or environmental deprivation*
- Memory impairment *related to neurologic disturbance*
- Self-esteem, chronic low
- Sensory or perceptual alteration (tactile)
- Social isolation *related to altered state of wellness*
- Spiritual distress, risk for
- Trauma, risk for *related to feelings of personal invulnerability*
- Trauma, risk for *related to internal factors*

Self-destructive behavior
- Anxiety *related to obsessive-compulsive behavior*
- Anxiety *related to situational crisis*
- Denial *related to fear or anxiety*
- Poisoning, risk for *related to external factors*
- Poisoning, risk for *related to internal factors (biological, psychological, developmental)*
- Self-esteem, chronic low
- Self-mutilation, risk for *related to emotional illness*
- Violence, risk for: Self-directed *related to suicide attempt*

Sepsis
- Confusion, acute
- Diarrhea *related to malabsorption, inflammation, or irritation of bowel*

- Growth and development alteration *related to perinatal insult or injury*
- Hyperthermia *related to infection*
- Hypothermia *related to cold, stress, or sepsis*
- Nutrition alteration: Less than body requirements *related to inability to digest or absorb nutrients because of biological factors*
- Pain *related to postpartum physiologic changes*
- Thermoregulation, ineffective *related to trauma or illness*
- Ventilation, spontaneous: Inability to sustain
- Ventilatory weaning response, dysfunctional *related to diminished ventilator support*

Sexual assault
- Posttrauma syndrome *related to assault*
- Posttrauma syndrome *related to incest*
- Rape-trauma syndrome
- Rape-trauma syndrome: Compound reaction
- Rape-trauma syndrome: Silent reaction
- Violence, risk for: Self-directed *related to suicide attempt*

Shaken baby syndrome
- Parenting alteration *related to lack of knowledge*
- Parenting alteration, risk for *related to lack of knowledge or ineffective role model*

Shock
- Airway clearance, ineffective *related to presence of tracheobronchial obstruction or secretions*
- Cardiac output, decreased *related to reduced stroke volume as a result of mechanical or structural problems*
- Fluid volume deficit *related to active loss*
- Fluid volume deficit *related to altered intake during labor*
- Gas exchange impairment *related to altered oxygen-carrying capacity of the blood*
- Infection, risk for *related to external factors*
- Oral mucous membrane alteration *related to dehydration*
- Tissue perfusion alteration (cardiopulmonary) *related to decreased cellular exchange*
- Tissue perfusion alteration (cerebral) *related to decreased cellular exchange*

• Tissue perfusion alteration (renal) *related to decreased cellular exchange*
• Ventilation, spontaneous: Inability to sustain

Sickle cell anemia
• Altered protection *related to myelosuppression and immunosuppression*
• Gas exchange impairment *related to altered oxygen-carrying capacity of the blood*
• Mobility impairment, physical *related to pain or discomfort*
• Pain *related to physical, biological, or chemical agents*
• Tissue perfusion alteration (peripheral) *related to reduced venous blood flow*
• Tissue perfusion alteration (renal) *related to decreased cellular exchange*

Sjögren's syndrome
• Oral mucous membrane alteration *related to pathologic condition*
• Pain *related to physical, biological, or chemical agents*
• Sensory or perceptual alteration (gustatory)

Somatic disorder
• Caregiver role strain *related to unpredictability of the care situation*

Spina bifida
• Latex allergy response
• Latex allergy response, risk for

Spinal cord defects
• Adjustment impairment *related to disability*
• Coping, family: Potential for growth *related to self-actualization needs*
• Growth and development alteration *related to physical disability or environmental deprivation*
• Incontinence, total *related to neuropathy, trauma, or disease affecting spinal nerves*
• Self-esteem, chronic low
• Urinary elimination alteration *related to sensory or neuromuscular impairment*

Spinal cord injury
• Activity intolerance *related to immobility*
• Adjustment impairment *related to disability*
• Airway clearance, ineffective *related to presence of tracheobronchial obstruction or secretions*

• Body image disturbance
• Constipation *related to GI obstruction*
• Constipation, risk of
• Development, altered, risk for
• Disuse syndrome, risk for
• Diversional activity deficit *related to long-term hospitalization or frequent, lengthy treatments*
• Dysreflexia *related to spinal cord trauma*
• Dysreflexia, risk for autonomic
• Fear *related to unfamiliarity*
• Grieving, dysfunctional *related to actual object loss*
• Growth and development alteration *related to effects of physical disability*
• Health maintenance alteration *related to lack of motor skills*
• Hopelessness *related to chronic illness*
• Incontinence, bowel *related to neuromuscular involvement*
• Incontinence, reflex *related to sensory or neuromuscular impairment*
• Incontinence, total *related to neurologic dysfunction*
• Incontinence, urinary urge, risk for
• Infection, risk for *related to external factors*
• Knowledge deficit *related to the Americans with Disabilities Act*
• Management of therapeutic regimen, ineffective: Individual *related to health beliefs*
• Mobility impairment, physical *related to neuromuscular impairment*
• Pain, chronic *related to physical disability*
• Posttrauma syndrome *related to accidental injury*
• Powerlessness *related to chronic illness*
• Self-care deficit *related to musculoskeletal impairment*
• Sensory or perceptual alteration
• Sexuality pattern alteration *related to illness or medical treatment*
• Skin integrity impairment, risk for
• Sleep deprivation
• Social isolation *related to altered state of wellness*
• Sorrow, chronic *related to change in physical, social, or psychological status*
• Transfer ability, impaired *related to neuromuscular dysfunction*
• Trauma, risk for *related to feelings of personal invulnerability*
• Trauma, risk for *related to internal factors*
• Urinary elimination alteration *related to sensory or neuromuscular impairment*
• Urinary retention *related to obstruction, sensory or neuromuscular impairment*

• Ventilation, spontaneous: Inability to sustain *related to home ventilation therapy*

Spinal tumor
• Breathing pattern, ineffective *related to decreased energy or fatigue*
• Dysreflexia *related to spinal cord trauma*
• Dysreflexia, risk for autonomic
• Incontinence, bowel *related to neuromuscular involvement*
• Incontinence, reflex *related to sensory or neuromuscular impairment*
• Incontinence, total *related to neurologic dysfunction*
• Incontinence, urinary urge, risk for
• Injury, risk for *related to external factors*
• Mobility impairment, physical *related to neuromuscular impairment*
• Self-care deficit *related to musculoskeletal impairment*
• Self-esteem, chronic low
• Self-esteem, situational low
• Sensory or perceptual alteration (kinesthetic)
• Sexual dysfunction *related to altered body structure or function*
• Skin integrity impairment, risk for
• Urinary elimination alteration *related to sensory or neuromuscular involvement*

Spouse abuse
• Posttrauma syndrome *related to assault*
• Rape-trauma syndrome
• Rape-trauma syndrome: Compound reaction
• Rape-trauma syndrome: Silent reaction
• Violence, risk for: Directed at others *related to excitement or antisocial behavior*

Streptococcal throat
• Hyperthermia *related to infection*
• Infection, risk for *related to external factors*
• Oral mucous membrane alteration *related to pathologic condition*

Substance abuse
• Altered family processes *related to dysfunctional behavior*
• Management of therapeutic regimen, ineffective: Community *related to drug and alcohol abuse among teenagers*
• Nutrition alteration: Less than body requirements *related to lack of resources or knowledge*
• Violence, risk for: Directed at others *related to excitement or antisocial behavior*

Suicidal behavior
• Anxiety *related to obsessive-compulsive behavior*
• Anxiety *related to situational crisis*
• Denial *related to fear or anxiety*
• Poisoning, risk for *related to external factors*
• Poisoning, risk for *related to internal factors (biological, psychological, developmental)*
• Self-esteem, chronic low
• Self-mutilation, risk for *related to emotional illness*
• Spiritual well-being, potential for enhanced *related to parish nursing*
• Violence, risk for: Self-directed *related to recurrent losses or changes in physical or mental condition*
• Violence, risk for: Self-directed *related to suicide attempt*

Syphilis
• Coping, ineffective community *related to increased levels of teen pregnancy*
• Infection, risk for *related to external factors*
• Infection, risk for *related to neonate's immature immune system*
• Injury, risk for *related to lack of awareness of environmental hazards*
• Knowledge deficit *related to lack of exposure*
• Sexuality pattern alteration *related to illness or medical treatment*

Tendinitis
• Activity intolerance *related to immobility*
• Mobility impairment, physical *related to pain or discomfort*
• Role performance alteration *related to ineffective coping*

Testicular cancer
• Body image disturbance
• Fear *related to unfamiliarity*
• Pain *related to physical, biological, or chemical agents*
• Sexual dysfunction *related to altered body structure or function*

Thoracic surgery
• Airway clearance, ineffective *related to presence of tracheobronchial obstruction or secretions*
• Breathing pattern, ineffective *related to pain*
• Fatigue
• Fear *related to unfamiliarity*

- Fluid volume deficit *related to active loss*
- Gas exchange impairment *related to altered oxygen supply*
- Infection, risk for *related to external factors*

Thrombophlebitis
- Gas exchange impairment *related to altered oxygen supply*
- Infection, risk for *related to home infusion therapy*
- Pain *related to physical, biological, or chemical agents*
- Pain *related to physiologic changes of pregnancy*
- Skin integrity impairment *related to internal (somatic) factors*
- Skin integrity impairment, risk for
- Skin integrity impairment, risk for *related to the aging process and impaired mobility*
- Tissue perfusion alteration (peripheral) *related to reduced arterial blood flow*

Tracheoesophageal fistula
- Aspiration, risk for *related to ineffective swallow reflex*
- Nutrition alteration: Less than body requirements *related to inability to absorb nutrients or insufficient intake*

Tracheostomy
- Nutrition alteration: Less than body requirements *related to inability to ingest foods*
- Skin integrity impairment *related to external (environmental) factors*
- Verbal communication impairment *related to physical barriers*

Transient ischemic attacks
- Confusion, acute
- Environmental interpretation syndrome, impaired
- Memory impairment *related to neurologic disturbance*
- Sensory or perceptual alteration (tactile)
- Tissue perfusion alteration (cerebral) *related to decreased cellular exchange*

Trauma
- Coping, ineffective family: Disabling *related to long-term illness*
- Coping, ineffective family: Disabling *related to unresolved emotional conflict between patient and family members*
- Death anxiety *related to terminal illness*
- Energy field disturbance

- Sensory or perceptual alteration (auditory) *related to illness or the aging process*
- Violence, risk for: Self-directed *related to recurrent losses or changes in physical or mental condition*
- Violence, risk for: Self-directed *related to suicide attempt*

Trigeminal neuralgia
- Anxiety *related to situational crisis*
- Knowledge deficit *related to lack of exposure*
- Nutrition alteration: Less than body requirements *related to inability to ingest foods*
- Pain *related to physical, biological, or chemical agents*

Tuberculosis
- Airway clearance, ineffective *related to presence of tracheobronchial obstruction or secretions*
- Breathing pattern, ineffective *related to decreased energy or fatigue*
- Dentition, altered
- Fatigue
- Fear *related to unfamiliarity*
- Gas exchange impairment *related to altered oxygen supply*
- Infection, risk for *related to increased incidence of tuberculosis*
- Loneliness, risk for
- Social isolation *related to altered state of wellness*

Urinary calculi
- Anxiety *related to situational crisis*
- Infection, risk for *related to external factors*
- Pain *related to physical, biological, or chemical agents*
- Tissue perfusion alteration (renal) *related to decreased cellular exchange*
- Urinary elimination alteration *related to obstruction*

Urinary diversion
- Breathing pattern, ineffective *related to pain*
- Constipation *related to inadequate intake of fluid and bulk*
- Grieving, anticipatory *related to perceived potential loss of significant object (such as person, job, possessions)*
- Infection *related to surgical incision*
- Pain *related to physical, biological, or chemical agents*

• Personal identity disturbance *related to lowered self-esteem*
• Sexual dysfunction *related to altered body structure or function*
• Sexuality pattern alteration *related to illness or medical treatment*
• Skin integrity impairment *related to external (environmental) factors*

Urinary incontinence

• Anxiety *related to situational crisis*
• Incontinence, functional *related to cognitive deficits*
• Incontinence, reflex *related to sensory or neuromuscular impairment*
• Incontinence, stress
• Incontinence, stress *related to weak pelvic musculature*
• Incontinence, total *related to neurologic dysfunction*
• Skin integrity impairment *related to external (environmental) factors*
• Social isolation *related to altered state of wellness*

Urinary tract infection

• Incontinence, stress
• Incontinence, stress *related to weak pelvic musculature*
• Incontinence, urge *related to decreased bladder capacity*
• Incontinence, urinary urge, risk for
• Infection, risk for *related to altered primary defenses during the postpartum period*
• Infection, risk for *related to external factors*
• Infection, risk for *related to labor and delivery*
• Pain *related to physical, biological, or chemical agents*
• Pain *related to physiologic changes of pregnancy*
• Urinary elimination pattern alteration *related to obstruction*

Uterine prolapse

• Body image disturbance
• Incontinence, stress
• Incontinence, stress *related to weak pelvic musculature*

Uterine rupture

• Fluid volume deficit *related to active loss*
• Pain *related to physical, biological, or chemical agents*

• Tissue perfusion alteration (cardiopulmonary) *related to decreased cellular exchange*
• Tissue perfusion alteration (cerebral) *related to decreased cellular exchange*
• Tissue perfusion alteration (renal) *related to decreased cellular exchange*

Vascular insufficiency

• Peripheral neurovascular dysfunction, risk for
• Tissue integrity impairment *related to peripheral vascular changes*

Viral hepatitis

• Fluid volume deficit *related to active loss*
• Infection, risk for *related to external factors*
• Nutrition alteration: Less than body requirements *related to inability to ingest foods*
• Skin integrity impairment *related to external (environmental) factors*
• Skin integrity impairment, risk for
• Social isolation *related to altered state of wellness*

GORDON'S FUNCTIONAL HEALTH PATTERNS

Gordon has described a functional health pattern system to help identify and formulate nursing diagnoses. Based on general categories, this system allows for easy organization of basic nursing information obtained during your initial assessment. Flexible and adaptable, these functional health patterns can be used for patients in various states of health and illness, in any age-group, and in any clinical specialty. Presented below is a brief outline of Gordon's functional health patterns.

Learning to incorporate Gordon's concepts into your assessment format may require time and practice; however, the rewards of understanding the patient and identifying specific areas where you can intervene are well worth the effort. When using the following health pattern categories, obtain the nursing history from the patient's perspective through a series of specific questions designed to elicit information in an organized manner.

1. Health perception and health management pattern
- General health
- Health practices
- Concerns about illness
- Responsibility for health restoration and maintenance

2. Nutritional and metabolic pattern
- Daily food and fluid intake
- Weight loss or gain
- Appetite
- Dietary restrictions
- Healing potential of skin wounds or lesions
- General body status or condition

3. Elimination pattern
- Bowel elimination pattern or problem
- Urinary elimination pattern or problem
- Perspiration pattern or problem

4. Activity and exercise pattern
- Energy level
- Exercise pattern

- Perceived ability for (use Functional level code* below):
_____ Bathing
_____ Bed mobility
_____ Cooking
_____ Dressing
_____ Feeding
_____ General mobility
_____ Grooming
_____ Home maintenance
_____ Shopping
_____ Toileting

5. Sleep and rest pattern
- Sleep problems
- Rested or not rested after sleep
- Use of sleep aids

6. Cognitive and perceptual pattern
- Sensory status: Visual, auditory, olfactory, tactile, gustatory
- Memory
- Intelligence
- Pain or discomfort

7. Self-perception and self-concept pattern
- Feelings about self
- Body image
- Self-esteem
- Emotional state

8. Role and relationship pattern
- Living arrangement
- Family or significant others
- Communication
- Role and responsibilities in family
- Socialization
- Finances

---

*Functional level code
0 = Completely independent
1 = Requires use of equipment or device
2 = Requires help, supervision, or teaching from another person
3 = Requires help from another person and equipment or device
4 = Dependent; does not participate in activity

9. Sexuality and reproductive pattern
- Sexual relations
- Sexual satisfaction or dissatisfaction
- Contraceptive use and problems
- Reproductive and menstrual history

10. Coping and stress-tolerance pattern
- Stressors
- Coping mechanisms
- Major life changes
- Problem management

11. Value and belief pattern
- Satisfaction with life
- Spirituality and religious beliefs
- Religious practices
- Conflicts

12. Other
- Concerns not already discussed

Nursing diagnoses and Gordon's functional health patterns

1. Health perception and health management pattern
- Altered protection
- Disuse syndrome, risk for
- Dysreflexia
- Health maintenance alteration
- Health-seeking behaviors
- Infection, risk for
- Injury, risk for
- Management of therapeutic regimen, effective: individual
- Management of therapeutic regimen, ineffective community
- Management of therapeutic regimen, ineffective: family
- Management of therapeutic regimen, ineffective: individual
- Noncompliance
- Poisoning, risk for
- Suffocation, risk for

2. Nutritional and metabolic pattern
- Body temperature alteration, risk for
- Breast-feeding, effective
- Breast-feeding, ineffective
- Breast-feeding, interrupted
- Fluid volume deficit
- Fluid volume deficit, risk for
- Fluid volume excess
- Hyperthermia
- Hypothermia
- Infant feeding pattern, ineffective
- Nutrition alteration: Less than body requirements
- Nutrition alteration: More than body requirements
- Nutrition alteration, risk for: More than body requirements
- Oral mucous membrane alteration
- Skin integrity impairment
- Skin integrity impairment, risk for
- Swallowing impairment
- Thermoregulation, ineffective
- Tissue integrity impairment

3. Elimination pattern
- Constipation
- Diarrhea
- Incontinence, bowel
- Incontinence, functional
- Incontinence, reflex
- Incontinence, stress
- Incontinence, total
- Incontinence, urge
- Urinary elimination pattern alteration
- Urinary retention

4. Activity and exercise pattern
- Activity intolerance
- Activity intolerance, risk for
- Airway clearance, ineffective
- Aspiration, risk for
- Breathing pattern, ineffective
- Cardiac output, decreased
- Diversional activity deficit
- Energy field disturbance
- Gas exchange impairment
- Home maintenance management impairment
- Intracranial adaptive capacity, decreased
- Mobility impairment (specify)
- Neglect, unilateral
- Perioperative positioning injury, risk for
- Peripheral neurovascular dysfunction, risk for
- Self-care deficit (specify)
- Tissue perfusion alteration (specify)
- Ventilation, spontaneous: Inability to sustain
- Ventilatory weaning response, dysfunctional

5. Sleep and rest pattern
- Fatigue
- Sleep pattern disturbance

6. Cognitive and perceptual pattern
- Confusion, acute
- Confusion, chronic
- Environmental interpretation syndrome, impaired
- Infant behavior, risk for disorganized
- Infant behavior, disorganized
- Infant behavior, potential for enhanced organization
- Memory impairment
- Knowledge deficit
- Pain
- Pain, chronic
- Sensory or perceptual alteration (specify)
- Thought process alteration

7. Self-perception and self-concept pattern
- Adjustment impairment
- Anxiety
- Body image disturbance
- Fear
- Grieving, anticipatory
- Hopelessness
- Personal identity disturbance
- Powerlessness
- Self-esteem, chronic low
- Self-esteem, situational low
- Self-esteem disturbance
- Self-mutilation, risk for
- Violence, risk for: Directed at others
- Violence, risk for: Self-directed

8. Role and relationship pattern
- Family process alteration
- Family process alteration: Alcoholism
- Grieving, anticipatory
- Grieving, dysfunctional
- Loneliness, risk for
- Parent-infant-child attachment alteration, risk for
- Parental role conflict
- Parenting alteration
- Parenting alteration, risk for
- Social interaction impairment
- Social isolation
- Verbal communication impairment
- Violence, risk for: Directed at others
- Violence, risk for: Self-directed

9. Sexuality and reproductive pattern
- Rape-trauma syndrome
- Sexual dysfunction
- Sexual pattern alteration

10. Coping and stress-tolerance pattern
- Caregiver role strain
- Caregiver role strain, risk for
- Coping, defensive
- Coping, family: Potential for growth
- Coping, ineffective community
- Coping, ineffective family: Compromised
- Coping, ineffective family: Disabling
- Coping, ineffective individual
- Coping, potential for enhanced community
- Decisional conflict
- Denial
- Grieving, dysfunctional
- Growth and development alteration
- Relocation stress syndrome

11. Value and belief pattern
- Spiritual distress
- Spiritual well-being, potential for enhanced

NURSING DIAGNOSES AND MASLOW'S HIERARCHY OF NEEDS

The diagram below depicts Maslow's hierarchy of needs. You can use this system when determining priorities for patient care. Shown at left is the ascending hierarchy of human needs; the definitions at right explain the five need categories.

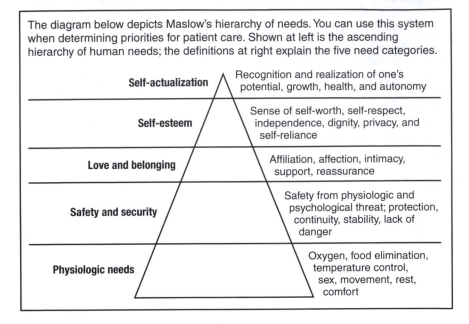

Self-actualization	Recognition and realization of one's potential, growth, health, and autonomy
Self-esteem	Sense of self-worth, self-respect, independence, dignity, privacy, and self-reliance
Love and belonging	Affiliation, affection, intimacy, support, reassurance
Safety and security	Safety from physiologic and psychological threat; protection, continuity, stability, lack of danger
Physiologic needs	Oxygen, food elimination, temperature control, sex, movement, rest, comfort

Maslow's hierarchy of needs is based on the idea that lower-level physiologic needs must be met before higher-level abstract needs can be met. Considering need categories as you identify patient problems will help you decide which nursing diagnoses to address first.

For example, a victim of physical abuse first needs his physical injuries treated (physiologic needs). Next, he may need protection from future episodes of abuse (safety and security). Moving up the hierarchy, you may then help the patient by providing support and reassurance (love and belonging). Long-term goals may include helping him build self-esteem. Keep in mind that a patient's need level may change throughout planning and intervention, so you'll have to continually reassess the patient and reevaluate his needs.

Self-actualization
• Growth and development alteration
• Health-seeking behaviors

• Knowledge deficit
• Spiritual distress
• Spiritual well-being, potential for enhanced

Self-esteem
• Adjustment impairment
• Body image disturbance
• Coping, defensive
• Coping, ineffective community
• Coping, ineffective family: Compromised
• Coping, ineffective family: Disabling
• Coping, ineffective individual
• Coping, potential for enhanced community
• Decisional conflict
• Denial
• Diversional activity deficit
• Energy field disturbance
• Hopelessness
• Noncompliance
• Personal identity disturbance
• Posttrauma response
• Powerlessness
• Rape-trauma syndrome

- Relocation stress syndrome
- Role performance alteration
- Self-esteem, chronic low
- Self-esteem, situational low
- Self-esteem disturbance
- Violence, risk for: Directed at others
- Violence, risk for: Self-directed

Love and belonging
- Caregiver role strain
- Caregiver role strain, risk for
- Coping, family: Potential for growth
- Coping, ineffective family: Compromised
- Coping, ineffective family: Disabling
- Family process alteration
- Family process alteration: Alcoholism
- Loneliness, risk for
- Parent-infant-child attachment alteration, risk for
- Parental role conflict
- Parenting alteration
- Social interaction impairment
- Social isolation

Safety and security
- Anxiety
- Confusion, acute
- Confusion, chronic
- Disuse syndrome, risk for
- Dysreflexia
- Environmental interpretation syndrome, impaired
- Fear
- Grieving, anticipatory
- Grieving, dysfunctional
- Health maintenance alteration
- Home maintenance management impairment
- Infection, risk for
- Injury, risk for
- Intracranial adaptive capacity, decreased
- Management of therapeutic regimen, effective: individual
- Management of therapeutic regimen, ineffective community
- Management of therapeutic regimen, ineffective: family
- Management of therapeutic regimen, ineffective: individual
- Memory impairment
- Neglect, unilateral
- Perioperative positioning injury, risk for
- Poisoning, risk for
- Self-mutilation, risk for
- Suffocation, risk for
- Trauma, risk for

- Verbal communication impairment

Physiologic needs
- Activity intolerance
- Airway clearance, ineffective
- Altered protection
- Aspiration, risk for
- Body temperature alteration, risk for
- Breast-feeding, effective
- Breast-feeding, ineffective
- Breast-feeding, interrupted
- Breathing pattern, ineffective
- Cardiac output, decreased
- Constipation, colonic
- Constipation, perceived
- Diarrhea
- Fatigue
- Fluid volume deficit
- Fluid volume excess
- Gas exchange impairment
- Hyperthermia
- Hypothermia
- Incontinence, bowel
- Incontinence, functional
- Incontinence, reflex
- Incontinence, stress
- Incontinence, total
- Incontinence, urge
- Infant feeding pattern, ineffective
- Mobility impairment (specify)
- Nutrition alteration: Less than body requirements
- Nutrition alteration: More than body requirements
- Oral mucous membrane alteration
- Pain
- Pain, chronic
- Peripheral neurovascular dysfunction, risk for
- Self-care deficit (specify)
- Sensory or perceptual alteration (specify)
- Sexual dysfunction
- Sexuality pattern alteration
- Skin integrity impairment
- Sleep pattern disturbance
- Swallowing impairment
- Thermoregulation, ineffective
- Thought process alteration
- Tissue integrity impairment
- Tissue perfusion alteration (specify)
- Urinary elimination pattern alteration
- Urinary retention
- Ventilation, spontaneous: Inability to sustain
- Ventilatory weaning response, dysfunctional

NURSING DIAGNOSES AND OREM'S UNIVERSAL SELF-CARE DEMANDS

Orem's concept of nursing focuses on self-care activities that individuals perform to maintain life, health, and well-being. In order to maintain integrated human functions, all individuals must meet *universal self-care demands*. If an individual is unable to satisfactorily meet these demands, the nurse intervenes by providing and managing care. According to Orem's theory, the goals of nursing include helping the patient to overcome circumstances that interfere with self-care and cause limitations and deficits. The list below uses Orem's universal self-care demands to group-related nursing diagnoses.

Air
- Airway clearance, ineffective
- Aspiration, risk for
- Breathing pattern, ineffective
- Gas exchange impairment
- Ventilation, spontaneous: Inability to sustain
- Ventilatory weaning response, dysfunctional

Water
- Cardiac output, decreased
- Fluid volume deficit
- Fluid volume deficit, risk for
- Fluid volume excess
- Tissue perfusion alteration (specify)

Food
- Breast-feeding, effective
- Breast-feeding, ineffective
- Breast-feeding, interrupted
- Infant feeding pattern, ineffective
- Nutrition alteration: Less than body requirements
- Nutrition alteration: More than body requirements
- Nutrition alteration, risk for: More than body requirements
- Oral mucous membrane alteration

Elimination
- Constipation
- Constipation, colonic

- Constipation, perceived
- Diarrhea
- Incontinence, bowel
- Incontinence, functional
- Incontinence, reflex
- Incontinence, stress
- Incontinence, total
- Incontinence, urge
- Skin integrity impairment
- Skin integrity impairment, risk for
- Urinary elimination pattern alteration
- Urinary retention

Activity and rest
- Activity intolerance
- Activity intolerance, risk for
- Disuse syndrome, risk for
- Diversional activity deficit
- Fatigue
- Loneliness, risk for
- Mobility impairment (specify)
- Neglect, unilateral
- Self-care deficit
- Sleep pattern disturbance

Solitude and social interaction
- Family process alteration
- Family process alteration: Alcoholism
- Parent-infant-child attachment alteration, risk for
- Parental role conflict
- Parenting alteration
- Parenting alteration, risk for
- Rape-trauma syndrome
- Role performance alteration
- Self-mutilation, risk for
- Sexual dysfunction
- Sexuality pattern alteration
- Social interaction impairment
- Social isolation
- Verbal communication impairment
- Violence, risk for: Directed at others
- Violence, risk for: Self-directed

Prevention of hazards
- Altered protection
- Body temperature alteration, risk for
- Dysreflexia

- Health maintenance alteration
- Health-seeking behaviors
- Home maintenance management impairment
- Hyperthermia
- Hypothermia
- Infection, risk for
- Injury, risk for
- Intracranial adaptive capacity, decreased
- Management of therapeutic regimen, ineffective community
- Management of therapeutic regimen, ineffective: family
- Management of therapeutic regimen, ineffective: individual
- Noncompliance
- Pain
- Pain, chronic
- Perioperative positioning injury, risk for
- Peripheral neurovascular dysfunction, risk for
- Poisoning, risk for
- Suffocation, risk for
- Swallowing impairment
- Thermoregulation, ineffective
- Tissue integrity impairment
- Trauma, risk for

Promotion of human functioning
- Adjustment impairment
- Anxiety
- Body image disturbance
- Caregiver role strain
- Caregiver role strain, risk for
- Confusion, acute
- Confusion, chronic
- Coping, defensive
- Coping, family: Potential for growth
- Coping, ineffective community
- Coping, ineffective family: Compromised
- Coping, ineffective family: Disabling
- Coping, ineffective individual
- Coping, potential for enhanced community
- Decisional conflict
- Denial
- Environmental interpretation syndrome, impaired
- Fear
- Grieving, anticipatory
- Grieving, dysfunctional
- Growth and development alteration
- Hopelessness
- Infant behavior, risk for disorganization
- Infant behavior, disorganized

- Infant behavior, potential for enhanced organization
- Knowledge deficit
- Management of therapeutic regimen, effective: individual
- Management of therapeutic regimen, ineffective community
- Management of therapeutic regimen, ineffective: family
- Management of therapeutic regimen, ineffective: individual
- Memory impairment
- Personal identity disturbance
- Posttrauma response
- Powerlessness
- Relocation stress syndrome
- Self-esteem, chronic low
- Self-esteem, situational low
- Self-esteem disturbance
- Sensory or perceptual alteration (specify)
- Spiritual distress
- Spiritual well-being, potential for enhanced
- Thought process alteration

N.A.N.D.A. NURSING DIAGNOSES

The North American Nursing Diagnosis Association's *Nursing Diagnoses: Definitions and Classifications,* organized around nine human response patterns, is the currently accepted classification system for nursing diagnoses. The complete taxonomic structure is listed below.

Pattern 1.
Exchanging: A human response pattern involving mutual giving and receiving

1.1.2.1	Altered nutrition: More than body requirements
1.1.2.2	Altered nutrition: Less than body requirements
1.1.2.3	Altered nutrition: Risk for more than body requirements
1.2.1.1	Risk for infection
1.2.2.1	Risk for altered body temperature
1.2.2.2	Hypothermia
1.2.2.3	Hyperthermia
1.2.2.4	Ineffective thermoregulation
1.2.3.1	Dysreflexia
1.2.3.2	Risk for autonomic dysreflexia
1.3.1.1	Constipation
1.3.1.1.1	Perceived constipation
1.3.1.1.2	Colonic constipation
1.3.1.2	Diarrhea
1.3.1.3	Bowel incontinence
1.3.1.4	Risk for constipation
1.3.2	Altered urinary elimination
1.3.2.1.1	Stress incontinence
1.3.2.1.2	Reflex urinary incontinence
1.3.2.1.3	Urge incontinence
1.3.2.1.4	Functional urinary incontinence
1.3.2.1.5	Total incontinence
1.3.2.1.6	Risk for urinary urge incontinence
1.3.2.2	Urinary retention
1.4.1.1	Altered tissue perfusion (specify type: renal, cerebral, cardiopulmonary, gastrointestinal, peripheral)
1.4.1.2	Risk for fluid volume imbalance
1.4.1.2.1	Fluid volume excess
1.4.1.2.2.1	Fluid volume deficit
1.4.1.2.2.2	Risk for fluid volume deficit
1.4.2.1	Decreased cardiac output
1.5.1.1	Impaired gas exchange
1.5.1.2	Ineffective airway clearance
1.5.1.3	Ineffective breathing pattern
1.5.1.3.1	Inability to sustain spontaneous ventilation
1.5.1.3.2	Dysfunctional ventilatory weaning response
1.6.1	Risk for injury
1.6.1.1	Risk for suffocation
1.6.1.2	Risk for poisoning
1.6.1.3	Risk for trauma
1.6.1.4	Risk for aspiration
1.6.1.5	Risk for disuse syndrome
1.6.1.6	Latex allergy response
1.6.1.7	Risk for latex allergy response
1.6.2	Altered protection
1.6.2.1	Impaired tissue integrity
1.6.2.1.1	Altered oral mucous membrane
1.6.2.1.2.1	Impaired skin integrity
1.6.2.1.2.2	Risk for impaired skin integrity
1.6.2.1.3	Altered dentition
1.7.1	Decreased adaptive capacity: Intracranial
1.8	Energy field disturbance

Pattern 2.
Communicating: A human response pattern involving sending messages

2.1.1.1	Impaired verbal communication

Pattern 3.
Relating: A human response pattern involving establishing bonds

3.1.1	Impaired social interaction
3.1.2	Social isolation
3.1.3	Risk for loneliness
3.2.1	Altered role performance
3.2.1.1.1	Altered parenting
3.2.1.1.2	Risk for altered parenting
3.2.1.1.2.1	Risk for altered parent-infant-child attachment
3.2.1.2.1	Sexual dysfunction
3.2.2	Altered family processes
3.2.2.1	Caregiver role strain
3.2.2.2	Risk for caregiver role strain
3.2.2.3.1	Altered family processes: Alcoholism
3.2.3.1	Parental role conflict
3.3	Altered sexuality patterns

Pattern 4.
Valuing: A human response pattern involving the assigning of relative worth

4.1.1	Spiritual distress (distress of the human spirit)
4.1.2	Risk for spiritual distress
4.2	Potential for enhanced spiritual well-being

Pattern 5.
Choosing: A human response pattern involving the selection of alternatives

5.1.1.1	Ineffective individual coping
5.1.1.1.1	Impaired adjustment
5.1.1.1.2	Defensive coping
5.1.1.1.3	Ineffective denial
5.1.2.1.1	Ineffective family coping: Disabling
5.1.2.1.2	Ineffective family coping: Compromised
5.1.2.2	Family coping: Potential for growth
5.1.3.1	Potential for enhanced community coping
5.1.3.2	Ineffective community coping
5.2.1	Ineffective management of therapeutic regimen: Individuals
5.2.1.1	Noncompliance (specify)
5.2.2	Ineffective management of therapeutic regimen: Families
5.2.3	Ineffective management of therapeutic regimen: Community
5.2.4	Effective management of therapeutic regimen: Individual
5.3.1.1	Decisional conflict (specify)
5.4	Health-seeking behaviors (specify)

Pattern 6.
Moving: A human response pattern involving activity

6.1.1.1	Impaired physical mobility
6.1.1.1.1	Risk for peripheral neurovascular dysfunction
6.1.1.1.2	Risk for perioperative positioning injury
6.1.1.1.3	Impaired walking
6.1.1.1.4	Impaired wheelchair mobility
6.1.1.1.5	Impaired transfer ability
6.1.1.1.6	Impaired bed mobility
6.1.1.2	Activity intolerance
6.1.1.2.1	Fatigue
6.1.1.3	Risk for activity intolerance
6.2.1	Sleep pattern disturbance
6.2.1.1	Sleep deprivation
6.3.1.1	Diversional activity deficit

6.4.1.1	Impaired home maintenance management
6.4.2	Altered health maintenance
6.4.2.1	Delayed surgical recovery
6.4.2.2	Adult failure to thrive
6.5.1	Feeding self-care deficit
6.5.1.1	Impaired swallowing
6.5.1.2	Ineffective breast-feeding
6.5.1.2.1	Interrupted breast-feeding
6.5.1.3	Effective breast-feeding
6.5.1.4	Ineffective infant feeding pattern
6.5.2	Bathing or hygiene self-care deficit
6.5.3	Dressing or grooming self-care deficit
6.5.4	Toileting self-care deficit
6.6	Altered growth and development
6.6.1	Risk for altered development
6.6.2	Risk for altered growth
6.7	Relocation stress syndrome
6.8.1	Risk for disorganized infant behavior
6.8.2	Disorganized infant behavior
6.8.3	Potential for enhanced organized infant behavior

Pattern 7.
Perceiving: A human response pattern involving the reception of information

7.1.1	Body image disturbance
7.1.2	Self-esteem disturbance
7.1.2.1	Chronic low self-esteem
7.1.2.2	Situational low self-esteem
7.1.3	Personal identity disturbance
7.2	Sensory or perceptual alterations (specify: visual, auditory, kinesthetic, gustatory, tactile, olfactory)
7.2.1.1	Unilateral neglect
7.3.1	Hopelessness
7.3.2	Powerlessness

Pattern 8.
Knowing: A human response pattern involving the meaning associated with information

8.1.1	Knowledge deficit (specify)
8.2.1	Impaired environmental interpretation syndrome
8.2.2	Acute confusion
8.2.3	Chronic confusion
8.3	Altered thought processes
8.3.1	Impaired memory

Pattern 9.
Feeling: A human response pattern involving the subjective awareness of information

9.1.1	Pain
9.1.1.1	Chronic pain
9.1.2	Nausea
9.2.1.1	Dysfunctional grieving
9.2.1.2	Anticipatory grieving
9.2.1.3	Chronic sorrow
9.2.2	Risk for violence: Directed at others
9.2.2.1	Risk for self-mutilation
9.2.2.2	Risk for violence: Self-directed
9.2.3	Posttrauma response
9.2.3.1	Rape-trauma syndrome
9.2.3.1.1	Rape-trauma syndrome: Compound reaction
9.2.3.1.2	Rape-trauma syndrome: Silent reaction
9.2.4	Risk for posttrauma syndrome
9.3.1	Anxiety
9.3.1.1	Death anxiety
9.3.2	Fear

NEW N.A.N.D.A.-APPROVED DIAGNOSES

The following section features care plans based on seven new diagnoses approved by the North American Nursing Diagnosis Association (NANDA) at the 2000 conference.

■ Falls, risk for

Definition
Increased susceptibility to falling that may cause physical harm

Assessment
- Age, increased risk with advancing age
- History of sensory or motor deficit, if present
- Health history, including cerebral function, mobility, sensory function, and use of adaptive devices
- Neurologic status, including level of consciousness, mental status, and orientation
- Physical impairment or limitation, including podiatry disorders, recent joint replacement, surgery, or illness
- Psychological status, including substance abuse, unfamiliarity with surroundings, mental status, coping skills, and self-concept
- Environmental hazards, such as throw rugs; carpet edges; stairways; slippery, wet, icy, or uneven surfaces, including tubs and showers; steps; unsteady handrails; inadequate lighting; cluttered living space; electrical wiring; unstable furniture; household layout; and improper use of assistive devices
- Medication use, including understanding of medications, compliance with prescribed regimen, use of over-the-counter medications, and interactions
- Knowledge, including understanding of safety precautions
- Medication history
- Pain or fatigue
- Inadequate footwear, such as those with slick leather soles and shoes lacking proper support
- Laboratory studies, including complete blood count and differential, and coagulation studies
- Diagnostic tests, including chest X-ray and cranial X-ray
- Sensory status, including hearing, vision, touch, and taste

Risk factors
Adults
- History of falls
- Use of wheelchair or assistive device (such as a walker or cane)
- Advanced age (age 65 or over)
- Lower limb prosthesis
- Physiologic factors (such as acute illness, postoperative conditions, visual or hearing difficulty, arthritis, and impaired physical mobility)
- Diminished mental status (such as confusion, delirium, dementia, and impaired reality testing)
- Use of medications
- Dangerous environmental conditions (such as inadequate lighting, wet floors, scatter rugs, and icy sidewalks)

Children
- Young age (less than age 2)
- Lack of auto restraints, gate on stairs, or window guard
- Bed located near window
- Unattended infant on bed, changing table, or sofa
- Lack of parental supervision

Associated medical diagnoses (selected)
Amputation, arthritis, brain tumors, cataracts, cerebral aneurysm, cerebrovascular accident, deafness, dehydration, dementia, detached retina, electrolyte imbalance, fever, fractures, glaucoma, head injury, heart failure, hypoglycemia, hypotension, impaired vision, joint replacement, malnutrition, osteoporosis, Parkinson's disease, recent surgical procedure, spinal injury, spinal tumor, transient ischemic attacks, vertigo

Expected outcomes

• Patient and family will identify factors that increase potential for injury.
• Patient and family will assist in identifying and applying safety measures to prevent injury.
• Patient and family will make necessary physical changes in environment to assure increased safety.
• Patient and family will develop strategies to maintain safety.
• Patient will optimize activities of daily living within sensorimotor limitations.

Interventions and rationales

• Identify factors that may cause or contribute to injury from a fall *to increase patient, family, and caregiver awareness.*
• Improve environmental safety as needed:
– Make changes in patient's environment that may cause or contribute to injury *to increase patient, family, and caregiver awareness.*
– Orient patient to environment. Assess patient's ability to use call bell, side rails, and bed positioning controls. Keep bed at lowest level, and watch closely at night. Remove throw rugs that may cause patient to slip. *These measures will help patient cope with unfamiliar surroundings.*
– Teach patient and family about need for safe illumination. Advise patient to wear sunglasses to reduce glare. Advise using contrast colors in household furnishings. *These measures will enhance visual discrimination.*
– For patient with hearing loss, encourage use of hearing aid *to minimize deficit.*
– Teach patient with unstable gait the correct use of assistive devices *to decrease potential risk for injury.*
• Provide additional patient teaching as needed such as household safety. Refer patient to appropriate resources (such as police, fire, and visiting nurses association) for more information. *Health education can help patient take steps to prevent injury.*

Evaluations for expected outcomes

• Patient and family identify and eliminate identified safety hazards that may increase risk for injury.
• Patient and family cooperate with nurse during assessment of environmental risks.

• Patient and family describe and demonstrate preventive measures to minimize potential for injury.

Documentation

• Statements by patient and family about potential for injury due to sensory or motor deficits
• Observation or knowledge of unsafe practices, lack of awareness, or disregard for safety hazards
• Interventions to decrease risk of injury to patient
• Patient's responses to nursing interventions
• Evaluations for expected outcomes

■ Powerlessness, risk for

related to chronic illness, illness-related regimen, or health care environment

Definition

Potential for perceived lack of control over a situation or for perceived inability to significantly affect an outcome

Assessment

• Nature of medical diagnosis
• Mobility
• Behavioral responses (verbal and nonverbal), including calmness, agitation, anger, anxiety, depression, independence or dependence, interest or apathy, satisfaction or dissatisfaction
• Usual coping strategies
• Past experiences with illness
• Knowledge, including current understanding of physical condition and physical, mental, and emotional readiness to learn
• Environment, including equipment and supplies, health care professionals and personnel, lighting, location of patient's personal belongings, noise, privacy, and space
• Number and types of stressors
• Social factors
• Spiritual beliefs and value system

Risk factors

• Acute or chronic illness (requiring hospitalization, intubation, ventilator, and suctioning)

• Acute injury or progressive debilitating disease (such as spinal cord injury or multiple sclerosis)
• Aging and its attendant reduction in physical strength and mobility
• Terminal illness
• Psychosocial factors (such as lack of knowledge of illness or healthcare system, lifestyle of dependency with inadequate coping patterns, decreased self-esteem, low or unstable body image)

Associated medical diagnoses (selected)

Conditions that are chronic or restrict or confine patients to a particular illness-related regimen or health care environment: acquired immunodeficiency syndrome, blindness, cancer, chronic renal failure, cystic fibrosis, diabetes mellitus, genital herpes, muscular dystrophy, panic disorder, paralysis, Parkinson's disease, psoriasis, spinal cord injury

Expected outcomes

• Patient will make decisions regarding course of treatment.
• Patient will decrease level of anxiety by changing response to stressors.
• Patient will participate in self-care activities (specify).
• Patient will describe modifications or adjustments to the environment that allow feelings of control.
• Patient will discuss factors in the illness-related regimen over which control can be maintained.
• Patient will demonstrate ability to plan for controllable factors.
• Patient will express feeling of maintaining control.
• Patient will accept and adapt to lifestyle changes.

Interventions and rationales

• Encourage patient to express feelings and concerns. Set aside time for discussions with patient about daily events. *This helps patient bring vaguely understood emotions into focus.*
• Try to be present during situations where feelings of powerlessness are likely to be greatest *to help patient cope.*
• Identify and develop patient's coping mechanisms, strengths, and resources for support. *By making use of coping skills, patient can reduce anxiety and fears and suc-*

cessfully undergo grieving necessary to come to terms with chronic illness.
• Discuss situations that provoke feelings of anger, anxiety, and powerlessness *to identify areas patient can control and to prevent anger from being inappropriately directed at himself or others.*
• Encourage participation in self-care. Provide positive reinforcement for patient's activities. Encourage patient to take active role as member of health care team. *This enhances patient's sense of control and reduces passive and dependent behavior.*
• Provide as many opportunities as possible for patient to make decisions with regard to self-care (such as positioning, choosing an injection site, and visiting) *to communicate respect for patient and enhance feelings of independence.*
• Help patient learn as much as possible about health condition, treatment, and prognosis *to help patient feel in control.*
• Modify environment when possible to meet patient's self-care needs *to promote patient's sense of control over the environment.*
• Acknowledge the importance of patient's space:
– Verbally delineate patient's space.
– Orient patient to space.
– If possible, allow patient to walk around the space and arrange personal belongings.
– If patient is immobilized, ask for instructions regarding placement of personal belongings. *These measures enhance patient's potential for regaining a sense of power.*
• Decrease unpredictable events by discussing rules, policies, procedures, and schedules with patient. *Fear of the unknown interferes with patient's ability to cope.*
• Encourage family members to support patient without taking control *to increase the patient's feelings of self-worth.*
• Reinforce patient's rights as stated in the Patients' Bill of Rights *to protect the patient's right to make decisions about health care treatment.*
• Identify and arrange to accommodate patient's spiritual needs. *Spirituality enables the patient to gain courage and resist despair.*

Evaluations for expected outcomes

• Patient verbalizes positive and negative feelings about current situation.
• Patient describes strategies for decreasing anxiety.

• Patient specifies preferences for care.
• Patient performs specified daily self-care measures.
• Patient identifies specific factors that he can control in the illness-related regimen and plans appropriate action.
• Patient demonstrates increased control by participating in decision making related to health care.
• Patient actively participates in planning and executing aspects of personal care and health care.

Documentation
• Patient's interest in surroundings, participation in self-care, verbalization of understanding, and demonstration of skill in relation to medical diagnosis and treatment and environment
• Observations and interactions related to disease process, treatment, and health care environment
• Patient's responses to opportunities to plan and participate in own care
• Patient's feelings about illness and situations that can't be changed
• Teaching and counseling to enhance patient's decision-making ability
• Interventions to help patient gain sense of control
• Patient's response to nursing interventions
• Evaluations for expected outcomes

■ Relocation stress syndrome, risk for

related to inadequate preparation for admission, transfer, or discharge

Definition
Potential for physiologic or psychosocial disturbance following transfer from one environment to another

Assessment
• Reason for transfer or relocation
• Past experiences with relocation
• Nature of relocation
• Physical and mental status of patient, including health condition, cognitive functioning, and functional abilities

• Financial resources
• Support systems, including family and friends, health care workers, and community services (including any possible changes in status related to relocation)
• Resources available to help prepare for relocation
• Conditions in original environment versus conditions in new environment, including structural differences, layout of facilities, need for presence of equipment or assistive devices, and availability of transportation
• Coping and problem-solving abilities, including educational level, past experiences with relocation, and participation in recreational activities or hobbies
• Perceived and actual implications for patient's future level of independence related to relocation

Risk factors
• Moderate to high degree of physical, ethnic, or cultural change
• Inadequate support system or group
• Feelings of powerlessness
• Moderate mental competence (alert enough to experience changes)
• Unpredictability of experiences
• Decreased psychosocial or physical health
• Lack of counseling before transfer
• Passive coping
• Current or recent loss

Associated medical diagnoses (selected)
Any change in physical, functional, or cognitive status that also requires a change in patient's environment, such as admission to hospital, transfer from one unit or institution to another, and discharge

Expected outcomes
• Patient will request information about new environment.
• Patient will communicate understanding of relocation.
• Patient and family will take steps to prepare for relocation.
• Patient will use available resources.
• Patient will express satisfaction with adjustment to new environment.

Interventions and rationales
• Assign a primary nurse to patient *to provide a consistent, caring, and accepting environment that enhances patient's adjustment and well-being.*

• If possible, include patient in decision-making process regarding potential locations, dates, and circumstances of relocation *to promote a feeling of participation in choices, which will allow feeling of control.*
• Help patient and family members prepare for relocation. Conduct group discussions, provide pictures of new setting, and communicate any additional information that will ease transition *to help patient cope with new environment.*
• If possible, allow patient and family members to visit new location and provide introductions to staff. *The more familiar the environment, the less stress patient will experience during relocation.*
• Assess patient's needs for additional health care services before relocation *to ensure that patient receives appropriate care in new environment.*
• Communicate all aspects of patient's discharge plan to appropriate staff at new location *to ensure continuity of care.*
• Educate family members about relocation stress syndrome and its potential effects *to encourage family members to provide needed emotional support throughout transition period.*
• Encourage patient to express emotions associated with relocation *to provide an opportunity to correct misconceptions, answer questions, and reduce anxiety.*
• Reassure patient that family members and friends know his new location and will continue to visit *to reduce feelings of abandonment and anxiety.*

Evaluations for expected outcomes
• Patient makes request for information about new environment.
• Patient expresses understanding of relocation process.
• Patient and family members complete preparation for relocation.
• Patient makes use of available resources to smooth transition to new environment.
• Patient expresses feelings associated with adjustment to new environment.

Documentation
• Evidence of patient's feelings regarding relocation
• Patient's participation in decision making
• Patient's needs in preparing for relocation
• Available resources and support systems

• Intervention to prepare patient and family members for relocation and patient's and family members' responses
• Coping strategies identified by nurse and family
• Family member's statements indicating intention to take action to minimize feelings of abandonment and anxiety, such as scheduling routine visits and moving familiar objects to new location
• Discharge plan instructions communicated to new staff
• Evaluations for expected outcomes

■ Self-esteem, situational low, risk for

related to anticipated or actual loss, illness, hospitalization, and forced dependence on health care team

Definition
Potential for developing a negative perception of self-worth in response to a current situation (specify)

Assessment
• Age
• Sex
• Developmental stage
• Cognitive ability
• Behavior
• Family status, including marital status, role in family, sibling position, or recent loss of spouse or significant other
• Reason for current health care visit or hospitalization
• Medical history, including chronic illnesses
• Mental status, including affect, general appearance, and mood; evidence of depression, hopelessness, or discouragement; preoccupation with bodily functions; and unrealistic fear of developing a serious disease
• Changes in physical appearance (including wrinkles, sagging skin, gray hair, aging spots, scoliosis, dowager's hump, and increased truncal fat), social status (including recent retirement [forced or voluntary]), or sleep patterns (including trouble falling asleep, frequent awakenings, and restless sleep)

Risk factors
- Developmental changes (specify)
- Disturbed body image
- Functional impairment (specify)
- Loss (specify)
- Social role changes (specify)
- History of learned helplessness, abuse, neglect, or abandonment
- Unrealistic self-expectations
- Behavior inconsistent with values
- Lack of recognition or rewards
- Failures or rejections
- Decreased power or control over environment
- Physical illness (specify)

Associated medical diagnoses (selected)
This nursing diagnosis can be used with any patient experiencing an anticipated or actual loss (body part, normal body function, control over environment, threat to life), diagnosis of a chronic or debilitating illness, or chronic use of medications whose adverse effects cause an alteration in body image or appearance. Diagnoses may include cataracts, cerebrovascular accident, conditions that necessitate chronic use of steroids or antirejection or anticonvulsant medications, end-stage cardiac disease, hypertension, impotence, infertility, myocardial infarction, obesity, seizure disorder, transplantation.

Expected outcomes
- Patient will participate in care.
- Patient will maintain eye contact and initiate conversations.
- Patient will maintain an upright and open posture.
- Patient's body language and speech content will be congruent.
- Patient will verbally appraise himself before current health problem.
- Patient will talk about feelings related to current situation and impact on lifestyle.
- Patient will express positive feelings about self (verbally or through behavior) that indicate acceptance of changes caused by health problem or situation.
- Patient will participate in decisions related to care and therapies.
- Patient will perform hygiene and self-care activities indicating attention to appearance.

Interventions and rationales
- Ask permission to enter patient's personal space. This may include areas around the bed, bedside tables, and closet. As patient's self-esteem decreases, significance of personal space increases. *Asking permission to enter personal space provides patient with a sense of control and raises self-esteem.*
- Encourage patient to wear own pajamas or gowns and robes *to contribute to a positive self-identity.*
- Arrange patient's personal items on the bedside stand so that they're within easy reach *to maintain patient's independence.*
- Incorporate appropriate exercise activities into patient's daily care *to enhance strength, endurance, and coordination and to improve self-esteem.*
- Encourage patient to express feelings about self (past and present). *Self-exploration encourages patient to consider future change.*
- Encourage patient to express feelings about health condition and fears about loss of independence and ability to participate in work and leisure activities. *This allows patient to gain insight and to rationally define problems and possible solutions.*
- Assess patient's mental status at least once each day through interview and observation. *If anxiety resulting from self-rejection becomes severe, patient may experience disorientation or psychotic symptoms.*
- Involve patient in the decision-making process. *Expressions of low self-esteem include ambivalence and procrastination.*
- Provide patient with positive feedback for verbal reports or behaviors indicating positive self-appraisal. *This gives patient feelings of approval and competence to cope effectively with stressful situations.*
- Provide information about appropriate support groups, and encourage interaction with individuals who have successfully adapted to illness or limitations *to increase patient's coping skills.*

Evaluations for expected outcomes
- Patient carries out activities of daily living while in hospital.
- Patient initiates conversations and maintains eye contact.
- Patient is open and receptive to others.
- Patient's speech and body language are congruent.
- Patient discusses feelings about aging, chronic illness, loss of independence, and diminished ability to participate in work and leisure activities.

• At least once each day, patient makes at least two statements reflecting positive self-esteem.

Documentation
• Mental status assessment (baseline and ongoing)
• Evidence of patient's feelings
• Available resources and support systems
• Coping strategies identified by nurse and family
• Interventions to support patient's self-esteem
• Patient's response to nursing interventions
• Evaluations for expected outcomes

■ Self-mutilation

related to emotional illness

Definition
Deliberate self-injurious behavior that causes tissue damage with the intent of causing nonfatal injury to attain relief of tension

Assessment
• Age
• Sex
• Developmental history
• Current stress level and coping behaviors
• Mental status, including judgment, thought content, and mood
• Family history, including abusive behavior
• Previous episodes of self-mutilation, and suicide attempts
• Substance abuse history
• Social history, including sexual activity and aggression within peer group
• History of depression and impulsiveness

Defining characteristics
• Cuts or scratches on body
• Picking at wounds
• Self-inflicted burns
• Ingestion or inhalation of harmful substances or objects
• Biting
• Abrading
• Severing
• Insertion of an object into body orifice
• Hitting

Associated medical diagnoses (selected)
Autism, borderline personality disorder, confusion and dementia, developmental disability, factitious disorder with physical symptoms, malingering, multiple personality disorder, sexual masochism, substance abuse

Expected outcomes
• Patient won't harm himself while in hospital.
• Patient will express increased sense of security.
• Patient will report being able to cope better with disorganization, aggressive impulses, anxiety, or hallucinations.
• Patient won't experience dissociative states or will experience fewer of them.
• Patient will participate in therapeutic milieu.
• Patient will report suicidal thoughts to staff.
• Patient will verbalize when beginning to experience feelings of lack of control.
• Patient will seek assistance from appropriate support persons who can help him refrain from self-abuse.
• Patient will contract not to harm self.
• Patient will demonstrate alternate ways to cope with stress and emotional problems.
• Patient will verbalize connection between feelings and self-mutilation behaviors.

Interventions and rationales
• Limit the number of staff members interacting with patient *to provide continuity of care and increase patient's sense of security.*
• Depending on seriousness of intent to do self-harm, have staff make frequent, short contacts with patient *to reassure patient without stifling independence.*
• Remove all dangerous objects from patient's environment *to promote safety.*
• Search patient's belongings and remove sharp objects, belts, matches, lighters, and medications that can be used for self-mutilation *to promote safety.*
• Make short-term verbal "contracts" with patient stating that patient won't harm self *to make patient aware that he's ultimately responsible for his own safety and that he's capable of guaranteeing it.*
• Administer psychotropic medications as ordered, *to reduce tension, impulsive behavior, hallucinations, and panic.*
• If patient enters a dissociative state or hallucinates, move him to a quiet room with re-

duced stimuli. If restraints must be used, remain with patient and provide reassurance *to calm patient and orient him to reality.*

• If hospitalized, patient can be asked to remain in areas within sight of staff and, depending upon seriousness of intent to do self-mutilation, should be observed continuously *to provide protection and increase patient's sense of security.*

• If patient is participating in therapeutic milieu, discuss patient's risk of self-harm with community members *to provide enhanced protection and psychological support.*

• If patient harms himself, care for injuries in a calm, nonjudgmental manner. Encourage patient to talk about feelings that prompted self-mutilation rather than focusing on act. *Discussion may help patient connect self-destructive behavior to feelings that preceded it. Discussion may also provide an opportunity to explore alternative ways of dealing with negative thoughts and feelings.*

• If self-destructive acts persist, consider developing a behavior-modification program where periods of self-control are rewarded through such benefits as personal attention or material items *to reinforce self-control.*

• Ask patient directly if he's thinking of suicide and, if so, what plan he has. *A self-destructive patient may become suicidal and therefore may require additional precautions.*

• Hold frequent treatment team meetings *to ensure consistent care that is appropriate to patient's current behavior.*

• Observe patient for verbal and nonverbal signs of increased helplessness, hopelessness, agitation, anxiety, and inability to interrupt thoughts about self-mutilation *to facilitate early intervention and patient remaining in least restrictive environment.*

• Work with patient when he's in a calm, nonagitated state, such as during a planned meeting, to identify events that trigger self-mutilation behavior *to enhance feelings of self-control and decrease feelings of powerlessness.*

• Document and communicate plan of care to all staff working with patient and seek cooperation *to insure consistency and predictability of treatment.*

• Take appropriate action to stop self-mutilation *to insure safety.*

• Promote emotional support for patient to identify feelings that lead to self-mutilation *as a means to prevent the act.*

• Observe patient's swallowing of medication *to reduce chance of "cheeking" medications and hoarding them for a self-destructive act.*

• Stay with patient during hygiene times *to promote safety or intervene during self-destructive acts.*

• Check at irregular times while patient sleeps *to promote safety or intervene during self-destructive acts.*

Evaluations for expected outcomes

• Patient doesn't incur injury.

• Patient expresses increased sense of security.

• Patient describes coping skills that enable him to deal better with disorganization, aggressive impulses, anxiety, or hallucinations.

• Patient experiences fewer dissociative states.

• Patient participates in therapeutic milieu.

• Patient tells staff member about suicidal thoughts.

• Patient can discuss strategies to maintain feelings of connectedness to self rather than experience dissociation and self-mutilation.

• Patient keeps terms of verbal "contracts" by stating that he won't harm himself.

• Patient can identify feelings and thoughts leading to self-mutilation acts before acting on such feelings and thoughts.

• Patient can talk about feelings rather than express feelings by acts of self-mutilation.

Documentation

• Nursing interventions performed and patient's response

• Contracts between patient and nurse

• Patient's responses to medication and behavioral modification program

• Revisions to treatment plan

• Drawing of self-inflicted injuries

• Evidence of suicidal ideation

• Patient feedback of effectiveness of various strategies

• Reduction in number of self-mutilation acts preintervention and postintervention

• Evaluations for expected outcomes

■ Suicide, risk for

Definition
At risk for self-inflicted, life-threatening injury

Assessment
- Age
- Sex
- Medical history
- Patient's life situation
- Recent stressors and coping behaviors
- Available support systems
- History of suicide attempts, including aggressiveness and lethality of attempts
- History of substance abuse: type and effects on mental status
- Reaction of family members
- Safety hazards
- Mental status, including abstract thinking, affect, content of thought, general information, insight, judgment, mood, orientation, recent and remote memory, and thought processes

Risk factors
- History of suicide attempt
- Threats of killing self
- Impulsive behaviors (such as buying a gun, stockpiling medication, making or changing a will, giving away possessions, and making a sudden and euphoric recovery from major depression)
- Marked changes in behavior, attitude, or school performance
- Situational factors (such as economic instability and loss of autonomy or independence)
- Adolescent living in nontraditional setting (such as juvenile detention center, prison, halfway house, or group home)
- Psychological factors (such as alcohol or substance abuse, psychiatric illness or disorder, childhood abuse, and family history of suicide)
- Terminal illness, debilitating disease, or chronic pain
- Social factors (such as loss of important relationship, disrupted family life, grief, inadequate support systems, loneliness, helplessness, legal or disciplinary problems, and cluster suicides)

Associated medical diagnoses (selected)
Any illness resulting in long-term disability or incapacity (terminal diseases, degenerative diseases, traumatic injury); bipolar disease (depressive phase); borderline personality disorder; depression; schizophrenia; self-destructive or suicidal behavior; sexual assault

Expected outcomes
- Patient won't harm self in hospital.
- Patient will recover from suicidal episode.
- Patient will discuss feelings that precipitated suicide attempt.
- Patient will consult mental health professional.
- Patient will describe available resources for crisis prevention and management.
- Patient will voice improvement in self-worth.

Interventions and rationales
- Observe patient closely and initiate suicide precautions protocol including checks every 15-minutes *to ensure that patient is protected and in a safe environment.*
- Ask patient directly: "Have you thought about killing yourself?" If he answers yes, ask him, "What do you plan to do?" *Suicide risk increases if patient has a definite plan.*
- Remove anything that could be used to inflict further self-injury (such as razor blades, belts, glass objects, pills, knives, cans, and mirrors) from patient's environment. *This helps to ensure patient's safety.*
- Make short-term contract with patient that he won't harm self during a specific time period. Continue negotiating until there is no evidence of suicidal ideation. *A contract gets the subject out in the open, places some responsibility for safety on patient, and conveys acceptance of patient as worthwhile person.*
- Supervise administration of prescribed medications. *Medications may be an appropriate alternative to verbal interventions.* Be aware of drug actions and adverse effects. Make sure patient doesn't hoard or "cheek" medications.
- Provide supervision (one-on-one observation when possible) of patient based on hospital policy. *This ensures compliance with legal requirements to protect patient and reassures patient of staff concern.*
- Use nonjudgmental manner *to show unconditional positive regard.*

• Listen carefully to patient and avoid challenging him *to communicate caring and support.*
• Demonstrate understanding but don't reinforce denial of current situation *because roots of suicidal feelings can be masked by denial.*
• Encourage patient to participate in group activities, especially those he enjoys, *to help build self-esteem.*
• Assist patient in recognizing inappropriate coping mechanisms and help identify those that enhance personal well-being *to use strengths and skills in preventing self-destructive behavior.*
• Make appropriate referrals to mental health professionals *to help patient work through suicidal feelings and develop healthier alternatives.*
• Help patient set goal for obtaining long-term psychiatric care. *Ambivalence about psychiatric care or refusal to consult with therapist marks suicidal patient's lack of insight and use of denial.*
• Provide patient with the necessary referral information about community centers, crisis centers, hot lines, and counselors. *Alternatives may ease anxiety about perceived threat of long-term psychotherapy.*

Evaluations for expected outcomes
• Patient's environment is free from potentially harmful objects.
• In the aftermath of initial suicide attempt, patient makes commitment not to act on suicidal thoughts.
• Patient states reasons for suicide attempt.
• Patient contacts mental health professional and makes appointment for continued therapy.
• Patient identifies crisis-prevention resources, such as hotline phone number, local crisis center, and name of therapist.
• Patient expresses positive feelings about self.

Documentation
• Patient's comments about the suicide attempt and current feelings about it
• Observations of patient's behavior
• Interventions to reduce or prevent self-destructive behavior
• Patient's observable responses to interventions
• Evaluations for expected outcomes

■ Wandering

Definition
Meandering, aimless, or repetitive locomotion that exposes the individual to harm and is frequently incongruent with boundaries, limits, or obstacles

Assessment
• Age
• Health history, including history of stressful life with wandering as a coping mechanism for handling stress; sleep habits; dietary and nutritional status; previous injuries, falls, or trauma; and medications
• Cardiovascular status, including dizziness and orthostatic hypotension
• Pain or discomfort
• Neurologic status, including cerebral function; sensory function; judgment; abstract thinking; general information; mood; affect; recent and remote memory; orientation to person, place, and time; confusion; cerebrovascular disease; and head injuries
• Psychological status, including coping skills; mental illness; history of restlessness associated with depression and anxiety; perceptions to external environmental stimuli (such as heat and cold); psychotropic medications; and illusions, delusions, and hallucinations
• Sensory status, including hearing; vision; touch; responses to touch or other stimuli; and somatic complaints
• Expression of wandering behavior, including continuous ambulation or pacing; attraction to random stimuli; self-stimulation, such as rocking, clapping, singing, and patting walls; constant searching for unattainable object or person (such as a deceased family member) or calling out for the object or person; constantly driven to engage in activities; walking a particular course or route without purpose or thought; and modeling behavior of others who leave room or home
• Communication skills, including reaction to interviews, body language, facial expressions, and gesturing
• Physical characteristics, including manner of dress, personal hygiene, posture, and gait
• Environmental status, including lights, location of personal belongings, noise, privacy, and space

Defining characteristics

• Frequent or continuous movement from place to place, often revisiting the same destinations
• Persistent locomotion in search of "missing" or unattainable people or places
• Locomotion that is haphazard, unauthorized, fretful, or without apparent destination that results in unintended leaving of the premises or that can't be easily dissuaded or redirected
• Inability to locate significant landmarks in a familiar setting
• Following behind or shadowing a caregiver's locomotion

Associated medical diagnoses (selected)

Cerebrovascular accident, mental retardation, multiple infarct dementia, senile dementia (Alzheimer's type), transient ischemic attack, traumatic brain injury

Expected outcomes

• Patient will participate in physical or other _____ (specify) activities to minimize wandering behavior.
• Patient and family members will anticipate patient's wandering behavior or ambulation patterns and provide gratification before onset of wandering behavior.
• Patient will remain free from physical injury.
• Patient will ambulate safely.
• Patient and family members will identify factors that contribute to wandering behavior.
• Patient won't have unplanned exits or elopements.

Interventions and rationales

• Assess occurrence of wandering behavior, including when, where, how, and with whom patient ambulates, *to explore severity of problem and plan interventions.*
• Assess reasons for specific behavioral patterns *to determine the type of wandering behavior, the need the behavior may be meeting, and possible triggers for wandering behaviors.*
• Determine how family members handle the wandering behavior *to provide a comprehensive database for planning care.*
• Assess patient's hobbies and previous social, leisure, and exercise activities and patterns *to assist in planning appropriate nursing interventions.*

• Provide a safe and structured daily routine and environment *to decrease wandering behavior and minimize caregiver stress.*
• Encourage participation in simple household chores, such as sweeping, folding laundry, and raking leaves, and encourage activities, such as dancing to familiar music or taking walks outdoors. *Exercise may reduce anxiety and restlessness.*
• Install door and window locks that aren't easily detected or manipulated *to prevent unsafe exits from the health care institution, home, or yard.*
• Use dead bolt locks on doors and keep a key accessible for quick exit *to prevent unplanned exits and to facilitate entrance and exit in an emergency situation.*
• Use fences or hedges around patios or yards and lock gates *to prevent unsafe exits.*
• Install electronic devices with buzzers or bells *to alert others when a door or window is opened.*
• Use pressure-sensitive doormats or chair or bed alarms *to alert caregivers of movement and prevent injury.*
• Avoid using physical or chemical restraints (sedatives) to control the patient's wandering behavior. *Restraints may increase agitation, anxiety, sensory deprivation, falls, complications of immobility, powerlessness, dependence on caregivers, and wandering behavior.*
• Notify neighbors, apartment doorman, and staff in residence or retirement communities about patient's condition. Keep a list of neighbor's names and phone numbers handy. Ask others to call if patient is seen outdoors without supervision. *Awareness by others can prevent patient from becoming lost and injured.*
• Notify local police department about patient's potential for wandering *to alert them in case unsafe exit occurs.*
• Alert all nursing staff in writing (in plan of care) and verbally (in shift reports) about patient's potential for elopement *to ensure continuity of care, prevent unplanned exits, and safeguard patient.*
• Utilize community resources, such as the Alzheimer's Association Safe Return Program, *to assist in the identification, location, and return of lost individuals with disorders characterized with wandering behaviors.*
• Check patient for hunger, thirst, pain, discomfort, or need for toileting. *These conditions may precipitate wandering.*

• Reduce noise levels where possible *to reduce confusion and sensory overload that may precipitate wandering.*
• Reassure patients who feel lost, abandoned, or disoriented *to help reduce anxiety and restlessness.*
• Utilize community resources and support groups *to help patient, family member, and caregivers cope with wandering behavior.*
• Survey immediate environment or neighborhood for dangerous areas, such as open stairwells, high balconies, open windows, unlocked doors, heavily traveled roads and streets, bus stops, and bodies of water, *to increase awareness of environmental hazards and to plan interventions to promote patient safety.*
• Utilize visual cues (such as large no exit sign), actual barriers (such as dead bolt locks), and safe items for manipulation (such as clothing to fold or put in drawers and plastic dishware to stack) *to create interest, provide stimulation, and prevent patient from leaving.*
• Incorporate regular physical exercise, walking, range-of-motion exercises, and stretching into daily structured routine. *These activities may decrease patient's need and desire to wander and prevent complications of immobility.*
• Prepare for possible wandering incident by keeping up-to-date identification information (patient's age, height, weight, hair color, identifying marks, medical condition, medications, allergies, blood type, dental work, and complexion):
– Keep several copies of a recent close-up photograph.
– Create a list of possible places the patient may go.
– Retain a piece of scented clothing that may be used by the police. Use plastic gloves to place an article of unwashed clothing in bag. Store bag where others won't disturb its contents. *These actions provide information for local police and other authorities to assist in finding a lost person.*
• Teach family members and caregivers to provide areas for walking. Instruct patient to use these designated areas in the home or health care institution. Reinforce need to remain indoors and not to leave or go outside. *These measures signify understanding that the patient needs to engage in wandering behavior and may prevent patient ur-*
gency to leave the home or health care institution.
• Evaluate the effectiveness of interventions taken *to determine whether actions increased or decreased wandering behavior.*

Evaluation for expected outcomes
• Patient participates in activities.
• Patient or family member identifies at least two triggers that precipitate wandering behavior.
• Patient cooperates with nurse during assessment of neurologic, cognitive, sensory, cardiovascular, and psychological status.
• Patient doesn't experience falls or injuries.
• Patient ambulates in specified areas without incident.
• Patient, family members, or caregiver verbalize methods to control wandering behavior
• Family members or caregiver demonstrate ability to anticipate wandering and take steps to prevent or minimize catastrophic reaction.
• Effectiveness of interventions and modifications is determined.

Documentation
• Type, frequency, and amount of patient participation in physical and other activities
• Observations about conditions, factors, and activities that precipitate or reduce wandering behavior
• All wandering patterns
• Patient reaction to environmental stimuli, including reaction to family members, caregivers, noise, and lights
• Effectiveness of interventions and modifications made
• Evaluations for expected outcomes

SELECTED REFERENCES

Behrman, R.E., et al. *Nelson Textbook of Pediatrics,* 16th ed. Edited by Nelson, W.E. Philadelphia: W.B. Saunders Co., 2000.

Boyd, M.W., and Tower, B.L. *Medical-Surgical Nursing,* 3rd ed. Springhouse Notes Series. Springhouse, Pa.: Springhouse Corp., 1997.

Craven, R.F., and Hirnle, C.J. *Fundamentals of Nursing: Human Health and Function,* 3rd ed. Philadelphia: Lippincott Williams & Wilkins, 2000.

Fuller, J., and Schaller-Ayers, J. *Health Assessment: A Nursing Approach,* 3rd ed. Philadelphia: Lippincott Williams & Wilkins, 2000.

Gordon, M. *Manual of Nursing Diagnosis,* 9th ed. St. Louis: Mosby–Year Book, Inc., 1999.

Handbook of Medical-Surgical Nursing, 2nd ed. Springhouse, Pa.: Springhouse Corp., 1998.

Ignatavicius, D.D., et al. *Medical-Surgical Nursing Across the Health Care Continuum,* 3rd ed. Philadelphia: W.B. Saunders Co., 1999.

Illustrated Handbook of Nursing Care. Springhouse, Pa.: Springhouse Corp., 1998.

Jaffe, M.S., and Melson, K.A. *Maternal-Infant Health Care Planning,* 3rd ed. Springhouse, Pa.: Springhouse Corp., 1999.

Johnson, M., et al. *Nursing Outcomes Classification (NOC) Iowa Outcomes Project,* 2nd ed. St. Louis: Mosby–Year Book, Inc., 2000.

Krupnick, S.L., and Wade, A.J. *Psychiatric Care Planning,* 2nd ed. Springhouse, Pa.: Springhouse Corp., 1999.

Lubkin, I.M. *Chronic Illness: Impact and Interventions,* 4th ed. Boston: Jones & Bartlett Pubs., Inc., 1998.

Maklebust J., and Sieggreen, M. *Pressure Ulcers: Guidelines for Prevention and Nursing Management,* 3rd ed. Springhouse, Pa.: Springhouse Corp., 2001.

Mastering Documentation, 2nd ed. Springhouse, Pa.: Springhouse Corp., 1999.

McCloskey, J.C., and Bulecheck, G.M. *Nursing Interventions Classification (NIC),* 3rd ed. St. Louis: Mosby–Year Book, Inc., 1999.

Meeker, M.H., and Rothrock, J.C., eds. *Alexander's Care of the Patient in Surgery,* 11th ed. St. Louis: Mosby–Year Book, Inc., 1999.

NANDA Nursing Diagnoses: Definitions & Classification, 1999-2000. Philadelphia: North American Nursing Diagnosis Association, 1999.

Nurse's Legal Handbook, 4th ed. Springhouse, Pa.: Springhouse Corp., 2000.

Pocket Guide to Home Care Standards. Springhouse, Pa.: Springhouse Corp., 2001.

Rantz, M.J., and LeMone, P., eds. *Classification of Nursing Diagnoses: Proceedings of the Thirteenth Conference of the North American Nursing Diagnosis Association.* Glendale, Calif.: CINAHL Information Systems, 2000.

Rubenfeld, M.G., and Scheffer, B.K. *Critical Thinking in Nursing: An Interactive Approach,* 2nd ed. Philadelphia: Lippincott Williams & Wilkins, 1999.

Taylor, C.M., and Sparks, S.M. *Nursing Diagnosis Cards,* 9th ed. Springhouse, Pa.: Springhouse Corp., 2000.

INDEX

WXYZ